Asthma, Health and Society

Andrew Harver • Harry Kotses
Editors

Asthma, Health and Society

A Public Health Perspective

Springer

Editors
Andrew Harver
Department of Public Health Sciences
UNC Charlotte
Charlotte, NC
USA

Harry Kotses
Department of Psychology
Ohio University
Athens, OH
USA

ISBN 978-0-387-78284-3 e-ISBN 978-0-387-78285-0
DOI 10.1007/978-0-387-78285-0
Springer New York Dordrecht Heidelberg London

Library of Congress Control Number: 2009939996

Printed on acid-free paper

Springer is part of Springer Science+Business Media (www.springer.com)

Preface

More is spent per person on health care in the United States than in any other nation in the world.[1] Healthcare spending is twice as great in the United Sates as compared to any other country on the planet, and accounts for roughly 15% of the country's Gross Domestic Product. Despite the reach and tangle of healthcare expenditures, the United States far from leads the world on key health-related indicators such as life expectancy, infant mortality, or breast cancer mortality. Debate has raged for decades over the access, efficiency, and quality purchased by the high sums spent. For example, the World Health Organization in 2000 ranked the US healthcare system first in both responsiveness and expenditure, but 37th in overall performance and 72nd by overall level of health (among 191 member nations included in the study).[2] Although the leading causes of death have shifted dramatically from the infectious diseases to the chronic diseases in the last 100 years, prevention and health promotion efforts account for less than 5% of all healthcare spending. Achieving the goals of Healthy People 2010 – to help individuals of all ages increase life expectancy and improve their quality of life; and to eliminate health disparities among different segments of the population – will require that individuals, communities, and policy makers take coordinated steps to ensure that good health, as well as long life, is enjoyed by all.[3] In other words, an integrated approach to the health of the population – one guided by an increased understanding of the health of individuals as well as the health of subgroups (minorities, ethnic groups, sexes), communities (neighborhoods, cities, regions), and functions (occupational groups, special groups, etc.) – is more likely to yield significant improvements in health and quality of life for a nation than one plagued by fragmentation and inequities.

This volume adopts a public health approach to asthma control that embraces the complex systems that guide care and access to care in the United States. Our population-based approach to improving asthma health outcomes relies on the social ecology model. The model emphasizes that individuals develop and live in social systems; and that people influence and are influenced by their families, their social networks, their communities, and their society. Interventions to improve health or to influence

[1] "Health Systems Resources" (Excel). *World Health Statistics 2008: Global Health Indicators*. World Health Organization. 2008. http://www.who.int/entity/whosis/whostat/4.xls. Retrieved on August 30, 2008.

[2] World Health Organization assesses the world's health system. Press Release WHO/44 21 June 2000. http://www.photius.com/rankings/who_world_health_ranks.html. Retrieved on March 25, 2009.

[3] *Healthy People 2010*. http://www.healthypeople.gov/default.htm. Retrieved on March 25, 2009.

health-related behavior can occur at any one or several of those levels. A full understanding of the interactions between health and behavior requires consideration of the separate levels and the interplay among them (i.e., the social ecology).

Asthma, Health and Society represents an effort to view asthma from a perspective of public health. It is divided into three sections: introduction, control of asthma, and the social ecology of asthma. The first section, the introduction, deals with basic aspects of asthma including its epidemiology, its pathogenesis, its genetic and environmental risk factors, its identification, and its role in society. Section II deals with asthma management. It includes discussions of medical and behavioral management of the disease and considerations of specific management questions concerning administration of steroid medication, home monitoring, and computer applications. Section III focuses on the problems of subpopulations of asthma patients, and how the disease impacts important societal institutions: the family, schools, and the workplace. It also includes chapters on barriers to asthma care and efforts to surmount them. Section III closes with a discussion of public policy as it relates to asthma. Together the three sections provide a comprehensive view of asthma as both an individual and societal problem, one deserving of a prominent place in discussions of public health policy.

Each contributor to this volume developed a highly original chapter with a broad public health audience in mind. We are grateful to them; this is their book.

Asthma, Health and Society was made possible, in part, by a grant (5R01HL068706) from the National Institutes of Health/National Heart, Lung, and Blood Institute to the senior editor and by support from The University of North Carolina at Charlotte and Ohio University.

Andrew Harver
Harry Kotses

Contents

III Asthma: A Social Ecological Perspective

Contributors

Andrea J. Apter, MD, MSc
Division of Pulmonary, Allergy, Critical Care, Hospital of the University of Pennsylvania, Philadelphia, PA, USA

Adam Atherly, PhD
Department of Health Systems, Management & Policy, Colorado School of Public Health, Aurora, CO, USA

Bruce G. Bender, PhD
Pediatric Behavioral Health, National Jewish Medical and Research Center, Denver, CO, USA

Larissa R. Brunner Huber, PhD
Department of Public Health Sciences, The University of North Carolina at Charlotte, Charlotte, NC, USA

Noreen M. Clark, PhD
Myron E. Wegman Distinguished University Professor, Center for Managing Chronic Disease, University of Michigan, Ann Arbor, MI, USA

Thomas L. Creer, PhD
Department of Psychology, Ohio University, Athens, OH, USA

Earl S. Ford, MD, MPH
Division of Adult and Community Health, National Center for Chronic Disease Prevention and Health Promotion, Centers for Disease Control and Prevention, Atlanta, GA, USA

Deborah Friedman, PhD
Bradley Hasbro Children's Research Center, Brown Medical School, Providence RI, USA

Denyse Gautrin, PhD
Center for Asthma in the Workplace, Hôpital du Sacré-Coeur de Montréal, Montreal, QC, Canada

Lynn B. Gerald, PhD, MSPH
Canyon Ranch Endowed Chair, Mel and Enid Zuckerman College of Public Health, University of Arizona, Tucson, AZ, USA

Peter J. Gergen, MD
National Institute for Allergy & Infectious Disease, National Institutes of Health, Atlanta, GA, USA

Andrew Harver, PhD
Department of Public Health Sciences, The University of North Carolina at Charlotte, Charlotte, NC, USA

Robert M. Kaplan, PhD
Fred W. and Pamela K. Wasserman Professor, Department of Health Services, UCLA School of Public Health, UCLA David Geffen School of Medicine, Los Angeles, CA, USA

Monroe J. King, DO
College of Medicine, University of South Florida, Tampa, FL, USA

Daphne Koinis-Mitchell, PhD
Bradley Hasbro Children's Research Center, Brown Medical School, Providence, RI, USA

Harry Kotses, PhD
Department of Psychology, Ohio University, Athens, OH, USA

James Krieger, MD, MPH
Epidemiology Planning and Evaluation Unit, Public Health – Seattle and King County, University of Washington Schools of Medicine and Public Health, Seattle, WA, USA

Karl J. Krobot, MD, PhD, MPH
Outcomes Research, MSD Sharp & Dohme GmbH, Haar, Germany

Manon Labrecque, MD, MSc
Center for Asthma in the Workplace, Hôpital du Sacré-Coeur de Montréal, Montreal, QC, Canada

Kim Lavoie, PhD
Center for Asthma in the Workplace, Hôpital du Sacré-Coeur de Montréal, Montreal, QC, Canada

Catherine Lemière, MD, MSc
Center for Asthma in the Workplace, Hôpital du Sacré-Coeur de Montréal, Montreal, QC, Canada

Jean-Luc Malo, MD
Center for Asthma in the Workplace, Hôpital du Sacré-Coeur de Montréal, Montreal, QC, Canada

Joan M. Mangan, PhD, MST
Lung Health Center, University of Alabama at Birmingham, Birmingham, AL, USA

David M. Mannino, MD
Division of Pulmonary, Critical Care, and Sleep Medicine, University of Kentucky Medical Center, Lexington, KY, USA

Elizabeth L. McQuaid, PhD
Bradley Hasbro Children's Research Center, Brown Medical School, Providence, RI, USA

Sarah Merkle, MPH
Division of Adolescent and School Health, Centers for Disease Control and Prevention, Atlanta, GA, USA

David R. Naimi, DO
Pediatrics, University of Washington, Seattle, WA, USA

Maeve O'Connor, MD, FAAAI
Carolina Asthma and Allergy Center, P.A., Charlotte, NC, USA
Department of Public Health Sciences, The University of North Carolina at Charlotte, Charlotte, NC, USA

Alexander N. Ortega, PhD
School of Public Health and Institute for Social Science Research, University of California Los Angeles, Los Angeles, CA, USA

Edith A. Parker, DrPH
Academic Affairs and Health Behavior and Health Education, University of Michigan School of Public Health, Ann Arbor, MI, USA

David B. Peden, MD, MS
The Center for Environmental Medicine, Asthma and Lung Biology, The University of North Carolina at Chapel Hill, Chapel Hill, NC, USA

Andrej Petrov, MD
Division of Pulmonary, Allergy and Critical Care Medicine, University of Pittsburgh School of Medicine, Pittsburgh, PA, USA

Melanie J. Rouse, MS
Department of Public Health Sciences, The University of North Carolina at Charlotte, Charlotte, NC, USA

Vasilisa Sazonov, MPharm, PhD
Global Outcomes Research, Reimbursement & Health Technology Assessment Department, Merck & Co. Inc., Whitehouse Station, NJ, USA

Richard Schwartzstein, MD
Division of Pulmonary and Critical Care Medicine, Beth Israel Deaconess Medical Center, Boston, MA, USA

Ross Shegog, PhD
Center for Health Promotion & Prevention Research, University of Texas Health Science Center – School of Public Health, Houston, TX, USA

Marianna M. Sockrider, MD, DrPH
Section of Pulmonology, Baylor College of Medicine, Houston, TX, USA
Pulmonary Medicine Clinics, Texas Children's Hospital, Houston, TX, USA

Tomas Tamulis, PhD
College of Public Health, Kent State University, Kent, OH, USA

Sam Walford, MA
School of Nursing, College of Health and Human Services, The University of North Carolina at Charlotte, Charlotte, NC, USA

Jan Warren-Findlow, PhD
Department of Public Health Sciences, The University of North Carolina at Charlotte, Charlotte, NC, USA

Sally E. Wenzel, MD
Division of Pulmonary, Allergy and Critical Care Medicine, University of Pittsburgh School of Medicine, Pittsburgh, PA, USA

Barbara P. Yawn, MD, MSc
Olmsted Medical Center, Rochester, MN, USA

Susie Yim Yeh, MD
Division of Pulmonary and Critical Care Medicine, Beth Israel Deaconess Medical Center, Boston, MA, USA

Part I
Asthma: An Introduction

Chapter 1
Considerations Regarding the Epidemiology and Public Health Burden of Asthma

Earl S. Ford and David M. Mannino

Epidemiologic Studies: An Introduction

Epidemiology has been defined as the study of the distribution and determinants of diseases and health. Commonly used epidemiological study designs are ecological studies, cross-sectional studies, case-control studies, prospective studies, and randomized trials. In an ecological study, levels of potential or actual risk factors are correlated with levels of disease across distinct geographically defined populations either among countries or within countries. In a cross-sectional study, a sample of participants is selected and subsequently those with a particular condition are compared with those who do not have that condition. Such studies provide solid information about the prevalence of a condition and the attendant risk factors. However, cross-sectional studies provide weaker evidence for potential associations between possible risk factors and outcomes than case-control or prospective studies. In a case-control study, people with a condition are selected and a separate control group is selected, and then the two groups are compared. These studies are usually performed to look for associations between potential risk factors and disease. Furthermore, case-control studies are a practical method to study associations for diseases that are relatively rare. In a prospective study (cohort study, panel study, longitudinal study), a sample of participants is selected and they are followed forward in time. These studies provide the most compelling evidence for possible causal relationships between potential risk factors and diseases, in part because the exposure of interest occurs prior to the outcome. Cross-sectional studies, case-control studies, and prospective studies are commonly referred to as observational studies. Each of these study designs is subject to various biases. Thus, the results from studies using these various study designs must be interpreted in the context of potential bias. In a randomized clinical trial, participants with a condition are selected, and they are then randomly assigned to one or more intervention groups or a control group. In a randomized community trial, communities are selected and randomly allocated to receiving an intervention or no or lower-level intervention. Such trials are generally considered to provide the most rigorous evidence supporting the causal relationship between a risk factor and disease or the usefulness of a specific treatment.

Public Health Burden of Asthma

A variety of measures can be used to assess the public health burden of asthma (Sennhauser et al. 2005; Bousquet et al. 2005). Prevalence is the proportion of people with asthma in a population, and incidence rate is a measure of the instantaneous force of asthma occurrence. Prevalence may be delineated into point prevalence (the proportion of people with asthma at a given point in time) and period prevalence (the proportion of people with asthma during a specified period of time such as the past 12 months). Incidence rate refers to the new onset of asthma during a specified period of time (number of new cases per unit of person-time), whereas cumulative incidence refers to the proportion of people initially free of disease who subsequently develop disease over a certain time span. Mortality

E.S. Ford (✉)
Division of Adult and Community Health, National Center for Chronic Disease Prevention and Health Promotion, Centers for Disease Control and Prevention, 4770 Buford Highway, MS K66, Atlanta, GA, 30341, USA
e-mail: eford@cdc.gov

A. Harver and H. Kotses (eds.), *Asthma, Health and Society: A Public Health Perspective*,
DOI 10.1007/978-0-387-78285-0_1, © Springer Science+Business Media, LLC 2010

rates provide an idea of how deadly the condition is and also an estimate of premature mortality through a calculation of years of productive life lost. Examining the number of physician office visits, emergency room visits, and hospitalizations yields important insights into the use of and need for medical resources and whether the capacity of the medical care sector is adequate to meet the need. Estimates of the direct and indirect costs of the disease provide critical insights into the dimensions of health care resources that are needed to combat this condition. Inherently tied to estimating indirect costs are the number of lost school days and lost workdays attributable to asthma. Measuring disability-adjusted life years and health-related quality of life of people with asthma provides another dimension of the burden of asthma.

Defining Asthma

Critical to the conduct of epidemiological studies and to examining the various facets of asthma is the availability of a case definition for asthma. In the Second Expert Panel Report of the Guidelines for the Diagnosis and Management of Asthma, asthma was defined as "a chronic inflammatory disorder of the airways in which many cells and cellular elements play a role, in particular, mast cells, eosinophils, T lymphocytes, neutrophils, and epithelial cells. In susceptible individuals, this inflammation causes recurrent episodes of wheezing, breathlessness, chest tightness, and cough, particularly at night and in the early morning. These episodes are usually associated with widespread but variable airflow obstruction that is often reversible either spontaneously or with treatment. The inflammation also causes an associated increase in the existing bronchial hyperresponsiveness to a variety of stimuli" (National Asthma Education and Prevention Program 1997). This definition is rooted in physiology and clinical considerations. For epidemiological purposes, however, a workable definition for use in often large-scale studies is a sine qua non.

Several approaches to defining asthma for epidemiologic use or developing case definitions have been taken (Table 1.1). The use of questionnaires is perhaps the most common approach. A single question or a series of questions is used to identify people with asthma. Examples from several large US surveys have been summarized elsewhere (Centers for Disease Control and Prevention 2009). Although this approach is conceptually attractive and is inexpensive, the validity and reliability of identifying people with asthma in this way need to be established. The simplicity of this approach can also lead to the creation of numerous such instruments that differ in minor or major ways, thus possibly compromising comparisons of study results. Consequently, attempts have been made to standardize asthma questionnaires to facilitate comparisons of the prevalence of asthma among populations as was done in the European Community Respiratory Health Survey (ECRHS 2007) and International Study of Asthma and Allergies in Childhood (ISAAC 1993). The development of such questionnaires requires a process of testing the validity and reliability of the questions (Venables et al. 1993; Jenkins et al. 1996; Galobardes et al. 1998; Sole et al. 1998; Wolf et al. 1999; Kilpelainen et al. 2001a; Aroni et al. 2004; Redline et al. 2004). This process may have to be repeated for special populations such as health-care workers (Delclos et al. 2006).

Table 1.1 Methods for determining asthma in epidemiological studies

Questionnaires
Diaries
Medical records
Administrative data bases
Pharmacy
Health maintenance organizations
Outpatient visits
Emergency room
Hospitalizations
Vital statistics
Provocation tests (bronchial hyperresponsiveness)
Methacholine challenge test
Histamine challenge
Adenosine 5′-monophosphate
Exercise challenge test
Cold air challenge
Hypertonic saline
Lung function tests
Spirometry
Peak expiratory flow rate variability
Exhaled nitric oxide
Eosinophilia
Blood sputum eosinophils

Asthma from Medical Records

Using medical records to identify people with asthma is another method of case ascertainment

(Wamboldt et al. 2002). The use of this technique depends heavily on the diagnosis made by clinicians. Although national or professional guidelines for diagnosing asthma have been developed, the degree to which clinicians adhere to these guidelines is not always clear. Thus, differences in diagnostic practices may occur among clinicians. In a sample of 182 children, the reliability and validity of coding asthma outcomes were good (Wamboldt et al. 2002).

Asthma from Administrative Databases

Large administrative databases are used for a variety of purposes including estimating the prevalence of disease, examining the use of medical resources (hospitalizations, physician-office visits, emergency room visits), performing pharmacoepidemiological studies, examining treatment patterns, following the prognosis of a disease, and studying compliance with guidelines (Blais et al. 2006). In the United States, examples include the National Hospital Discharge System, Nationwide Inpatient Sample, the National Ambulatory Care Medical Survey, National Hospital Ambulatory Medical Care Survey, National Disease and Therapeutic Index, Medicare, Medicaid, and health maintenance organization databases. For many of these databases, conditions are often coded using the International Classification of Diseases. In addition, large pharmacy databases can be used to identify people who use asthma medications (Allen-Ramey et al. 2006).

Bronchial Hyperreactivity Testing

Determining the presence of asthma using questionnaires was not considered a rigorous method; measuring airway hyperresponsiveness was considered a more physiologic approach. However, several considerations limit the use of this method. It is time-consuming, resource-intensive, and carries a small risk for an adverse event. Some proportion of people with asthma do not have airway hyperresponsiveness as determined by bronchial hyperreactivity testing. Thus, this approach may underestimate people with asthma, especially those with mild asthma. For example, approximately 30% of children with asthma may not have bronchial hyperreactivity, whereas approximately 15% of children who have never wheezed may have a positive bronchial hyperreactivity test (Phelan 1994).

Nevertheless, bronchial hyperreactivity is often used as a "hard measure" of asthma. Testing for bronchial hyperreactivity may involve the use of metacholine, histamine, adenosine, cold air, hypertonic saline solution, and exercise as triggers (de Meer et al. 2004).

Furthermore, different protocols exist for various stimulants that could yield somewhat different findings in studies. The relative merit of these protocols is still being investigated (Haby et al. 1995).

Death Certificates

Because deaths from asthma are a relatively rare occurrence, the use of death certificates for case-definitions of asthma is usually confined to studies of mortality trends. Diagnostic practices for asthma may show geographical and temporal variation, and it is, therefore, helpful to understand the validity of death certificates when comparing study results (Subcommittee of the BTA Research Committee 1984; Sears et al. 1986; Campbell et al. 1992; Jenkins et al. 1992; Hunt et al. 1993; Wright et al. 1994; Guite and Burney 1996; Sidenius et al. 2000).

Exhaled Nitric Oxide

The recognition that inflammation of the airways is an important component of asthma provides a rationale to attempt to diagnose asthma by measuring the underlying inflammation. One such test is the measurement of exhaled nitric oxide (Dupont et al. 2003; Deykin et al. 2002; Smith et al. 2004; Berkman et al. 2005; Zitt 2005). Patients perform a slow expiratory vital capacity maneuver with a constant flow rate. The optimal cutoff point of exhaled nitric oxide still needs to be established. Thus far, measuring exhaled nitric oxide has not been commonly used in epidemiologic studies.

Summary

A number of methods exist to identify asthma in patients and study participants, each of which has advantages and disadvantages. Because there is no "gold standard" to assess asthma, the validity of the different methods is difficult to establish. A clinical diagnosis of asthma derived by following professional guidelines is often used as the "gold standard." The choice of which test to incorporate in a study will be based on the perceived accuracy of a test as well as on practical considerations involving cost, invasiveness, complexity, and patient acceptability. Attempts have been made to assess the validity of different methods in diagnosing asthma (Hunter et al. 2002; Yurdakul et al. 2005). The findings of inconsistent rates of asthma across four different data sources used routinely for surveillance purposes in the United Kingdom sound a note of caution about the use of such data (Hansell et al. 2003).

Prevalence of Asthma

Estimates of the prevalence of asthma show tremendous temporal and spatial variation (Pearce and Douwes 2006). In the United States, several data systems provide information about the prevalence of asthma including National Health and Nutrition Examination Surveys, National Health Interview Surveys (NHIS), Behavioral Risk Factor Surveillance System (BRFSS), and ISAAC. Estimates from these surveys are all based on the results from questionnaires. Data from the NHIS show that the prevalence of asthma, based on a household member having had asthma during the previous 12 months, in the US population rose from <4% to approximately 5.5% in 1996 (Mannino et al. 2002). In 2004, 9.9% of US adults representing an estimated 21.3 million people had ever had asthma, and 6.4% or approximately 14.4 million still had asthma (Centers for Disease Control and Prevention 2006a). In 2004, 12.2% of US children representing an estimated 8.9 million children were ever diagnosed with asthma, and 5.4% or 4 million children had experienced an attack in the past 12 months (Centers for Disease Control and Prevention 2005). Data from the BRFSS administered to participants aged 18+ years showed a steady rise in the prevalence of lifetime asthma ("Did a doctor ever tell you that you had asthma?") from 10.4% in 2000 to 13.3% in 2004 and that of current asthma ("Do you still have asthma?") from 7.2% to 8.1% (Fig. 1.1) (Centers for Disease Control and Prevention 2004a). In contrast, the prevalence of ever having asthma or having an asthma attack in the past 12 months among children varied only slightly from 1997 through 2004, according to NHIS data (Fig. 1.2) (Centers for Disease Control and Prevention 2005; Centers for Disease Control and Prevention 2002a, b; Centers for Disease Control and Prevention 2003a, b, c; Centers for Disease Control and Prevention 2004b; Centers for Disease Control and Prevention 2006b). Previously, the prevalence of having asthma during the previous 12 months in children increased from 3.6% in 1980 to 6.2% in 1996 (Akinbami and Schoendorf 2002).

Age, Sex, and Race or Ethnicity

In general, the prevalence of ever having asthma and having an asthma attack in the past 12 months increases progressively during childhood (Fig. 1.3). In addition, during childhood, the prevalence of ever having asthma and having an asthma attack in the past 12 months is higher among males than females (Fig. 1.4), whereas among adults the prevalence of lifetime asthma and current asthma is generally higher among females than males (Fig. 1.5). US data from the 2004 NHIS show somewhat varying patterns in the prevalence of ever having asthma with respect to age (Figs. 1.3 and 1.6). The prevalence of ever having asthma is highest among those aged 12–17 years. Among adults, relatively little variation in the prevalence of ever having asthma by age group is present. In contrast, the prevalence of still having asthma increases gradually with age through ages 65–74 years. Of the three major racial or ethnic groups, the prevalence of ever having asthma is highest among African American children and lowest among Hispanic children (Fig. 1.7) (McDaniel et al. 2006). Racial or ethnic differences among adults were similar to those among children except that the difference between whites and African Americans was less pronounced (Fig. 1.8).

Geographic Variability Within Countries

BRFSS data for the United States show significant variation among the fifty states and two territories

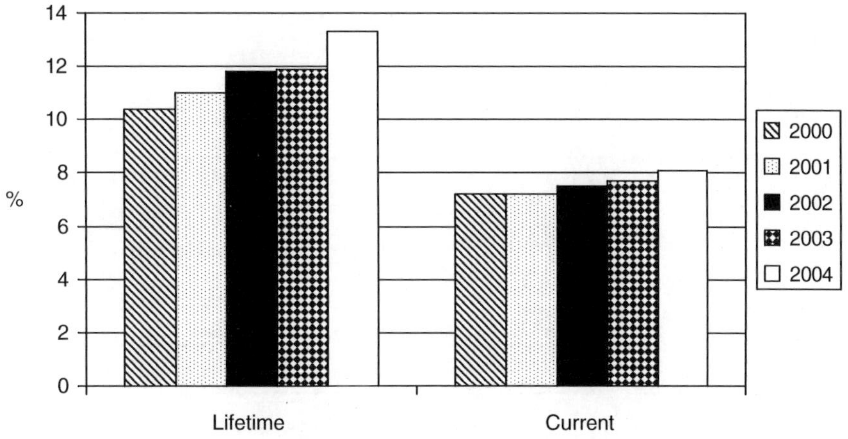

Fig. 1.1 Trend in the prevalence of asthma among US adults aged ≥18 years with asthma, Behavioral Risk Factor Surveillance System, 2000–2004

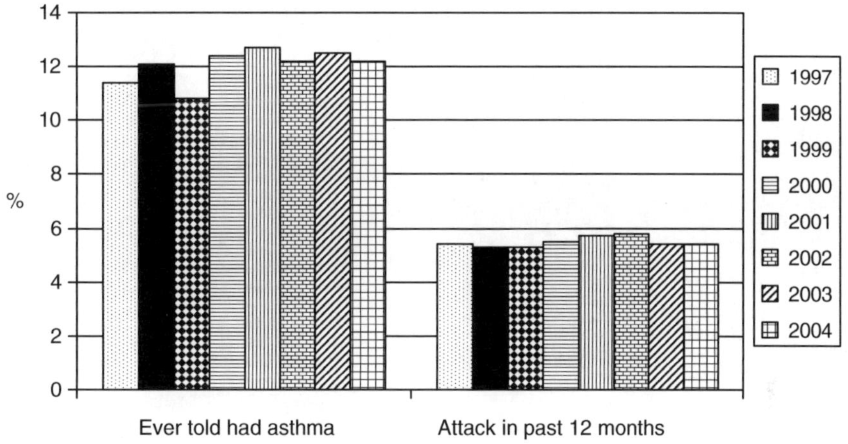

Fig. 1.2 Trend in the prevalence of asthma among US children aged <18 years with asthma, National Health Interview Survey, 1997–2004

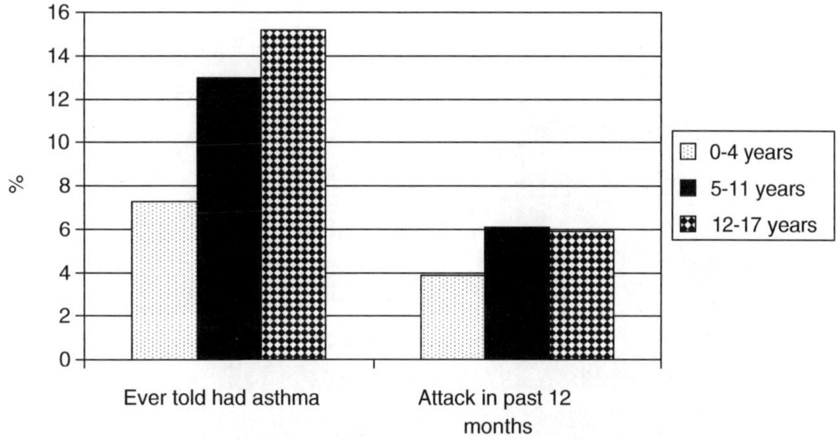

Fig. 1.3 Age-specific percentage of US children aged <18 years with asthma, National Health Interview Survey, 2004

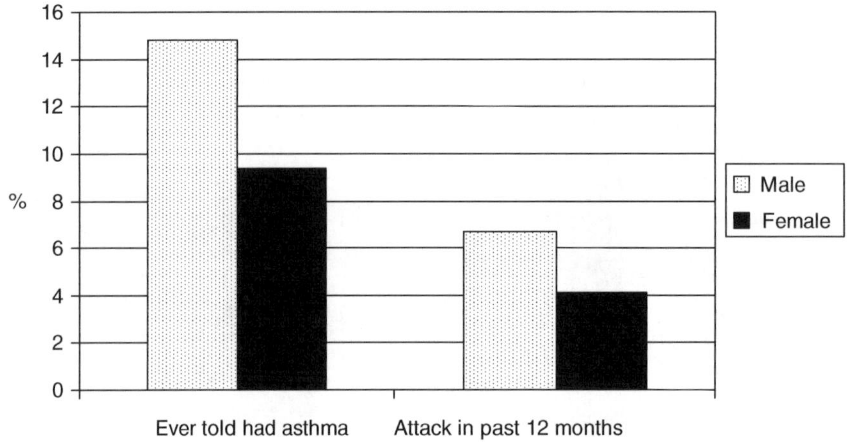

Fig. 1.4 Age-adjusted percentage of US children aged <18 years with asthma, by gender, National Health Interview Survey, 2004

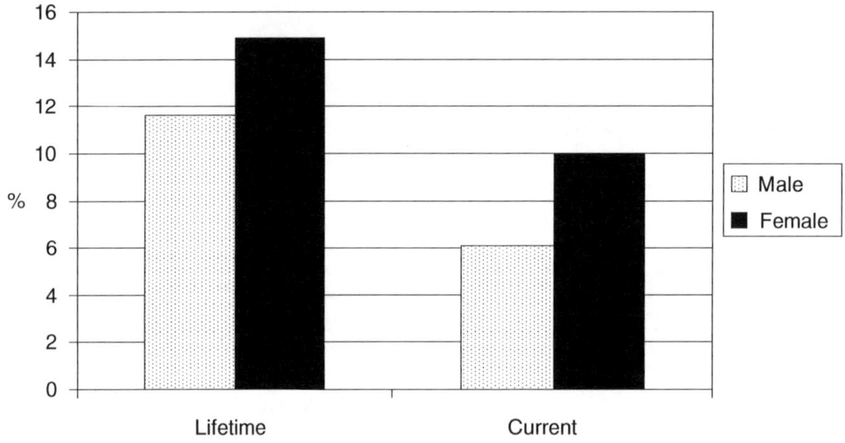

Fig. 1.5 Age-adjusted percentage of US adults aged ≥18 years with asthma, by gender, Behavioral Risk Factor Surveillance System, 2004

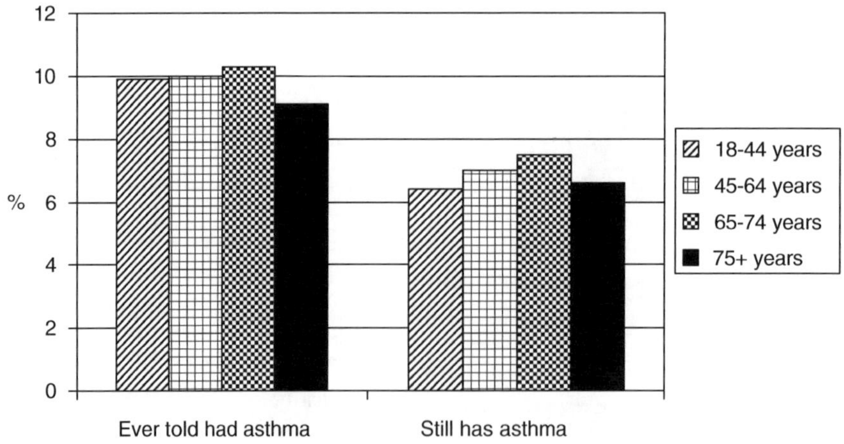

Fig. 1.6 Age-specific percentage of US adults with asthma, National Health Interview Survey, 2004

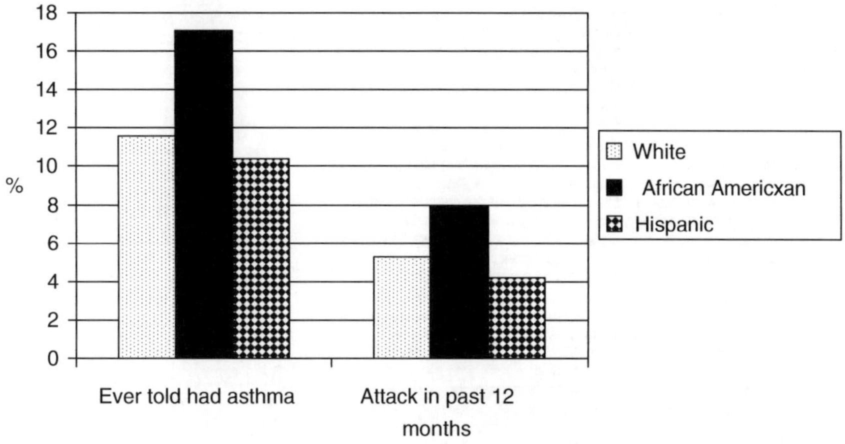

Fig. 1.7 Age-adjusted percentage of US children aged <18 years with asthma, by race or ethnicity, National Health Interview Survey, 2004

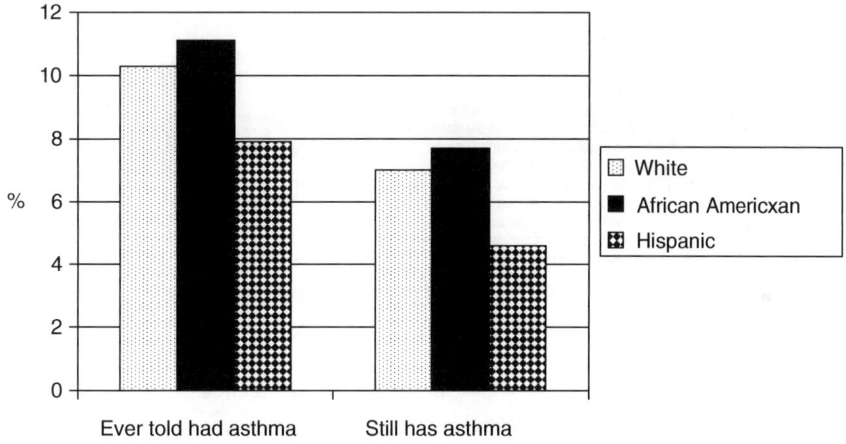

Fig. 1.8 Age-adjusted percentage of US adults aged ≥18 years with asthma, by race or ethnicity, National Health Interview Survey, 2004

(Figs. 1.9 and 1.10). In 2004, the lifetime prevalence of asthma ranged from 10.3% in South Dakota and the Virgin Islands to 16.3% in Oregon and 18.8% in Puerto Rico, whereas the prevalence of current asthma ranged from 4.6% in the Virgin Islands to 10.3% in New Hampshire (Centers for Disease Control and Prevention 2004a). In addition, data from ISAAC also show significant variation within other countries such as Brazil, India, Italy, Spain, and the United Kingdom (ISAAC Steering Committee 1998).

Geographic Variability Among Countries

ISAAC was conducted in 56 countries among children aged 13–14 years using standardized techniques (ISAAC Steering Committee 1998). The results showed enormous variation in the prevalence of 12-month asthma ranging from 1.6% in Indonesia to 36.8% in the United Kingdom. Other data reviewed by Pearce and Douwes show equally dramatic variation in the prevalence of asthma across the world

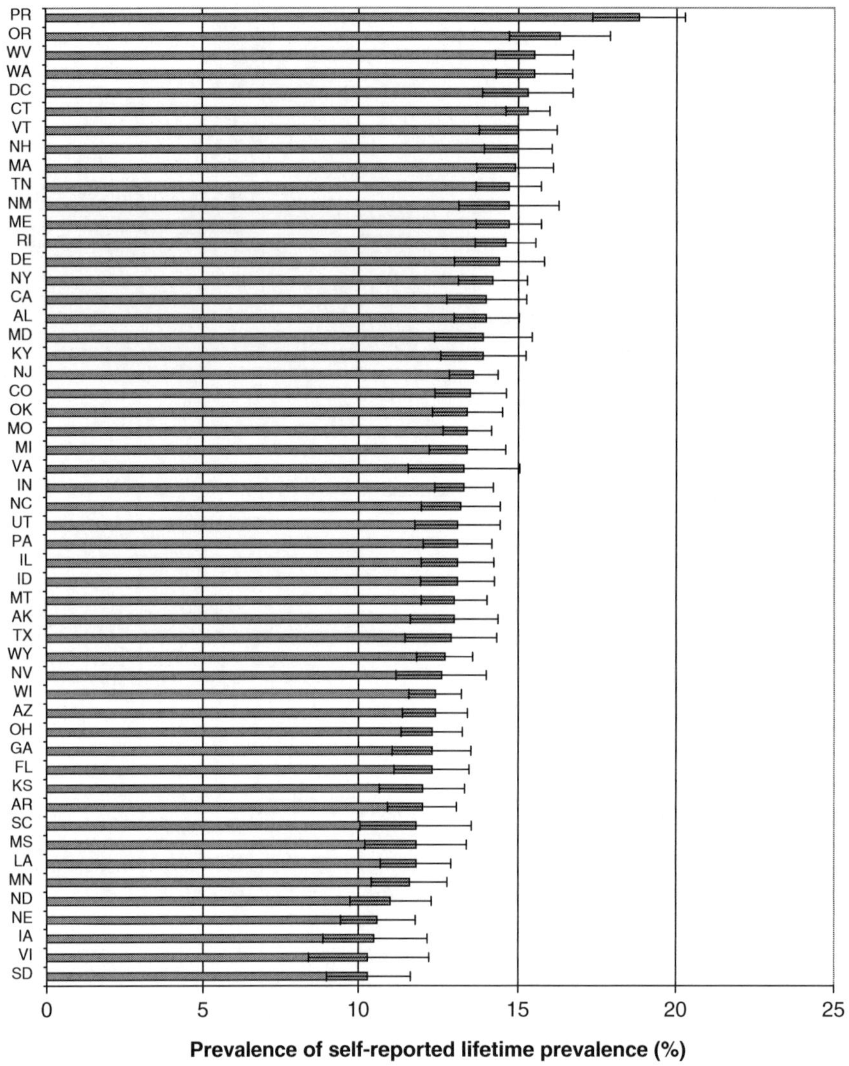

Fig. 1.9 Prevalence of self-reported lifetime asthma (percent, 95% confidence interval), by state or territory, Behavioral Risk Factor Surveillance System, 2004

(Pearce and Douwes 2006). Among children, adolescents, and young adults, the prevalence ranges from 0% in Papua, New Guinea during 1973–1984 to 33.9% in the United Kingdom during 1991–1998. Furthermore, the European Community Respiratory Health Survey conducted among participants aged 20–44 years showed that estimates of diagnosed asthma ranged from 2% in Tartu, Estonia to 8.4% in Cambridge, United Kingdom during the early 1990s (ECRHS 1996).

Temporal Trends

Studies from the 1950s to the 1990s found increases in prevalence of asthma and asthma symptoms in many countries (Robertson et al. 1991; von Mutius 1998). However, in the last 10–15 years, the prevalence of asthma or asthma symptoms has either reached a plateau or decreased in several countries (Robertson et al. 2004). Many of these studies documenting the trends used questionnaires. However, increases in

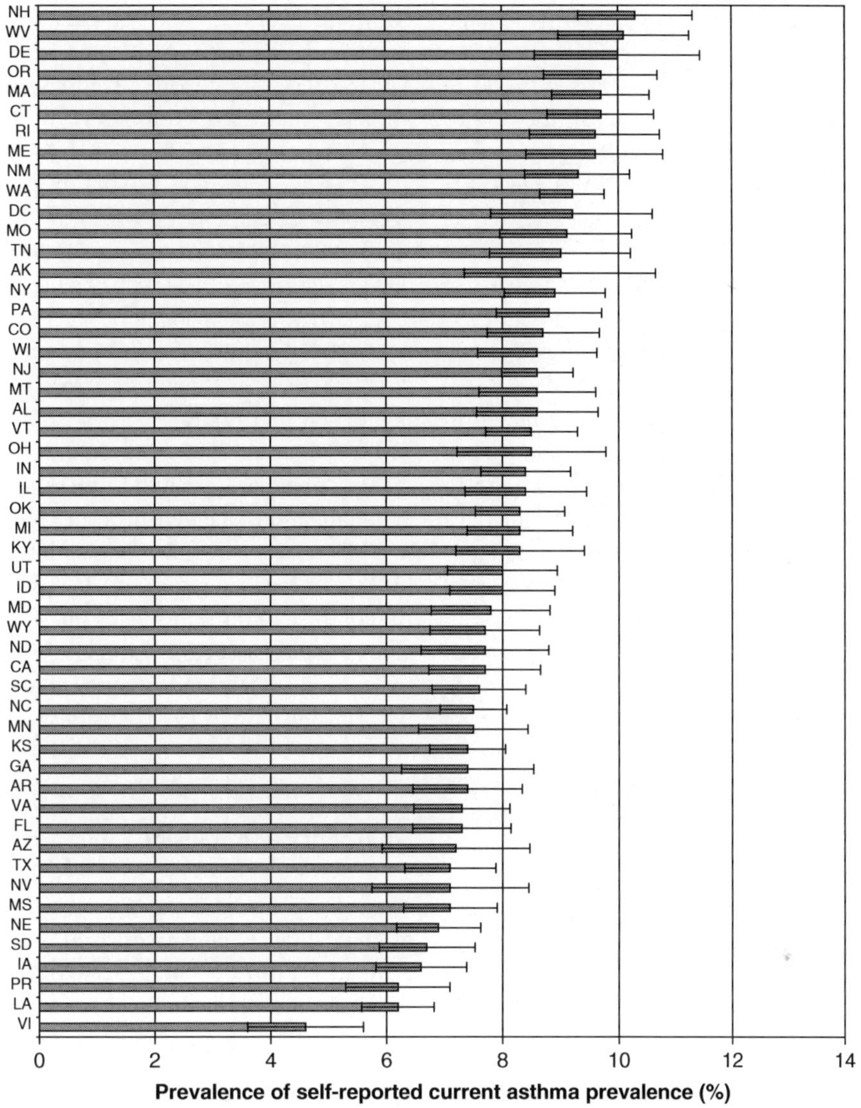

Fig. 1.10 Prevalence of self-reported current asthma (percent, 95% confidence interval), by state or territory, Behavioral Risk Factor Surveillance System, 2004

bronchial hyperreactivity in children over time have been documented as well (Burr et al. 1989; Peat et al. 1994).

Incidence of Asthma

Incidence data at the national level is difficult to come by. However, numerous cohort studies provide some insights into the incidence of this disease. In a recent review of 40 prospective studies from 13 countries, the incidence of asthma ranged from 0.6 to 29.5 per 1,000 persons (King et al. 2004).

Medical Care Utilization

Hospitalizations

Despite some instability in the annual rates of hospitalization for asthma in the United States, the estimated rate generally decreased from 1985 to 1999 (from 19.7 to 17.6 per 10,000 population) (Mannino et al. 2002). Because of a growing population, however, the number of such hospitalizations was 408,000 in 1980 and 478,000 in 1999. The trend in the rate of hospitalization differed by sex, ethnicity, and age. The highest rates in men occurred in 1980 and 1985, whereas among women the highest rate occurred in 1995. The highest rate occurred in 1997 among those aged <4 years, in 1995 in those aged 5–34 years, in 1980 among those aged 35–64 years, and in 1985 among those aged 65+ years. Among whites, the rate peaked in 1985 before decreasing (15.6 per 10,000 population in 1985 to 10.6 per 10,000 population in 1999), whereas in African Americans, the rate peaked in 1995 (from 40.7 per 10,000 population in 1985 to 35.6 per 10,000 population in 1999). In all years, rates were higher in women than men, in African Americans than whites, and were highest in those aged ≤4 years and lowest in those aged 15–34 years. More recent data through 2002 show further decreases in hospitalization rates among whites but not African Americans (Getahun et al. 2005).

In other countries, rates of hospitalization for asthma have varied in time as well. In Scotland, the rate of hospitalization increased overall between 1981 and 1997 (from 106.7 to 236.7 per 100,000 population) (Morrison and McLoone 2001). However, among those aged <15 years, the rates peaked in 1992 and then decreased progressively through 1997. In contrast, rates continued to increase in those aged 15+ years. Furthermore, trends differed between males and females. In northeastern Israel, the rate of first hospital admission for asthma increased, but that of readmission decreased among children aged <18 years from 1990 to 1999 (Rottem et al. 2005). In Norway, the rate of admissions increased among children aged <15 years during the 1980s before decreasing and stabilizing (29.5 per 10,000 during 1980–1985, 36.3 per 10,000 during 1986–1990, and 33.0 per 10,000 during 1991–1995) (Jonasson et al. 2000). After peaking in 1984 and 1985, rates of readmissions decreased. In addition, the age at admission and length of hospital stay decreased. In Athens, Greece, the admission rate for children aged <15 years rose by 271% from 1978 to 2000 (Priftis et al. 2005). Admission rates were higher among children aged <4 years than among those aged 5–14 years. In Eastern Finland, hospital admissions for asthma among children aged ≤16 years increased from 1.2 per 1000 in 1988 to 2.7 per 1,000 in 1997 (Korhonen et al. 2002). The readmission rate decreased, however. At a nationwide institution in Mexico, the rate of hospitalizations among people of all ages increased from 1991 to 1996 and then decreased progressively through 2001 (Vargas et al. 2004). Although some variability was present in the age-specific trends, the rates in all age groups decreased since 1999. In Victoria, Australia, the admission rates decreased from 3.11 per 1000 population in 1993–1994 to 2.15 per 1,000 population in 1999–2000 (Ansari et al. 2003). A decrease in hospitalization rates was also observed in Singapore (from 21.7 per 10,000 population in 1991 to 15.4 per 10,000 population in 1998) (Ng et al. 2003) and in Ontario from 1988 to 2000 (Crighton et al. 2001). Interestingly, the rate of hospitalization changed little in Quebec from 1988 to 1989 (1.76 per 1,000 population) to 1994–1995 (1.75 per 1,000 population) (Laurier et al. 1999). In contrast, admission rates in Taiwan increased among children aged 2–14 years from 1990 to 1998 (Kao et al. 2001) and among children from South Africa from 1986 to 1996 (MacIntyre et al. 2001).

Emergency Room Visits

The number of visits to the emergency room for asthma in the United States increased steadily, from an estimated 1,467,000 in 1992 to 1,997,000 in 1999, whereas the rate of these visits was lowest in 1992 (56.8 per 10,000 population) and bounced between 70 and 75 per 10,000 population between 1995 and 1999 (Mannino et al. 2002). Rates were markedly higher in African Americans than whites (in 1995 over four times higher), and more modestly so among women than men. In addition, rates were highest among children ≤4 years. In a Mexican nationwide institution, the rate of emergency room visits increased from 1991 to 1996 and then decreased steadily through 2001 (Vargas et al. 2004).

Physician-Office Visits

The annual number of office visits to physicians for asthma in the United States also increased over time from approximately 5,921,000 in 1980 to 13,853,000 in 1998 and 10,808,000 in 1999 (Mannino et al. 2002).

The rate of these visits increased from 26.1 per 1,000 population in 1980 to 51.5 per 1,000 population in 1998. The differential between African Americans and whites was much less pronounced, whereas the rate among women was consistently higher than that among men. In addition, the rate was highest among those aged 5–14 years. In a Mexican nationwide institution, the rate of office visits to family physicians increased from 1991 to 1995, was stable in 1996 and 1997, and then decreased through 2001 (Vargas et al. 2004).

Economic Impact

The estimated direct and indirect costs of asthma have continued to escalate in the United States. The costs of asthma were calculated to be $4.5 billion in 1985 (Weiss et al. 2000), $6.2 billion in 1990 (Weiss et al. 1992), $10.7 billion in 1994 (Weiss et al. 2000), $12.7 billion in 1998 (Weiss and Sullivan 2001), and $19.7 billion in 2009 (American Lung Association 2009). Estimates have also been generated in other countries. For example, the indirect and direct costs of asthma were estimated at $32 million in 1992/1993 dollars in Singapore (Chew et al. 1999), CAN$810-954 million in Canada in 1990 (Krahn et al. 1996), 2.74 billion euros in Germany during in 1999 (Stock et al. 2005), 1.252 billion Swiss franks in Switzerland in 1997 (Szucs et al. 1999), 1.9 billion Danish kronen in 2000 (Mossing and Nielsen 2003), and 0.9–1.2 billion euros in Spain (Nieto et al. 2001). In addition, direct costs were 2.1 million euros in Estonia in 1997 or approximately 1.4% of direct health care costs (Kiivet et al. 2001). Finally, the costs for children aged <15 years living in one of the 25 countries in Europe were approximately 3 billion in 2004 euros (van den Akker-van Marle et al. 2005).

Asthma Mortality

In the United States, the race-, sex-, and age-adjusted mortality rate for asthma increased from 1980 until about the mid 1990s and then decreased through 1998 (Mannino et al. 2002). Since then, the number of deaths for which asthma was listed as the underlying cause was 4,657 in 1999, 4,487 in 2000, 4,269 in 2001, and 4,261 in 2002. During these 4 years, the age-adjusted mortality rate dropped from 1.3 to 1.2 per 100,000 population in males and from 2.0 to 1.7 per 100,000 population in females. The mortality rate increased with age and reached a maximum for those aged 85+ years. The mortality rate decreased among both whites (from 1.4 to 1.2 per 100,000) and African Americans (from 3.9 to 3.4 per 100,000) but remained approximately 2.8 to 3.0 times higher among African Americans.

A comparison of mortality rates from asthma for populations aged 5–34 years from 14 countries from 1970 through the mid 1980s showed large variation in mortality rates and in most countries increases in the mortality rates (Jackson et al. 1988). In the United Kingdom, the mortality rates from asthma during the period from 1983 to 1995 declined in age groups younger than 75 years (Campbell et al. 1997). For those aged 75 years and older, rates were either roughly stationary or increased. In Denmark, mortality trends for those aged 1–19 years increased from 1973 until about 1983–1987 for most age groups before decreasing though 1993–1994 (Jorgensen et al. 2000). Furthermore, mortality rates decreased in Capetown, South Africa in all racial groups between 1980 and 1997 (Zar et al. 2001). In contrast, mortality rates from asthma remained relatively stable between 1980 and 1997 among Israelis aged 5–34 years (Picard et al. 2002).

Comparing mortality rates among countries is complicated by coding practices in countries, changes in International Classification of Diseases codes over time (ICD-8, ICD-9, and ICD-10), and changes in diagnostic practices by clinicians. It appears, however, that mortality rates have fallen in many countries, although the time points when the decreases commenced may have differed.

Disability-Adjusted Life-Years (DALY)

The World Health Organization (WHO) defines the DALY as “a health gap measure that extends the concept of potential years of life lost due to premature death (PYLL) to include equivalent years of ‘healthy’ life lost by virtue of being in states of poor health or disability. The DALY combines in one measure the time lived with disability and the time lost due to premature mortality. One DALY can be thought of as one lost year of 'healthy' life and the burden of disease as a measurement of the gap between current health status and an ideal situation where everyone lives into old age free of disease and disability" (World Health Organization 2009). Thus, the DALY is a measure of the state of health of a population that reflects both the loss of quality of life and loss of life years (Murray 1994). One DALY reflects the loss of one healthy life year. In 2001, WHO attributed approximately 15 million DALYs to asthma worldwide, or approximately 1% of the total DALYs for all causes that were considered (World Health Organization 2002).

Risk Factors

Numerous epidemiological studies have examined a host of factors as predictors of asthma incidence or correlates of prevalence. A number of these are listed in Table 1.2. Because subsequent chapters will provide a detailed look at these factors, we will content ourselves with some general remarks. Despite a lengthy list of potential risk factors, few have been subjected to systematic review.

The distinction between a risk factor and trigger in studies of asthma etiology is not always straightforward. Although a particular factor could be both, it is also possible that it could be one or the other. Furthermore, another distinction needs to be drawn between a risk factor and a risk marker. The former implies that the factor is causally related to the disease, whereas the latter predicts disease but is not causally related to the disease. The distinction is important because a risk factor is potentially amenable to intervention, whereas a risk marker is not. Nevertheless, risk markers may still be useful in identifying groups of people at increased risk of developing asthma.

Some studies have suggested complex interactions between risk factors and the risk of asthma or asthma symptoms. Examples of reported interactions between factors include atopy and smoking (Sunyer et al. 1997), age and exposure to pets (Apelberg et al. 2001), atopic heritability and home dampness (Kilpelainen et al. 2001b), parental history of asthma and exposure to pets (Celedon et al. 2002), gender and smoking status and/or exposure to pets (Chen et al. 2002), genetic factors and environmental factors (Bisgaard 2004), and diet and indoor allergen exposure (Kim et al. 2005).

Table 1.2 Purported risk and protective factors for asthma

Risk factors
Sociodemographic
Age
Gender
Ethnicity
Acculturation
Socioeconomic status
Infections
Host factors
Atopy
Allergies
House mites
Cockroaches
Pollen
Pets
Environmental
Indoor air pollution
Outdoor air pollution
Environmental tobacco smoke
Bio-aeroallergens
Lifestyle
Smoking
Exercise
Nutrition
Obesity
Developmental
Low birth weight
Breastfeeding
Occupational exposures
Genetics
Protective factors
Breastfeeding
Menopause
Daycare attendance
Pet ownership
Parasites

Determinants of early-onset asthma may also differ from those of late-onset asthma. Because the bulk of asthma among children and adolescents occurs at a young age, studies of risk factors in pediatric populations have to be done among young children (Weiss 2001).

Finally, although some risk factors may be strongly related to asthma, as evidenced by large measures of association (i.e., odds ratios, relative risks, or hazard ratios), they may occur relatively rarely. Conversely, some risk factors for asthma may be more modestly associated with asthma incidence yet occur much more frequently in the population. The population attributable risk, also known by several other names, combines estimates of relative risk and prevalence into a single measure. This statistic is, therefore, important from a public health perspective because it can help to prioritize prevention strategies and allocate resources appropriately.

References

(1984) Accuracy of death certificates in bronchial asthma. Accuracy of certification procedures during the confidential inquiry by the British Thoracic Association. A subcommittee of the BTA Research Committee. Thorax 39:505–509

(1996) Variations in the prevalence of respiratory symptoms, self-reported asthma attacks, and use of asthma medication in the European Community Respiratory Health Survey (ECRHS). Eur Respir J 9:687–695

(1998) Worldwide variation in prevalence of symptoms of asthma, allergic rhinoconjunctivitis, and atopic eczema: ISAAC. The International Study of Asthma and Allergies in Childhood (ISAAC) Steering Committee. Lancet 351:1225–1232

Akinbami LJ, Schoendorf KC (2002) Trends in childhood asthma: prevalence, health care utilization, and mortality. Pediatrics 110:315–322

Allen-Ramey FC, Bukstein D, Luskin A, Sajjan SG, Markson LE (2006) Administrative claims analysis of asthma-related health care utilization for patients who received inhaled corticosteroids with either montelukast or salmeterol as combination therapy. J Manag Care Pharm 12:310–321

American Lung Association. Asthma in adults fact sheet. Available from http://www.lungusa.org/site/apps/nl/content3.asp?c=dvLUK9O0E&b=2058817&content_id=%7b39966A20-AE3C-4F85-B285-68E23EDC6CA8%7d&notoc=1

Ansari Z, Haby MM, Henderson T, Cicuttini F, Ackland MJ (2003) Trends and geographic variations in hospital admissions for asthma in Victoria. Opportunities for targeted interventions. Aust Fam Physician 32:286–288

Apelberg BJ, Aoki Y, Jaakkola JJ (2001) Systematic review: Exposure to pets and risk of asthma and asthma-like symptoms. J Allergy Clin Immunol 107:455–460

Aroni R, Goeman D, Stewart K, Thien F, Sawyer S, Abramson M, Douglass J (2004) Enhancing validity: what counts as an asthma attack? J Asthma 41:729–737

Berkman N, Avital A, Breuer R, Bardach E, Springer C, Godfrey S (2005) Exhaled nitric oxide in the diagnosis of asthma: comparison with bronchial provocation tests. Thorax 60:383–388

Bisgaard H (2004) The Copenhagen Prospective Study on Asthma in Childhood (COPSAC): design, rationale, and baseline data from a longitudinal birth cohort study. Ann Allergy Asthma Immunol 93:381–389

Blais L, Lemiere C, Menzies D, Berbiche D (2006) Validity of asthma diagnoses recorded in the medical services database of Quebec. Pharmacoepidemiol Drug Saf 15:245–252

Bousquet J, Bousquet PJ, Godard P, Daures JP (2005) The public health implications of asthma. Bull World Health Organ 83:548–554

Burr ML, Butland BK, King S, Vaughan-Williams E (1989) Changes in asthma prevalence: two surveys 15 years apart. Arch Dis Child 64:1452–1456

Campbell DA, McLennan G, Coates JR, Frith PA, Gluyas PA, Latimer KM, Martin AJ, Roder DM, Ruffin RE, Yellowlees PM (1992) Accuracy of asthma statistics from death certificates in South Australia. Med J Aust 156:860–863

Campbell MJ, Cogman GR, Holgate ST, Johnston SL (1997) Age specific trends inasthma mortality in England and Wales, 1983–95: results of an observational study. BMJ 314:1439–1441

Celedon JC, Litonjua AA, Ryan L, Platts-Mills T, Weiss ST, Gold DR (2002) Exposure to cat allergen, maternal history of asthma, and wheezing in first 5 years of life. Lancet 360:781–782

Centers for Disease Control and Prevention (2002a) Summary Health Statistics for U.S. Children: National Health Interview Survey, 1997. Vital Health Stat Series 10:1–46

Centers for Disease Control and Prevention (2002b) Summary Health Statistics for U.S. Children: National Health Interview Survey, 1998. Vital Health Stat Series 10:1–46

Centers for Disease Control and Prevention (2003a) Summary Health Statistics for U.S. Children: National Health Interview Survey, 1999. Vital Health Stat Series 10:1–50

Centers for Disease Control and Prevention (2003b) Summary Health Statistics for U.S. Children: National Health Interview Survey, 2000. Vital Health Stat Series 10:1–48

Centers for Disease Control and Prevention (2003c) Summary Health Statistics for U.S. Children: National Health Interview Survey, 2001. Vital Health Stat Series 10:1–54

Centers for Disease Control and Prevention. 2004 Adult asthma data: prevalence tables and maps. Available from http://www.cdc.gov/asthma/brfss/04/brfssdata.htm

Centers for Disease Control and Prevention (2004b) Summary Health Statistics for U.S. Children: National Health Interview Survey, 2002. Vital Health Stat Series 10:1–78

Centers for Disease Control and Prevention (2005) Summary Health Statistics for U.S. Children: National Health Interview Survey, 2003. Vital Health Stat Series 10:1–78

Centers for Disease Control and Prevention (2006a) Summary Health Statistics for U.S. Adults: National Health Interview Survey, 2004. Vital Health Stat Series 10:1–153

Centers for Disease Control and Prevention (2006b) Summary Health Statistics for U.S. Children: National Health Interview Survey, 2004. Vital Health Stat Series 10:1–85

Chen Y, Dales R, Tang M, Krewski D (2002) Sex-related interactive effect of smoking and household pets on asthma incidence. Eur Respir J 20:1162–1166

Chew FT, Goh DY, Lee BW (1999) The economic cost of asthma in Singapore. Aust NZ J Med 29:228–233

Crighton EJ, Mamdani MM, Upshur RE (2001) A population based time series analysis of asthma hospitalisations in Ontario, Canada: 1988 to 2000. BMC Health Serv Res 1:7

de Meer G, Marks GB, Postma DS (2004) Direct or indirect stimuli for bronchial challenge testing: what is the relevance for asthma epidemiology? Clin Exp Allergy 34:9–16

Delclos GL, Arif AA, Aday L, Carson A, Lai D, Lusk C, Stock T, Symanski E, Whitehead LW, Benavides FG,

Anto JM (2006) Validation of an asthma questionnaire for use in healthcare workers. Occup Environ Med 63:173–179
Deykin A, Massaro AF, Drazen JM, Israel E (2002) Exhaled nitric oxide as a diagnostic test for asthma: online versus offline techniques and effect of flow rate. Am J Respir Crit Care Med 165:1597–1601
Dupont LJ, Demedts MG, Verleden GM (2003) Prospective evaluation of the validity of exhaled nitric oxide for the diagnosis of asthma. Chest 123:751–756
Galobardes B, Sunyer J, Anto JM, Castellsague J, Soriano JB, Tobias A (1998) Effect of the method of administration, mail or telephone, on the validity and reliability of a respiratory health questionnaire. The Spanish Centers of the European Asthma Study. J Clin Epidemiol 51:875–881
Getahun D, Demissie K, Rhoads GG (2005) Recent trends in asthma hospitalization and mortality in the United States. J Asthma 42:373–378
Guite HF, Burney PG (1996) Accuracy of recording of deaths from asthma in the UK: the false negative rate. Thorax 51:924–928
Haby MM, Peat JK, Mellis CM, Anderson SD, Woolcock AJ (1995) An exercise challenge for epidemiological studies of childhood asthma: validity and repeatability. Eur Respir J 8:729–736
Hansell A, Hollowell J, McNiece R, Nichols T, Strachan D (2003) Validity and interpretation of mortality, health service and survey data on COPD and asthma in England. Eur Respir J 21:279–286
Hunt LW Jr, Silverstein MD, Reed CE, O'Connell EJ, O'Fallon WM, Yunginger JW (1993) Accuracy of the death certificate in a population-based study of asthmatic patients. JAMA 269:1947–1952
Hunter CJ, Brightling CE, Woltmann G, Wardlaw AJ, Pavord ID (2002) A comparison of the validity of different diagnostic tests in adults with asthma. Chest 121:1051–1057
Jackson R, Sears MR, Beaglehole R, Rea HH (1988) International trends in asthma mortality: 1970 to 1985. Chest 94:914–918
Jenkins MA, Rubinfeld AR, Robertson CF, Bowes G (1992) Accuracy of asthma death statistics in Australia. Aust J Public Health 16:427–429
Jenkins MA, Clarke JR, Carlin JB, Robertson CF, Hopper JL, Dalton MF, Holst DP, Choi K, Giles GG (1996) Validation of questionnaire and bronchial hyperresponsiveness against respiratory physician assessment in the diagnosis of asthma. Int J Epidemiol 25:609–616
Jonasson G, Lodrup Carlsen KC, Leegaard J, Carlsen KH, Mowinckel P, Halvorsen KS (2000) Trends in hospital admissions for childhood asthma in Oslo, Norway, 1980–95. Allergy 55:232–239
Jorgensen IM, Bulow S, Jensen VB, Dahm TL, Prahl P, Juel K (2000) Asthma mortality in Danish children and young adults, 1973–1994: epidemiology and validity of death certificates. Eur Respir J 15:844–848
Kao CC, See LC, Yan DC, Ou LS, Huang JL (2001) Time trends and seasonal variations in hospital admissions for childhood asthma in Taiwan from 1990 to 1998. Asian Pac J Allergy Immunol 19:63–68
Kiivet RA, Kaur I, Lang A, Aaviksoo A, Nirk L (2001) Costs of asthma treatment in Estonia. Eur J Public Health 11:89–92
Kilpelainen M, Terho EO, Helenius H, Koskenvuo M (2001a) Validation of a new questionnaire on asthma, allergic rhinitis, and conjunctivitis in young adults. Allergy 56:377–384
Kilpelainen M, Terho EO, Helenius H, Koskenvuo M (2001b) Home dampness, current allergic diseases, and respiratory infections among young adults. Thorax 56:462–467
Kim JL, Elfman L, Mi Y, Johansson M, Smedje G, Norback D (2005) Current asthma and respiratory symptoms among pupils in relation to dietary factors and allergens in the school environment. Indoor Air 15:170–182
King ME, Mannino DM, Holguin F (2004) Risk factors for asthma incidence. A review of recent prospective evidence. Panminerva Med 46:97–110
Korhonen K, Reijonen TM, Malmstrom K, Klaukka T, Remes K, Korppi M (2002) Hospitalization trends for paediatric asthma in eastern Finland: a 10-yr survey. Eur Respir J 19:1035–1039
Krahn MD, Berka C, Langlois P, Detsky AS (1996) Direct and indirect costs of asthma in Canada, 1990. CMAJ 154:821–831
Laurier C, Kennedy W, Malo JL, Par M, Labb D, Archambault A (1999) Rate and cost of hospitalizations for asthma in Quebec: An analysis of 1988/89, 1989/90 and 1994/95 data. Chronic Dis Can 20:82–88
MacIntyre UE, de Villiers FP, Owange-Iraka JW (2001) Increase in childhood asthma admissions in an urbanising population. S Afr Med J 91:667–672
Mannino DM, Homa DM, Akinbami LJ, Moorman JE, Gwynn C, Redd SC (2002) Surveillance for asthma – United States, 1980–1999. MMWR Surveill Summ 51:113
McDaniel M, Paxson C, Waldfogel J (2006) Racial disparities in childhood asthma in the United States: evidence from the National Health Interview Survey, 1997 to 2003. Pediatrics 117:e868–e877
Morrison DS, McLoone P (2001) Changing patterns of hospital admission for asthma, 1981–97. Thorax 56:687–690
Mossing R, Nielsen GD (2003) Cost-of-illness of asthma in Denmark in the year 2000. Ugeskr Laeger 165:2646–2649
Murray CJ (1994) Quantifying the burden of disease: the technical basis for disability-adjusted life years. Bull World Health Organ 72:429–445
National Asthma Education and Prevention Program (1997) Guidelines for the Diagnosis and Management of Asthma. National Institutes of Health, Bethesda, MD NIH Publication No. 98-4051
Ng TP, Niti M, Tan WC (2003) Trends and ethnic differences in asthma hospitalization rates in Singapore, 1991 to 1998. Ann Allergy Asthma Immunol 90:51–55
Nieto A, Alvarez-Cuesta E, Boquete M, Mazon A, de la Torre F (2001) The cost of asthma treatment in Spain and rationalizing the expense. J Investig Allergol Clin Immunol 11:139–148
Pearce N, Douwes J (2006) The global epidemiology of asthma in children. Int J Tuberc Lung Dis 10:125–132
Peat JK, van den Berg RH, Green WF, Mellis CM, Leeder SR, Woolcock AJ (1994) Changing prevalence of asthma in Australian children. BMJ 308:1591–1596
Phelan PD (1994) Asthma in children: epidemiology. BMJ 308:1584–1585

Picard E, Barmeir M, Schwartz S, Villa Y, Goldberg S, Virgilis D, Kerem E (2002) Rate and place of death from asthma among different ethnic groups in Israel: national trends 1980 to 1997. Chest 122:1222–1227

Priftis K, Panagiotopoulou-Gartagani P, Tapratzi-Potamianou P, Zachariadi-Xypolita A, Sagriotis A, Saxoni-Papageorgiou P (2005) Hospitalizations for childhood asthma in Athens, Greece, from 1978 to 2000. Pediatr Allergy Immunol 16:82–85

Redline S, Gruchalla RS, Wolf RL, Yawn BP, Cartar L, Gan V, Nelson P, Wollan P (2004) Development and validation of school-based asthma and allergy screening questionnaires in a 4-city study. School Nurse News 21:12–14

Robertson CF, Heycock E, Bishop J, Nolan T, Olinsky A, Phelan PD (1991) Prevalence of asthma in Melbourne schoolchildren: Changes over 26 years. BMJ 302:1116–1118

Robertson CF, Roberts MF, Kappers JH (2004) Asthma prevalence in Melbourne schoolchildren: have we reached the peak? Med J Aust 180:273–276

Rottem M, Zitansky A, Horovitz Y (2005) Hospital admission trends for pediatric asthma: results of a 10 year survey in Israel. Isr Med Assoc J 7:785–789

Sears MR, Rea HH, de Boer G, Beaglehole R, Gillies AJ, Holst PE, O'Donnell TV, Rothwell RP (1986) Accuracy of certification of deaths due to asthma. A national study. Am J Epidemiol 124:1004–1011

Sennhauser FH, Braun-Fahrlander C, Wildhaber JH (2005) The burden of asthma in children: a European perspective. Paediatr Respir Rev 6:2–7

Sidenius KE, Munch EP, Madsen F, Lange P, Viskum K, Soes-Petersen U (2000) Accuracy of recorded asthma deaths in Denmark in a 12-months period in 1994/95. Respir Med 94:373–377

Smith AD, Cowan JO, Filsell S, McLachlan C, Monti-Sheehan G, Jackson P, Taylor DR (2004) Diagnosing asthma: comparisons between exhaled nitric oxide measurements and conventional tests. Am J Respir Crit Care Med 169:473–478

Sole D, Vanna AT, Yamada E, Rizzo MC, Naspitz CK (1998) International Study of Asthma and Allergies in Childhood (ISAAC) written questionnaire: validation of the asthma component among Brazilian children. J Investig Allergol Clin Immunol 8:376–382

Stock S, Redaelli M, Luengen M, Wendland G, Civello D, Lauterbach KW (2005) Asthma: prevalence and cost of illness. Eur Respir J 25:47–53

Sunyer J, Anto JM, Kogevinas M, Soriano JB, Tobias A, Munoz A (1997) Smoking and bronchial responsiveness in nonatopic and atopic young adults. Spanish Group of the European Study of Asthma. Thorax 52:235–238

Szucs TD, Anderhub H, Rutishauser M (1999) The economic burden of asthma: direct and indirect costs in Switzerland. Eur Respir J 13:281–286

van den Akker-van Marle ME, Bruil J, Detmar SB (2005) Evaluation of cost of disease: assessing the burden to society of asthma in children in the European Union. Allergy 60:140–149

Vargas MH, az-Mejia GS, Furuya ME, Salas J, Lugo A (2004) Trends of asthma in Mexico: an 11-year analysis in a nationwide institution. Chest 125:1993–1997

Venables KM, Farrer N, Sharp L, Graneek BJ, Newman Taylor AJ (1993) Respiratory symptoms questionnaire for asthma epidemiology: validity and reproducibility. Thorax 48: 214–219

von Mutius E (1998) The rising trends in asthma and allergic disease. Clin Exp Allergy 28(Suppl 5):45–49 discussion 50–1: 45–49

Wamboldt FS, Price MR, Hume LA, Gavin LA, Wamboldt MZ, Klinnert MD (2002) Reliability and validity of a system for coding asthma outcomes from medical records. J Asthma 39:299–305

Weiss ST (2001) Epidemiology and heterogeneity of asthma. Ann Allergy Asthma Immunol 87:5–8

Weiss KB, Sullivan SD (2001) The health economics of asthma and rhinitis. I. Assessing the economic impact. J Allergy Clin Immunol 107:3–8

Weiss KB, Gergen PJ, Hodgson TA (1992) An economic evaluation of asthma in the United States. N Engl J Med 326:862–866

Weiss KB, Sullivan SD, Lyttle CS (2000) Trends in the cost of illness for asthma in the United States, 1985–1994. J Allergy Clin Immunol 106:493–499

Wolf RL, Berry CA, O'Connor T, Coover L (1999) Validation of the Brief Pediatric Asthma Screen. Chest 116:224S–228S

World Health Organization (2002) World Health Report 2002. Reducing risks, promoting healthy life. World Health Organization, Geneva, Switzerland

Wright SC, Evans AE, Sinnamon DG, MacMahon J (1994) Asthma mortality and death certification in Northern Ireland. Thorax 49:141–143

Yurdakul AS, Dursun B, Canbakan S, Cakaloglu A, Capan N (2005) The assessment of validity of different asthma diagnostic tools in adults. J Asthma 42:843–846

Zar HJ, Stickells D, Toerien A, Wilson D, Klein M, Bateman ED (2001) Changes in fatal and near-fatal asthma in an urban area of South Africa from 1980–1997. Eur Respir J 18:33–37

Zitt M (2005) Clinical applications of exhaled nitric oxide for the diagnosis and management of asthma: a consensus report. Clin Ther 27:1238–1250

Centers for Disease Control and Prevention. Asthma survey questions. Available from http://www.cdc.gov/asthma/questions.htm

European Community Respiratory Health Survey. Questionnaires, Protocols and Instructions. Available from http://www.ecrhs.org/quests.htm

International Study of Asthma and Allergies in Childhood. Study instruments. Available from http://isaac.auckland.ac.nz/PhaseOne/Manual/Section7/Sec7Frame.html

World Health Organization (2009) Definitions. Available from http://www.who.int/hac/about/definitions/en/index.htmll

Chapter 2
Asthma: Pathophysiology and Diagnosis

Susie Yim Yeh and Richard Schwartzstein

Introduction

Although asthma is a common disorder affecting approximately 7.8% of the United States population (Schiller et al. 2006) or 23 million Americans, the pathogenesis of this disease remains to be fully elucidated. Extensive research over the last few decades has yielded a better understanding of asthma. We know that the basic features of asthma include episodic airways inflammation, airways hyperresponsiveness, and mucous hypersecretion. Although we understand the basic clinical features of asthma, the links between symptoms, physical signs, and underlying pathophysiological mechanisms are still being delineated. Asthma is a heterogeneous disease process with varying phenotypes and presentations. In this chapter, we will briefly explore some major theories of asthma pathogenesis, both new and old. We will also explore how understanding the pathophysiology of asthma can help us to understand the symptoms and presentation of asthma, as well as the best strategies for diagnosing this disease.

Pathology and Histology

What Do the Lungs Look Like in Asthma?

The autopsies of patients who have died of asthma gave researchers the first clues as to the possible etiology of this disease. Although there have been many advances in the treatment of asthma, death from this airways disease is still an unfortunate outcome in a minority of patients. Before describing the abnormal features of the asthmatic airway, we must first briefly describe the basic features of the normal airway.

Asthma is thought to be a disease of the small airways. If one thinks of the lungs as a series of tubes that continues to divide, the tubes get smaller and smaller until they end in small air sacks (called alveoli), where the exchange of gas occurs. The characteristics of the larger tubes as compared to the smaller tubes are very different. In the lung, the larger tubes such as the trachea and main bronchus are supported by both cartilaginous rings and smooth muscle. However, as the tubes get smaller, these cartilaginous rings disappear and only a layer of smooth muscle remains (Fig. 2.1). These smaller tubes are called bronchi and bronchioles. Without the support of cartilage, when smooth muscle contracts, the airways become increasingly narrow. Smooth muscle surrounds other tubular structures in the human body, such as arteries, where smooth muscle contraction dictates the flow of blood to vital organs. Similarly, in the lungs, contraction of smooth muscle in the bronchioles determines the air flow. The cross-sectional area of all the bronchioles is much larger than the cross-sectional area of the biggest airway. Therefore, contraction of smooth muscle can greatly increase airway resistance and diminish the flow of air into the lungs by decreasing size of the small airways.

The cells that line the respiratory tract are known as *the respiratory epithelium.* These cells vary in appearance and function. Some cells have hair-like structures (cilia), while other cells produce mucous. Beneath these cells lie connective tissue and more glands that secrete mucous. In the trachea, cartilage, and smooth

S. Yim Yeh (✉)
Harvard Program in Pulmonary and Critical Care Medicine, Beth Israel Deaconess Medical Center, 330 Brookline Avenue, Boston, MA, 02215, USA
e-mail: syim@bidmc.harvard.edu

A. Harver and H. Kotses (eds.), *Asthma, Health and Society: A Public Health Perspective*,
DOI 10.1007/978-0-387-78285-0_2, © Springer Science+Business Media, LLC 2010

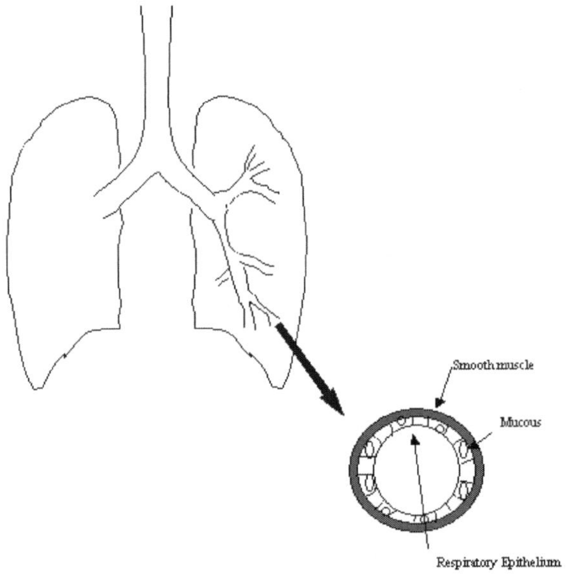

Fig. 2.1 The basic structure of the respiratory bronchiole. The bronchiole differs from the larger airways in that it is surrounded only by smooth muscle without cartilage support. Also note the cells lining the airways consist of mucous secreting cells

muscle is present beneath these glands. As the airways become increasingly smaller, the amount of cartilage starts to decrease and smooth muscle becomes more prominent. In the smallest airways, such as the bronchioles, there is no longer any cartilage. The connective tissue and glands decrease and smooth muscle lies beneath the respiratory epithelium. There are also many small blood vessels that lie beneath the airway supplying nutrients to both the respiratory epithelium and smooth muscle cells. In asthma, these blood vessels can become leaky, allowing the infiltration of inflammatory cells and fluid, which can cause edema.

Asthma, at its core, is an inflammatory disease. In response to a variety of stimuli, some in the environment such as allergens, and some reflecting changes within the body as occurs with exercise, a cascade of reactions that we characterize as inflammation is triggered. Autopsies of patients with fatal asthma have shown many derangements consistent with inflammation in the structure of the airways. In addition, mucous plugs fill the airways. The cells that produce mucus appear larger and are more numerous than in patients without asthma. The bronchioles also appear edematous with an increased number of inflammatory cells (such as eosinophils, neutrophils, and mast cells) that infiltrate the airways. The connective tissue is thickened and the respiratory epithelium is denuded. In addition, the amount of smooth muscle that surrounds the airways is increased (Fig. 2.2); whether this is due to muscle contraction and hypertrophy or is another process secondary to inflammation is still up for debate. It was thought that these dramatic changes were specific to patients with fatal asthma; bronchoscopic biopsies of patients with mild asthma, however, have demonstrated some of the same features. Although these findings can be patchy, biopsies of patients with mild to moderate asthma have shown a significant amount of inflammation as demonstrated by denuded epithelium, thickened basement membrane, and infiltration of inflammatory cells including mast cells, lymphocytes, and eosinophils (Busse and Lemanske 2001).

Another hallmark of asthma is that it represents a potentially reversible disease process. Between asthma attacks or during mild attacks, the airways can appear normal (Barrios et al. 2006). If asthma continues to progress, however, these changes become more permanent. This process is termed *airway remodeling*, and is

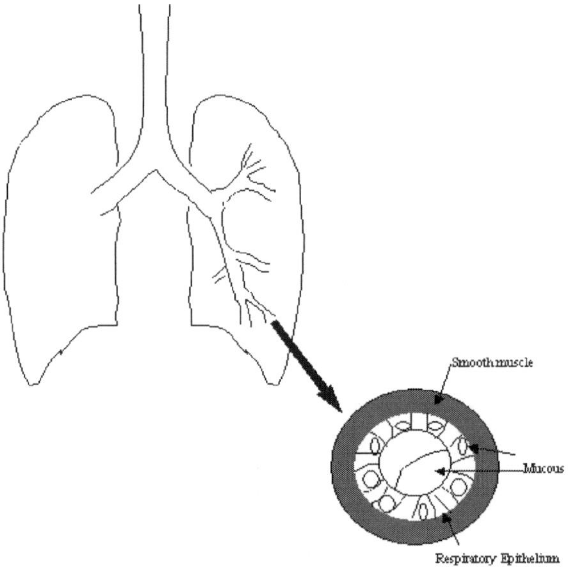

Fig. 2.2 Schematic of the respiratory bronchiole during an asthma attack. The airway is lined by the respiratory epithelium which is made of ciliated and mucous producing cells. These mucous producing cells increase mucous production. Mucous then plugs up the airway, making it harder for the asthmatic to breathe. Underneath the respiratory epithelium lies a layer of smooth muscle. When the smooth muscle contracts, the airway becomes smaller, decreasing airflow

thought to be due to persistent airway inflammation (Holgate et al. 1999). Patients with airway remodeling have thickened airway walls, with an increase in the amount of tissue directly under the respiratory epithelium, and larger smooth muscle mass (Busse and Lemanske 2001). Once remodeling has occurred, the medications used to reverse obstruction of the airways become less effective and symptoms may be more chronic.

Pathogenesis

Introduction

As mentioned earlier, the three basic features of asthma are airways inflammation, airways hyperresponsiveness, and mucous hypersecretion. These three features lead to bronchoconstriction and airflow obstruction, which manifest as wheezing and dyspnea in the patient with asthma. The challenge for most researchers has been to uncover triggers of airways inflammation in the patient with asthma. Several theories have emerged such as the TH2 hypothesis, the Hygiene hypothesis, the infectious causes hypothesis, and the Dutch hypothesis. What these theories have in common is that in the susceptible individual, there is an exuberant immune response after exposure to a substance whether it be an allergen, a virus, or something else. This increased immune response leads to airways inflammation and bronchoconstriction. Why this occurs is still debatable.

Allergy and the Immune System

Many researchers have tried to identify the main causes of airways inflammation. Abnormalities of the immune system, which protects our bodies from infection, have been thought to be major contributors to the development of asthma. More specifically, allergic responses have been considered to be the main determinants of the asthma phenotype. Extensive research over the years, however, has shown that there are different phenotypes of asthma and not all are mediated by allergies. Even so, we will first explore the allergy-driven *TH2 hypothesis* before describing some of the other theories of asthma pathogenesis.

The immune system is an intricate and complicated structure, the details of which are too complex to explore here. However, to understand asthma, one must have some understanding of how the immune system works. In order to fight infection, the human body has developed a complex system to identify foreign intruders and to "remember" them in case of further invasions. This is called the *adaptive immune response*. That way, the body can be ready immediately for the next attack. Yet to exist in this world, the immune system cannot recognize everything foreign as being dangerous or else we would not be able to smell flowers or eat food without coughing, sneezing, or developing fevers. Life would be unbearable. The immune system, therefore, has developed a way to distinguish between benign and malignant foreign particles or *antigens*. There are times, however, for unclear reasons, when the immune system recognizes benign antigens such as dust, animal dander, or food as being "dangerous." When this occurs, we say that the person has an "allergy." When the human body develops allergies, the bronchospasm, cough, and wheeze that develop is an exaggerated response to a benign particle.

What are the steps involved from being exposed to a piece of dust to developing wheezing? It is clear that this process does not happen to everyone and that only susceptible individuals have this problem. Over the last several decades there have been several basic immune mechanisms described including antibody-mediated and cell-mediated immunity, that are thought to be responsible for airways inflammation and obstruction in response to an allergic stimulus.

Antibody-Mediated Immunity

One of the most important immune cells is called the *lymphocyte*. These cells are the building blocks of the immune system. There are two types of lymphocytes, the *B-cell* and the *T-cell*. When activated, some B-cells differentiate into *plasma cells* which then produce antibodies that are released in the blood. When an antibody recognizes a foreign pathogen or *antigen*, the antibody attaches to the antigen and neutralizes it. In allergic diseases, a benign particle, or *allergen*, acts as an antigen. Another immune cell called the *macrophage*, then recognizes the antibody–antigen or antibody–allergen complex, absorbs the complex and destroys it. The human body makes several different types of antibodies that have slightly different functions. They are subdivided in to five classes of isotypes called IgA, IgM, IgG, IgD, and IgE. The antibody most important to asthma is the IgE isotype. IgE differs from the other isotypes in that instead of circulating freely in the blood and extracellular fluid, IgE is bound to *mast cells*. Mast cells reside in the airways and are loaded with enzymes that are released once the mast cell is stimulated by the IgE–allergen complex. In developing countries, the IgE-mediated immune response is important in fighting and killing parasites. However, in developed countries, IgE-mediated immune responses are most responsible for allergic reactions.

The *immediate hypersensitivity response* is IgE-mediated and is one of the most important causes of asthma. When IgE recognizes an antigen (or in this case *allergen*), a cascade of events occur that cause the degranulation and release of toxic inflammatory molecules from these mast cells (including proteolytic enzymes and histamine), which were meant to destroy foreign intruders (Wills-Karp 1999). Even when no such intruders are present, these toxic molecules cause the airways to become inflamed. The toxic molecules attract more immune cells to the area, thereby worsening the inflammation. Blood vessels become engorged and leaky, thereby allowing cells to migrate out of the blood stream and into the tissues. In asthma, the mast cells attract white blood cells called *eosinophils* to the area. They also initiate the production of inflammatory chemicals, *leukotrienes*, that are important in asthma. Leukotrienes have been implicated in inducing airway hyperresponsiveness, eosinophilia, and mucous hypersecretion (Bochner and Busse 2005).

Asthmatics typically have two phases during an asthma attack, the early and late response. It is thought that when the allergen activates IgE and mast cells, the histamine, leukotrienes, and cytokines released cause immediate constriction of smooth muscles that can resolve in approximately 1 h. However, 4–6 h later, another bout of airways obstruction can occur. This late reaction is thought to be due to different cytokines that are being released by the mast cells, eosinophils, macrophages, and lymphocytes (Busse and Lemanske 2001). The late response is responsible for prolonged asthma attacks.

Cell-Mediated Immunity

The T-cell differs from B-cells in the kind of antigen to which they respond. B-cell antibodies identify whole molecules. T-cells, on the other hand, do not rely on antibodies but rather develop receptors that recognize small pieces of a molecule. This makes it easier to recognize and destroy very small particles such as viruses. T-cells also differ from B-cells in their diversity. There are several different types of T-cells called cytotoxic T-cells, type 1 helper T-cell (TH1 cells) and the type 2 helper T-cell (TH2 cells). The roles of all these different T-cell types are too involved to explain here. In general the TH1 and TH2 cells differ in the types of immune reactions that they promote. In asthma, the TH2 cells often recognize the same allergens as B-cell antibodies do and help to activate the B-cell. The cytokines that the TH2 cell secretes to "help" the B-cell often contribute to the development of airways inflammation in the patient with asthma.

The TH2 cell does not rely on IgE antibodies but instead recognizes the allergen directly through its own receptor. The TH2 cell then activates and releases the cytokines to attract and activate more immune cells. This process was discovered when it was recognized that antibody-deficient mice (who do not make IgE molecules) were able to develop asthma (Corry et al. 1998). In this scenario, when TH2 cells are activated, the release of cytokines act directly on airway smooth muscle to induce airway bronchospasm (Corry et al. 1998; Wills-Karp et al. 1998). These cytokines also increase mucous secretions, airway inflammation and eosinophilia in the same way that leukotrienes do, but through a different mechanism.

To further complicate matters, the cytokines (such as IL-4) released by the TH2 cells also contribute indirectly to the immediate hypersensitivity response. IL4 is a key player in mast cell maturation (Madden et al. 1991), IgE secretion (Finkelman et al. 1988) and eosinophil recruitment to the lung (Corry et al. 1998). These immune responses, therefore, potentiate each other, showing how asthma can be the result of several different simultaneous processes.

TH2 Hypothesis

The observation that TH1 and TH2 cells promote different types of immunity generated the idea that perhaps one type of immunity is dominant in a particular individual. Specifically, that in one person, the TH1 cell-mediated immunity could be more active than the TH2 cell-mediated immunity. Because TH2 cell-mediated immunity has been associated with allergen-induced inflammation, it was thought that individuals who had predominantly TH2 cell-mediated immunity would be more prone to asthma and allergy. This is the basis for the TH2 hypothesis.

Further research has suggested that TH1 and TH2 cells regulate each other. For example if the TH2 cell is more active, it will release chemicals to suppress the TH1 cell and vice versa. When tested in the lab, chemicals from TH1 cells were found to decrease production of TH2 cells (Scott 1991). The question then becomes, what determines which TH cell mediated immunity dominates in an individual?

Hygiene Hypothesis

As the TH2 hypothesis gained popularity, the idea that the environment may determine which TH response dominates in a particular individual began to emerge. Exposures to certain pathogens or allergens at a young age (or even during the neonatal period) could determine if a person would have a TH1 or a TH2-mediated immunity (Table 2.1). Furthermore, if a person had a predominantly TH2-mediated immunity, then that person would be more susceptible to allergic diseases and/or asthma. This hypothesis has been dubbed the "hygiene hypothesis." However, the idea that immunity is either TH1 or TH2 mediated is too simplistic as evidence has shown there is a complicated interaction between these two that is still being explored. That being said, we will explore briefly the hygiene hypothesis and the rationale behind this intriguing idea.

Table 2.1 Factors promoting TH1 and TH2 phenotype

Factors promoting TH1 phenotype	Factors promoting TH2 phenotype
Endotoxin exposure	Use of antibiotics
Rural or farm setting	Western lifestyle
Older siblings	Urban setting
Daycare	
Infections (Hepatitis A, HSV 1, tuberculosis, toxoplasma)	

Asthma is more common in Western countries (The International Study of Asthma and Allergies in Childhood (ISAAC) Steering Committee 1998), suggesting there may be an environmental reason for the increased prevalence of the disease in these areas. The term "hygiene hypothesis" alludes to the idea that perhaps it is the decreased exposure to infections and allergens in the Western world that promotes TH2-mediated immunity. Furthermore, use of antibiotics has been associated with increased risk of asthma perhaps by decreasing exposure to infections that would promote the TH1 mediated immunity (Cohet et al. 2004; Droste et al. 2000). Interestingly, asthma is more prevalent in urban settings when compared to rural or farm settings (von Mutius 2000). Intense epidemiological research has looked at why this may be true. Several studies have looked at how exposure to *endotoxin* early in life could affect development of wheezing and asthma. Endotoxin, a component of (gram-negative) bacterial cell walls, can induce inflammation and cause bronchoconstriction when inhaled by asthmatics (Michel et al. 1989). Interestingly, endotoxin promotes TH1-mediated response and has been found to increase production of TH1-related cytokines (D'Andrea et al. 1992; Gereda et al. 2000; Lapa e Silva et al. 2000; Le et al. 1986). It appears that endotoxin is more abundant in farm settings, likely due to increased exposure to livestock, than in nonfarm settings (von Mutius et al. 2000). Although in decreased quantities, endotoxin can also be found in common household dust. Researchers have asked whether it is the exposure to endotoxin that predicts the development of asthma thereby explaining the differences in asthma prevalence between urban and rural/farm settings.

Litonjua et al. (2002) studied children from Boston, MA who were less than 5 years old. The results of this study, which was conducted over 4 years, showed that children who were exposed to higher endotoxin levels initially had increased wheezing during the first year of life. However, as the children became older, they had a progressive decline in wheezing. By age 5–9 years, children who had higher endotoxin exposure had less wheezing when compared to children who had lower endotoxin exposure. This paradoxical relationship whereby increased endotoxin exposure increases risk of wheezing early in life, but decreases risk of wheezing later in life, suggests that exposure to endotoxin may have "protective" effects. By enhancing TH1-mediated immunity, endotoxin exposure may decrease the development of asthma and/or allergy in susceptible individuals.

When studying other exposures that may enhance the TH1-mediated response it has been shown that previous exposure to *Mycobacterium tuberculosis*, hepatitis A, *Toxoplasma gondii*, Herpes Simplex 1 and the common cold have been associated with decreased risk of allergy or asthma. Viruses and bacteria activate cell-mediated immunity (TH1 response). The German Multicenter Allergy Study studied children from birth to 7 years of age and found that children who had more colds with a runny nose had less wheezing (Illi et al. 2001). Similarly, the Tucson Children's Respiratory Study, which followed children from birth, found that children who had more siblings or attended daycare from an early age were more likely to have wheezing at age 2 but increasingly less likely to have asthma as they became older (at age 6, 8, 11, and 13) (Ball et al. 2000).

The hygiene hypothesis, however, has remained very controversial. As stated earlier, the simple TH1 versus TH2 model does not hold true in many instances. For example, in rural Africa where parasitic diseases are common, infection with certain parasites (*Shistosoma* species) (van den Biggelaar et al. 2000) and Ascaris hook-worm (Scrivener et al. 2001) was associated with decreased prevalence of asthma and allergy. Parasitic diseases activate the TH2 response and require IgE to fight off these infections. Therefore, one might think that factors favoring the TH2 phenotype would increase the incidence of asthma and allergy. However, on closer inspection, it is thought that another factor may be "bypassing" the TH2 response in parasitic diseases. Another group of T-cells called *regulatory T-cells* that produce a cytokine called Interleukin-10 (IL-10), may be increasingly active during parasitic infections. It is thought that these regulatory T-cells can override the TH2 response. In a mouse experiment, injection with IL-10 producing T-cells decreased the allergic response in these animals (Cottrez et al. 2000). In other experiments, IL-10 in combination with IL-4 caused B lymphocytes to produce IgG instead of IgE (Jeannin et al. 1998). This line of research is promising in further clarifying the immune responses that are contributing to the asthma and allergy phenotype.

Lastly, the hygiene hypothesis does not explain the cause-effect relationships that occur later in life. In other words, once an individual has established an allergic response, repeated exposures do not decrease this response. In the endotoxin example, individuals with established asthma have increased airways inflammation, bronchoconstriction, and susceptibility to viral illnesses when exposed to endotoxin (Reed and Milton 2001). Endotoxin exposure is a common cause of asthma in the workplace and repeated exposures in asthmatic individuals leads to chronic bronchitis and emphysema (Reed and Milton 2001). Instead of mitigating the allergic reaction, repeated exposures to endotoxin in the person who already has asthma causes worsening disease. This example suggests that the hygiene hypothesis may only be relevant early in life and cannot be extrapolated to the adult setting.

Viral/Bacterial Infections

Since the 1970s there has been a well-established relationship between asthma and respiratory tract infections (Blasi et al. 2001). Many patients with asthma have worsening of their symptoms in the setting of a respiratory infection. In children, studies have shown up to 45% of asthma exacerbations are related to respiratory infections (Mertsola et al. 1991). Likewise, in adults, up to 37% of asthma exacerbations were associated with respiratory infections (Teichtahl et al. 1997). However, whether these infections are involved in the etiology of asthma or the progression of disease has remained unclear. There is also interest in whether respiratory infections play a significant role in the TH1/TH2 or hygiene hypotheses as well. Although more commonly associated with viruses, several specific bacteria such as *Chlamydia pneumoniae* and *Mycoplasma pneumoniae* have been increasingly associated with asthma.

C. pneumoniae and *M. pneumoniae* are two common bacterial respiratory infections and are typically associated with pneumonia. *C. pneumoniae* is different from most other bacteria in that it must invade cells, such as respiratory epithelial cells and macrophages, in order to replicate. However, because *C. pneumoniae* does not have to destroy the cell that it invades; it can persist as a latent infection by allowing infected cells to proliferate. Latent infections can be quiescent without causing symptoms. If triggered, however, they can erupt into an acute infection. Cold sores, for example, are due to latent infection with Herpes

Simplex virus that develops into an acute infection from time to time. *C. pneumoniae* has been implicated in acute exacerbations of asthma (Allegra et al. 1994) and chronic asthma (Black et al. 2000).

C. pneumoniae has been associated with asthma since the 1970s. Since then, efforts to quantify this association have been attempted. Several studies have measured antibodies against *C. pneumoniae* in the blood of asthma patients and found an increase in certain types of antibodies (IgA) to *C. pneumoniae* when compared to controls (Berkovich et al. 1970; Gencay et al. 2001; Huhti et al. 1974). Antibody studies, however, are difficult to interpret since the presence of antibodies does not confirm whether an infection is past, latent, or acute. It has been suggested that chronic infection with *C. pneumoniae* is more prevalent in asthmatics (Biscione et al. 2004; Gencay et al. 2001). When using methods to directly test for presence of the bacteria in nasal aspirates of asthmatics and their non-asthmatic spouses over a 2 month period, it was found that 22% of the asthmatics and 9% of the spouses had presence of the organism at least once during the study period (Biscione et al. 2004). However, it was still unclear as to whether the increase in positive tests for *C. pneumoniae* in asthmatics truly represents active infection or colonization.

It is logical to ask that if *C. pneumoniae* infection is associated with asthma, then does treatment with antibiotics improve symptoms and outcome? Unfortunately the results have been mixed. Several studies have shown that treatment of asthmatics with antibiotics for 6–8 weeks have shown decreases in eosinophil counts (Amayasu et al. 2000) and improvements in peak expiratory flows (PEF) (Black et al. 2001) but that the effect on pulmonary function tests were modest at best. Most recently, a double-blinded, randomized, placebo-controlled trial attempted to more accurately assess the effect of antibiotics (against *C. pneumoniae* and *M. pneumoniae*) in the setting of an acute asthma exacerbation (Johnston et al. 2006). Patients with an acute asthma exacerbation were randomized to take placebo or an antibiotic for 10 days in addition to regular asthma treatment. Although asthma symptoms improved in the antibiotic group, there was no difference in PEF. Interestingly, 61% of the subjects studied had evidence of infection from either *C. pneumoniae* or *M. pneumoniae* or both but unfortunately there was no correlation between antibiotic response and history of infection in this study.

Results have been similar with *M. pneumoniae*, a common bacteria responsible for "atypical" or "walking" pneumonia. Like *C. pneumoniae*, it has been implicated in the etiology, progression, and clinical course of asthma, but treatment with antibiotics has not yielded significant improvements. It is the smallest free-living organism and is different from other bacteria in that it does not have a cell wall. It infects the respiratory epithelium and disables the ciliated cells responsible for clearing mucus and foreign particles from the airways. Like *C. pneumoniae*, *M pneumoniae* can persist as a chronic infection. Although it does not enter cells like *C. pneumoniae*, it can burrow between cells, evading host defenses and establishing residence in the airways.

Despite unclear results in small clinical trials assessing the effectiveness of treatment with antibiotics in asthmatics, there is still much interest in what role these bacterial infections play in the development of asthma. As discussed earlier, the hygiene hypothesis suggests that exposures to certain infections early in life may induce a TH1-mediated immunity resulting in a decreased propensity for asthma. However, once the allergic phenotype is established, recurrent exposures to a pathogen or allergen exacerbates the disease. Researchers looked at this phenomenon in an allergic-asthma mouse model. Chu and colleagues exposed mice to *M. pneumoniae* at different times and observed the response (Chu et al. 2003). When they infected the mice before exposure to an allergen, the mice had significantly less bronchial hyperresponsiveness, and lung inflammation and had increased production of cytokines associated with the TH1 response. Conversely, when they infected the mice after exposure to an allergen, they developed increased bronchial hyperresponsiveness, and lung inflammation, and produced cytokines associated with the TH2 response (IL-4). This line of research is very interesting and suggests that both *C. pneumoniae* and *M. pneumoniae* may have varying importance in the development and progression of asthma based on when the infection occurs.

Although we have been discussing the role of bacterial infections in asthma pathogenesis, viral infections have been implicated in the etiology of asthma as well. Viral infections during infancy have been associated with the development of asthma. This has been most convincing in studies of *Respiratory Syncytial Virus* (RSV). Most children are infected with RSV by 2 years of age (Simoes 1999) and many are hospitalized.

RSV can cause respiratory distress, wheezing, and fever. It can cause a "bronchiolitis," inflammation of the respiratory bronchioles described earlier. Many have observed that children who suffered from RSV bronchiolitis as an infant had a higher propensity to wheeze for years after the infection (Stein et al. 1999). Sigurs and colleagues (2005) studied a group of children who were hospitalized with RSV bronchiolitis as infants (<1 year old). They compared this group, which was followed until age 13, to a group of children who had never been hospitalized with RSV bronchiolitis. These researchers found that children in the RSV group had increased wheezing and airways obstruction. What was also interesting was that these children had increased allergies to common inhaled allergens. This research suggests there may be a relationship between early RSV infection and the development of asthma and allergies later on in life. However, other studies have shown that infants infected with RSV "outgrew" their wheezing and did not go on to develop asthma in adolescence (Taussig et al. 2003). Whether RSV is merely a risk factor for asthma or is a causative agent in asthma pathogenesis remains unclear.

In addition to being implicated in asthma pathogenesis, viral infections are commonly associated with asthma exacerbations (Venarske et al. 2006). Often, when a person develops an asthma attack, there is usually an inciting factor or "trigger" associated with the attack. For many asthmatics, the common cold can precipitate an attack. In fact, viruses have been associated with up to 85% of asthma exacerbations in children (Johnston et al. 1995) and 60% of exacerbations in adults (Nicholson et al. 1993). It has been shown that during times when viral syndromes are "going around" there are increased admissions to area hospitals with asthma exacerbations (Johnston et al. 1996).

The reason why upper respiratory viruses have been associated with asthma exacerbations, however, has remained unclear. *Rhinovirus*, one of the viruses responsible for the common cold, has been most frequently associated with asthma exacerbations. One study found that infection with rhinovirus was associated with an increase in asthma-related hospitalizations (Venarske et al. 2006). Some have suggested that viruses may potentiate the inflammatory response to allergens causing bronchospasm and airways obstruction in asthma patients (Busse and Lemanske 2001; Calhoun et al. 1991). Others have proposed that asthma may cause abnormalities in the immune system that makes it harder to fight viral infections in the airway (Papi and Johnston 1999). The role of rhinovirus and other viral illnesses (such as *influenza, parainfluenza, and coronavirus*) in causing or contributing to asthma exacerbations needs to be further clarified.

Dutch Hypothesis

Before delving into what the Dutch Hypothesis is, we must first briefly explain the differences between asthma and chronic obstructive pulmonary disease (COPD). As we have been discussing, asthma is characterized by reversible airflow obstruction, airways hyperresponsiveness, and increased mucous secretion. Typically, asthma does not cause progressive loss of lung function and the lung parenchyma itself remains intact. Usually, asthma presents in childhood or young adulthood. On the other hand, COPD, a term used to describe chronic bronchitis, emphysema, and a variety of less common conditions such as bronchiectasis, is commonly associated with smoking and presents in older adulthood. Even though COPD is also characterized by airflow obstruction, it is usually irreversible or only partially reversible. There is also progressive loss of lung function. Asthma and COPD are commonly thought of as distinctly different diseases. Asthma has been described as an inflammatory airway disease mediated by a dysregulated immune response (as described by the TH2 hypothesis). COPD, on the other hand, is thought to occur when destructive enzymes damage the lung in response to some inflammatory stimulus (i.e., cigarette smoke).

The Dutch Hypothesis was first proposed in the 1960s and is one of the older but still relevant theories on asthma/COPD pathogenesis. During that time, tuberculosis was the most common respiratory illness but as effective treatment for tuberculosis became available, Drs. Orie and Sluiter began to notice that obstructive lung diseases were very common with similar characteristics in both younger and older patients (Postma and Boezen 2004). They proposed, in the first Bronchitis Symposium held in Groningen, Netherlands, that obstructive airways diseases such as asthma, chronic bronchitis, and emphysema should be considered not as different diseases but as different manifestations of one disease entity, which they called *chronic nonspecific lung disease* (CNSLD) (Postma and Boezen 2004).

They hypothesized that both genetic and environmental factors contribute to the pathogenesis of CNSLD and that it is the interaction between these two that determines what phenotype a person will develop. One example of an interaction between a person and his/her environment is smoking. Tobacco smoke has been highly associated with COPD. However, only 10% of smokers get COPD suggesting that there is a genetic propensity for a person to develop COPD in response to cigarette smoke. There has also been an association between passive smoke exposure and the development of asthma in children. According to the Dutch hypothesis, the time of tobacco smoke exposure, whether in childhood or adulthood, and the type of exposure, passive or active, determines if a person with genetic susceptibility develops the asthma or COPD phenotype.

The Dutch hypothesis, as it is now known as, has been controversial. Efforts to try and test this hypothesis have been flawed as study designs do not lend to testing a process that spans a lifetime. Also, current studies of asthma and COPD have had strict inclusion criteria that try to eliminate subjects who have aspects of both, which limits our ability to determine if the pathogenesis of the two is similar. Over the years, however, there has been some evidence to support the Dutch hypothesis. Clinically, there are populations of asthma patients who have loss of lung function similar to COPD (Jeffery 2000; Ulrik et al. 1995). Similarly, there are patients with COPD who have reversible airflow obstruction (Bousquet et al. 1996). These observations suggest that there is considerable overlap between asthma and COPD.

Other observations have contributed to the blurring between asthma and COPD. There is evidence to suggest that both conditions are secondary to lung inflammation. In the past, different types of inflammation were described in patients with asthma and COPD. In asthma, it was thought that the inflammatory process was confined to the airway and that in COPD, the inflammatory process was confined to the lung parenchyma. However, there have been some studies that have shown that there are inflammatory cells, such as eosinophils and neutrophils, within the lung tissue in some subjects with asthma (Kraft et al. 1996; Wenzel et al. 1999). Additionally, biopsies of COPD subjects have shown high numbers of eosinophils in the airways especially during acute exacerbations (Saetta et al. 1994). Asthma and COPD share histologic features suggesting that there is substantial overlap between these two disease processes.

There have been several other features of both diseases that suggest a common pathogenesis. For example, the airways of asthma and COPD patients are similar. Both have an increase in mucous secreting cells lining the airways. Increases in smooth muscle surround the airways, however, was thought to be unique to asthma. Recent studies have shown that there is also an increase in smooth muscle among COPD patients as well (Jeffery 2000). Finally, changes in the lung parenchyma itself have shown some similarity among asthma and COPD subjects. Typically, as already mentioned, asthma is thought to be strictly an airways disease that does not affect the lung parenchyma or alveoli. However, the destructive enzymes found in COPD lungs have also been found in biopsies of asthma lungs as well (Atkinson and Senior 2003; Bousquet et al. 1996).

Studies are ongoing to further assess whether asthma and COPD are two distinct diseases or different presentations of the same disease. Over the years, the popularity of the Dutch Hypothesis has waxed and waned. However, there has been growing scientific evidence to support this hypothesis, which highlights that asthma is indeed a complex and heterogeneous disease process.

Asthma Subtypes

Although the majority of asthma is initially triggered by allergies, there are several different phenotypes of asthma that have different characteristics from the common allergy-induced asthma. "Intrinsic asthma," aspirin-induced asthma (AIA), and exercise-induced asthma (EIA) are a few asthma subtypes that have unique characteristics not readily associated with allergens. There are, however, several other subtypes of asthma, such as gastroesophageal reflux associated asthma, obesity-related asthma, menstrual cycle-related asthma, and nocturnal asthma that are also included in the asthma syndromes, but will not be discussed here.

Intrinsic Asthma

The term "intrinsic asthma" has been used to describe patients who suffer from asthma but do not have typical features of atopy or allergies. This is in contrast to the allergy-induced ("extrinsic") asthma we have been discussing. Patients with "intrinsic" asthma do not have allergies, family histories of atopy, abnormal serum IgE levels, or hypersensitivity reactions to skin prick-tests. The clinical course of patients with intrinsic asthma differs as well. Usually, patients with intrinsic asthma tend to be older, have later onset of asthma, and more severe disease (Ulrik et al. 1995). For many years, it was believed that "intrinsic" asthma represented a different pathological process leading to asthma and that the distinction between "intrinsic" and "extrinsic" (allergy-induced) asthma was very apparent. More recently, however, the differences between "intrinsic" and "extrinsic" asthma have become less clear. In one study, lung biopsies of patients with extrinsic asthma were compared to patients with intrinsic asthma (Humbert et al. 1996). Both had similar inflammatory cells and cytokines present, suggesting that a similar process was occurring in both forms of asthma regardless of whether the patient had allergies or not. These findings have prompted researchers to view "intrinsic" asthma differently. Instead of thinking of "intrinsic" asthma as being different from "extrinsic" asthma, there may only be differences in the triggers leading to the same causative pathways for asthma (Humbert et al. 1999). For example, some have suggested that intrinsic asthma may be a form of autoimmunity, triggered by a respiratory viral illness. In other words, antibodies made to the initial viral illness may now be initiating a cascade of inflammation leading to asthma (Humbert et al. 1999). Others believe that patients with "intrinsic" asthma are actually allergic to something that researchers have not yet been able to identify (Humbert et al. 1999). The pathogenesis of "intrinsic" asthma has not been elucidated and may reflect a heterogeneous process rather than a single disease entity. Although similarities between "intrinsic" and "extrinsic" asthma exist, the concept that asthma does not necessarily represent a solely allergy-related disease is important and speaks to the complexity of asthma.

Aspirin-Induced Asthma

One could consider AIA a kind of "intrinsic" asthma for which we know the trigger. Aspirin is one of the most widely taken medications in the world. In the United States alone, over 80 billion tablets per year are consumed. As such, the recognition of AIA is important as AIA may represent 10–20% of the asthma population (Sturtevant 1999). The AIA syndrome usually includes a triad of symptoms: nasal polyps and nasal congestion, sinusitis, and asthma with chronic symptoms. Patients with AIA often have chronic severe asthma with acute symptoms triggered after ingestion of aspirin or a similar drug (such as ibuprofen). Many times, symptoms can begin within 3 h after ingestion of aspirin with a profuse runny nose, swollen eyes, and flushing of the face in addition to wheezing. Breathing can become severely impaired, requiring hospitalization, and can progress to respiratory failure.

Although symptoms begin shortly after exposure to aspirin, AIA is not an allergic reaction per se. Skin prick tests with aspirin are usually negative, indicating that an antibody to aspirin does not exist in patients with AIA (Babu and Salvi 2000). Instead, aspirin blocks enzymes and, by doing so, causes increased production of cytokines called leukotrienes. These leukotrienes, in turn, promote inflammation and asthma in the susceptible individual. AIA is an example of how different mechanisms can lead to asthma.

Exercise-Induced Asthma

Like AIA, EIA is also not allergen mediated. It is very common with reports of 40–90% of asthmatics affected (Bundgaard 1981; Tan and Spector 2002). Many asthmatics experience increased airways resistance during exercise. Because of the dyspnea experienced during exercise, many patients with asthma often do not pursue aerobic activities as much as their non-asthmatic counterparts and are less fit as a result (Garfinkel et al. 1992). EIA, therefore, is important to recognize and treat so that patients with asthma can become more involved in exercise. Patients with asthma often feel better when they are physically fit (Ram et al. 2005). It is also thought that EIA may be triggered by moving large amounts of air in and out of the lungs. If asthmatics are more fit, they may breathe less heavily with mild to moderate exercise thereby decreasing the triggers for EIA (Ram et al. 2005).

The mechanism for EIA is debated. Two of the most common theories are the *osmotic hypothesis* and the *thermal hypothesis*. The thermal hypothesis suggests that bronchoconstriction during exercise is due to changes in temperature and water content of the airways (McFadden and Gilbert 1994). As large volumes of air move in and out of the lungs, the airways warm and humidify that air (also known as conditioning). Although the airways warm and heat air continuously (regardless of whether we are exercising or not) when we are quietly breathing with low tidal volumes, only a portion of the airways heat and humidify the air. During exercise, however, ventilation can increase by a factor of 20. As ventilation increases, the conditioning of air moves from the upper airways to the lower airways where more movement of heat and water from the airway cells is required to heat and humidify the air (McFadden and Gilbert 1994). When exercise stops and ventilation decreases, the airways rewarm quickly as they are no longer losing heat and water to the air. This cycle of cooling and rewarming is associated with airway narrowing and bronchoconstriction. Breathing warm humidified air ameliorates exercise-induced bronchoconstriction and breathing cold dry air worsens it (Bundgaard et al. 1982). It is not entirely clear why the airways narrow in response to rapid cooling and rewarming although increased blood flow and subsequent airway edema is thought to play a role (McFadden and Gilbert 1994; McFadden et al. 1986).

The osmotic hypothesis, on the other hand, suggests that airway dehydration during exercise causes a series of events leading to airway smooth muscle contraction and increased airways resistance (Anderson 1984). Proponents of the osmotic hypothesis argue that it is water loss, not changes in temperature that lead to bronchoconstriction. During exercise, large volumes of air move in and out of the lungs as respiratory rate and tidal volume increase. This movement of air is thought to cause evaporation of water in the airways. It is thought that the water loss causes an increase in osmolarity, which then triggers cells to release inflammatory chemicals, which in turn act on smooth muscle to contract. The loss of water in the lungs is also thought to cause an increase in blood flow to the lungs that can cause edema of the airways and even worsening airway constriction (Anderson and Daviskas 2000). Observations that EIA occurs when subjects breath gases of varying temperature but similar water content supports the osmotic hypothesis (Ingenito et al. 1988). Treatment of EIA usually consists of using a bronchodilator before exercise

Physiology

Until now, we have discussed the pathogenesis of asthma and possible mechanisms for increased airways inflammation. This inflammation in turn leads to air flow obstruction and airway hyperresponsiveness. But what does this mean in terms of how asthma manifests clinically? How does this lead to symptoms of shortness of breath? What happens to respiratory physiology when asthma occurs?

The hallmark of asthma is reversible airways obstruction. As the airways become narrowed during an asthma attack, resistance of the airways increases and airflow into the lungs is diminished at the same level of respiratory effort. One could imagine this by comparing the difference between blowing into a large straw versus a small straw. If one blows the same volume of air through the large and small straw, it will take a significantly longer time to blow out all the air through the small straw because flow is greatly diminished. The lungs are more complex than the one straw system, however, as smaller and smaller branching airways have differing lengths, compliances, and different types of air flow (laminar and turbulent). Because of this, there comes a point when no matter how hard one blows, flow will not increase. This is called airflow limitation.

One of the most common complaints in patients with asthma is that they have difficulty breathing in. There are several reasons for this. With increased bronchoconstriction there is diminished air flow and increased airways resistance. In order to compensate for the increase in airways resistance, the inspiratory muscles must generate greater tension. Imagine that instead of blowing through the small straw, that one tries to breathe in through the small straw. The amount of effort required to take in a breath will increase. However, it turns out that the increased work of breathing associated with inhalation is complicated by a second factor, hyperinflation of the lungs and chest wall. Furthermore, inhalation is an active process; muscle activity is required. Exhalation, on the other hand, is typically passive during quiet breathing. The normal elastic properties of the lungs and chest wall push air out of the lungs during exhalation.

Now imagine trying to blow out through the small straw and then continue to breathe in and out through this small straw. Although one may not be aware of it, as one continues to breathe in and out through that small straw, a process called "dynamic hyperinflation" is occurring. In other words, because it takes longer to exhale out all the air when air flow is decreased, one may initiate the next breath before all the air is exhaled from the last breath. The volume of the lung and chest wall then increases. The next breath is even harder to take in because at higher lung volumes, the inspiratory muscles operate at a shorter length and are less able to generate tension. In addition, the compliance of the lungs and chest wall is reduced at higher lung volumes. This means that the respiratory system is stiffer and more work is required to take in a breath. You can try to experience this by taking a breath in before you have fully exhaled the last breath. When a group of patients with mild asthma were given medication to induce bronchoconstriction, hyperinflation was the greatest indicator of how short of breath they felt (Lougheed et al. 1993). Surprisingly, an increase in airways resistance did not correlate with how dyspneic the subjects felt. This points to the importance of hyperinflation as a cause of dyspnea in the asthmatic patient.

Hyperinflation can also induce "length-tension inappropriateness" another mechanism that may contribute to dyspnea in asthma. If tension is generated in the muscle but it does not shorten appropriately because of the mechanical load on the system (similar to when trying to lift a weight that is too heavy), there is a discrepancy between the tension generated in the muscle and the degree to which it shortens (Campbell and Howell 1963). This concept has been broadened to include discrepancies between the neurological output to the muscles and the mechanical response of the respiratory system (neuromechanical dissociation). If the inspiratory muscle force generated does not match the expected change in lung volume, feelings of breathlessness may occur (Campbell and Howell 1963). Hyperinflation contributes to neuromechanical dissociation in several ways. The hyperinflated lung places the respiratory muscles at a mechanical disadvantage making these muscles less effective in creating tension. Therefore, even though the brain is sending out a message to the respiratory muscles to contract, the force generated and the change in lung volume may not match what the brain expects, causing neuromechanical dissociation. Hyperinflation also creates an inspiratory load that the respiratory muscles have to overcome before flow into the lungs can occur. This phenomenon is called "auto PEEP" or positive end expiratory pressure. What this means is that if the lungs have residual air in them because one could not fully exhale, there is still positive pressure in the lungs at the end of the breath. Normally, exhalation is a passive process akin to letting air out of a balloon. When we exhale, the pressure in our lungs equilibrates to atmospheric pressure. If one does not fully exhale, however, there may be a few centimeters of H_2O pressure left in the lungs before inhalation begins. The flow of air travels from areas of low pressure to high pressure. In auto PEEP, the inspiratory respiratory muscles must first overcome this pressure gradient to equilibrate to atmospheric pressure, and only after that can negative pressure be generated so that air can flow into the lungs. Thus, there is a period of time when the respiratory muscles are firing but no air is flowing into the lungs and, therefore, there is no change in lung volume. Imagine walking about while breathing through a mouthpiece that is connected to a valve that does not open until you generate a negative pressure of 5 or 7 cm H_2O with your inspiratory muscles. It is not surprising that individuals with auto-PEEP complain of shortness of breath.

However, there are many patients with mild asthma who complain of chest tightness or difficulty breathing with only mild bronchoconstriction, levels of airways obstruction not associated with hyperinflation. These symptoms cannot be readily explained by increased work of breathing alone. Several studies have elucidated what may be occurring in this groups of patients. Taguchi et al. (1991) tested subjects by having them inhale a medication that causes bronchoconstriction and compared the respiratory sensation associated with an asthma-type reaction in the lungs to what the subjects felt when breathing through a high resistance (like our straw example). Although the degree of hyperinflation was the same in both conditions, subjects felt more short of breath when they were given a medication that caused bronchoconstriction. This sensation of shortness of breath was relieved when the subjects breathed in lidocaine (a topical anesthetic). This study suggests that there are nerve receptors in the lungs that contribute to the sensation of breathlessness during bronchoconstriction. Binks et al. (2002) tried to clarify further the mechanism behind the chest "tightness" often described by asthmatics during an attack. They gave patients inhaled medication to provoke bronchoconstriction. They then placed these patients on a mechanical ventilator thereby eliminating the effort required by the patient to inhale by having a machine breathe for them. Even though the patients felt like it required less effort to breathe on the ventilator, they still experienced the sensation of chest tightness. They then put subjects without bronchoconstriction on a mechanical ventilator and increased the end expiratory volume to mimic hyperinflation. Even though their lungs were hyperinflated, the subjects did not experience chest tightness. This experiment suggests that the feeling of chest tightness is separate from the effort of breathing during an asthma attack. Although the effort to breathe is related to bronchoconstriction and the resultant increased work of breathing, tightness may be caused by changes within the airway itself that lead to stimulation of pulmonary receptors, which may send messages to the brain creating the sensation of tightness.

Bronchoconstriction may also affect the delivery of oxygen into the lungs. If airflow to the lungs is diminished, it is hard to get air in and out and, therefore, the movement of oxygen into the lungs and carbon dioxide out of the lungs is impaired. The human body, however, has developed an interesting system to deal with changes in airflow and oxygen delivery to the lungs. The body has a tremendous ability to constrict blood flow to areas of the lung that have low oxygen levels. This phenomenon is called hypoxic vasoconstriction. In response to low oxygen levels in the lungs, the body will decrease flow of blood to these areas and divert blood to areas of the lung with normal oxygen levels. Because asthma is a heterogeneous disease process, some areas of the lung will experience inflammation and bronchoconstriction while other areas of the lung will be relatively normal. Therefore, the body usually can maintain adequate oxygen levels even in the face of mild to moderate asthma attacks.

Another mechanism that contributes to near normal oxygen levels during an asthma attack is hyperventilation. During a mild or moderate asthma attack, the patient will typically hyperventilate. Possible reasons for hyperventilation include stimulation of pulmonary receptors as well as behavioral factors (shortness of breath and anxiety can lead to hyperventilation). The rapid replacement of oxygen in the alveoli during hyperventilation helps to maintain normal oxygen levels in the blood.

In patients with fatal or near-fatal asthma, however, hypoxemia may blunt the sensation of dyspnea or uncomfortable breathing, making it more difficult for individuals to recognize the severity of their problem, thereby leading to a delay in seeking medical treatment. Although hypoxemia is not a common feature of asthma, the body's attempts to divert blood to normal lung is insufficient when bronchoconstriction becomes severe. If there is little normal lung to which to divert blood, oxygen levels will start to decrease. In people without asthma (Chronos et al. 1988), or with other lung diseases such as COPD (Lane et al. 1987), hypoxemia itself can provoke shortness of breath. Unfortunately, when patients with asthma become hypoxemic, the ability to feel short of breath or chest tightness may diminish (Eckert et al. 2004).

Diagnosis

Symptoms

Just as the pathogenesis of asthma is relatively complex, the signs and symptoms of asthma can be confusing as well. Asthma can present with a paucity or overabundance of symptoms, and can coexist with other illnesses. There are also many disease processes that can mimic asthma, thereby confusing health care providers. Finally, because asthma is an episodic disease, patients can have normal exams and pulmonary function tests between "attacks," which makes diagnostic studies insensitive to the presence of asthma. According to the National Heart Lung and Blood Institute, the diagnosis of asthma should be considered in anyone who has episodic airways obstruction, reversible (or at least partially reversible) airways obstruction, and in whom other diagnoses have been excluded (Teichtahl et al. 1997). We will review the presenting symptoms of asthma, the role of diagnostic studies (such as pulmonary function tests, peak flow, and methacholine challenge tests (MCT)) and the conditions that may mimic asthma and which should be considered in difficult cases.

Many patients with asthma will initially present with wheezing, a high pitched sound usually heard during exhalation. As the airways narrow and airways resistance increases, there is more turbulent flow causing vibrations that we hear as a "wheeze." Some have argued that the opening and closing of airways also contributes to this vibration. However, a lack of wheezing does not exclude the diagnosis of asthma.

First, because asthma is an episodic disease, wheezing is not always present; patients who present to their health care provider during an asymptomatic period can have a completely normal exam. Second, the sound of wheezing actually decreases if airways resistance becomes severe. If airways resistance becomes so high that air flow is severely reduced, as in cases of extreme bronchoconstriction, turbulent flow can no longer be heard. Therefore, a patient who presents with a severe asthma attack can initially have wheezing that subsequently quiets down or stops. Instead of interpreting the lack of wheezing as an improvement in asthma, one must be vigilant that this does not signify a worsening of airways obstruction. Similarly, complete absence in breath sounds, or a "quiet chest" can also signify worsening airways obstruction and impending respiratory failure.

Some patients never develop wheezing as a symptom of asthma. There are many patients whose initial symptom is cough. This phenomenon has been termed "cough-variant" asthma. Gastroesophageal reflux disease (GERD), postnasal drip, and asthma are the three most common causes of chronic cough (Irwin et al. 1990). Because asthma is so common in the diagnosis of chronic cough, empiric treatment with bronchodilators (beta-agonists, which cause smooth muscle relaxation) is a common diagnostic test to evaluate if asthma is the cause of chronic cough. However, there is complex relationship between GERD and asthma. Acid reflux can cause bronchoconstriction through a neural reflex that leads to increased airways resistance. Postnasal drip also has many associations with asthma as both can be presentations of the allergic phenotype. Therefore, GERD, postnasal drip, and asthma often coexist and treatment of all three conditions may be needed to resolve chronic cough. Asthma, however, can present as cough alone and should be considered as a diagnosis in those individuals who present with chronic cough.

Dyspnea and shortness of breath are common symptoms of asthma (Table 2.2). Many respiratory diseases, however, present with feelings of dyspnea; distinguishing asthma from other diseases, such as COPD, can be difficult when based on symptoms of dyspnea alone. To complicate matters, the perception of dyspnea in patients with asthma is variable and does not necessarily correlate with objective measurements of lung function. Most concerning are those patients whose perception of dyspnea is "blunted" despite having severe airways obstruction as measured by the forced expiratory volume in 1 s (FEV1). Briefly, the FEV1 is the volume of air exhaled in the 1st second of a forced expiration after a maximal inhalation. In other words, it is the amount of air exhaled after the patient is asked to take a deep breath in and blow out as hard as she can. The FEV1 is reported as a percent predicted, when compared to patients of the same height, age, sex, and race. A reduction in FEV1 is associated with increased airways resistance in patients with asthma. Several studies have shown that patients with substantial airways resistance have minimal symptoms. Furthermore, symptoms in general do not correlate with objective measures of lung function (Foo and Sly 1991; Hewson et al. 1996; Molema et al. 1989; Teeter and Bleecker 1998). Asking whether dyspnea is present or absent or even asking about the intensity of dyspnea may not be specific enough to assess the presence or severity of asthma. What may be more useful is understanding the language of dyspnea. Different respiratory diseases have distinct characteristics to their shortness of breath. This is not unlike cardiovascular disease and chest pain. Over the years, we have come to recognize different representations of ischemic chest pain and that not all patients present with the typical left-sided chest pain. We have now come to recognize jaw pain, arm numbness, indigestion, belching, and chest pressure as anginal equivalents. Similarly, dyspnea has many diverse characteristics and varying presentations.

Table 2.2 Common symptoms of asthma

Common symptoms of asthma
Wheezing
Cough
Shortness of breath
Dyspnea
Chest tightness
Mucous production

Researchers have compiled a group of phrases used to describe shortness of breath by patients with different lung and heart diseases that are listed in Table 2.3 (Simon et al. 1990). They found that patients experiencing an asthma attack chose phrases describing increased "work/effort" and "tightness" when asked to describe their dyspnea (Mahler et al. 1996). Further research has tried to assess the use of specific descriptors of dyspnea in assessing severity of an asthma attack. Moy et al. (1998) asked patients, in the midst of an asthma attack, to describe their feelings of shortness of breath (using Table 2.3) when they first presented to an emergency room and after treatment with bronchodilators. These patients were also asked to rate the severity of their dyspnea and were given breathing tests to objectively assess lung function. What was interesting was that these patients reported improvement in their feelings of shortness of breath after treatment with bronchodilators even if they had no improvement in their FEV1, an objective measure. Importantly, some aspects of their breathing discomfort improved more than others. For example, patients reported persistent feelings of increased "work" or "effort" of breathing, which better correlated with the severity of their diseases. In contrast, the sense of chest tightness improved after administration of bronchodilators. Moy et al. (1998) hypothesized that chest "tightness" may reflect bronchoconstriction, whereas "work" or "effort" may reflect ongoing inflammation and airways obstruction present during the later stages of an asthma attack. Therefore, medications that immediately dilate the airways by relaxing smooth muscles (such as bronchodilators) would provide relief from chest "tightness." However, the "work" of breathing would persist because of obstruction due to ongoing airways inflammation. Unaware of these relationships between dyspnea and asthma, doctors may discharge patients from the emergency room or hospital before their lung function has improved (Salmeron et al. 2001). In a study of asthma management in French emergency rooms, 24% of patients with severe asthma were discharged 2 h after presentation when lung function was still poor (Salmeron et al. 2001). This may be because patients reported improvements in symptoms despite persistent airway resistance. Practitioners, therefore, should be cautious when interpreting the patient's perception of dyspnea, and should attempt to distinguish between changes in chest tightness and the work or effort of breathing. Objective measures of lung function should be used routinely to manage patients in the midst of an acute exacerbation.

Table 2.3 Descriptors of dyspnea

Descriptors of dyspnea
I feel that my breathing is rapid
My breath does not go out all the way
My breath does not go in all the way
My breathing is shallow
My breathing requires effort
My breathing requires more work
I feel that I am smothering
I feel that I am suffocating
I feel a hunger for more air
I feel out of breath
I cannot get enough air
My chest feels tight
My chest is constricted
My breathing is heavy
I feel that I am breathing more

From Moy et al. (1998)

Finally, the patterns of symptoms may help to diagnose asthma. For example, many asthmatics may have worse symptoms during certain seasons when allergies are increasingly prevalent. Others may have increased difficulty breathing at night or upon awakening in the early morning and may have improvements of their symptoms during the day. It is important to try and establish whether symptoms are persistent or episodic and whether certain triggers can be identified.

Diagnostic Tools

Medical History

The medical history is one of the most important tools in diagnosing asthma. As mentioned earlier, common symptoms of asthma include episodic wheezing, cough, shortness of breath, chest tightness, increased work or effort of breathing, and difficulty inhaling. These symptoms, however, can occur with other respiratory illnesses, and taking a detailed history may help to support or refute the diagnosis of asthma. Going back to previous discussions on asthma pathogenesis, we outlined several hypotheses including the TH2 hypothesis, the hygiene hypothesis, the role of viral and bacterial illnesses, and the Dutch hypothesis. Understanding these hypotheses helps the clinician recognize factors that support the likelihood of asthma in an individual (Table 2.4). For example childhood onset of wheezing in association with other allergic symptoms would suggest TH2-mediated immune dysregulation and asthma. A family history of asthma and/or COPD could suggest a genetic propensity to develop respiratory disease in response to a particular insult as suggested by the Dutch hypothesis. Alternatively, a childhood history of RSV disease

Table 2.4 Asthma pathogenesis hypotheses and possible corresponding medical histories

Possible mechanisms for asthma pathogenesis	Possible associated medical history
TH2 hypothesis	• Childhood onset • History of allergies, sinusitis, rhinitis, or nasal polyps • Association with allergy seasons, mold exposure, animal fur/dander
Hygiene hypothesis	• Childhood onset • History of allergies, sinusitis, rhinitis, or nasal polyps • Home environment (dust exposure) • Childhood environment (urban vs. farm, presence or absence of siblings, etc)
Viral/bacterial infections	• History of severe respiratory illness as a child (possibly RSV) • Frequent common colds
Dutch hypothesis	• Family history of respiratory diseases • Exposure to passive/active smoke • Disease progression
Other associations	• GERD • Exposures to exhaust, perfumes, strong smells • Strong emotions • Exercise-induced • Cold air exposure • Aspirin-induced

requiring hospitalization could suggest asthma as the etiology of his/her symptoms.

Physical Exam

Often times the physical exam can be normal, especially if the patient is not having any symptoms of asthma. In those cases, one must rely on the medical history to help establish the diagnosis. If, however, a patient is experiencing symptoms at the time of the physical exam, there are some findings that increase the likelihood of asthma. For example, if airways obstruction is so significant that the patient cannot exhale all the air out before taking another breath, the lungs can become "hyperexpanded." When hyperexpansion occurs, it is more difficult to breathe because the chest wall is at a mechanical disadvantage. Patients will begin to use "accessory muscles" to breathe. These muscles are not commonly utilized in quiet breathing, but if breathing becomes more labored they are recruited to assist in the movement of the chest wall. These accessory muscles include the neck muscles and abdominal muscles. Also, the activity of the intercostals muscles between the ribs can become more apparent during labored breathing. If breathing becomes more difficult, some patients will hunch over or assume the "tripod" position with their hands on their knees, leaning forward while sitting; this position transforms the pectoralis muscles, normally used to move the arms, into breathing muscles that elevate the chest wall.

After observing how the patient is breathing, auscultation of the chest can be informative as well. As discussed earlier, wheezing is a common sound of early airways obstruction. Usually a wheeze is heard on exhalation. With increasing airways resistance, however, inspiratory wheezes can be heard as well. The inspiratory to expiratory, or "I:E," ratio is also reduced, meaning the expiratory phase is prolonged during airways obstruction. Usually, when listening to a patient's chest, the clinician instructs the patient to breathe deeply, which results in an I:E ratio of 1:1. If airways obstruction is present, however, the I:E ratio can decrease to 1:2 because the lungs take longer to empty.

In cases of severe asthma attacks, a phenomenon called "pulsus paradoxus" can occur. The term "pulsus paradoxus" describes what happens to the pulse or systolic blood pressure during inspiration. Normally there is a slight weakening of the pulse during inhalation and a slight strengthening of the pulse during exhalation. This happens because of the small pressure swings in the chest that occur when we inhale and exhale and the effect that these slight changes of pressure have on the heart's ability to pump blood. During a severe asthma attack, the work of breathing increases tremendously and the pressure swings in the chest become more pronounced. A person can generate −70 to −100 cm of H_2O pressure (normal is between −2 and −5 cm of H_2O pressure) which causes a severe strain on the heart's ability to pump effectively. The pulse then becomes very weak during inspiration and returns during exhalation. This physical finding is called "pulsus paradoxus" and is a sign of severe airways obstruction and possible impending respiratory failure.

The rest of the physical exam can help to identify if the patient is prone to allergies. For example, examination of the nose may reveal mucosal swelling or nasal polyps to suggest allergic rhinitis. Similarly the eyes may be itchy, red, and teary. Skin exam may review rashes, such as hives or eczema, indicative of an allergic skin disorder. Taken together, if the physical exam is consistent with allergies in the context of shortness of breath and wheezing, the likelihood of asthma is increased.

Imaging

Most imaging will be normal in patients with asthma. In some cases, one might see evidence of hyperinflation on a chest X-ray (CXR) with flattening of the diaphragm. The main purpose of imaging, however, is to assess the patient for other conditions that may mimic asthma such as chronic eosinophilic pneumonia, bronchiectasis, cryptogenic organizing pneumonia, and emphysema among other diseases. Additionally, a chest CT may be useful if the CXR is unrevealing but the suspicion of asthma is still suspect. Chest CT's can more accurately show abnormalities of the airways, such as foreign bodies or tracheomalacia, which may be the cause of wheezing. It can also better image chronic bronchitis or bronchiectasis that may not be readily evident on a CXR. We recommend starting with a CXR in a patient newly diagnosed with asthma to exclude other possible causes of his/her symptoms.

Pulmonary Function Tests

Pulmonary function tests can be very helpful in diagnosing asthma. As mentioned earlier, measurement of FEV1 is important in diagnosing airflow obstruction. FEV1 is the amount of air exhaled during the 1st second of a forced exhalation after maximal inhalation. The forced vital capacity (FVC) is the amount of air exhaled in total after the patient blows out for as long as possible (at least 6 s); the air remaining in the lungs after such a maneuver is the residual volume (RV). If the FEV1/FVC ratio is less than what would be predicted for that person, then airflow obstruction is present. However, diseases such as chronic bronchitis, emphysema, or cystic fibrosis, all present with airflow obstruction. What increases the likelihood of asthma is the reversibility of the airflow obstruction. Often times in the lab, when we suspect that a person has asthma, we will assess the FEV1 and FVC before and after a bronchodilator. If the FEV1 increases by as least 12% and 200 cc, the patient has a significant response to bronchodilators suggestive of asthma. Wide variations in FEV1 over time with repeated pulmonary function testing are also suggestive of asthma. However, because these tests are very effort dependent, fluctuations in FEV1 can be due to patient effort rather than true reversible airways disease. In moderate to severe asthma, the patient may not be able to exhale fully during the vital capacity maneuver. The result is a diminished FVC and an elevated RV.

There are many instances when patients will not be experiencing airflow obstruction during pulmonary function testing, making it harder to diagnose asthma. Another strategy is to ask the patient to measure his PEF at home at various times during the day. This can be accomplished by asking the patient to use an inexpensive peak flow meter. Similar to the FEV1 measurement, the PEF assesses the rate at which air exits the lung during a forced expiration after maximal inspiration. In asthma, PEF is usually lowest in the morning and highest between noon and 2 p.m. (Quackenboss et al. 1991). The patient makes PEF measurements several times a day and a 20% difference in values between the highest and lowest flow measurements is suggestive of asthma.

If, after obtaining the history, physical exam, CXR, and pulmonary function tests, the diagnosis of asthma is still in doubt, a bronchoprovocation test to induce airways obstruction may help to establish or exclude the diagnosis. Commonly, a bronchoprovocation test is useful when conventional therapies for asthma do not resolve the patient's symptoms. The physician must decide whether to intensify the medical regimen or question the diagnosis of asthma. A MCT can help confirm or exclude a diagnosis of asthma and guide further therapy (Fig. 2.3).

The hallmark of asthma is bronchial hyperresponsiveness, meaning that the airways constrict robustly in response to an irritant or other stimulus. Methacholine is a medication that causes constriction of the smooth muscles around the airways. When given in high enough doses, a person with normal airways can have bronchoconstriction with methacholine. In asthmatics, however, the airways will constrict with very small doses that usually do not affect the normal airway. The MCT is administered in a monitored setting. The subject inhales a solution of methacholine in increasing doses. After each inhalation, FEV1 and FVC are measured. If there is a decrease of 20% in the FEV1 after an inhalation of a certain dose of methacholine, the test is stopped. This is called the PC20, the provocation

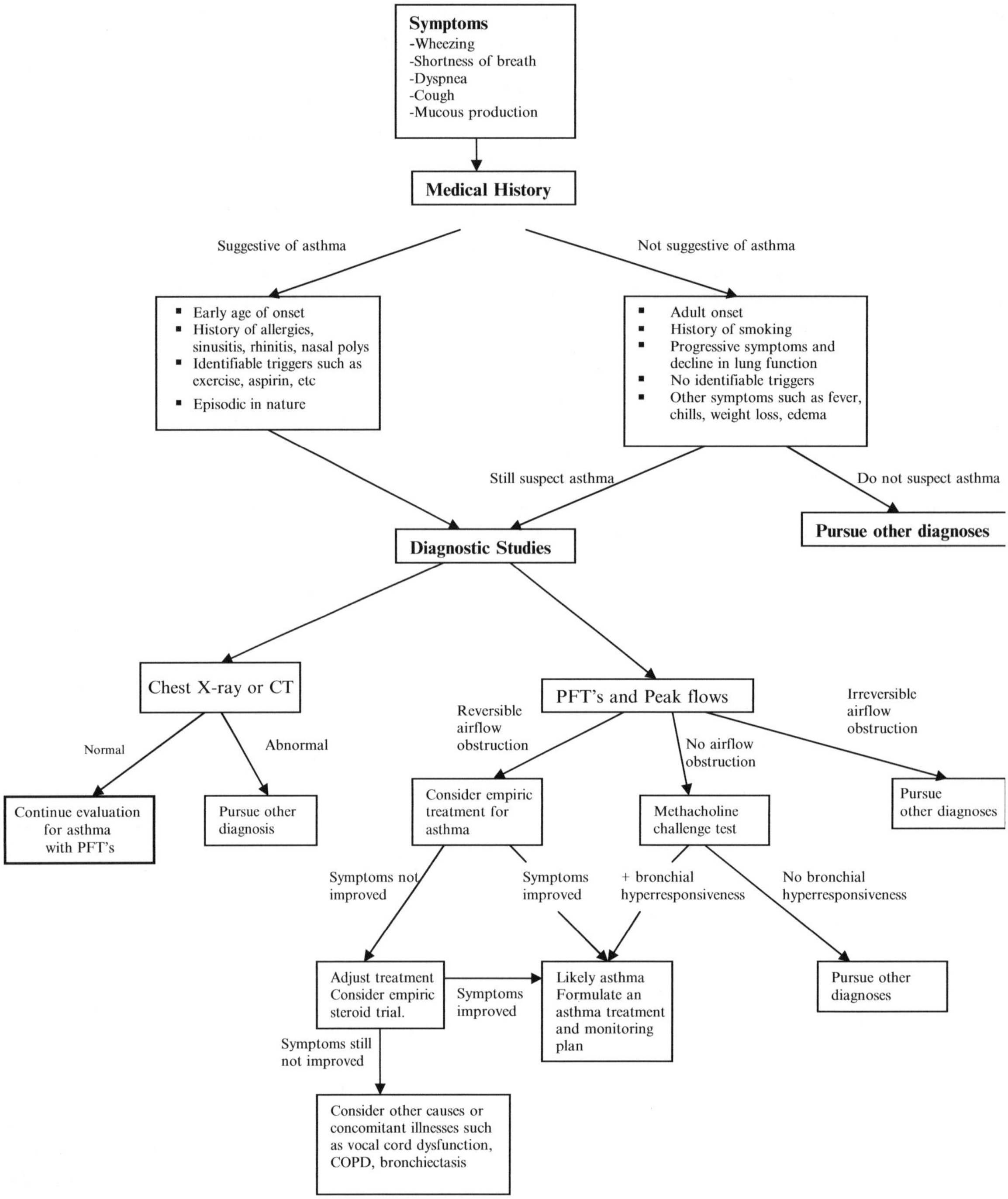

Fig. 2.3 Algorithm for asthma diagnosis

concentration that is required to decrease the FEV1 by 20%. As outlined in the Table 2.5, the degree of bronchial hyperresponsiveness depends on how much methacholine is required to cause significant bronchoconstriction. The MCT is a useful test for diagnosing asthma but the results must be interpreted in the context of all the information known about the patient. It is not 100% diagnostic.

Table 2.5 Degree of bronchial hyperreponsiveness after administration of methacholine

Methacholine challenge test	
PC20 (mg/ml)	Bronchial hyperresponsiveness
>16	Normal
4.0–16	Borderline
1.0–4.0	Mild
<1.0	Moderate to severe

From ATS AJRCCM 2000 (Crapo et al. 2000)

Although the MCT is not a foolproof test, it is helpful in trying to obtain the correct diagnosis in a patient with asthma-like symptoms. In a study of patients evaluated for dyspnea and cough who did not improve with asthma treatment, 82.5% had negative MCT (Chevalier and Schwartzstein 2001). As a result of these negative tests, bronchodilators were discontinued and other causes for dyspnea and cough were pursued and then treated. Other studies have shown that even a previous history of asthma did not reliably predict a positive MCT (Pratter et al. 1989). The MCT, therefore, is a powerful tool to help establish the diagnosis of asthma in some cases and exclude it in others, thereby allowing the patient to receive the treatment she needs.

Mimickers of Asthma

All that wheezes is not always asthma. Often times, in difficult cases, other diagnoses should be explored if the diagnosis of asthma is in question. These are usually cases in which the patient does not respond to treatment or has a physical exam or history that seems inconsistent with asthma. The mimickers of asthma can be categorized into diseases affecting the large airways, small airways, and lung parenchyma. Non-pulmonary causes should also be considered.

One of the most difficult diagnoses to make is vocal cord dysfunction (VCD). VCD can present like asthma and patients usually have a history of asthma that has not been responsive to steroids or bronchodilators. Because they continue to wheeze despite therapy, these patients can be exposed to large doses of steroids and bronchodilators putting them at risk for complications of these medications. Although the etiology of VCD is not fully elucidated, it is more common in young adults with psychiatric disorders. It occurs when the vocal cords adduct (come together in the midline) during inhalation and exhalation creating airflow limitation at the level of the vocal cords. The lungs and airways themselves, however, are normal. The patient adducts the vocal cords subconsciously and can often appear to be in respiratory distress. VCD presents with similar symptoms and signs as asthma, such as shortness of breath and wheezing. In extreme cases, however, patients with VCD can hypoventilate and be intubated for respiratory failure. Unlike asthma, however, wheezes cease after intubation because the endotracheal tube bypasses the vocal cords, the site of obstruction. After intubation, the patient with VCD is easily ventilated and can be removed from mechanical support within 24 h.

Definitive diagnosis of this disorder can be difficult and usually requires direct visualization of the vocal cords during symptomatic episodes. Physical exam during an episode usually reveals a monophonic wheeze heard loudest over the throat. Patients may have trouble vocalizing while wheezing and symptoms can come on suddenly without warning. Treatment requires intense speech therapy during which these patients learn techniques for relaxed throat breathing. With treatment, patients with VCD can come off steroids and bronchodilator therapy and live a better quality of life. In extreme cases, a tracheostomy is performed to bypass the site of recurrent obstruction.

Other problems of the large airways that can cause wheezing included foreign bodies in the large airways. Aspiration of nuts or other food products can cause foreign bodies to get trapped in a large airway. In severe cases, these foreign bodies can act as a ball-valve causing hyperinflation and eventual respiratory distress. Immediate removal of the foreign body by a trained bronchoscopist is required. Besides aspirated objects, congenital abnormalities, such as vascular rings or laryngeal webs, can cause obstruction of the trachea and lead to wheezing and shortness of breath. Other masses, such as tumors, can cause obstruction of the airways as well and with similar presenting symptoms. Lung cancer and carcinoid tumors may cause focal airway obstruction. In patients who have had prior intubations, tracheal stenosis as a late complication of endotracheal intubation can also present like asthma. A bronchoscopy to inspect the airway is usually required to make this diagnosis. Even if the airway is normal, structures outside of the airway can be abnormal and can cause compression resulting in obstruction. Lymph nodes, vascular structures, or tumor can impinge upon the large airways in this manner. Often times, a chest CT is helpful in making this diagnosis.

Sometimes the airways can be affected by other disease processes such as bronchiectasis. Bronchiectasis is a common disorder that can present with signs and symptoms similar to asthma. Patients with bronchiectasis have distorted and abnormal airways usually due to an infectious process. People can develop bronchiectasis as a sequelae of a severe necrotizing lung infection or toxic gas exposure. In necrotizing pneumonia, the abnormal airways usually are confined to the region of the lung where the original infection took place, whereas toxic gas exposure can cause more diffuse bronchiectasis. Because the airways are abnormal, it becomes more difficult to clear infections from bronchiectatic lung and recurrent infections occur. Some patients develop bronchiectasis after aspirating a foreign object that gets lodged in the airway. The object makes it difficult to clear pus, creating recurrent persistent infections and progressive damage to the airway. Other patients may develop bronchiectasis as a result of an underlying condition that makes the patient prone to lung infections and impairs the ability of the body to clear infections despite appropriate antibiotics. Such conditions include cystic fibrosis (a genetic disorder causing thick mucous plugs that are difficult clear) and immunodeficiency states. Regardless of the underlying cause for bronchiectasis, the presentation is similar with daily cough productive of purulent sputum, recurrent pulmonary infections, shortness of breath, and wheezing. The wheezing associated with bronchiectasis may be due to airflow obstruction associated with mucous plugging or distorted airways. Unlike asthma, the airflow obstruction is not completely reversible. Asthma, however, can also exist concomitantly with bronchiectasis. If a patient with wheezing has recurrent pulmonary infections or daily cough productive of purulent sputum, the diagnosis of bronchiectasis should be considered. Chest imaging can determine if the airways are distorted or abnormal to confirm the diagnosis of bronchiectasis.

Other airway diseases can also mimic asthma. In children, congenital abnormalities such bronchopulmonary dysplasia should be considered. In adults, diseases such as sarcoidosis can cause wheezing, cough, and dyspnea as well. Sarcoidosis is a disease of unclear etiology in which non-caseating granulomas affect the lymph nodes and airways. Airway or lymph node biopsy is often required to make the diagnosis. Diseases such as COPD are also common in adults and can mimic asthma as well. Occasionally, asthma and COPD can coexist.

Diseases that affect the lung parenchyma can cause wheezing, cough, and shortness of breath. Chronic eosinophilic pneumonia, in which eosinophils infiltrate the peripheral lung parenchyma, can present with wheezing and usually requires high doses of steroids to treat. Hypersensitivity pneumonitis is also a disease of the lung parenchyma, usually affecting the upper lobes and precipitated by exposure to some inhaled substance such as mold, flour, bird allergens, etc. Hypersensitivity pneumonitis can present acutely with fevers, cough, and dyspnea or less acutely with cough, wheezing, and shortness of breath. Other diseases that affect the lungs, such as pulmonary emboli or pneumonia, can also mimic asthma. Imaging, careful history, and physical exam may help to distinguish these conditions from asthma.

Processes that affect the pulmonary vasculature can also present as asthma does. As noted above pulmonary embolism can present with shortness of breath and wheezing. Although wheezing is not a common symptom of pulmonary embolism, it has been reported in the medical literature (Calvo-Romero et al. 2003). Although the etiology of wheezing in pulmonary embolism is not clear, possible mechanisms include an inflammatory reaction resulting from the embolism or the release of chemicals such as bradykinin that may lead to bronchoconstriction and wheezing. Congestive heart failure can also cause dyspnea, cough, and wheezing (often termed cardiac asthma) due to pulmonary edema. When the heart fails to pump adequately, fluid builds up in the pulmonary lymphatics and pulmonary venous capillaries, which then causes edema of the lungs and can promote wheezing.

Other conditions that may mimic asthma include reactions to medications such as angiotensin converting enzyme I inhibitors (ACE-I), which can cause chronic cough. GERD can also cause both cough and bronchoconstriction as mentioned earlier. Aspiration can cause wheezing and cough due to inflammation of the airways. In cases of GERD, the patient may be unaware of these episodes. In severe cases, if routine treatment of GERD (including proton pump inhibitors and behavioral modification) does not alleviate the problem, procedures to tighten the lower esophageal sphincter are needed to prevent reflux.

A careful history, physical exam, and clinical acumen are required to identify when a diagnosis of asthma just doesn't seem right. Clues, such as poor response to asthma therapy, persistent instead of episodic symptoms, or constitutional symptoms (weight loss, fever, nausea/vomiting), can be useful in stimulating a search for non-asthma diagnoses. Chest imaging can be helpful in excluding diseases of the lung parenchymal, and bronchoscopic imaging may further help diagnose large airways obstruction.

Summary

We have briefly reviewed general theories of asthma pathogenesis including the TH2 hypothesis, the hygiene hypothesis, the Dutch hypothesis, and the role of infectious diseases in asthma. These theories demonstrate that asthma is a heterogeneous disease with multiple causative mechanisms in susceptible individuals. We reviewed the physiology of asthma and its relationship to symptoms such as dyspnea. We outlined a diagnostic approach to asthma based on symptoms, history and physical exam. In cases in which the asthma diagnosis is still in question, a MCT may help to support or exclude the diagnosis. Finally, an awareness of conditions that mimic asthma is important when confronted with a patient who may have atypical features or who fails to respond to therapy.

References

Allegra L, Blasi F, Centanni S, Cosentini R, Denti F, Raccanelli R, Tarsia P, Valenti V (1994) Acute exacerbations of asthma in adults: role of Chlamydia pneumoniae infection. Eur Respir J 7(12):2165–2168

Amayasu H, Yoshida S, Ebana S, Yamamoto Y, Nishikawa T, Shoji T, Nakagawa H, Hasegawa H, Nakabayashi M, Ishizaki Y (2000) Clarithromycin suppresses bronchial hyperresponsiveness associated with eosinophilic inflammation in patients with asthma. Ann Allergy Asthma Immunol 84(6):594–598

Anderson SD (1984) Is there a unifying hypothesis for exercise-induced asthma? J Allergy Clin Immunol 73(5 Pt 2): 660–665

Anderson SD, Daviskas E (2000) The mechanism of exercise-induced asthma is. J Allergy Clin Immunol 106(3):453–459

Atkinson JJ, Senior RM (2003) Matrix metalloproteinase-9 in lung remodeling. Am J Respir Cell Mol Biol 28(1):12–24

Babu KS, Salvi SS (2000) Aspirin and asthma. Chest 118(5): 1470–1476

Ball TM, Castro-Rodriguez JA, Griffith KA, Holberg CJ, Martinez FD, Wright AL (2000) Siblings, day-care attendance, and the risk of asthma and wheezing during childhood. N Engl J Med 343(8):538–543

Barrios RJ, Kheradmand F, Batts L, Corry DB (2006) Asthma: pathology and pathophysiology. Arch Pathol Lab Med 130(4):447–451

Berkovich S, Millian SJ, Snyder RD (1970) The association of viral and mycoplasma infections with recurrence of wheezing in the asthmatic child. Ann Allergy 28(2):43–49

Binks AP, Moosavi SH, Banzett RB, Schwartzstein RM (2002) "Tightness" sensation of asthma does not arise from the work of breathing. Am J Respir Crit Care Med 165(1): 78–82

Biscione GL, Corne J, Chauhan AJ, Johnston SL (2004) Increased frequency of detection of Chlamydophila pneumoniae in asthma. Eur Respir J 24(5):745–749

Black PN, Blasi F, Jenkins CR, Scicchitano R, Mills GD, Rubinfeld AR, Ruffin RE, Mullins PR, Dangain J, Cooper BC, David DB, Allegra L (2001) Trial of roxithromycin in subjects with asthma and serological evidence of infection with Chlamydia pneumoniae. Am J Respir Crit Care Med 164(4):536–541

Black PN, Scicchitano R, Jenkins CR, Blasi F, Allegra L, Wlodarczyk J, Cooper BC (2000) Serological evidence of infection with Chlamydia pneumoniae is related to the severity of asthma. Eur Respir J 15(2):254–259

Blasi F, Cosentini R, Tarsia P, Capone P, Allegra L (2001) Atypical pathogens and asthma: can they influence the natural history of the disease? Monaldi Arch Chest Dis 56(3):276–280

Bochner BS, Busse WW (2005) Allergy and asthma. J Allergy Clin Immunol 115(5):953–959

Bousquet J, Lacoste JY, Chanez P, Vic P, Godard P, Michel FB (1996) Bronchial elastic fibers in normal subjects and asthmatic patients. Am J Respir Crit Care Med 153(5):1648–1654

Bundgaard A (1981) Incidence of exercise-induced asthma in adult asthmatics. Allergy 36(1):23–26

Bundgaard A, Ingemann-Hansen T, Schmidt A, Halkjaer-Kristensen J (1982) Influence of temperature and relative humidity of inhaled gas on exercise-induced asthma. Eur J Respir Dis 63(3):239–244

Busse WW, Lemanske RF Jr (2001) Asthma. N Engl J Med 344(5):350–362

Calhoun WJ, Swenson CA, Dick EC, Schwartz LB, Lemanske RF Jr, Busse WW (1991) Experimental rhinovirus 16 infection potentiates histamine release after antigen bronchoprovocation in allergic subjects. Am Rev Respir Dis 144(6): 1267–1273

Calvo-Romero JM, Perez-Miranda M, Bureo-Dacal P (2003) Wheezing in patients with acute pulmonary embolism with and without previous cardiopulmonary disease. Eur J Emerg Med 10(4):288–289

Campbell EJ, Howell JB (1963) The sensation of breathlessness. Br Med Bull 19:36–40

Chanez P, Vignola AM, O'Shaugnessy T, Enander I, Li D, Jeffery PK et al (1997) Corticosteroid reversibility in COPD is related to features of asthma. Am J Respir Crit Care Med 155(5):1529–1534

Chevalier B, Schwartzstein R (2001) The role of the methacholine inhalation challenge: avoiding a misdiagnosis of asthma. J Respir Dis 22:153–160

Chronos N, Adams L, Guz A (1988) Effect of hyperoxia and hypoxia on exercise-induced breathlessness in normal subjects. Clin Sci (Lond) 74(5):531–537

Chu HW, Honour JM, Rawlinson CA, Harbeck RJ, Martin RJ (2003) Effects of respiratory Mycoplasma pneumoniae infection on allergen-induced bronchial hyperresponsiveness and lung inflammation in mice. Infect Immun 71(3):1520–1526

Cohet C, Cheng S, MacDonald C, Baker M, Foliaki S, Huntington N, Douwes J, Pearce N (2004) Infections, medication use, and the prevalence of symptoms of asthma, rhinitis, and eczema in childhood. J Epidemiol Community Health 58(10):852–857

Corry DB, Grunig G, Hadeiba H, Kurup VP, Warnock ML, Sheppard D, Rennick DM, Locksley RM (1998) Requirements for allergen-induced airway hyperreactivity in T and B cell-deficient mice. Mol Med 4(5):344–355

Cottrez F, Hurst SD, Coffman RL, Groux H (2000) T regulatory cells 1 inhibit a Th2-specific response in vivo. J Immunol 165(9):4848–4853

Crapo RO, Casaburi R, Coates AL, Enright PL, Hankinson JL, Irvin CG, MacIntyre NR, McKay RT, Wanger JS, Anderson SD, Cockcroft DW, Fish JE, Sterk PJ (2000) Guidelines for methacholine and exercise challenge testing-1999. This official statement of the American Thoracic Society was adopted by the ATS Board of Directors, July 1999. Am J Respir Crit Care Med 161(1):309–329

D'Andrea A, Rengaraju M, Valiante NM, Chehimi J, Kubin M, Aste M, Chan SH, Kobayashi M, Young D, Nickbarg E, Chizzonite R, Wolf SF, Trinchieri G (1992) Production of natural killer cell stimulatory factor (interleukin 12) by peripheral blood mononuclear cells. J Exp Med 176(5): 1387–1398

Droste JH, Wieringa MH, Weyler JJ, Nelen VJ, Vermeire PA, Van Bever HP (2000) Does the use of antibiotics in early childhood increase the risk of asthma and allergic disease? Clin Exp Allergy 30(11):1547–1553

Eckert DJ, Catcheside PG, Smith JH, Frith PA, McEvoy RD (2004) Hypoxia suppresses symptom perception in asthma. Am J Respir Crit Care Med 169(11):1224–1230

Finkelman FD, Katona IM, Urban JF Jr, Holmes J, Ohara J, Tung AS, Sample JV, Paul WE (1988) IL-4 is required to generate and sustain in vivo IgE responses. J Immunol 141(7):2335–2341

Foo AL, Sly PD (1991) Pulmonary function in a hospital population of asthmatic children. J Asthma 28(4):273–280

Garfinkel SK, Kesten S, Chapman KR, Rebuck AS (1992) Physiologic and nonphysiologic determinants of aerobic fitness in mild to moderate asthma. Am Rev Respir Dis 145(4 Pt 1):741–745

Gencay M, Rudiger JJ, Tamm M, Soler M, Perruchoud AP, Roth M (2001) Increased frequency of Chlamydia pneumoniae antibodies in patients with asthma. Am J Respir Crit Care Med 163(5):1097–1100

Gereda JE, Leung DY, Thatayatikom A, Streib JE, Price MR, Klinnert MD, Liu AH (2000) Relation between house-dust endotoxin exposure, type 1 T-cell development, and allergen sensitisation in infants at high risk of asthma. Lancet 355(9216):1680–1683

National Asthma Education and Prevention Program (1997) Guidelines for the diagnosis and management of asthma. NIH Publication No. 97-4051. National Institutes of Health, Bethesda, MD

Hewson PH, Tippett EA, Jones DM, Maddern JP, Higgs P (1996) Routine pulmonary function tests in young adolescents with asthma in general practice. Med J Aust 165(9):469–472

Holgate ST, Lackie PM, Davies DE, Roche WR, Walls AF (1999) The bronchial epithelium as a key regulator of airway inflammation and remodelling in asthma. Clin Exp Allergy 29(Suppl 2):90–95

Huhti E, Mokka T, Nikoskelainen J, Halonen P (1974) Association of viral and mycoplasma infections with exacerbations of asthma. Ann Allergy 33(3):145–149

Humbert M, Durham SR, Ying S, Kimmitt P, Barkans J, Assoufi B, Pfister R, Menz G, Robinson DS, Kay AB, Corrigan CJ (1996) IL-4 and IL-5 mRNA and protein in bronchial biopsies from patients with atopic and nonatopic asthma: evidence against "intrinsic" asthma being a distinct immunopathologic entity. Am J Respir Crit Care Med 154(5):1497–1504

Humbert M, Menz G, Ying S, Corrigan CJ, Robinson DS, Durham SR, Kay AB (1999) The immunopathology of extrinsic (atopic) and intrinsic (non-atopic) asthma: more similarities than differences. Immunol Today 20(11):528–533

Illi S, von Mutius E, Lau S, Bergmann R, Niggemann B, Sommerfeld C, Wahn U (2001) Early childhood infectious diseases and the development of asthma up to school age: a birth cohort study. BMJ 322(7283):390–395

Ingenito E, Solway J, Lafleur J, Lombardo A, Drazen JM, Pichurko B (1988) Dissociation of temperature-gradient and evaporative heat loss during cold gas hyperventilation in cold-induced asthma. Am Rev Respir Dis 138(3):540–546

Irwin RS, Curley FJ, French CL (1990) Chronic cough. The spectrum and frequency of causes, key components of the diagnostic evaluation, and outcome of specific therapy. Am Rev Respir Dis 141(3):640–647

Jeannin P, Lecoanet S, Delneste Y, Gauchat JF, Bonnefoy JY (1998) IgE versus IgG4 production can be differentially regulated by IL-10. J Immunol 160(7):3555–3561

Jeffery PK (2000) Comparison of the structural and inflammatory features of COPD and asthma. Giles F. Filley Lecture. Chest 117(5 Suppl 1):251S–260S

Johnston SL, Blasi F, Black PN, Martin RJ, Farrell DJ, Nieman RB (2006) The effect of telithromycin in acute exacerbations of asthma. N Engl J Med 354(15):1589–1600

Johnston SL, Pattemore PK, Sanderson G, Smith S, Campbell MJ, Josephs LK, Cunningham A, Robinson BS, Myint SH, Ward ME, Tyrrell DA, Holgate ST (1996) The relationship between upper respiratory infections and hospital admissions for asthma: a time-trend analysis. Am J Respir Crit Care Med 154(3 Pt 1):654–660

Johnston SL, Pattemore PK, Sanderson G, Smith S, Lampe F, Josephs L, Symington P, O'Toole S, Myint SH, Tyrrell DA, Holgate ST (1995) Community study of role of viral infections in exacerbations of asthma in 9–11 year old children. BMJ 310(6989):1225–1229

Kraft M, Djukanovic R, Wilson S, Holgate ST, Martin RJ (1996) Alveolar tissue inflammation in asthma. Am J Respir Crit Care Med 154(5):1505–1510

Lane R, Cockcroft A, Adams L, Guz A (1987) Arterial oxygen saturation and breathlessness in patients with chronic obstructive airways disease. Clin Sci (Lond) 72(6):693–698

Lapa e Silva JR, Possebon da Silva MD, Lefort J, Vargaftig BB (2000) Endotoxins, asthma, and allergic immune responses. Toxicology 152(1–3):31–35

Le J, Lin JX, Henriksen-DeStefano D, Vilcek J (1986) Bacterial lipopolysaccharide-induced interferon-gamma production: roles of interleukin 1 and interleukin 2. J Immunol 136(12): 4525–4530

Lemanske RF Jr, Dick EC, Swenson CA, Vrtis RF, Busse WW (1989) Rhinovirus upper respiratory infection increases airway hyperreactivity and late asthmatic reactions. J Clin Invest 83(1):1–10

Litonjua AA, Milton DK, Celedon JC, Ryan L, Weiss ST, Gold DR (2002) A longitudinal analysis of wheezing in young children: the independent effects of early life exposure to house dust endotoxin, allergens, and pets. J Allergy Clin Immunol 110(5):736–742

Lougheed MD, Lam M, Forkert L, Webb KA, O'Donnell DE (1993) Breathlessness during acute bronchoconstriction in asthma. Pathophysiologic mechanisms. Am Rev Respir Dis 148(6 Pt 1):1452–1459

Madden KB, Urban JF Jr, Ziltener HJ, Schrader JW, Finkelman FD, Katona IM (1991) Antibodies to IL-3 and IL-4 suppress helminth-induced intestinal mastocytosis. J Immunol 147(4):1387–1391

Mahler DA, Harver A, Lentine T, Scott JA, Beck K, Schwartzstein RM (1996) Descriptors of breathlessness in cardiorespiratory diseases. Am J Respir Crit Care Med 154(5):1357–1363

McFadden ER Jr, Gilbert IA (1994) Exercise-induced asthma. N Engl J Med 330(19):1362–1367

McFadden ER Jr, Lenner KA, Strohl KP (1986) Postexertional airway rewarming and thermally induced asthma. New insights into pathophysiology and possible pathogenesis. J Clin Invest 78(1):18–25

Mertsola J, Ziegler T, Ruuskanen O, Vanto T, Koivikko A, Halonen P (1991) Recurrent wheezy bronchitis and viral respiratory infections. Arch Dis Child 66(1):124–129

Michel O, Duchateau J, Sergysels R (1989) Effect of inhaled endotoxin on bronchial reactivity in asthmatic and normal subjects. J Appl Physiol 66(3):1059–1064

Molema J, van Herwaarden CL, Folgering HT (1989) Effects of inhaled budesonide on the relationships between symptoms, lung function indices and airway hyperresponsiveness in patients with allergic asthma. Pulm Pharmacol 1(4):179–185

Moy ML, Lantin ML, Harver A, Schwartzstein RM (1998) Language of dyspnea in assessment of patients with acute asthma treated with nebulized albuterol. Am J Respir Crit Care Med 158(3):749–753

Nicholson KG, Kent J, Ireland DC (1993) Respiratory viruses and exacerbations of asthma in adults. BMJ 307(6910):982–986

Papi A, Johnston SL (1999) Rhinovirus infection induces expression of its own receptor intercellular adhesion molecule 1 (ICAM-1) via increased NF-kappaB-mediated transcription. J Biol Chem 274(14):9707–9720

Postma DS, Boezen HM (2004) Rationale for the Dutch hypothesis. Allergy and airway hyperresponsiveness as genetic factors and their interaction with environment in the development of asthma and COPD. Chest 126(2 Suppl): 96S–104S; discussion 159S–161S

Pratter MR, Curley FJ, Dubois J, Irwin RS (1989) Cause and evaluation of chronic dyspnea in a pulmonary disease clinic. Arch Intern Med 149(10):2277–2282

Quackenboss JJ, Lebowitz MD, Krzyzanowski M (1991) The normal range of diurnal changes in peak expiratory flow rates. Relationship to symptoms and respiratory disease. Am Rev Respir Dis 143(2):323–330

Ram FS, Robinson SM, Black PN, Picot J (2005) Physical training for asthma. Cochrane Database Syst Rev (4):CD001116

Reed CE, Milton DK (2001) Endotoxin-stimulated innate immunity: a contributing factor for asthma. J Allergy Clin Immunol 108(2):157–166

Saetta M, Di Stefano A, Maestrelli P, Turato G, Ruggieri MP, Roggeri A, Calcagni P, Mapp A, Ciaccia A, Fabbri LM (1994) Airway eosinophilia in chronic bronchitis during exacerbations. Am J Respir Crit Care Med 150(6 Pt 1): 1646–1652

Salmeron S, Liard R, Elkharrat D, Muir J, Neukirch F, Ellrodt A (2001) Asthma severity and adequacy of management in accident and emergency departments in France: a prospective study. Lancet 358(9282):629–635

Schiller J, Martinez M, Barnes P (2006) Early release of selected estimates based on data from the 2005 National Health Interview Survey. National Center for Health Statistics. http://www.cdc.gov/nchs/nhis.htm

Scott P (1991) IFN-gamma modulates the early development of Th1 and Th2 responses in a murine model of cutaneous leishmaniasis. J Immunol 147(9):3149–3155

Scrivener S, Yemaneberhan H, Zebenigus M, Tilahun D, Girma S, Ali S, McElroy P, Custovic A, Woodcock A, Pritchard D, Venn A, Britton J (2001) Independent effects of intestinal parasite infection and domestic allergen exposure on risk of wheeze in Ethiopia: a nested case-control study. Lancet 358(9292):1493–1499

Simoes EA (1999) Respiratory syncytial virus infection. Lancet 354(9181):847–852

Simon PM, Schwartzstein RM, Weiss JW, Fencl V, Teghtsoonian M, Weinberger SE (1990) Distinguishable types of dyspnea in patients with shortness of breath. Am Rev Respir Dis 142(5):1009–1014

Stein RT, Sherrill D, Morgan WJ, Holberg CJ, Halonen M, Taussig LM, Wright AL, Martinez FD (1999) Respiratory syncytial virus in early life and risk of wheeze and allergy by age 13 years. Lancet 354(9178):541–545

Sturtevant J (1999) NSAID-induced bronchospasm – a common and serious problem. A report from MEDSAFE, the New Zealand Medicines and Medical Devices Safety Authority. N Z Dent J 95(421):84

Taguchi O, Kikuchi Y, Hida W, Iwase N, Satoh M, Chonan T, Takishima T (1991) Effects of bronchoconstriction and external resistive loading on the sensation of dyspnea. J Appl Physiol 71(6):2183–2190

Tan RA, Spector SL (2002) Exercise-induced asthma: diagnosis and management. Ann Allergy Asthma Immunol 89(3): 226–235; quiz 235–227, 297

Taussig LM, Wright AL, Holberg CJ, Halonen M, Morgan WJ, Martinez FD (2003) Tucson Children's Respiratory Study: 1980 to present. J Allergy Clin Immunol 111(4):661–675; quiz 676

Teeter JG, Bleecker ER (1998) Relationship between airway obstruction and respiratory symptoms in adult asthmatics. Chest 113(2):272–277

Teichtahl H, Buckmaster N, Pertnikovs E (1997) The incidence of respiratory tract infection in adults requiring hospitalization for asthma. Chest 112(3):591–596

Ulrik CS, Backer V (1999) Nonreversible airflow obstruction in life-long nonsmokers with moderate to severe asthma. Eur Respir J 14(4):892–896

Ulrik CS, Backer V, Dirksen A, Pedersen M, Koch C (1995) Extrinsic and intrinsic asthma from childhood to adult age: a 10-yr follow-up. Respir Med 89(8):547–554

van den Biggelaar AH, van Ree R, Rodrigues LC, Lell B, Deelder AM, Kremsner PG, Yazdanbakhsh M (2000) Decreased atopy in children infected with Schistosoma haematobium: a role for parasite-induced interleukin-10. Lancet 356(9243):1723–1727

Venarske DL, Busse WW, Griffin MR, Gebretsadik T, Shintani AK, Minton PA, Peebles RS, Hamilton R, Weisshaar E, Vrtis R, Higgins SB, Hartert TV (2006) The relationship of rhinovirus-associated asthma hospitalizations with inhaled corticosteroids and smoking. J Infect Dis 193(11):1536–1543

von Mutius E (2000) The environmental predictors of allergic disease. J Allergy Clin Immunol 105(1 Pt 1):9–19

von Mutius E, Braun-Fahrlander C, Schierl R, Riedler J, Ehlermann S, Maisch S, Waser M, Nowak D (2000) Exposure to endotoxin or other bacterial components might protect against the development of atopy. Clin Exp Allergy 30(9): 1230–1234

Wenzel SE, Schwartz LB, Langmack EL, Halliday JL, Trudeau JB, Gibbs RL, Chu HW (1999) Evidence that severe asthma can be divided pathologically into two inflammatory subtypes with distinct physiologic and clinical characteristics. Am J Respir Crit Care Med 160(3):1001–1008

Wills-Karp M (1999) Immunologic basis of antigen-induced airway hyperresponsiveness. Annu Rev Immunol 17:255–281

Wills-Karp M, Luyimbazi J, Xu X, Schofield B, Neben TY, Karp CL, Donaldson DD (1998) Interleukin-13: central mediator of allergic asthma. Science 282(5397): 2258–2261

(1998) Worldwide variation in prevalence of symptoms of asthma, allergic rhinoconjunctivitis, and atopic eczema: ISAAC. The International Study of Asthma and Allergies in Childhood (ISAAC) Steering Committee. Lancet 351(9111): 1225–1232

Chapter 3
Genetic and Environmental Factors in Asthma

David B. Peden

Introduction

Asthma and other allergic diseases are among the most common disorders in the United States, with asthma being a leading cause for hospitalization and lost school days for children. Asthma is a complex disease, characterized by eosinophilic inflammation, mucus cell hypertrophy and hypersecretion, airway reactivity and bronchoconstriction. Linkage analyses have identified loci on chromosomes 1–7, 11–13, 16, 19 and 20 that are associated with various phenotypes consistent with asthma (Ober and Moffatt 2000; Ober and Hoffjan 2006). Given the biological complexity of asthma, it is not surprizing that a wide variety of genes have been associated with this syndrome.

However, despite the large number of genes associated with asthma, this disease increased at an alarming rate beginning approximately 50 years ago. The sudden increase in asthma suggests that changes in both environmental exposures and lifestyle factors are a major reason for the increase in disease (Eder et al. 2006). Initially, this increase was most notable in North America, Western Europe, Australia and New Zealand. However, increased incidence of asthma has more recently been reported in Hong Kong, Taiwan, Singapore and Korea, with many speculating that this is linked with adoption of an increasingly Western lifestyle. This chapter will examine many environmental factors which influence asthma development and exacerbation, genetic factors which have been identified as risk factors for developing asthma, and examples of gene-by-environment interactions in expression of this disease.

D.B. Peden (✉)
The Center for Environmental Medicine, Asthma and Lung Biology, School of Medicine, The University of North Carolina at Chapel Hill, 104 Mason Farm Road, CB#7310, Chapel Hill, NC, 27599-7310, USA
e-mail: peden@med.unc.edu

Environmental Factors Associated with Increased Asthma and Allergy

Lifestyle

Many biological agents that contribute to airway inflammation in asthma include allergens from house dust mite and mold. Nonspecific irritants derived from microbes such as endotoxin from gram-negative bacteria and 1,3 beta-glucans from molds may also impact airway inflammation in both atopic and non-atopic subjects (Zeldin et al. 2006; Rylander and Holt 1998; Rylander et al. 1998). Additionally, volatile organic compounds produced by micro-organisms may also have an impact on human health (Etzel and Rylander 1999). House dust mites, molds and environmentally encountered bacteria all thrive in humid environments, suggesting that high relative humidity in indoor environments is linked to increased adverse health effects (Zeldin et al. 2006). Several European studies demonstrate that asthma is increased in association with high indoor humidity or in homes with water damage. Asthma and respiratory tract infections are increased in schools with increased humidity and mold spore counts (Taskinen et al. 1999) and measures of airway obstruction, variability in peak flow rates and peripheral blood eosinophils and mold allergy have been reported to be increased in children living in more humid homes. (Taskinen et al. 1997)

There are conflicting observations regarding the relationship between increased humidity and endotoxin

A. Harver and H. Kotses (eds.), *Asthma, Health and Society: A Public Health Perspective*,
DOI 10.1007/978-0-387-78285-0_3, © Springer Science+Business Media, LLC 2010

levels. However, even when humidity and dampness are examined independently of an association with endotoxin, decreased levels of humidity are associated with decreased severity of asthma (van Strien et al. 1994; van Strien et al. 2004a; Tavernier et al. 2006). Although house dust mite allergen as well as mold growth are optimal in humid environments, the effect of humidity in asthma cannot be ascribed to its impact on mite allergen alone. Nicolai et al. (2003) identified 234 children with active asthma out of a large cohort of 4th graders (5% of the total cohort), and measured lung function and nonspecific airway reactivity in 155 of these children 3 years later. Increased night-time wheeze and shortness of breath were associated with dampness, but not persisting asthma. Risk factors for bronchial hyperreactivity in adolescence included allergen exposure and damp housing conditions. Mite antigen levels were examined from homes of 70% of the asthma cohort and found to significantly correlate with dampness and bronchial hyperreactivity. However, the effect of dampness was not due to mite allergen alone, as bronchial hyperreactivity remained significantly correlated with humidity even when adjusting for mite allergen levels.

It has recently been reported that use of mechanical ventilation systems can minimize indoor humidity. While it has been reported that such systems do not modify mite allergen levels, other studies suggest air-handling systems, which impact humidity, may mitigate increased levels of mite allergen and airway dysfunction. Homes that have mechanical ventilation systems are significantly less humid, with decreased numbers of mites and Der p 1 concentrations in bedroom spaces compared to homes without such systems (Warner et al. 2000). Nonspecific responses to histamine were improved in a nearly significant number of patients ($p=0.085$) living in homes with mechanical ventilation systems. Likewise, in studies of indoor air quality interventions in schools, reports of asthma symptoms are decreased in students attending school buildings randomly selected to have increased air-exchange rates. This was associated with reductions of relative humidity and concentration of several airborne pollutants relative to schools employing standard ventilation protocols (Smedje et al. 1997). Differences in modes of heating homes in rural and urban settings may also impact atopy. In studies of homes in rural and urban Germany, use of wood and coal burning furnaces in rural settings is associated with decreased asthma and atopy prevalence of rural children (von Mutius et al. 1996). This may be due to lower indoor and bedroom temperatures in these homes (von Mutius et al. 1996). Dampness and water damage have also been associated with increased expression of allergic disease, and may be modified by wood and coal use (Spengler et al. 2004).

Perhaps the most intriguing example of overall lifestyle modulation of development of atopy is the prevalence of asthma and atopy in children from eastern and western Germany at various times following political reunification of that nation. Shortly after reunification in 1990, children from the East were less likely to have atopy, had fewer positive skin tests, and had a lower prevalence of asthma than their Western counterparts (von Mutius et al. 1994). This could not be ascribed to allergen exposure as indoor allergen exposures (especially to house dust mite allergen) were not found to be notably different between eastern and western children (von Mutius et al. 1994; Hirsch 1999). However, there were a number of differences in other lifestyle and environmental conditions observed between these regions immediately after reunification. Compared to children in the west, eastern German children were more likely to be placed in communal day care, consume lower dietary fat, and be exposed to particulate air pollutants, rather than ozone (von Mutius et al. 1994; Nicolai and von Mutius 1996; von Mutius et al. 1995).

In a remarkably short period of years after reunification, there has been a notable increase in prevalence of atopy and allergic diseases in children born in the formerly communist regions of Germany. This has been associated with development of a more "westernized" lifestyle in the East, including decreased use of coal in industry, increased automobile use, and increased availability of high fat foods. Similar observations have been made between other previously Eastern bloc and Western countries, as well as comparison of asthma in rural vs. urban Africa, New Zealand and Australia, and Asia. Likewise, the problem of asthma in inner city minority populations suggests a role for urbanization in expression of atopy.

Nutritional factors may also influence asthma outcomes. It has been recently reported that a number of vitamins with antioxidant or anti-inflammatory actions may influence asthma development. Litonjua et al. reported that maternal intake of vitamin E and Zn were associated with a significantly decreased risk of wheeze at age 2 (Litonjua et al. 2006). Likewise, Devereux et al. examined questionnaire data from 1,253 individuals, including 700 who underwent skin prick testing and 478 who underwent spirometry. Maternal vitamin E intake during pregnancy was negatively associated with wheeze in the previous year, ever having asthma, and persistent wheezing. Maternal plasma α-tocopherol during pregnancy was positively associated with post-bronchodilator FEV_1 in 5-year-old children, while there was no association between the children's vitamin consumption and asthma or wheeze.

Omega-3 fatty acids have also been examined for their role in decreasing occurrence of allergy in infants and as a complementary treatment for asthma in adults (Dunstan and Prescott 2005; Dunstan et al. 2004; Dunstan et al. 2003; Mickleborough 2005; Mickleborough and Rundell 2005; Mickleborough et al. 2004; Oddy et al. 2004; Prescott and Calder 2004). Though there are few well-controlled clinical trials of this modality in asthma or allergy, a clinical trial conducted in Australia provides interesting insights into the possible role of omega-3 fatty acids in allergic disease. In that trial 98 atopic, pregnant women were randomized to received fish oil (3.7 g n-3 polyunsaturated fatty acids/day) or placebo from 20 weeks' gestation until delivery, with 83 completing the trial. Fish oil supplementation ($n=40$) resulted in increased tissue stores of n-3 PUFA as determined by measures in erythrocyte membranes as well as trend for decreases in all neonatal cytokine (IL-5, IL-13, IL-10, and IFN-gamma) responses of peripheral blood monocytic cells to allergen, which were significant in the treated group for cat induced IL-10 response. The fish oil group was also three times less likely to have a positive skin prick test to egg at 1 year of age (Oddy et al. 2004). Vitamin C has also been suggested as an adjunct treatment for asthma as well (Romieu et al. 2002; Romieu and Trenga 2001). While much remains to be learned about dietary factors and asthma pathogenesis, these studies do suggest a potential role for such interventions.

Overall, urbanization has emerged as a key feature in the development of asthma and atopy. It has been proposed that urban environments result in changes in gene expression, which allow for expression of an atopic phenotype. Delineation of the specific features of urban lifestyle, which allow the atopic phenotype to be expressed, is incomplete. However, candidate influences include allergen exposure, the hygiene hypothesis, as well as exposure to indoor and outdoor air pollutants.

Allergen Exposure, Development of Atopy, and Development of Asthma

Given that a majority of asthma cases in children (and a significant proportion of asthma cases in adults) is associated with development of IgE responses to allergens, it has been argued that decreased exposure to allergens would be linked to decreased occurrence of asthma. Indeed, many studies have shown that sensitization to indoor allergens predicts asthma severity. This idea was supported by Rosenstreich et al. (1997) who examined a cohort of 476 children with asthma (age, 4–9 years) recruited from eight inner-city areas in the United States. These children underwent allergen skin testing and levels of environmental allergen for cockroach (Bla g 1), dust mites (Der p 1 and Der f 1), and cat dander (Fel d 1) were assessed. 36.8% of the children were allergic to cockroach allergen, 34.9% to dust-mite allergen, and 22.7% to cat allergen. Cockroach-sensitized children who were exposed to high levels of this allergen had increased annual rates of hospitalization (0.37 hospitalization a year), vs. 0.11 for the other children ($p=0.001$). Other measures of asthma morbidity were also increased in cockroach-allergic asthmatics. Increased levels of mite and cat allergen were not linked to increased asthma morbidity, suggesting that at least in the inner city cockroach allergy was a critical environmental exposure.

In a larger inner-city study (Gruchalla et al. 2005), 937 inner-city children 5–11 years old were skin-tested, with sensitization to cockroach (69%), dust mites (62%), and molds (50%) being the most common in this group. However, there were clearly geographically distinct patterns of sensitization, with cockroach allergy being greatest in the Bronx, New York, and Dallas (81.2%, 78.7%, and 78.5%, respectively), and dust mite sensitivity was highest in Dallas and Seattle (83.7% and 78.0%, respectively). Bedroom dust samples were evaluated for Der p 1, Der f 1, Bla g 1, Fel d 1, and Can f 1 and the relationship among allergen exposure, skin test reactivity and asthma morbidities was assessed. Again it was found that cockroach-sensitized children exposed to cockroach had increased morbidity. This effect was not observed with other allergens, and the authors concluded that cockroach allergen appears to have a greater effect on asthma morbidity than dust mite or pet allergen in these children. Together, these studies show that allergen exposure is a key determinant of disease, especially in cockroach-allergic people.

However, while most authorities agree that decreased exposure to allergen decreases asthma morbidity in allergic asthmatics, it is unclear if allergen exposure in early life alone is a determining risk factor for asthma development. A multicenter prospective study of 1,314 infants was undertaken in five German cities in 1990 to assess the relationship between early life allergen exposure and development of asthma (Lau et al. 2000; Lau et al. 2002). 939 of these children were available for follow-up at age 7 years for assessment of spirometry and nonspecific airway reactivity. Levels of serum IgE directed against food and inhalant allergens were assessed at age 6 months, 18 months, 36 months and 7 years, as were levels of indoor allergen levels. Not surprisingly, sensitization to indoor allergens was associated with asthma, wheeze, and increased airway reactivity. However, the degree of neonatal allergen exposure was not associated with these asthma features, suggesting that factors other than (or in addition to) allergen exposure was necessary to develop allergic asthma.

The data are mixed concerning the effectiveness of environmental control maneuvers inside homes, especially when studies are focused on a specific intervention. However, there is a growing body of evidence that comprehensive and customized approaches to improving indoor air quality result in significant decreases in asthma symptoms and severity. Also notable was that a multipronged environmental intervention strategy was tested in the second inner-city asthma study noted above. This approach accounted for each relevant allergen and irritant for an individual and was found to be effective in decreased asthma morbidity (Morgan et al. 2004). More recently, a multifaceted approach to primary prevention of allergic disease has been undertaken, and found to be effective in decreasing disease occurrence. These approaches include decreased exposure to allergen using allergen-specific methodologies as well as pollutants such as tobacco smoke (Morgan et al. 2004; Chan-Yeung et al. 2005; Eggleston et al. 2005). Taken together, these studies suggest that allergen exposure is an important feature of allergen disease, but other factors also contribute to development of the allergic phenotype.

Hygiene Hypothesis

The "Hygiene Hypothesis" was suggested by Strachan in 1989, when he suggested that allergic rhinitis was less prevalent in children who had many older siblings or experienced day care (Strachan 1989). He suggested that exposure of younger siblings to infections present in older siblings during early protected against the development of atopy. Since then, there have been a great number of reports demonstrating that exposure of infants and young children to either a large number of siblings or a cohort of children in day-care settings is associated with decreased incidence of asthma and other allergic diseases (Eder et al. 2006; Liu and Leung 2006; Martinez 2001; Weiss 2002). Whether this is actually due to increased occurrence of infection in younger siblings (with the influence that has on immune development) or other factors is not clear. Nonetheless, these observations have led to an explosion of studies examining the role of bacterial exposures on development of atopy.

The hygiene hypothesis has been extended to include the examination of the effect of a large number of microbial and immune exposures on development of asthma, including exposure to environmental endotoxin and animals. Perhaps the most avidly studied of these factors is the relationship between environmental endotoxin exposure and asthma. In a series of studies, von Mutius and colleagues have reported that rural lifestyle has been associated with decreased occurrence of atopy and allergic disease (Eder et al. 2006; Braun-Fahrlander and Lauener 2003; Braun-Fahrlander 2001; van Strien et al. 2004b). Among the many environmental exposures which are increased in rural settings is endotoxin. It has been proposed that endotoxin exposure skews immune development away from development of IgE and other TH2 characteristics and towards development of TH1 responses. This was very clearly delineated in a study in which endotoxin content of mattress dust was determined and compared to the likelihood of developing allergic disease during childhood. Those children exposed to increased levels of endotoxin had decreased development of atopy and atopic wheeze (Braun-Fahrlander et al. 2002).

Many other studies have found that increased incidence of allergic diseases in children with decreased exposure to environmental endotoxin and other microbial exposures. Douwes et al. found an inverse relationship between levels of endotoxin, 1-3 beta glucans and extracellular fungal polysaccharides from the genera Penicillium and Aspergillus and doctor diagnosed asthma (Douwes et al. 2006). A study by Perkin and Strachan (Perkin and Strachan 2006) examined the occurrence of asthma and atopy in a cohort children who underwent skin testing and had environmental endotoxin levels assessed as well as assessment of consumption of unpasteurized milk. They observed that farm children had decreased airway allergic diseases and that drinking unpasteurized milk (in either farm or nonfarm children) was associated with decreased atopy as well as increased circulating γ-IFN levels.

A number of animal studies suggest that endotoxin exposure in early life may protect against development of IgE and eosinophilic responses following experimental sensitization with model allergens (Liu and Leung 2006; Cochran et al. 2002; Gerhold et al. 2006; Holt 1987; Liu 2002; Tulic et al. 2002; Tulic et al. 2000; Watanabe et al. 2003). Gereda et al. reported that endotoxin exposure was linked to decreased atopy and TH1 skewing of lymphocytes in exposed children (Gereda et al. 2000), and more recently Ege at al (Ege et al. 2006) examined a subset of children from the Prevention of Allergy Risk Factors for Sensitization in Children Related to Farming and Anthroposophic Life Style study and found that maternal exposure during pregnancy to environmental microbial products was associated with decreased occurrence of allergic disease and enhanced gene expression for CD14, TLR2 and TLR4 in mRNA from blood samples of children. These studies highlight the biological plausibility that microbial exposures modulate immune response in infants in a fashion which may protect against the development of atopy.

However, there are also a number of reports which suggest that domestic endotoxin exposure might also increase atopic disease or wheeze in children and adults. Michel et al. reported that levels of endotoxin in house dust correlated better with asthma symptoms than did levels of mite allergen (Michel et al. 1991; Michel et al. 1996). Studies have shown that house dust levels of endotoxin are linked with wheezing in infants, though it is unclear if this is due to IgE mediated asthma (Litonjua et al. 2002; Park et al. 2001). Gillispie et al. (2006) examined the relationship between environmental endotoxin exposure at 3 months of age and subsequent expression of allergic symptoms at 15 months of age in a cohort of 881 children in New Zealand, and found that endotoxin was associated with increased airway and skin symptoms. Likewise, Thorne et al. reported that indoor endotoxin levels were associated with increased risk for wheeze in a study based in the US (Thorne et al. 2005), as did Tavernier et al. in British homes (Tavernier et al. 2006). In a study which recruited 301 Dominican and African American inner city study participants, Perzanowski et al. reported that children in homes with higher endotoxin concentration were less likely to have eczema at age 1 year, but more likely to wheeze at age 2 years, especially if there was a maternal history of asthma (Perzanowski et al. 2006).

Another intriguing aspect of the hygiene hypothesis is the role of pet exposure on development of atopy in children. While it is well accepted that exposure of already sensitized persons to dog or cat allergen will increase IgE mediated inflammation and associated diseases, recent studies suggest that exposure to these animals may decrease the likelihood of developing asthma or other allergic diseases. One of the earliest reports to suggest this was from a study in Detroit, in which 835 children were recruited at 1 year of age with 474 available to follow-up at ages 6 or 7 (Ownby et al. 2002). The number of pets present in the home at age 1 was determined as well as numbers of positive skin tests and serum IgE levels, and it was found that the presence of two or more dogs or cats in the home at age 1 was associated with decreased atopy at ages 6 and 7. Likewise, Campo et al. examined a cohort of 532 children in Cincinnati and observed that dog ownership coupled with increased endotoxin exposure was linked to decreased wheezing in infancy (Campo et al. 2006), Gern also observed that dog exposure in early life was linked to decreased atopy and increased secretion of IL-10 and IL-13 by circulating monocytes (Gern et al. 2004). While some have made similar observations regarding cat exposures and asthma, there is more variability regarding the role of cat exposure in asthma, with many studies suggesting that cat allergen exposure may worsen disease. It is also not clear whether the effect of pets in the house-during early exerts effects due to allergen exposure, or primarily due to the effect of endotoxin, which is increased in homes with pets (Liu 2002; Simpson and Custovic 2003; Kaiser 2004; Renz and Herz 2002).

Taken together, these reports provide substantial support for the hygiene hypothesis, though they also demonstrate that the impact of bacterially stimulated innate immunity on development of allergic disease is very complex, and likely depends on exposure duration, dose, and genetic factors.

Indoor Air and Environmental Tobacco Smoke

Biomass burning of wood, plant-derived fuels, and tobacco is an important source of indoor air pollution, (Brims and Chauhan 2005; Gupta et al. 2006; Mishra 2003; Schei et al. 2004) which results in production of particulates rich in polyaromatic hydrocarbons, and other organic molecules which exert oxidant stress (Gilmour et al. 2006). In a study of 11 restaurants in a Kentucky town, the mean PM2.5 concentration in smoking areas was 177 $\mu g/m^3$ vs. 87 $\mu g/m^3$ in the non-smoking section, which in turn was 29 times higher than that in smoke-free air and six times higher than local outdoor air in Paducah (Jones et al. 2006). Endotoxin levels of indoor particulates are also increased in locations where smoking occurs (Larsson et al. 2004). Burning of wood in indoor stoves and fireplaces also generates on indoor particulates and gases, and is associated with increased respiratory tract illness. As shown in the example above, use of tobacco or wood fuel inside the home is an important determinant of indoor air quality.

Nitrogen dioxide (NO_2) is an important component of indoor and outdoor ambient air pollution. Oxides of nitrogen (NOx, including NO_2) are precursors for production of ambient air ozone (Committee of the Environmental and Occupational Health Assembly of the American Thoracic Society 1996). van Strien et al. (2004c) examined a cohort of infants living in New England that had at least one older sibling with asthma (suggesting increased genetic risk for asthma in this cohort). Infants exposed to >17.4 ppb NO_2 had significantly increased risk for respiratory disease compared to those experiencing low level (<5.1 ppb) NO_2 exposure. This finding is consistent with a 2003 report by McConnell et al. (2003) showing that outdoor NO_2 exposure is associated with bronchitic symptoms in asthmatic children in Southern California. Chauhan et al. (2003) observed that increased indoor NO_2 exposure was associated with increased severity of viral-induced exacerbation of asthma. Together, these studies and others show that NO_2 is a risk factor for exacerbation of asthma.

NO_2 derives from use of natural gas appliances, especially if they are poorly maintained or vented, and in indoor settings it exerts a direct effect on asthma. Increased levels of NO_2 inside dwellings correlates with increased respiratory symptoms in children (Brunekreef et al. 1990). These studies also link increased reports of cough, wheeze, phlegm, and bronchitis with the annual average household NO_2 concentration as well as an enhancement of the effect of viral infection in asthma (van Strien et al. 2004c; Chauhan et al. 2003; Brunekreef et al. 1990; Neas et al. 1991; Chauhan and Johnston 2003).

Environmental tobacco smoke (ETS) is clearly a significant factor in exacerbating airway illnesses affecting airway mucosa. The evidence is overwhelming that ETS is a cause of airway disease, with numerous reviews detailing the role of ETS in asthma exacerbation and development of allergy (Brims and Chauhan 2005; Gilmour et al. 2006; Alberg et al. 2005; Chan-Yeung and Dimich-Ward 2003; Delfino 2002; Dhala et al. 2006; Eisner 2005; Etzel 2003; Gergen 2001; Gold 2000; Singh and Davis 2002). Mechanistic studies by Seymour and colleagues have shown that mice exposed to ETS have increased levels of the TH2 cytokines IL-4 and IL-10 and eosinophils following allergen challenge, suggesting that ETS may directly contribute to development of allergic disease (Seymour et al. 2003). Diaz-Sanchez and colleagues also report ETS has a strong adjuvant action, facilitating sensitization with ovalbumin (OVA) (Rumold et al. 2001). These investigators examined the effect of ETS challenge on nasal responses to allergen in humans, and found a marked enhancement of allergen-induced specific IgE and IgG4, increased IL-4, IL-5 and IL-13, with decreased levels of γ-interferon, and increased amounts of post-allergen histamine in nasal lavage fluid (Diaz-Sanchez et al. 2006). It is notable that polyaromatic hydrocarbons are an important component of both DEP and ETS. Taken together, these studies provide initial mechanistic support to the epidemiological reports suggesting that ETS exposure enhances development of atopy and asthma (Gilmour et al. 2006; Bernstein et al. 2004; Nel et al. 2001).

Outdoor Air Pollutants

Air pollutants that cause adverse human health effects include those regulated by the US EPA under the Clean Air Act (including NO_2, O_3 and particulate matter

Table 3.1 Primary national ambient air quality standards, United States

Carbon monoxide	Lead	NO_2	Ozone	Sulfur oxides	PM_{10}	PM_{10} (1997 proposed standards)
9 ppm (8-h average)	1.5 μg/m^3 (quarterly average)	0.053 (annual mean)	0.08 ppm (8-h standard)	0.14 (24-h mean)	50 μg/m^3 (annual mean)	15 μg/m^3 (annual mean)
35 ppm (1-h average)			0.12 ppm (1-h average)	0.03 (annual mean)	50 μg/m^3 (24-h mean)	65 μg/m^3 (24-h mean)

(PM), see Table 3.1) (Peden 2003), as well as organic carbon and volatile organic compounds (McConnell et al. 2003; McConnell et al. 1999; McConnell et al. 2002). Monitoring of these pollutants is conducted primarily at the state and local level, and generally relies on fixed monitoring stations, providing an overview of air quality for a given area (Peden 2003).

Increased ambient air particulate levels have been linked to asthma exacerbation. An example of this is seen in the need for asthma medication in a cohort of asthmatics studied in Utah (Pope 1991; Pope 1989). Hospitalization for asthma in Seattle was found to occur in conjunction with increases in airborne particulate matter (Schwartz et al. 1993), with similar observations having been made in other locations as well, including Germany, the Czech Republic and Mexico City, and other locations (Peters et al. 1996; Peters et al. 2000; Peters et al. 1997a; Peters et al. 1997b). Several studies, too numerous to detail here, also show that occupational exposure to PM components, including metals and biologicals such as endotoxin contribute to wheezing and asthma exacerbation (Bernstein et al. 2004).

Studies performed in the Utah Valley offer a unique opportunity to link the effect of particulates to the work activity of a local steel mill (Pope 1991; Pope 1989). These investigations examined respiratory disease episodes (asthma exacerbation, hospital admission for respiratory complaints, etc.) that occurred during the year that the mill was closed due to a labor dispute, as well as the years preceding and following the strike. Respiratory morbidities and the level of particulates were both markedly decreased during the strike year, demonstrating a link between levels of ambient air particulates and occurrence of disease exacerbation in asthma and bronchitis.

Vehicular traffic is also an important source of pollutants that have health effects. Gauderman and colleagues (Gauderman et al. 2004) studied 1,759 10-year-old children from 12 Southern California cities until age 18 and examined the effect of exposure to a number of products of vehicle fuel combustion (O_3, NO_2, acid vapor, PM10, PM2.5 and elemental carbon) on lung function. Of these, NO_2, acid vapor, PM2.5 and elemental carbon exposure were all significantly correlated with decreased lung function. Using PM2.5 as an example, the percentage of children with a FEV1 <80% of the predicted value was 1.6% with exposure to nearly 5 mg/m^3 air vs. 7.9% at an exposure over 20 mg/m^3. This level of impairment is similar to that found in children of smoking mothers.

Further evidence of the impact of vehicular traffic on asthma is found in studies of the effects of proximity to a roadway on health. In a study of children aged 5 or less in Birmingham UK (Edwards et al. 1994), it was found that those admitted to a hospital with a diagnosis of asthma were more likely to reside in a high traffic exposure area (>24,000 vehicles/24 h at the nearest segment of main road) than either children admitted for nonrespiratory reasons ($p<0.02$) or well children ($p<0.002$). Traffic exposure (vehicles/24 h) correlated well with admission in those living <500 m from a road ($p<0.006$). Compared to well children, those admitted for respiratory reasons were more likely to live within 200 m of a main road ($p<0.02$).

In a German study (Nicolai et al. 2003), a group of 7,509 school children were randomly selected to participate in a survey of traffic exposure on asthma and allergy outcomes, with 83% participating. Allergen skin testing, assessment of serum IgE, and lung function testing was conducted, and traffic exposure was estimated by traffic counts and an emission model which predicted soot, benzene and nitrogen dioxide (NO_2) exposure. Traffic counts correlated with active asthma, cough and wheeze, and in children exposed to ETS, having a positive skin test. Pollutant exposure was also linked to cough, wheeze, and asthma.

A case/control study in Erie County, NY children aged 0–14 years ($n=417$ and 461, respectively) indicated that exposure to high truck volume within a 200 m distance was associated with increased risk for hospitalization due to asthma (Lin et al. 2002). In US Veterans, there is a reported 1.7 relative risk of wheeze associated with living within 50 m of a heavily traveled road compared to those living more than 400 m from a road (Garshick et al. 2003). Other health outcomes, most notably myocardial infarction, have also been associated with proximity to vehicular traffic (Peters et al. 2004).

Like PM, ozone causes increased asthma and respiratory tract morbidity, including ER visits, hospitalizations, and rescue medication use (Bernstein et al. 2004; Peden 2003). White et al. reported increased ER visits by school children in Atlanta for asthma when 1 h ozone levels exceeded 0.11 ppm (White et al. 1994), with similar observations having been made in Mexico City and Los Angeles (Peden 2003; Romieu et al. 1995; Romieu et al. 1996; Romieu et al. 1997). A 2003 report by Gent et al. involving 271 children in southern New England demonstrated that levels of ozone below the current 1 and 8 h ozone standard (0.12 and 0.085 ppm respectively) were also associated with exacerbation of asthma (Gent et al. 2003).

A cohort of 3,535 children with no history of asthma from schools in 12 cities in Southern California was studied for up to 5 years (McConnell et al. 2002). During this period, 265 children developed a newly recognized diagnosis of asthma. It was observed that participation in outdoor sports (presumably associated with increased minute ventilation) in areas of increased ozone concentration was a risk factor for asthma. McDonnell and colleagues prospectively studied a cohort of 3,091 adult nonsmokers. Over a 15-year interval, new diagnoses of asthma by a physician occurred in 3.2% of men and 4.3% of women. In the men (but not the women) with newly diagnosed asthma, the 20-year mean 8-h average for ambient ozone levels was a significant risk factor associated with new asthma (relative risk of 2.09 for a 27 ppb increase in ambient air ozone) (McDonnell et al. 1999). These data suggest that long-term exposure to ambient ozone may be associated with development of asthma in both children and adults.

Genetic Factors and Gene/Environment Interactions in Asthma and Allergy

Studies of the development of asthma in monozygotic (MZ) and dizygotic (DZ) twin pairs were some of the first assessments of genetic factors in development of asthma and allergy. In two such studies, there was much greater concordance of disease between MZ than DZ twins, with one study revealing that MZ twins were 19.8% concordant for asthma compared to 4.8% in DZ twins. A second study involving 2,902 twin pairs revealed 30% vs. 12% concordance in MZ vs. DZ twins. In studies using atopy as the primary endpoint, 50–60% concordance has been reported in twin pairs. However, it is notable that monozygotic twins did not have a 100% concordance for asthma or allergy, despite having identical genomes. These and other observations emphasize that gene-by-environment interactions, not just genetic factors alone, determine the expression of an atopic or asthma phenotype (Blumenthal 2004; Colilla et al. 2003; Cozen et al. 2004; Duffy et al. 1998; Peden 2000).

The most commonly used approaches to identification of gene discovery in asthma include family-based linkage studies and positional cloning to identify regions in the genome, which associate with a specific asthma phenotype and gene association studies, in which a candidate gene is examined within a population to determine its effect on a particular asthma phenotype. It is important to note that phenotype definition is central to either process. Several phenotypic definitions have been used in asthma studies, including asthma, adult asthma, wheeze, bronchial hyperreactivity, atopy, FEV1, and total IgE. In a review by Ober and Hoffjan of over 500 publications, 100 genes were reported to be associated with an asthma relevant phenotype, with 25 having been identified in at least six different populations and an additional 54 having been identified in two to five different populations (Ober and Hoffjan 2006). Asthma genes have been identified on chromosomes 1p, 2p, 3p, 4q, 5p, 5q, 6q, 7p, 11q, 13q, 16p, 16q, 17q, and 19q, though some chromosomal regions are more involved than others. An example of an especially rich chromosomal region is the 5q region at which 15 genes have been identified which associate with one or more asthma phenotypes. These include the *IL3, CSF, IRF1, IL5, IL13, IL4, CD14, UGFR1, SPINK5, ADRB2, IL12B, HAVCR1, HAVCR2, CYFIP2,* and *LTC4S* genes, many of which code for important TH2 proteins. Table 3.2 lists genes which have been associated with asthma phenotypes in multiple studies. The reader is referred to a number of excellent reviews for a more in depth review of the genetics of asthma.

Table 3.2 Genes associated with asthma in >10 populations (adapted from Ober and Hoffjan(2006))

Gene symbol	Gene name	Function	Chromosome location
ADAM33	ADAM metallopeptidase domain 33	Metalloprotease	20p13
ADRβ2	Adrenergic, beta-2-receptor surface	Beta2 receptor	5p31
CD14	CD14 molecule	LPS receptor	5q31
FCERI	Fc fragment of IgE, high affinity I receptor for alpha polypeptide	IgE receptor subunit	1q23
HLADRB1	Major histocompatibility complex, class II, DR beta 1	Antigen presentation molecule	6p21.3
HLADQB1	Major histocompatibility complex, class II, DQ beta 1	Antigen presentation molecule	6p21.3
IL4	IL-4	TH2 cytokine	5q31
IL4RA	IL4 receptor	IL4 receptor	16p12.1-p11.2
IL13	IL-13	TH2 cytokine	5q31
TNF	Tumor necrosis factor	TNF	6p21.3

CD14, Asthma and Allergy

The CD14 gene is located on the 5q region and has been identified in over 10 study populations, making it a significant candidate gene for modulation of asthma. Baldini et al. (1999) reported that increased levels of serum levels of soluble CD14-recovered children were associated with decreased production of IgE, and that a specific polymorphism, the C-159T single nucleotide polymorphism in the CD14 promoter region was linked with CD14 levels, with the TT homozygote state being associated with increased expression of sCD14. Since that time, over 200 articles (as identified by a PubMed search) have been published examining the role that CD14 plays in development of atopy and asthma. As noted in previous sections, environmental endotoxin exposure in early life has been linked to decreased development of atopy, eczema, allergic rhinitis, and allergic asthma. The vast majority of studies have linked the TT homozygote state with decreased risk for development of atopy and allergic diseases, consistent with the initial observation by Baldini et al. 1999 and extensively reviewed by others (Liu 2002; Baldini et al. 2002; Feijen et al. 2000; Kleeberger and Peden 2005; Koppelman 2006; Koppelman and Postma 2003; Liu and Redmon 2001).

However, more recent studies indicate that the relationship between the C-159T SNP for CD14, and development of asthma or allergy is more complex and dependent on the level of endotoxin present in the environment. Ober et al. (2000), in a study of 693 Hutterites, suggested that the T allele of the CD14 gene promoter was linked with increased IgE, or was in linkage disequilibrium with an as yet unknown genetic determinate of allergy. Woo et al. (2003) studied patients with asthma and food allergy as well as normal controls and found that the TT homozygote state was linked with a 4.4-fold increased risk for food allergy and a 3.1-fold increased risk for nonatopic asthma. Zambelli-Weiner et al. (2005) examined the role of the TT genotype for the CD14 gene and observed that it was protective against asthma development with low-level house dust endotoxin levels, but was a risk factor which favored asthma pathogenesis with high endotoxin levels. Williams et al. (2006) examined the effect of the C-260T single nucleotide polymorphism for the CD14 gene promoter on the effect of environmental endotoxin exposure on serum IgE levels in 517 adults in a 2006 study, reporting that with lower levels of endotoxin exposure, the CC genotype was associated with higher IgE levels, whereas with higher levels of endotoxin exposure, TT individuals had the highest IgE levels (see Fig. 3.1, which demonstrates an excellent example of a gene-by-environment interaction). Simpson and colleagues (Simpson et al. 2006) examined 447 children (33% of which were atopic) for CD14 genotype, IgE levels, and presence of wheeze. They found no effect of the TT or CT genotypes on IgE responses or on risk of non-atopic wheeze. However, they did find increased risk of non-atopic wheeze and decreased risk for allergen sensitization and eczema in the CC homozygotes. Taken together, these studies demonstrate both the importance of phenotype definition and the complexity of the interaction between the CD14 gene, degree of endotoxin exposure and development of symptoms consistent with asthma or another allergic disease.

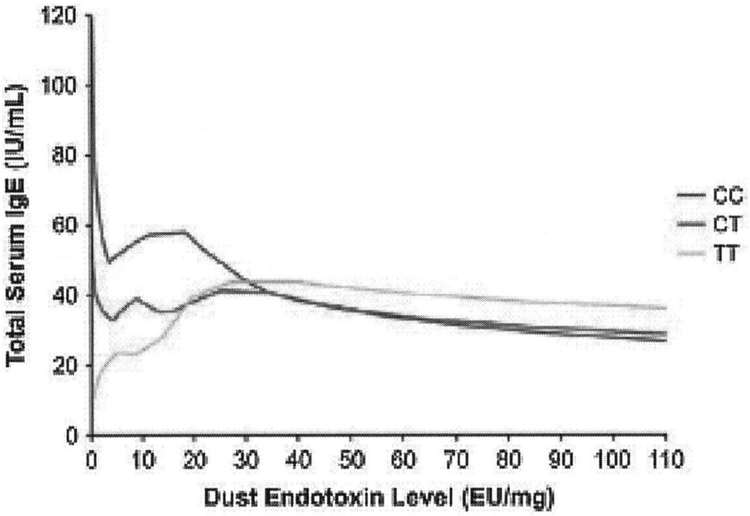

Fig. 3.1 Example of a gene-by-environment interaction depicting the relationship between endotoxin and IgE levels stratified by genotype for CD14 (adapted from Williams et al (2006))

Evidence for Genetic Susceptibility to Oxidizing Pollutants

Regulation of oxidant stress (ROS) is also achieved to a great extent by activation of the Antioxidant Response Element (ARE) genes with subsequent production of phase II enzymes which interact in a variety of ways to handle ROS. These enzymes include NQO1, GSTM1, GSTP1, HO-1 and a variety of others (Gilliland et al. 2004). A common feature of these ARE genes is that they are activated at a nuclear level by translocation of NRF2 to the nucleus (after oxidative attack of critical-SG residues of KEAP1) (Kensler et al. 2006; Kong et al. 2001; Lee and Surh 2005). Note that GSTM1 and GSTP1 are both genes associated with asthma in over 6 study populations. The importance of NRF2 is highlighted by a series of studies in which lung injury due to exposure to allergen (IgE mediated), virus infection, LPS (CD14/TLR4), bleomycin, hyperoxia, and ozone are all markedly enhanced in NRF2 knock-out animals (Kensler et al. 2006; Biswal et al. 2006; Osburn et al. 2006; Rangasamy et al. 2005; Rangasamy et al. 2004; Thimmulappa et al. 2006). Furthermore, epidemiological, animal, and human challenge studies demonstrate that defects in NRF2-derived enzymes (GSTM1, NQO1, selenoproteins like GPX1–3) are associated with environmental asthma, viral injury of the lung, and response to PAHs (Gilliland et al. 2004) and O_3 (Gilliland et al. 2004; David et al. 2003; Romieu et al. 2004).

Of the individual genes activated by NRF2, perhaps the best studied are those which influence cellular glutathione. Glutathione-S-transferase M1 (*GSTM1*), is a member of the μ family of GSTs. GSTM1 has a null allele (GSTM1*0) which results in no protein expression with resultant decreases in antioxidant capability. Approximately 40% of the population is affected by this allele. Another GST of interest is the GSTP1, in which the single nucleotide polymorphisms at the 105 position are important. Glutathione-S-Transferase genes play a role in lung growth, as shown in a study of a large cohort of 1,954 schoolchildren in Southern California, in which children with the *GSTM1* null allele or a *GSTP1* val105/val105 genotype have decreased lung function growth over a 4 year period (Gilliland et al. 2002a). Studies of children in Mexico City have examined the risk for asthma relative to lifetime ozone exposure. These studies indicate that expression of GST proteins is an important determinant of asthma severity. GSTM1 null children with asthma have decreased lung function associated with ozone exposure compared to those who are GSTM1 sufficient. Interestingly, within this group, if one also screens for a second antioxidant SNP (the Pro187Ser single nucleotide polymorphism for Nicotinamide adenine dinucleotide (phosphate) reduced:quinone oxidoreductase (NQO1)), those with the Pro/Pro allele genotype for NQO1 have significantly reduced asthma risk ascribed to ozone exposure, compared to GSTM1 null children with other NQO1 genotypes (David et al. 2003). Thus, while GSMT1 null state is associated with risk for ozone-induced asthma exacerbation, this risk may be mitigated by other protective genes. These investigators also studied the ability of dietary supplementation of vitamin C and E to protect asthmatics from ozone-induced exacerbation of disease. Overall, there was a significant protective effect observed in the entire group of asthmatics, but this effect was much more apparent in those children with the GSTM1 null genotype (Romieu et al. 2004).

In a Southern California study, children with the GSTM1 null genotype and born to mothers who smoked during pregnancy also have increased occurrence of early onset asthma, persistent asthma, exercise-induced wheeze, need for rescue medication use, and emergency room visits for asthma compared to children with protective GST alleles or born to nonsmoking mothers (Gilliland et al. 2002b). A German study from a cohort of 3,504 children revealed that exposure to ETS was associated with a markedly increased risk of asthma and asthma symptoms in GSTM1 null individuals (Kabesch et al. 2004). GSTM1 and GSTT1 insufficient children exposed to in utero ETS were also found to be at increased risk for decreased lung function. Taken together, these studies suggest that specific SNPs of GST genes modulate the response of asthmatics to a variety of oxidizing air pollutants.

Diesel exhaust challenge and ETS have been shown to induce production of IgE and, like O_3, act as adjuvants for increased response to allergen. It has recently been reported that the adjuvant effect of diesel exhaust on response to ragweed challenge of the nasal airway is greater in subjects having either the GSTM1 null or GSTP1 105 wildtype genotypes (Gilliland et al. 2004; Bastain et al. 2003). A similar genetic influence on the effect of ETS has also been observed. NFR2, a regulatory nuclear factor which activates phase II antioxidant pathways (including GSTM1 expression), has also been found to protect macrophages and epithelial cells from the adverse effects of diesel exhaust particles, demonstrating the role of GSTM1-related antioxidants in protection from the effects of diesel exhaust.

Summary

The past 50 years has seen a marked increase in allergic diseases and asthma. Over 100 genes have been identified which are associated with a phenotypic feature of asthma. However, the presence of these genes alone does not explain the rapid increase in asthma prevalence. Changes in environmental exposures, which have occurred over the past 50 years result in differential expression of asthma genes. Indeed, the gene-by-environment interactions identified in asthma and other allergic diseases can be very complex, with the effect of a gene allele on asthma phenotype shifting across an environmental gradient. It is only with a full appreciation of the gene-by-environment interactions that exist in asthma that a full understanding of asthma biology will be attained. With this understanding, novel pharmaceutical and nutritional approaches will be developed to decrease asthma development. Likewise, knowledge of gene-by-environment interactions in asthma will guide rational environmental intervention strategies that can be developed to decrease the development of asthma, which ultimately may be the most effective public health approach to this disease.

References

(1996) Health effects of outdoor air pollution. Committee of the Environmental and Occupational Health Assembly of the American Thoracic Society. Am J Respir Crit Care Med 153(1):3–50

Alberg AJ, Brock MV, Samet JM (2005) Epidemiology of lung cancer: looking to the future. J Clin Oncol 23(14):3175–3185

Baldini M, Lohman IC, Halonen M, Erickson RP, Holt PG, Martinez FD (1999) A Polymorphism* in the 5' flanking region of the CD14 gene is associated with circulating soluble CD14 levels and with total serum immunoglobulin E. Am J Respir Cell Mol Biol 20(5):976–983

Baldini M, Vercelli D, Martinez FD (2002) CD14: an example of gene by environment interaction in allergic disease. Allergy 57(3):188–192

Bastain TM, Gilliland FD, Li YF, Saxon A, Diaz-Sanchez D (2003) Intraindividual reproducibility of nasal allergic responses to diesel exhaust particles indicates a susceptible phenotype. Clin Immunol 109(2):130–136

Bernstein JA, Alexis N, Barnes C, Bernstein IL, Bernstein JA, Nel A et al (2004) Health effects of air pollution. J Allergy Clin Immunol 114(5):1116–1123

Biswal S, Rangasamy T, Tuder RM (2006) Modifier role of Nrf2 in cigarette smoke-induced emphysema. Proc Am Thorac Soc 3(6):543a

Blumenthal MN (2004) New thoughts regarding the genetics of atopy. Am J Respir Crit Care Med 169(5):555–556

Braun-Fahrlander C (2001) The role of the farm environment and animal contact for the development of asthma and allergies. Clin Exp Allergy 31(12):1799–1803

Braun-Fahrlander C, Lauener R (2003) Farming and protective agents against allergy and asthma. Clin Exp Allergy 33(4):409–411

Braun-Fahrlander C, Riedler J, Herz U, Eder W, Waser M, Grize L et al (2002) Environmental exposure to endotoxin and its relation to asthma in school-age children. N Engl J Med 347(12):869–877

Brims F, Chauhan AJ (2005) Air quality, tobacco smoke, urban crowding and day care: modern menaces and their effects on health. Pediatr Infect Dis J 24(11 Suppl):S152–S156, discussion

Brunekreef B, Houthuijs D, Dijkstra L, Boleij JS (1990) Indoor nitrogen dioxide exposure and children's pulmonary function. J Air Waste Manage Assoc 40(9):1252–1256

Campo P, Kalra HK, Levin L, Reponen T, Olds R, Lummus ZL et al (2006) Influence of dog ownership and high endotoxin on wheezing and atopy during infancy. J Allergy Clin Immunol 118(6):1271–1278

Chan-Yeung M, Dimich-Ward H (2003) Respiratory health effects of exposure to environmental tobacco smoke. Respirology 8(2):131–139

Chan-Yeung M, Ferguson A, Watson W, Dimich-Ward H, Rousseau R, Lilley M et al (2005) The Canadian Childhood Asthma Primary Prevention Study: outcomes at 7 years of age. J Allergy Clin Immunol 116(1):49–55

Chauhan AJ, Johnston SL (2003) Air pollution and infection in respiratory illness. Br Med Bull 68:95–112

Chauhan AJ, Inskip HM, Linaker CH, Smith S, Schreiber J, Johnston SL et al (2003) Personal exposure to nitrogen dioxide (NO2) and the severity of virus-induced asthma in children. Lancet 361(9373):1939–1944

Cochran JR, Khan AM, Elidemir O, Xue H, Cua B, Fullmer J et al (2002) Influence of lipopolysaccharide exposure on airway function and allergic responses in developing mice. Pediatr Pulmonol 34(4):267–277

Colilla S, Nicolae D, Pluzhnikov A, Blumenthal MN, Beaty TH, Bleecker ER et al (2003) Evidence for gene-environment interactions in a linkage study of asthma and smoking exposure. J Allergy Clin Immunol 111(4):840–846

Cozen W, Diaz-Sanchez D, James GW, Zadnick J, Cockburn MG, Gill PS et al (2004) Th1 and Th2 cytokines and IgE levels in identical twins with varying levels of cigarette consumption. J Clin Immunol 24(6):617–622

David GL, Romieu I, Sienra-Monge JJ, Collins WJ, Ramirez-Aguilar M, del Rio-Navarro BE et al (2003) Nicotinamide adenine dinucleotide (phosphate) reduced:quinone oxidoreductase and glutathione S-transferase M1 polymorphisms and childhood asthma. Am J Respir Crit Care Med 168(10): 1199–1204

Delfino RJ (2002) Epidemiologic evidence for asthma and exposure to air toxics: linkages between occupational, indoor, and community air pollution research. Environ Health Perspect 110(Suppl 4):573–589

Dhala A, Pinsker K, Prezant DJ (2006) Respiratory health consequences of environmental tobacco smoke. Clin Occup Environ Med 5(1):139–156

Diaz-Sanchez D, Rumold R, Gong H Jr (2006) Challenge with environmental tobacco smoke exacerbates allergic airway disease in human beings. J Allergy Clin Immunol 118(2):441–446

Douwes J, van Strien R, Doekes G, Smit J, Kerkhof M, Gerritsen J et al (2006) Does early indoor microbial exposure reduce the risk of asthma? The Prevention and Incidence of Asthma and Mite Allergy birth cohort study. J Allergy Clin Immunol 117(5):1067–1073

Duffy DL, Mitchell CA, Martin NG (1998) Genetic and environmental risk factors for asthma: a cotwin-control study. Am J Respir Crit Care Med 157(3 Pt 1):840–845

Dunstan JA, Prescott SL (2005) Does fish oil supplementation in pregnancy reduce the risk of allergic disease in infants? Curr Opin Allergy Clin Immunol 5(3):215–221

Dunstan JA, Mori TA, Barden A, Beilin LJ, Taylor AL, Holt PG et al (2003) Maternal fish oil supplementation in pregnancy reduces interleukin-13 levels in cord blood of infants at high risk of atopy. Clin Exp Allergy 33(4):442–448

Dunstan JA, Mori TA, Barden A, Beilin LJ, Holt PG, Calder PC et al (2004) Effects of n-3 polyunsaturated fatty acid supplementation in pregnancy on maternal and fetal erythrocyte fatty acid composition. Eur J Clin Nutr 58(3):429–437

Eder W, Ege MJ, von Mutius E (2006) The asthma epidemic. N Engl J Med 355(21):2226–2235

Edwards J, Walters S, Griffiths RK (1994) Hospital admissions for asthma in preschool children: relationship to major roads in Birmingham, United Kingdom. Arch Environ Health 49(4):223–227

Ege MJ, Bieli C, Frei R, van Strien RT, Riedler J, Ublagger E et al (2006) Prenatal farm exposure is related to the expression of receptors of the innate immunity and to atopic sensitization in school-age children. J Allergy Clin Immunol 117(4):817–823

Eggleston PA, Butz A, Rand C, Curtin-Brosnan J, Kanchanaraksa S, Swartz L et al (2005) Home environmental intervention in inner-city asthma: a randomized controlled clinical trial. Ann Allergy Asthma Immunol 95(6):518–524

Eisner MD (2005) Environmental tobacco smoke and adult asthma. Exp Lung Res 31(Suppl 1):8–14

Etzel RA (2003) How environmental exposures influence the development and exacerbation of asthma. Pediatrics 112(1 Pt 2):233–239

Etzel R, Rylander R (1999) Indoor mold and children's health. Environ Health Perspect 107(Suppl 3):463

Feijen M, Gerritsen J, Postma DS (2000) Genetics of allergic disease. Br Med Bull 56(4):894–907

Garshick E, Laden F, Hart JE, Caron A (2003) Residence near a major road and respiratory symptoms in U.S. Veterans. Epidemiology 14(6):728–736

Gauderman WJ, Avol E, Gilliland F, Vora H, Thomas D, Berhane K et al (2004) The effect of air pollution on lung development from 10 to 18 years of age. N Engl J Med 351(11):1057–1067

Gent JF, Triche EW, Holford TR, Belanger K, Bracken MB, Beckett WS et al (2003) Association of low-level ozone and fine particles with respiratory symptoms in children with asthma. JAMA 290(14):1859–1867

Gereda JE, Leung DY, Thatayatikom A, Streib JE, Price MR, Klinnert MD et al (2000) Relation between house-dust endotoxin exposure, type 1 T-cell development, and allergen sensitisation in infants at high risk of asthma. Lancet 355 (9216):1680–1683

Gergen PJ (2001) Environmental tobacco smoke as a risk factor for respiratory disease in children. Respir Physiol 128(1):39–46

Gerhold K, Avagyan A, Seib C, Frei R, Steinle J, Ahrens B et al (2006) Prenatal initiation of endotoxin airway exposure prevents subsequent allergen-induced sensitization and airway inflammation in mice. J Allergy Clin Immunol 118(3):666–673

Gern JE, Reardon CL, Hoffjan S, Nicolae D, Li Z, Roberg KA et al (2004) Effects of dog ownership and genotype on immune development and atopy in infancy. J Allergy Clin Immunol 113(2):307–314
Gillespie J, Wickens K, Siebers R, Howden-Chapman P, Town I, Epton M et al (2006) Endotoxin exposure, wheezing, and rash in infancy in a New Zealand birth cohort. J Allergy Clin Immunol 118(6):1265–1270
Gilliland FD, Gauderman WJ, Vora H, Rappaport E, Dubeau L (2002a) Effects of glutathione-S-transferase M1, T1, and P1 on childhood lung function growth. Am J Respir Crit Care Med 166(5):710–716
Gilliland FD, Li YF, Dubeau L, Berhane K, Avol E, McConnell R et al (2002b) Effects of glutathione S-transferase M1, maternal smoking during pregnancy, and environmental tobacco smoke on asthma and wheezing in children. Am J Respir Crit Care Med 166(4):457–463
Gilliland FD, Li YF, Saxon A, Diaz-Sanchez D (2004) Effect of glutathione-S-transferase M1 and P1 genotypes on xenobiotic enhancement of allergic responses: randomised, placebo-controlled crossover study. Lancet 363(9403):119–125
Gilmour MI, Jaakkola MS, London SJ, Nel AE, Rogers CA (2006) How exposure to environmental tobacco smoke, outdoor air pollutants, and increased pollen burdens influences the incidence of asthma. Environ Health Perspect 114(4):627–633
Gold DR (2000) Environmental tobacco smoke, indoor allergens, and childhood asthma. Environ Health Perspect 108(Suppl 4):643–651
Gruchalla RS, Pongracic J, Plaut M, Evans R III, Visness CM, Walter M et al (2005) Inner City Asthma Study: relationships among sensitivity, allergen exposure, and asthma morbidity. J Allergy Clin Immunol 115(3):478–485
Gupta D, Aggarwal AN, Chaudhry K, Chhabra SK, D'Souza GA, Jindal SK et al (2006) Household environmental tobacco smoke exposure, respiratory symptoms and asthma in non-smoker adults: a multicentric population study from India. Indian J Chest Dis Allied Sci 48(1):31–36
Hirsch T (1999) Indoor allergen exposure in west and East Germany: a cause for different prevalences of asthma and atopy? Rev Environ Health 14(3):159–168
Holt PG (1987) Current trends in research on the etiology and pathogenesis of byssinosis. Am J Ind Med 12(6):711–716
Jones SC, Travers MJ, Hahn EJ, Robertson H, Lee K, Higbee C et al (2006) Secondhand smoke and indoor public spaces in Paducah, Kentucky. J Ky Med Assoc 104(7):281–288
Kabesch M, Hoefler C, Carr D, Leupold W, Weiland SK, von Mutius E (2004) Glutathione S transferase deficiency and passive smoking increase childhood asthma. Thorax 59(7):569–573
Kaiser HB (2004) Risk factors in allergy/asthma. Allergy Asthma Proc 25(1):7–10
Kensler TW, Waka0bayashi N, Biswal S (2006) Cell survival responses to environmental stresses via the Keap1-Nrf2-ARE pathway. Annu Rev Pharmacol Toxicol
Kleeberger SR, Peden D (2005) Gene-environment interactions in asthma and other respiratory diseases. Annu Rev Med 56:383–400
Kong AN, Owuor E, Yu R, Hebbar V, Chen C, Hu R et al (2001) Induction of xenobiotic enzymes by the MAP kinase pathway and the antioxidant or electrophile response element (ARE/EpRE). Drug Metab Rev 33(3–4):255–271
Koppelman GH (2006) Gene by environment interaction in asthma. Curr Allergy Asthma Rep 6(2):103–111
Koppelman GH, Postma DS (2003) The genetics of CD14 in allergic disease. Curr Opin Allergy Clin Immunol 3(5):347–352
Larsson L, Szponar B, Pehrson C (2004) Tobacco smoking increases dramatically air concentrations of endotoxin. Indoor Air 14(6):421–424
Lau S, Illi S, Sommerfeld C, Niggemann B, Bergmann R, von Mutius E et al (2000) Early exposure to house-dust mite and cat allergens and development of childhood asthma: a cohort study. Multicentre Allergy Study Group. Lancet 356(9239):1392–1397
Lau S, Nickel R, Niggemann B, Gruber C, Sommerfeld C, Illi S et al (2002) The development of childhood asthma: lessons from the German Multicentre Allergy Study (MAS). Paediatr Respir Rev 3(3):265–272
Lee JS, Surh YJ (2005) Nrf2 as a novel molecular target for chemoprevention. Cancer Lett 224(2):171–184
Lin S, Munsie JP, Hwang SA, Fitzgerald E, Cayo MR (2002) Childhood asthma hospitalization and residential exposure to state route traffic. Environ Res 88(2):73–81
Litonjua AA, Milton DK, Celedon JC, Ryan L, Weiss ST, Gold DR (2002) A longitudinal analysis of wheezing in young children: the independent effects of early life exposure to house dust endotoxin, allergens, and pets. J Allergy Clin Immunol 110(5):736–742
Litonjua AA, Rifas-Shiman SL, Ly NP, Tantisira KG, Rich-Edwards JW, Camargo CA Jr et al (2006) Maternal antioxidant intake in pregnancy and wheezing illnesses in children at 2 y of age. Am J Clin Nutr 84(4):903–911
Liu AH (2002) Endotoxin exposure in allergy and asthma: reconciling a paradox. J Allergy Clin Immunol 109(3):379–392
Liu AH, Leung DY (2006) Renaissance of the hygiene hypothesis. J Allergy Clin Immunol 117(5):1063–1066
Liu AH, Redmon AH Jr (2001) Endotoxin: friend or foe? Allergy Asthma Proc 22(6):337–340
Martinez FD (2001) The coming-of-age of the hygiene hypothesis. Respir Res 2(3):129–132
McConnell R, Berhane K, Gilliland F, London SJ, Vora H, Avol E et al (1999) Air pollution and bronchitic symptoms in Southern California children with asthma. Environ Health Perspect 107(9):757–760
McConnell R, Berhane K, Gilliland F, London SJ, Islam T, Gauderman WJ et al (2002) Asthma in exercising children exposed to ozone: a cohort study. Lancet 359(9304):386–391
McConnell R, Berhane K, Gilliland F, Molitor J, Thomas D, Lurmann F et al (2003) Prospective study of air pollution and bronchitic symptoms in children with asthma. Am J Respir Crit Care Med 168(7):790–797
McDonnell WF, Abbey DE, Nishino N, Lebowitz MD (1999) Long-term ambient ozone concentration and the incidence of asthma in nonsmoking adults: the AHSMOG Study. Environ Res 80(2 Pt 1):110–121
Michel O, Ginanni R, Duchateau J, Vertongen F, Le Bon B, Sergysels R (1991) Domestic endotoxin exposure and clinical severity of asthma. Clin Exp Allergy 21(4):441–448
Michel O, Kips J, Duchateau J, Vertongen F, Robert L, Collet H et al (1996) Severity of asthma is related to endotoxin in house dust. Am J Respir Crit Care Med 154(6 Pt 1):1641–1646
Mickleborough TD (2005) Dietary omega-3 polyunsaturated fatty acid supplementation and airway hyperresponsiveness in asthma. J Asthma 42(5):305–314

Mickleborough TD, Rundell KW (2005) Dietary polyunsaturated fatty acids in asthma- and exercise-induced bronchoconstriction. Eur J Clin Nutr 59(12):1335–1346

Mickleborough TD, Ionescu AA, Rundell KW (2004) Omega-3 Fatty acids and airway hyperresponsiveness in asthma. J Altern Complement Med 10(6):1067–1075

Mishra V (2003) Effect of indoor air pollution from biomass combustion on prevalence of asthma in the elderly. Environ Health Perspect 111(1):71–78

Morgan WJ, Crain EF, Gruchalla RS, O'Connor GT, Kattan M, Evans R III et al (2004) Results of a home-based environmental intervention among urban children with asthma. N Engl J Med 351(11):1068–1080

Neas LM, Dockery DW, Ware JH, Spengler JD, Speizer FE, Ferris BG Jr (1991) Association of indoor nitrogen dioxide with respiratory symptoms and pulmonary function in children. Am J Epidemiol 134(2):204–219

Nel AE, Diaz-Sanchez D, Li N (2001) The role of particulate pollutants in pulmonary inflammation and asthma: evidence for the involvement of organic chemicals and oxidative stress. Curr Opin Pulm Med 7(1):20–26

Nicolai T, von Mutius E (1996) Respiratory hypersensitivity and environmental factors: East and West Germany. Toxicol Lett 86(2–3):105–113

Nicolai T, Carr D, Weiland SK, Duhme H, von Ehrenstein O, Wagner C et al (2003) Urban traffic and pollutant exposure related to respiratory outcomes and atopy in a large sample of children. Eur Respir J 21(6):956–963

Ober C, Hoffjan S (2006) Asthma genetics 2006: the long and winding road to gene discovery. Genes Immun 7(2):95–100

Ober C, Moffatt MF (2000) Contributing factors to the pathobiology. The genetics of asthma. Clin Chest Med 21(2):245–261

Ober C, Tsalenko A, Parry R, Cox NJ (2000) A second-generation genomewide screen for asthma-susceptibility alleles in a founder population. Am J Hum Genet 67(5):1154–1162

Oddy WH, de Klerk NH, Kendall GE, Mihrshahi S, Peat JK (2004) Ratio of omega-6 to omega-3 fatty acids and childhood asthma. J Asthma 41(3):319–326

Osburn WO, Wakabayashi N, Misra V, Nilles T, Biswal S, Trush MA et al (2006) Nrf2 regulates an adaptive response protecting against oxidative damage following diquat-mediated formation of superoxide anion. Arch Biochem Biophys 454(1):7–15

Ownby DR, Johnson CC, Peterson EL (2002) Exposure to dogs and cats in the first year of life and risk of allergic sensitization at 6 to 7 years of age. JAMA 288(8):963–972

Park JH, Gold DR, Spiegelman DL, Burge HA, Milton DK (2001) House dust endotoxin and wheeze in the first year of life. Am J Respir Crit Care Med 163(2):322–328

Peden DB (2000) Development of atopy and asthma: candidate environmental influences and important periods of exposure. Environ Health Perspect 108(Suppl 3):475–482

Peden DB (2003) Air pollution: indoor and outdoor. In: Adkinson NF Jr, Yunginger JW, Busse WW, Bochner BS, Holgate SK, Simons FE (eds) Middleton's allergy: principles and practice. Mosby, Philadelphia, PA, pp 515–528

Perkin MR, Strachan DP (2006) Which aspects of the farming lifestyle explain the inverse association with childhood allergy? J Allergy Clin Immunol 117(6):1374–1381

Perzanowski MS, Miller RL, Thorne PS, Barr RG, Divjan A, Sheares BJ et al (2006) Endotoxin in inner-city homes: associations with wheeze and eczema in early childhood. J Allergy Clin Immunol 117(5):1082–1089

Peters A, Goldstein IF, Beyer U, Franke K, Heinrich J, Dockery DW et al (1996) Acute health effects of exposure to high levels of air pollution in eastern Europe. Am J Epidemiol 144(6):570–581

Peters A, Wichmann HE, Tuch T, Heinrich J, Heyder J (1997a) Respiratory effects are associated with the number of ultrafine particles. Am J Respir Crit Care Med 155(4):1376–1383

Peters A, Dockery DW, Heinrich J, Wichmann HE (1997b) Short-term effects of particulate air pollution on respiratory morbidity in asthmatic children. Eur Respir J 10(4):872–879

Peters A, Liu E, Verrier RL, Schwartz J, Gold DR, Mittleman M et al (2000) Air pollution and incidence of cardiac arrhythmia. Epidemiology 11(1):11–17

Peters A, von Klot S, Heier M, Trentinaglia I, Hormann A, Wichmann HE et al (2004) Exposure to traffic and the onset of myocardial infarction. N Engl J Med 351(17):1721–1730

Pope CA III (1989) Respiratory disease associated with community air pollution and a steel mill, Utah Valley. Am J Public Health 79(5):623–628

Pope CA III (1991) Respiratory hospital admissions associated with PM10 pollution in Utah, Salt Lake, and Cache Valleys. Arch Environ Health 46(2):90–97

Prescott SL, Calder PC (2004) N-3 polyunsaturated fatty acids and allergic disease. Curr Opin Clin Nutr Metab Care 7(2):123–129

Rangasamy T, Cho CY, Thimmulappa RK, Zhen L, Srisuma SS, Kensler TW et al (2004) Genetic ablation of Nrf2 enhances susceptibility to cigarette smoke-induced emphysema in mice. J Clin Invest 114(9):1248–1259

Rangasamy T, Guo J, Mitzner WA, Roman J, Singh A, Fryer AD et al (2005) Disruption of Nrf2 enhances susceptibility to severe airway inflammation and asthma in mice. J Exp Med 202(1):47–59

Renz H, Herz U (2002) The bidirectional capacity of bacterial antigens to modulate allergy and asthma. Eur Respir J 19(1):158–171

Romieu I, Trenga C (2001) Diet and obstructive lung diseases. Epidemiol Rev 23(2):268–287

Romieu I, Meneses F, Sienra-Monge JJ, Huerta J, Ruiz VS, White MC et al (1995) Effects of urban air pollutants on emergency visits for childhood asthma in Mexico City. Am J Epidemiol 141(6):546–553

Romieu I, Meneses F, Ruiz S, Sienra JJ, Huerta J, White MC et al (1996) Effects of air pollution on the respiratory health of asthmatic children living in Mexico City. Am J Respir Crit Care Med 154(2 Pt 1):300–307

Romieu I, Meneses F, Ruiz S, Huerta J, Sienra JJ, White M et al (1997) Effects of intermittent ozone exposure on peak expiratory flow and respiratory symptoms among asthmatic children in Mexico City. Arch Environ Health 52(5):368–376

Romieu I, Sienra-Monge JJ, Ramirez-Aguilar M, Tellez-Rojo MM, Moreno-Macias H, Reyes-Ruiz NI et al (2002) Antioxidant supplementation and lung functions among children with asthma exposed to high levels of air pollutants. Am J Respir Crit Care Med 166(5):703–709

Romieu I, Sienra-Monge JJ, Ramirez-Aguilar M, Moreno-Macias H, Reyes-Ruiz NI, Estela del Rio-Navarro B et al (2004) Genetic polymorphism of GSTM1 and antioxidant supplementation influence lung function in relation to ozone exposure in asthmatic children in Mexico City. Thorax 59(1):8–10

Rosenstreich DL, Eggleston P, Kattan M, Baker D, Slavin RG, Gergen P et al (1997) The role of cockroach allergy and exposure to cockroach allergen in causing morbidity among inner-city children with asthma. N Engl J Med 336(19):1356–1363

Rumold R, Jyrala M, Diaz-Sanchez D (2001) Secondhand smoke induces allergic sensitization in mice. J Immunol 167(8):4765–4770

Rylander R, Holt PG (1998) (1–>3)-beta-D-glucan and endotoxin modulate immune response to inhaled allergen. Mediators Inflamm 7(2):105–110

Rylander R, Norrhall M, Engdahl U, Tunsater A, Holt PG (1998) Airways inflammation, atopy, and (1–> 3)-beta-D-glucan exposures in two schools. Am J Respir Crit Care Med 158(5 Pt 1):1685–1687

Schei MA, Hessen JO, Smith KR, Bruce N, McCracken J, Lopez V (2004) Childhood asthma and indoor woodsmoke from cooking in Guatemala. J Expo Anal Environ Epidemiol 14(Suppl 1):S110–S117

Schwartz J, Slater D, Larson TV, Pierson WE, Koenig JQ (1993) Particulate air pollution and hospital emergency room visits for asthma in Seattle. Am Rev Respir Dis 147(4):826–831

Seymour BW, Schelegle ES, Pinkerton KE, Friebertshauser KE, Peake JL, Kurup VP et al (2003) Second-hand smoke increases bronchial hyperreactivity and eosinophilia in a murine model of allergic aspergillosis. Clin Dev Immunol 10(1):35–42

Simpson A, Custovic A (2003) Early pet exposure: friend or foe? Curr Opin Allergy Clin Immunol 3(1):7–14

Simpson A, John SL, Jury F, Niven R, Woodcock A, Ollier WE et al (2006) Endotoxin exposure, CD14, and allergic disease: an interaction between genes and the environment. Am J Respir Crit Care Med 174(4):386–392

Singh N, Davis GS (2002) Review: occupational and environmental lung disease. Curr Opin Pulm Med 8(2):117–125

Smedje G, Norback D, Edling C (1997) Asthma among secondary schoolchildren in relation to the school environment. Clin Exp Allergy 27(11):1270–1278

Spengler JD, Jaakkola JJ, Parise H, Katsnelson BA, Privalova LI, Kosheleva AA (2004) Housing characteristics and children's respiratory health in the Russian Federation. Am J Public Health 94(4):657–662

Strachan DP (1989) Hay fever, hygiene, and household size. BMJ 299(6710):1259–1260

Taskinen T, Meklin T, Nousiainen M, Husman T, Nevalainen A, Korppi M (1997) Moisture and mould problems in schools and respiratory manifestations in schoolchildren: clinical and skin test findings. Acta Paediatr 86(11):1181–1187

Taskinen T, Hyvarinen A, Meklin T, Husman T, Nevalainen A, Korppi M (1999) Asthma and respiratory infections in school children with special reference to moisture and mold problems in the school. Acta Paediatr 88(12):1373–1379

Tavernier G, Fletcher G, Gee I, Watson A, Blacklock G, Francis H et al (2006) IPEADAM study: indoor endotoxin exposure, family status, and some housing characteristics in English children. J Allergy Clin Immunol 117(3):656–662

Thimmulappa RK, Lee H, Rangasamy T, Reddy SP, Yamamoto M, Kensler TW et al (2006) Nrf2 is a critical regulator of the innate immune response and survival during experimental sepsis. J Clin Invest 116(4):984–995

Thorne PS, Kulhankova K, Yin M, Cohn R, Arbes SJ, Zeldin DC (2005) Endotoxin exposure is a risk factor for asthma – The National Survey of Endotoxin in United States Housing. Am J Respir Crit Care Med 172(11):1371–1377

Tulic MK, Wale JL, Holt PG, Sly PD (2000) Modification of the inflammatory response to allergen challenge after exposure to bacterial lipopolysaccharide. Am J Respir Cell Mol Biol 22(5):604–612

Tulic MK, Holt PG, Sly PD (2002) Modification of acute and late-phase allergic responses to ovalbumin with lipopolysaccharide. Int Arch Allergy Immunol 129(2):119–128

van Strien RT, Verhoeff AP, Brunekreef B, van Wijnen JH (1994) Mite antigen in house dust: relationship with different housing characteristics in The Netherlands. Clin Exp Allergy 24(9):843–853

van Strien RT, Gehring U, Belanger K, Triche E, Gent J, Bracken MB et al (2004a) The influence of air conditioning, humidity, temperature and other household characteristics on mite allergen concentrations in the northeastern United States. Allergy 59(6):645–652

van Strien RT, Engel R, Holst O, Bufe A, Eder W, Waser M et al (2004b) Microbial exposure of rural school children, as assessed by levels of N-acetyl-muramic acid in mattress dust, and its association with respiratory health. J Allergy Clin Immunol 113(5):860–867

van Strien RT, Gent JF, Belanger K, Triche E, Bracken MB, Leaderer BP (2004c) Exposure to NO2 and nitrous acid and respiratory symptoms in the first year of life. Epidemiology 15(4):471–478

von Mutius E, Martinez FD, Fritzsch C, Nicolai T, Roell G, Thiemann HH (1994) Prevalence of asthma and atopy in two areas of West and East Germany. Am J Respir Crit Care Med 149(2 Pt 1):358–364

von Mutius E, Sherrill DL, Fritzsch C, Martinez FD, Lebowitz MD (1995) Air pollution and upper respiratory symptoms in children from East Germany. Eur Respir J 8(5):723–728

von Mutius E, Illi S, Nicolai T, Martinez FD (1996) Relation of indoor heating with asthma, allergic sensitisation, and bronchial responsiveness: survey of children in south Bavaria. BMJ 312(7044):1448–1450

Warner JA, Frederick JM, Bryant TN, Weich C, Raw GJ, Hunter C et al (2000) Mechanical ventilation and high-efficiency vacuum cleaning: a combined strategy of mite and mite allergen reduction in the control of mite-sensitive asthma. J Allergy Clin Immunol 105(1 Pt 1):75–82

Watanabe J, Miyazaki Y, Zimmerman GA, Albertine KH, McIntyre TM (2003) Endotoxin contamination of ovalbumin suppresses murine immunologic responses and development of airway hyper-reactivity. J Biol Chem 278(43):42361–42368

Weiss ST (2002) Eat dirt–the hygiene hypothesis and allergic diseases. N Engl J Med 347(12):930–931

White MC, Etzel RA, Wilcox WD, Lloyd C (1994) Exacerbations of childhood asthma and ozone pollution in Atlanta. Environ Res 65(1):56–68

Williams LK, McPhee RA, Ownby DR, Peterson EL, James M, Zoratti EM et al (2006) Gene-environment interactions with CD14 C-260T and their relationship to total serum IgE levels in adults. J Allergy Clin Immunol 118(4):851–857

Woo JG, Assa'ad A, Heizer AB, Bernstein JA, Hershey GK (2003) The -159 C–>T polymorphism of CD14 is associated with nonatopic asthma and food allergy. J Allergy Clin Immunol 112(2):438–444

Zambelli-Weiner A, Ehrlich E, Stockton ML, Grant AV, Zhang S, Levett PN et al (2005) Evaluation of the CD14/-260 polymorphism and house dust endotoxin exposure in the Barbados Asthma Genetics Study. J Allergy Clin Immunol 115(6):1203–1209

Zeldin DC, Eggleston P, Chapman M, Piedimonte G, Renz H, Peden D (2006) How exposures to biologics influence the induction and incidence of asthma. Environ Health Perspect 114(4):620–626

Chapter 4
Screening for Asthma

Robert M. Kaplan

Introduction

Asthma is the most common chronic disease found in children in the United States. Many people believe that asthma is like other chronic diseases such as cancer and heart disease, which may progress slowly over the course of time. It is widely believed that early identification of these chronic disease processes will lead to early treatment and the prevention of some disease consequences. The purpose of this chapter is to explore the value of screening for disease and to evaluate the need to screen children for asthma.

The public is exposed to conflicting opinions about the value of screening for asthma. By screening, we mean population-based efforts to identify cases in people who are not currently exhibiting symptoms. The American Academy of Pediatrics (http://www.aap.org) and the National Institute of Allergies and Infectious Diseases (http://www.niaid.nih.gov) each suggest that no screening tests are currently available for asthma. Instead, asthma diagnosis begins when asthma symptoms are present. Nevertheless, the American College of Allergy, Asthma, and Immunology offers free screenings for asthma. In 2004, they launched an aggressive campaign to encourage screening programs. The public was told that asthma is a serious medical condition that could be life-threatening. Further, concern was raised because most people are exposed to irritants in the air. Reporters, such as Emily Senay, MD, MPH Health and Medical Correspondent for the CBS Early Show, argued that breathing the air "can be deadly." Senay's reports noted that death rates from asthma exceed 5,000 per year and that there are 500,000 asthma hospitalizations per year. She attributed 2 million emergency room visits to asthma and suggested that early identification of cases was necessary. The American College of Allergy, Asthma, and Immunology told the general public that asthma can be stimulated by allergens such as pollen, mold, pet dander, drugs or food additives, viral respiratory infections, exercise, and second-hand smoke. Those who ever experience shortness of breath were urged to see their physicians. Although most organizations suggest that screening is unnecessary, some controversy remains.

R.M. Kaplan (✉)
Department of Health Services, UCLA School of Public Health, P.O. Box 951772 Los Angeles, CA, 90095-1772, USA
e-mail: rmkaplan@ucla.edu

Related Controversies Relevant to Lung Disease Screening

Controversies about screening for lung diseases have a long history. Perhaps the most interesting one concerns studies on screening for lung cancer. It is widely believed that early detection is the best approach to cancer control. The goal of screening is to detect cancer early while tumors are still small. Screening clearly does detect more cases. However, the goal of screening is not simply to detect tumors. It is to save lives. Identifying cancers early does not make much difference if people who have their cancers detected early do not live any longer than those who are not screened.

A widely cited study on cancer screening conducted by the Mayo clinic is at the heart of the controversy. In the Mayo Lung Project (MLP), 9,211 male smokers were randomly assigned to either chest x-ray and sputum cytology every 4 months or to usual-care. Six years later, the screened subjects were no less likely to

A. Harver and H. Kotses (eds.), *Asthma, Health and Society: A Public Health Perspective*,
DOI 10.1007/978-0-387-78285-0_4, © Springer Science+Business Media, LLC 2010

die of lung cancer than those who were not screened. The investigators then extended follow-up through 1996 to allow a median follow-up time of 20.5 years. At the end of the extended follow-up, the lung cancer mortality was 4.4 deaths per 1,000 person-years in the screened group and 3.9 in the usual-care group. Although the differences were not statistically significant, the screened group actually had a higher lung cancer death rate. Screening did lead to the identification of many more cases, and to significant increases in lung surgery (Marcus et al. 2000). It was suggested that screening may have led to the identification of some cancers that would not have been clinically important if left undetected and other tumors for which treatment was not effective.

The study challenges our belief that all cancers must be treated. In fact, there may be many cancers that will not become life-threatening (Welch 2004). Two recent studies exemplify the controversy. The first study, reported in the *New England Journal of Medicine*, evaluated nearly 31,000 people for lung cancer using spiral CT technology (Henschke et al. 2006). The screening identified 484 patients with lung cancer and among these 80% survived for 10 years. This was a remarkable finding because the 10-year survival rate for lung cancer patients has been reported to be only 10%. The paper stimulated interest in spiral CT scanning and led to significant promotion of screening promotions. However, there are problems. First, CT technology is very powerful and it can find many cases that other methods would have missed. The 80% survival includes many people with very minor cases that may not have caused death if left untreated.

The other recent study, published in the *Journal of the American Medical Association*, also considers the screening of about 3,200 people. In this report, 144 had lung cancer and among these 38 died of lung cancer. In other words, the survival rate was about the same as expected without screening (Bach et al. 2007). The studies differed in several important ways. First, the *JAMA* study had a higher detection rate because the patients were older. Second, the study had a longer period of follow up. Part of the reason that survival looks so much better in the *New England Journal* article is that the denominator was inflated by detected cases were that not likely to become life-threatening. Thus, the percentage survival looks better (Black and Baron 2007). Overall the interpretation depends on the outcome measures. Since screening identifies cases earlier, it looks like it improves survival. However, when RCTs compare how many people are alive years after screening, those who have been tested have no advantage. The JAMA paper concluded that screening is not only ineffective, but it may be harmful because it leads to treatment that does not extend the life expectancy.

Part of the controversy about screening for asthma may be similar. Many children who are identified as at risk for asthma may do well without intervention. If they are screened and identified as at risk, they are likely to get treatment. However, it is not clear that the good health they have later in life can be attributed to the early intervention for asthma.

Conceptual Model: The Disease Reservoir Hypothesis

The purpose of health care is to improve health. Health outcomes can be defined in terms of only two concepts: quantity and quality of life. A successful treatment is one that makes people live longer and/or improves quality of life (Kaplan and Wingard 2000; Kaplan 1994). If a treatment neither extends life expectancy nor improves life quality, we must challenge whether it has benefit. Many people express their level of wellness in terms of numbers given by common medical tests, such as the forced expiratory volume in 1 s (FEV_1) or peak flow. These numbers have earned their importance because they are related to the chances of having a shorter life or of developing disabling illness in the future. Other biological markers are less clearly related to meaningful clinical outcomes. Tests or biomarkers should only be considered important if they are correlated with either quality of quantity of life.

It is becoming increasingly clear that there are also huge reservoirs of undiagnosed disease in human populations. As diagnostic technology improves, the healthcare system will be challenged because these common problems will be identified in many individuals who may not benefit from treatment because their length of life or quality of life will never be affected. The problem has been fiercely debated in relation to cancer screening tests such as mammography and prostate specific antigen (PSA) (Welch and Black 1997a; Welch et al. 2000).

According to the American Cancer Society, screening and early detection of cancers save lives (Kaplan and Groessl 2002). It is believed that the reservoir of undetected disease that might be eliminated through more aggressive intervention. Screening guidelines have been proposed and compliance to guidelines is now used as evidence for high quality medical care (McGlynn et al. 2003). Further, test rates are increasing because there are now financial incentives for physicians of offer specific tests, such as mammography (Epstein et al. 2004).

In order to better appreciate the problem, it is necessary to understand the natural history of disease. Public health campaigns assume that disease is binary; either a person has the "diagnosis," or they do not. However, most diseases are processes. It is likely that chronic disease begins long before it is diagnosed. For example, autopsy studies consistently show that most young adults who died early in life from noncardiovascular causes have fatty streaks in their coronary arteries indicating the initiation of coronary disease (Strong et al. 1999). Not all people who have a disease will ultimately suffer from the problem. With many diseases, most of those affected will never even know they are sick. For example, autopsy studies show that nearly half of men who die in their 1970s or 1980s have prostate cancer, (Gosselaar et al. 2005) and that as many as 40% of older women had some evidence of breast cancer at the time they died (Welch and Black 1997b). However, most of these people were never tested for these cancers and never knew of these problems. Diagnosis and treatment could have resulted in complications but are unlikely to have improved health (Welch and Black 1997a).

Among those who do have problems, some may not benefit from treatment. For example, if smokers are screened for lung cancer, many cases can be identified (Klingler 2004). However, clinical trials have shown that the course of the disease is likely to be the same for those who are screened and those not subjected to screening, even though screening leads to more diagnosis and treatment (Marcus et al. 2000). The harder we look, the more likely it is that cases will be found. Advanced MRI technology has revealed surprisingly high rates of undiagnosed stroke. One cross-sectional study of 3,502 men and women over age 65 found that 29% had evidence of mild stokes and that 75% had plaque in their carotid arteries (Manolio et al. 1999).

Black and Welch make the distinction between disease and pseudodisease (Black and Welch 1997). Pseudodisease is disease that will not affect life duration or quality of life at any point in a patient's lifetime. A diagnosis followed by surgical treatment may have consequences, often leaving the patient with new symptoms or problems as complications of the treatment. Outcomes researchers consider the benefits of screening and treatment from the patient's perspective (Kaplan 2000).

What is Disease?

The dictionary defines disease as "… the lack of ease: a pathological condition of the body that presents a group of clinical signs, symptoms and laboratory findings peculiar to it and setting the condition apart as an abnormal entity differing from other normal more pathological conditions." Disease, quite literally, is the lack of ease.

The dictionary definition of disease raises several important questions. Do we have disease if there is no lack of ease? In other words, what do we do about conditions that do not cause signs or symptoms? The answer is fairly clear. Pathological conditions that will cause signs or symptoms at some future time must qualify as disease. For example, high blood pressure is associated with the increased probability of stroke or heart attacks in the future (MacMahon 2000). Even though a condition does not cause symptoms or dysfunction now, it must be of concern if it will cause early death, dysfunction or symptoms in the future. But, let's take this one step further. Suppose that a condition does not cause symptoms or dysfunction now and it will never cause early death, dysfunction or symptoms. Does the condition qualify as a disease?

In modern medicine, we know of many conditions that represent genuine pathology of a tissue, but may never cause early death, dysfunction, or symptoms. In fact, this may be so for the majority of cases of prostate cancer (Black 1999). In addition, the substantial majority of cases of low-grade breast cancer, known as ductal carcinoma in situ, would never affect people's lives if they had not been diagnosed. Autopsy studies suggest as many as 60% of men die with prostate cancer while only about 3% of men die of prostate cancer. Similarly, autopsy studies have shown that nearly 40% of older women may have DCIS at the time of death. However, only about 3% of women die of breast cancer (Welch and Black 1997b).

Is there a Disease Reservoir for Asthma?

Definition of Asthma

One of the biggest challenges in epidemiologic studies of asthma is how the condition is defined. Ford and Mannino (this volume) acknowledged the difficulty in defining asthma. Citing the Second Expert Panel Report of the Guidelines for the Diagnosis and Management of Asthma, they endorsed the definition of asthma as, "a chronic inflammatory disorder of the airways in which many cells and cellular elements play a role, in particular, mast cells, eosinophils, t-lymphocytes, neutrophils, and epithelial cells. In susceptible individuals, this inflammation causes recurrent episodes of wheezing, breathlessness, chest tightness, and cough, particularly at night and in the early morning. These episodes are usually associated with widespread but variable air flow obstruction that is often reversible either spontaneously or with treatment. The inflammation also causes an associated increase in the existing bronchial hyper-responsiveness to a variety of stimuli" (National Asthma Education and Prevention Program. Guidelines for the Diagnosis and Management of Asthma. Bethesda, MD, National Institutes of Health, NIH Publication no. 98–4051, 1997).

Evidence from the Behavioral Risk Factors Surveillance System suggests that there is an asthma epidemic. Cases of asthma have systematically increased between the year 2000 and 2004. There are at least two explanations for this trend. First, there may be a genuine epidemic. The second explanation is that the real rate of asthma in the population is about the same but more aggressive screening leads to an increase in the number of diagnosed cases. We believe the second explanation is a true possibility, given the greater attention to asthma screening in the populations.

Case Detection

The most common method for identifying asthma in epidemiologic studies involves questionnaires. The reliability and validity of these questionnaires have been challenged in a variety of studies (Peat et al. 1992). An alternative approach involves estimation of asthma rates from reviews of medical records. The difficulty with this approach is that it depends upon the reliability of physician assessment of asthma. We know there is remarkable variability in the rate of diagnosis of asthma and this may, in part, be attributable to the application of different standards by different clinicians. The use of administrative databases has also been considered, but these approaches suffer from the same types of biases.

In response to these concerns, it has been suggested that measures of bronchial hyperactivity be used for screening. The difficulty is that bronchial hyperactivity, even though considered to be a physiological standard, is not synonymous with asthma. There are false negatives. For example, one study estimated that 30% of children with asthma do not have bronchial hyperactivity (Phelan 1994). The same study showed that at least 15% of children who never show any other signs of asthma have positive results on the bronchial hyperactivity.

The issue of exercise-induced airway hyperresponsiveness has been studied by a variety of authors. In studies that exclude patients with a known diagnosis of asthma, the prevalence of exercise-induced bronchospasm has been reported to be 19% in a group of fitness center members (Mannix et al. 2003), and 29% among adolescents (Rupp et al. 1992). Among athletes, exercise-induced asthma rates between 11% and 50% have been reported (Parsons and Mastronarde 2005). Among athletes with a history of asthma, the rate has been reported to be as high as 90% (McFadden and Gilbert 1994). The United States Olympic Committee noted that 11.2% of all athletes who competed in the 1984 Winter Olympics experienced exercise-induced bronchospasm (Voy 1986). A similar study conducted as part as the 1996 Summer Olympic Games used questionnaires to identify which athletes had a previous diagnosis of asthma or used asthma medications. The study found that 16.7% reported the use of asthma medication or had a previous diagnosis of asthma. About 4% of the athletes were taking medication for asthma at the time of the Olympic games. Endurance athletic activities may provoke bronchospasm, and as a result, increase the diagnosis rate. In the 1996 Olympics, 50% of the participants in cycling and mountain biking had a previous diagnosis of asthma or were taking asthma medications (Weiler et al. 1998).

One study of high school athletes not involved in elite competitions noted an airway hyperactivity rate of 38% (Mannix et al. 2004).

Population-based studies using methacholine challenge are rare. However, the few that have been completed raise interesting issues. Population studies suggest that the prevalence of symptomatic asthma in the US population is about 4–7%. We would expect that some people are asymptomatic. This might inflate the expected number of people with reactive airways up to about 10%.

Weiler and colleagues are among the few who have done methacholine bronchial provocation (MBP) tests on asymptomatic people. As professors at the University of Iowa, who set up a challenge for the University of Iowa football team prior the teams' appearance in the 1982 Rose bowl football contest. To their surprise, 76 of 151 healthy athletes (50%) had positive tests. Among athletes with some respiratory symptoms, 76% had positive results.

Wyler and Ryan performed a similar study in relation to the 1998 winter Olympic games. Athletes were asked about past history of asthma, medication use and symptoms. A high percentage (22.4%) reported asthma medication use, a diagnosis of asthma, or both. Among Nordic, cross country, or short track events, the rate was 60.7%.

Athletes are more likely to be tested because they have good access to medical care. A diagnosis can get them medication that could enhance performance. If we were to look as aggressively in other populations, it is likely that higher asthma rates would be observed. It is likely that there is a large reservoir of undetected airway reactivity. Many of these cases will be labeled as asthma.

Psychological Distress and Diagnosis of Asthma

Asthma is the most common chronic illness during childhood in the United States. Further, there are substantial disparities in the rate of asthma. African-American children and adolescents have the highest burden of asthma. Latino children also have high rates of asthma. Figure 4.1, based on our California Health Interview Survey, shows the highest rates for American Indian/Alaska Native groups and African-Americans

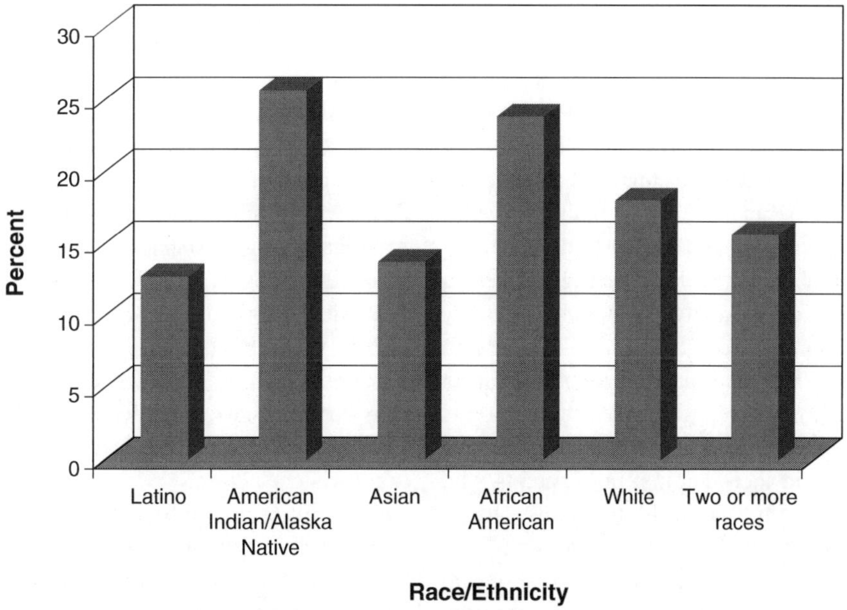

Fig. 4.1 Percent Ever Diagnosed With Asthma by Race/Ethnicty: California Health Interview Survey (CHIS), 2005

and the lowest rates for Latinos. However, the Latinos can be divided into various sub-groups, and when they are disaggregated Puerto Rican children have higher rates of asthma than African-American children. The California study is misleading because only a small portion of California Latinos are Puerto Rican. One study suggested that the rate of asthma among Puerto Rican children is 26%. By contrast, the rate of asthma among Mexican-American children is only 10% (Lara et al. 2006). Studies conducted on the island of Puerto Rico suggest that one in three individuals experience asthma during their lifetime (Ortega et al. 2002). Studies in primary care clinics among mainland Puerto Rican children suggest that nearly half experience asthma (Cloutier et al. 2002). In addition to case finding, evidence suggests that Puerto Rican children in the east Bronx experience a higher degree of functional limitations associated with asthma than do other ethnic groups. For example, they miss more school days and experience more asthma exacerbations (Findley et al. 2003).

The initial reaction to these differences may be that they represent genetic influences. However, there are other explanations. Since much of the diagnosis of asthma is based on self-report, the question of whether or not cultural issues may play a role needs to be explored. For example, there may be cultural difference in the way individuals describe symptoms. Feldman and colleagues (2006) argued that there is substantial co-morbidity between asthma attacks and internalizing disorders among Puerto Rican children. Studying 5–18-year-olds living on the island of Puerto Rico, they used the Diagnostic Interview Schedule for children to assess internalizing disorders. At baseline they evaluated whether or not the children had a lifetime history of asthma. Then, they followed the children 1 year later to determine whether or not they had internalized psychiatric or psychological problems. The results suggested that emotional problems may have been expressed as breathing problems similar to asthmatic symptoms. In other words, the high rate of asthma-like symptom reporting may have been an expression of psychological stress. Other studies have suggested that parents with mental health problems are more likely to report asthma symptoms in their children than parents who have not experienced mental health problems (Ortega et al. 2004a). Since many of the studies in Puerto Rico have used parent report of symptoms, the relationship between asthma and parental interpretation of symptoms is important. One evaluation of 1891 children between the ages of 4 and 17 noted that the diagnosis of asthma was associated with the diagnosis of depression and a symptom of separation anxiety. These results, again, challenge the use of parental reports that are common in epidemiologic studies of asthma (Ortega et al. 2004b). They also raise the question of whether the recorded diagnosis of asthma represents a consistent underlying pathology.

As a result of these concerns, it is very difficult to determine a reliable number for the proportion of children with asthma. However, we do know that there is rather remarkable variation, as pointed out in the Ford and Mannino chapter (this volume). For example, a study of worldwide variation in the prevalence of asthma symptoms (The International Study of Asthma and Allergies in Childhood (ISAAC) Steering Committee 1998) suggested that the 12-month prevalence of asthma was as low as 1.6% in Indonesia and as high as 36.8% in the United Kingdom. Although genetic and environmental factors affect asthma symptoms, it is unlikely that variations these large can be totally explained by these factors. Differences in asthma detection are likely to play an important role.

Deaths and Hospital Discharges

The disease reservoir hypothesis argues that more surveillance will lead to the identification of more cases of low threshold asthma, or more cases of pseudo-asthma. Thus the hypothesis suggests that the incidence of new cases should increase, but that the rate of serious problems should be unaffected. In order to investigate this, we used data from several sources. First, we considered an analysis completed by the American Lung Association. They examined asthma mortality rates standardized to two populations: 1940 (lower line of Fig. 4.2) and 2000 (upper line of Fig. 4.2). The International Classification of Diseases was revised in 1979 and again in1996. The figure considers the years 1979 through 2003. The changes in asthma death rates may reflect changes in the classification systems. Prior to 1996, asthma was grouped with emphysema and chronic bronchitis to form the category chronic obstructive pulmonary disease (COPD). It is likely that emphysema was increasing between 1979 and 1996. Overall, the best estimate is that asthma deaths have been relatively steady.

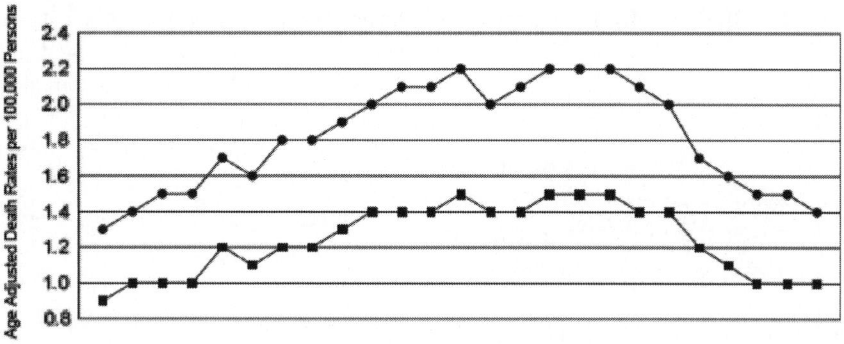

Fig. 4.2 Asthma age adjusted death rates based on the 1940 and 2000 Standard Population, 1979-2003

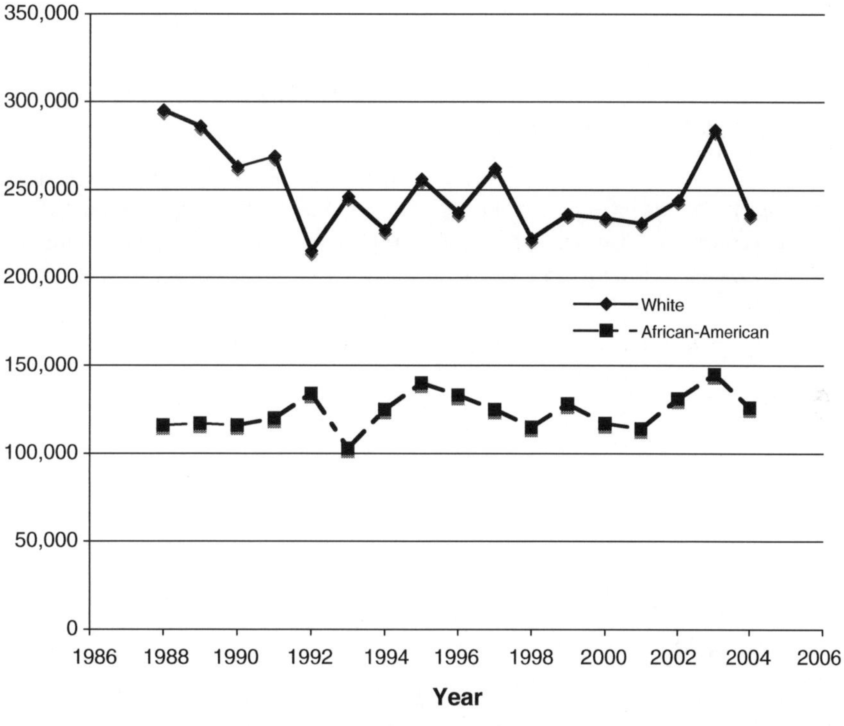

Fig. 4.3 Asthma Hospital Discharges/10,000 Population by Year and Race. Data from NHIS National Hospital Discharge Survey

Further evidence comes from the study of hospital discharges. If there was really an epidemic of serious asthma, we would expect that there would be an increase in the number of people admitted to hospitals with asthma. Figure 4.3 uses data from the National Center for Health Statistics, National Hospital Discharge Survey to explore this issue. For both White and African-Americans, the rate of hospital discharges per 10,000 persons in the populations remained relatively steady between 1989 and 2004. The finding that there are more incident cases of asthma, but not more serious outcomes is consistent with the disease reservoir hypotheses predictions. More screening finds more cases, but many of these cases will not have serious health consequences.

What Happens to Undetected Cases?

To appraise the value of screening, we must know the natural history of the condition. Unlike some cancers that are expected to progress over the course of time, evidence does not clearly show that cases of asthma progress from mild to moderate to more severe conditions. For example, if asthma goes undetected and it is a progressive disease, we would expect it to emerge at latter ages. Thus, it would be predicted that the number of cases would increase with age. Figure 4.4, using data from the population-based.California Health Interview Survey shows that the proportion diagnosed with asthma does increase until about age 17. Thereafter, it declines and levels off. Failure to detect asthma early in life does not appear to lead to an increase in new cases later in life.

The Advantages of Early Intervention

Early identification of asthma would be important if early treatment changed the course of disease. It remains unclear whether early treatment has an important impact on the course of the disease. Systematic clinical trials have been used to address this issue. For example, Bisgaard and colleagues (2006) studied 1-month-old infants. They randomly assigned the infants to a 2-week course of inhaled bedesonide (400 UG/day) or to a placebo. All of the infants had demonstrated a 3-day episode of the wheezing prior to entering the study. Children were followed for 3 years to determine the number of symptom-free days. This study showed that infants treated with active medication were symptom-free on 83% of the days while those treated with placebo were symptom-free on 82% of days. These differences were nowhere near statistically significant. Further, a number of children who had persistent wheezing in the active medication group (24%) did not significantly differ from the percentage of children who experienced wheezing in the placebo group (21%). Overall, the study offered no evidence that early intervention affected the course of the disease.

Criteria for Screening

A variety of groups have proposed guidelines for screening. On an international level, Wilson and Jungner proposed the most commonly cited criteria (Feldman et al. 2006). According to these authors, ten criteria should be met in order to justify a screening test. The World Health Organization has adopted these

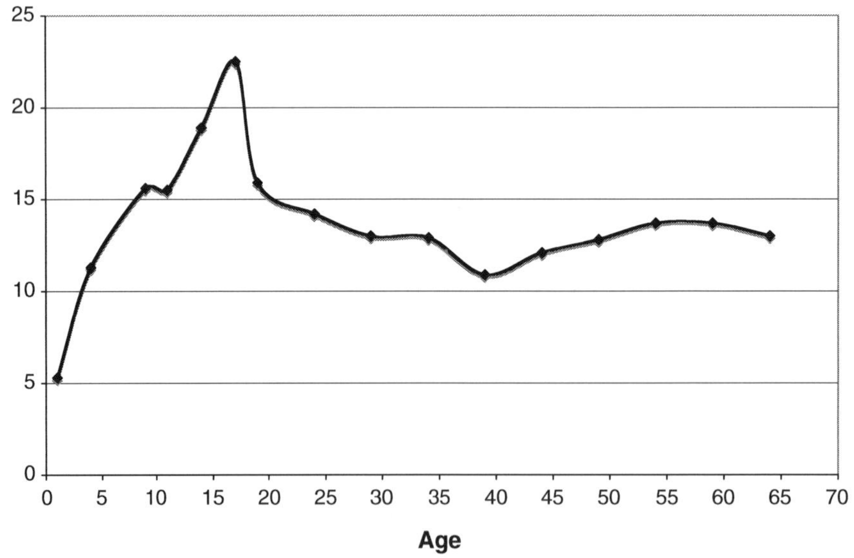

Fig. 4.4 Percent Asthma Diagnosis by Age: CHIS 2005

Table 4.1 Wilson proposed ten criteria for screening and the decision to screen for asthma

Criterion	Met	Comment	Reference
The condition should pose an important health problem	Yes	Asthma is an important health problem. There is an apparent epidemic of asthma in children	Cloutier et al. 2002
The natural history of the disease should be well understood	Unclear	Although the natural history of asthma has been studied, considerable controversy remains about what happens to asthma and reactive airways if they are untreated. NHIS data suggest that prevalence declines with age	Fig. 4.4
There should be a recognizable early, latent, pre-symptomatic stage	No	Asthma typically emerges as a symptomatic disease. There is not sufficient evidence suggesting that early intervention modifies the disease process	Bisgaard et al. 2006
Treatment of disease in the early stages should be of more benefit than treatment in a later stage	No	Emerging evidence questions whether or not early treatment for asthma provides benefit	Bisgaard et al. 2006
There should be a suitable test	No	A variety of methods are available to test for asthma. Many epidemiologic studies are based on self report-questionnaires. The reliability of these questionnaires has been challenged	Peat et al. 1992
The test should be acceptable to the population	No	Although questionnaires are minimally invasive, they are also less reliable. Challenge tests involve expense and are less acceptable to the population	Peat et al. 1992
There should be adequate facilities for the diagnosis and treatment of abnormalities detected	No	Increasingly, asthma is a disease of low-income children. These are the same populations that tend to have inadequate access to healthcare. Further, treatment of asthma is moving toward high expense medications	Phelan 1994
There should be an agreed policy on who to treat	Unclear	Over the last few years, treatment guidelines for the management of asthma have immerged. Thus, there is a growing consensus on who should be treated for symptomatic asthma. On the other hand, there appears to be no clear consensus on the management of children with the early stages of asthma or those in the pre-symptomatic stages	
Case finding should be continuous	No	Screening must be repeated at intervals. If screening is undertaken, it needs to be repeated on a regular basis. There have been significant challenges to the notion that we should screen for asthma. Thus, it is unclear that regular interval screening should be applied	Gerald and Sockrider 2007
The costs of screening should be economical in relation to total healthcare – all costs must be balanced against benefits	No	The costs of screening may be substantial, however the benefits of screening are not well understood. At this time, it does not appear that benefits exceed costs	Screening not studied. Optimal treatment (Simonella et al. 2006)

criteria and they are summarized in Table 4.1. The Table also comments on whether each criterion is met for asthma screening. For example, asthma is clearly an important public health problem, and there is accepted treatment for those recognized with the disease. On the other hand, several of the criteria are not met. For example, it is not clear that we understand the natural history of the disease. Further, it is not clearly understood that there is a latent or early symptomatic stage other than truly symptomatic expression of asthma symptoms. Further, it is not clear that there is a suitable screening test that is acceptable to the population.

Gerald and associates, on behalf of the Behavioral Science Committee of the American Thoracic Society, considered the issue of screening for asthma (Gerald and Sockrider 2007). They systematically worked through the WHO guidelines and concluded that the adoption of population-based asthma case detection is not appropriate at this time. The statement is in contrast to the American College of Allergy, Asthma, and Immunology who argue that systematic screening may be of value to children. The ATS committee challenged the evidence supporting the position. However, they noted that too little was known about asthma phenotypes and the natural history of asthma to recommend systematic screening. Further, the cost-effectiveness of asthma screening remains unknown.

Summary

Screening for disease is an attractive alternative. If a disease progresses slowly, early identification may lead to early treatment and the prevention of adverse health effects. Criteria have been established to help decide whether screening for disease is meaningful. This chapter challenges the value of screening for several diseases. Further, we explore the potential of screening children for asthma. At this point, few of the criteria for screening are met. We conclude that there is not sufficient evidence to screen children for asthma. Further, it is suggested that screening may not be a valuable use of health care resources.

References

(1998) Worldwide variation in prevalence of symptoms of asthma, allergic rhinoconjunctivitis, and atopic eczema: ISAAC. The International Study of Asthma and Allergies in Childhood (ISAAC) Steering Committee. Lancet 351(9111): 1225–1232

Bach PB, Jett JR, Pastorino U, Tockman MS, Swensen SJ, Begg CB (2007) Computed tomography screening and lung cancer outcomes. JAMA 297(9):953–961

Bisgaard H, Hermansen MN, Loland L, Halkjaer LB, Buchvald F (2006) Intermittent inhaled corticosteroids in infants with episodic wheezing. N Engl J Med 354(19):1998–2005

Black WC (1999) Should this patient be screened for cancer? Eff Clin Pract 2(2):86–95

Black WC, Baron JA (2007) CT screening for lung cancer: spiraling into confusion? JAMA 297(9):995–997

Black WC, Welch HG (1997) Screening for disease. AJR Am J Roentgenol 168(1):3–11

Cloutier MM, Wakefield DB, Hall CB, Bailit HL (2002) Childhood asthma in an urban community: prevalence, care system, and treatment. Chest 122(5):1571–1579

Epstein AM, Lee TH, Hamel MB (2004) Paying physicians for high-quality care. N Engl J Med 350(4):406–410

Feldman JM, Ortega AN, McQuaid EL, Canino G (2006) Comorbidity between asthma attacks and internalizing disorders among Puerto Rican children at one-year follow-up. Psychosomatics 47(4):333–339

Findley S, Lawler K, Bindra M, Maggio L, Penachio MM, Maylahn C (2003) Elevated asthma and indoor environmental exposures among Puerto Rican children of East Harlem. J Asthma 40(5):557–569

Gerald LB, Sockrider MM, Grad R, Bender BG, Boss LP, Galant SP, et al. (2007) An official ATS workshop report: issues in screening for asthma in children. Proc Am Thorac Soc, 4(2):133–141

Gosselaar C, Roobol MJ, Schroder FH (2005) Prevalence and characteristics of screen-detected prostate carcinomas at low prostate-specific antigen levels: aggressive or insignificant? BJU Int 95(2):231–237

Henschke CI, Yankelevitz DF, Libby DM, Pasmantier MW, Smith JP, Miettinen OS (2006) Survival of patients with stage I lung cancer detected on CT screening. N Engl J Med 355(17):1763–1771

Kaplan RM (1994) The Ziggy theorem – toward an outcomes-focused health psychology. Health Psychol 13(6):451–460

Kaplan RM (2000) Two pathways to prevention. Am Psychol 55(4):382–396

Kaplan RM & Groessl EJ (2002) Applications of cost-effectiveness methodologies in behavioral medicine. Journal Of Consulting And Clinical Psychology 70(3):482–493

Kaplan RM, Wingard DL (2000) Trends in breast cancer incidence, survival, and mortality. Lancet 356(9229):592–593

Klingler K (2004) Early detection of lung cancer by CT-screening. Eur J Cancer ECJ Suppl 2(1):23

Lara M, Akinbami L, Flores G, Morgenstern H (2006) Heterogeneity of childhood asthma among Hispanic children: Puerto Rican children bear a disproportionate burden. Pediatrics 117(1):43–53

MacMahon S (2000) Blood pressure and the risk of cardiovascular disease. N Engl J Med 342(1):50–52

Mannix ET, Roberts M, Fagin DP, Reid B, Farber MO (2003) The prevalence of airways hyperresponsiveness in members of an exercise training facility. J Asthma 40(4):349–355

Mannix ET, Roberts MA, Dukes HJ, Magnes CJ, Farber MO (2004) Airways hyperresponsiveness in high school athletes. J Asthma 41(5):567–574

Manolio TA, Burke GL, O'Leary DH et al (1999) Relationships of cerebral MRI findings to ultrasonographic carotid atherosclerosis in older adults: the Cardiovascular Health Study. CHS collaborative research group. Arterioscler Thromb Vasc Biol 19(2):356–365

Marcus PM, Bergstralh EJ, Fagerstrom RM et al (2000) Lung cancer mortality in the Mayo Lung Project: impact of extended follow-up. J Natl Cancer Inst 92(16):1308–1316
McFadden ER Jr, Gilbert IA (1994) Exercise-induced asthma. N Engl J Med 330(19):1362–1367
McGlynn EA, Asch SM, Adams J et al (2003) The quality of health care delivered to adults in the United States. N Engl J Med 348(26):2635–2645
Ortega AN, Huertas SE, Canino G, Ramirez R, Rubio-Stipec M (2002) Childhood asthma, chronic illness, and psychiatric disorders. J Nerv Ment Dis 190(5):275–281
Ortega AN, Goodwin RD, McQuaid EL, Canino G (2004a) Parental mental health, childhood psychiatric disorders, and asthma attacks in island Puerto Rican youth. Ambul Pediatr 4(4):308–315
Ortega AN, McQuaid EL, Canino G, Goodwin RD, Fritz GK (2004b) Comorbidity of asthma and anxiety and depression in Puerto Rican children. Psychosomatics 45(2):93–99
Parsons JP, Mastronarde JG (2005) Exercise-induced bronchoconstriction in athletes. Chest 128(6):3966–3974
Peat JK, Salome CM, Toelle BG, Bauman A, Woolcock AJ (1992) Reliability of a respiratory history questionnaire and effect of mode of administration on classification of asthma in children. Chest 102(1):153–157
Phelan PD (1994) Asthma in children: epidemiology. BMJ 308(6944):1584–1585
Rupp NT, Guill MF, Brudno DS (1992) Unrecognized exercise-induced bronchospasm in adolescent athletes. Am J Dis Child 146(8):941–944
Simonella L, Marks G, Sanderson K, Andrews G (2006) Cost-effectiveness of current and optimal treatment for adult asthma. Intern Med J 36(4):244–250
Strong JP, Malcom GT, McMahan CA et al (1999) Prevalence and extent of atherosclerosis in adolescents and young adults: implications for prevention from the Pathobiological Determinants of Atherosclerosis in Youth Study. JAMA 281(8):727–735
Voy RO (1986) The U.S. Olympic Committee experience with exercise-induced bronchospasm, 1984. Med Sci Sports Exerc 18(3):328–330
Weiler JM, Layton T, Hunt M (1998) Asthma in United States olympic athletes who participated in the 1996 summer games. J Allergy Clin Immunol 102(5):722–726
Welch HG, Black WC (1997) Using autopsy series to estimate the disease "reservoir" for ductal carcinoma in situ of the breast: how much more breast cancer can we find? Ann Intern Med 127(11):1023–1028
Welch HG, Schwartz LM, Woloshin S (2000) Do increased 5-year survival rates in prostate cancer indicate better outcomes? JAMA 284(16):2053–2055
Welch HG (2004) Should I be tested for cancer? Berkeley, CA: Universlty of California Press

Chapter 5
Ecology and Asthma

Barbara P. Yawn

Introduction

Ecology is the study of patterns of relationships between organisms and their environment (Green et al. 2001). When applied to asthma, investigators have taken several different approaches to the "environment," usually by studying the effect of the environment on the "organism" defined as people with asthma (Harper 2004; Hart and Whitehead 1990; Stoloff 2000; Lanphear et al. 2001; Gold and Wright 2005; Bousquet et al. 2005; Milton et al. 2004; Parkes et al. 2003; Redd 2002). The exact approach depends on the expertise of the investigator from anthropologist to health services researcher to atmospheric scientist. In each case, the environment is seen through the lenses of the specific scientific discipline. In this regard, few authors have viewed the 'asthma environment' through the lens of the patient or family dealing with asthma. Such a view requires knowledge of the social ecology of asthma that has been addressed most commonly in children with asthma as the nested arrangement of family, school, neighborhood, and community (Earls and Carlson 2001; Klinnert et al. 2002). In this chapter, the work published under the key terms of asthma and ecology will be reviewed and when possible integrated into a holistic approach. The perspective of the person (organism) with asthma will be emphasized. It is the patient centered ecology of asthma that becomes pertinent, and highly relevant to the people who live with work with and suffer from asthma (Fig. 5.1).

B.P. Yawn (✉)
Olmsted Medical Center, 210 Ninth Street SE, Rochester, MN, 55904, USA
e-mail: yawnx002@umn.edu

Cultural, Social and Economic Environment

In the United States, asthma prevalence as well as the burden of asthma morbidity and mortality is higher in communities of color, such as those of African American or Caribbean American descent (Gold and Wright 2005; Mannino 2004). The reasons for the differences have been suggested to be genetic, such as the levels of genetic markers (e.g., arginine/arginine) believed to be important in metabolizing and utilization beta agonists (Nelson et al. 2006; Israel 2005) as well as social, cultural, economic, and environmental factors. From the ecology perspective, it is all of these factors plus the interaction of each factor with the other factors that result in the complex bio-psycho-social construct called asthma. For example, people of color are more likely to deal daily with the economic and social stresses of poverty and near poverty (Shanawani 2006) that yield limited time for addressing the management of a chronic illness (Hendrika et al. 2003; Kean et al. 2006; Rydstrom et al. 2004). But racial disparities are not just a consequence of lack of a family's time or access to health care. In a study of people with asthma who participated in managed care plans (Krishnan et al. 2001), African Americans were significantly less likely than Whites to report they had been offered or received education for self-management and avoidance of asthma triggers. Why was a racial subset of the managed care patients treated differently? The answer may be based on the interaction of health professionals' personal experience, and available resources deal with the economic, cultural and life-chaos realities of poor African-American that has evolved into a generalized perception of people of color. Or perhaps it is based on health professionals'

A. Harver and H. Kotses (eds.), *Asthma, Health and Society: A Public Health Perspective*,
DOI 10.1007/978-0-387-78285-0_5, © Springer Science+Business Media, LLC 2010

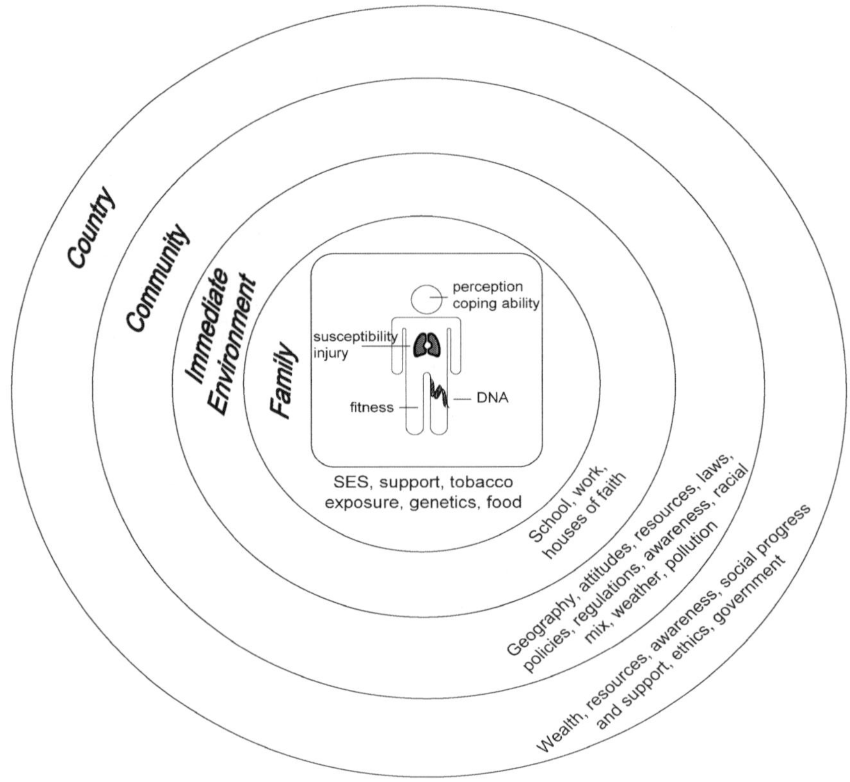

Fig. 5.1 The person with asthma in their socio-physiological-cultural environment

assumptions that asthma education is not accepted, understood, or acted upon even when presented in a manner that is clear to the educator and meets the health professional's needs (Couturaud et al. 2002; Cowie et al. 2002; Neri et al. 2001). Such professional biases are not uncommon and can occur when educational materials ignore the patient's and families' cultural and health beliefs (Becker et al. 1978).

Cultural or ethnic beliefs or practices often influence how asthma is perceived and internalized for both the person with asthma as well as their family members (Pachter and Weller 1993; Kleinman et al. 1978). Among Latino communities, asthma is viewed as a "cold" illness amenable to "hot" treatment (Risser and Mazur 1995; Pachter et al. 2002). An inhaler may be viewed as "cold" therapy since the rapid thrust of the drug against the back of the throat may feel cool and therefore viewed as unlikely to help. Simply suggesting that the inhaler be used after a cup of hot tea, soup or water will not interfer with the efficacy of the inhaler, but may greatly improve the inhaler's effectiveness by increasing inhaler use. Distrust of Western medicine, the medical profession, or even Caucasian professionals in general must also be considered a factor in the total ecology of the asthma patient, especially those living in communities of color (Bearison et al. 2002; George et al. 2003; Halbert and Isonaka 2006). There is a need for improved understanding of how ethno-cultural practices, independent of socioeconomic variables, may influence asthma care and the use of health care services and therapies. Open-ended questions such as "In your community, what does having asthma mean?" can elicit informative responses. Understanding, validating, and incorporating a person's ethno-cultural beliefs may ease the patient and family's job of adding the management of a chronic illness to their daily routine (Hendrika et al. 2003; Kean et al. 2006; Rydstrom et al. 2004). It can also make working with the family and patient less frustrating, more satisfying and ultimately more successful.

However, the importance of cultural beliefs does not stop with just the symptoms of asthma and whether or not those symptoms are hot or cold, or due to congestion of the lungs or stress. Among health care professionals, asthma is considered a chronic disease (National Heart, Lung, and Blood Institute 2007). For people with moderate or severe asthma who experience daily symptoms, the concept of asthma as a chronic disease agrees with their experience. However, only 75–80% of people do not have daily symptoms and may therefore, may not easily accept the concept of asthma as a chronic disease (Apter 2003). It is difficult for the professional and frightening for the patient to suggest that a disease is continuing to affect your lungs even when you have no symptoms. Such suggestions may trigger images of cancer, often the only condition to be accepted as chronic and present without symptoms. The difficulty of advancing the image of asthma as a chronic disease is pervasive. Consider the large number of health care professionals who fail to comply with guidelines recommending daily anti-inflammatory medications for people with persistent asthma (Rastogi et al. 2006).

Health Communication

We communicate about our environments primarily through language. Language discordance between the person with asthma and the group of people explaining and guiding asthma education and management may affect the ability and the desire of the person with asthma to adhere to recommended and appropriate use of health care services (Manson 1988; Halterman et al. 2000). For example, Spanish immigrant parents cited language as the greatest barrier to health care access for their children even in communities with bi-lingual health professionals (Flores 2000). In some languages such as Somali, there is no word for asthma or the constellation of asthma symptoms. Other languages may have many terms that describe several asthma-related symptoms such as wheeze or breathlessness, but fail to have a word that puts these concepts together to form a chronic disease. (Yawn et al. 1999) Asthma related terms may be both gender- and-age dependent. In preschool children the diagnosis of asthma can be difficult and terms such as "bronchitis," "reactive airway disease," or "wheezy bronchitis" are used in culture where males must be strong, asthma may continued to be described by symptoms (Gautrin et al. 1994a, b; Weinberger et al. 2002).

The community environment affects language, and language impacts the environment in which health care professionals attempt to diagnose and treat asthma. A medical interpreter should be used when there is language discordance between clinician and patient (Flores 2004; Baker et al. 1996). On these occasions, the medical interpreter also becomes a cultural interpreter and must therefore be knowledgeable in areas of languages, health terminology, and cultural beliefs to effectively express the questions and answers of both parties in the medical communication. In addition, the interpreter must be willing to share patient-reported cultural and health beliefs with the health care professional rather than "edit" the patient's responses to fit the assumed beliefs of the health care professional (Woloshin et al. 1995).

Not all ethno-cultural beliefs can be so obviously tied to racial or language differences. Few who have traveled throughout the United States would suggest that there are no regional differences between the ethos or culture of Maine, Southern California, and Texas. Undoubtedly, some of the differences are due to the Spanish settlers in Texas, and the Northern Europeans and puritan settlers of Maine. But the differences are also influenced by geography, oceans, mountains, climate and natural and unnatural resources such as timber, oil, minerals, and smog. Those differences impact the prevalence of asthma, the age of asthma onset, the impact of therapy, the seasonality of symptoms, and even the acceptance of the concept of asthma as a chronic condition. Minnesota farmers experience periods of airborne triggers from planting, using herbicides and harvesting grain crops. But they also often have a dislike of conditions that suggest they personally have need for outside support – conditions like asthma that require regular care and affect a crucial body function (breathing). It is not unusual to hear them discuss the need to "work through" the breathing problems and to not become dependent on inhalers. The combination of external and internal environmental factors can make asthma management challenging even in those whose ethno-culture background may superficially appear similar to the majority of US physicians who are White and Anglo Saxons (Yawn et al. 1993).

Expectations and Health Beliefs

Expectations are another part of the intellectual or belief environment that affects asthma management. Many Americans, particularly people of color, accept suboptimal levels of asthma control perhaps because they are unaware of the possibilities of improved asthma management and its ability to enhance their quality of life (Pearlman et al. 2006). Several large asthma studies have described the current level of asthma symptoms that appear to be tolerated by American of all ages, both genders, and many cultures (Yawn et al. 2002; Halm et al. 2006; Riekert et al. 2003; Children and Asthma in America 2006). This lack of high expectations may be affirmed by physicians who often fail to assess the burden of asthma during asthma-related visits (Cabana et al. 2003; Yawn 2004; Stoloff and Boushey 2006; Yawn 2008). The failure of health care professionals, especially in pediatrics, family medicine and internal medicine to inquire about the frequency and severity of symptoms may affirm for the patient that symptom burden is not important, not amendable to treatment and that only "attacks" should be monitored and treated. Such low expectations regarding the ability to address the everyday burden of asthma may be what drive the lack of adherence to daily anti-inflammatory therapy and other self-management behaviors (Halm et al. 2006; Riekert et al. 2003). Recognizing the combination of low expectations and fears about the side-effects of daily inhaled steroids highlights how knowing the ecology of asthma can clarify the underlying patterns of overuse of rescue medications or avoidance of activities to avoid symptoms (George et al. 2003; Leickly et al. 1998; Mansour et al. 2000; Van Sickle and Wright 2001).

Health Literacy

To the social ecology surrounding asthma, we must add health and reading literacy. One in four American adults cannot read and comprehend most written health material (Kirsch 1993; Doak et al. 1996) due to limitations in reading abilities and health literacy. Simply targeting educational materials to a fifth grade reading level as determined by an Anglo American scoring tool is insufficient. Most tools that assess reading levels have limited ability to differentiate between common health-related words such as pneumonia that may be familiar from complex concepts represented by words of the same length and number of syllables. To date we have no computer-based tools that are easy to use to determine the health literacy level of any materials let alone the cultural acceptability of written materials. With this is mind, it may be appropriate to consider written materials as the last resort rather than the panacea for all patient education (Neri et al. 1996; Kelso et al. 1996; Patel and Potter 2004; Williams et al. 1998). Pictures, videos and even cartoon drawings may be more useful than pamphlets full of text (Paasche-Orlow et al. 2005). What are we adding to the ecological mix when we introduce materials that cannot be read or understood or are in direct contradiction to a common community health belief?

For the researcher, disentangling the impact of economic stress from cultural imperatives is often important. Assigning causality requires this separation. However, for the health care professional trying to provide care for asthma, the separation may be less useful. Attempting to understand how to provide care, education, and support is more about identifying barriers and finding solutions than attributing those barriers to poverty or ethnicity or religion or culture. Few studies have addressed the identification of barriers in the context of assessing and improving adherence to medical care for asthma. This would be an appropriate application of the social and medical ecology of asthma to health care.

Using Ecology to Improve Asthma Outcomes

In medical parlance, most of the topics discussed so far in this chapter would fall under the concerns regarding adherence or non-adherence to therapy and control of asthma (Rand 2005; Bender 2006; Adams et al. 2004; Suissa et al. 2000; Williams et al. 2004; Weinstein 2005). Adherence is a measure of how well we as health care professionals advise and offer therapy considered important and doable by the patient and their families. We appear to have limited success in our efforts to incorporate these factors into our education and treatment plans since even in clinical trial settings medication adherence often falls to less than 50% of doses within weeks to months of treatment initiation (Jonasson et al. 2000; Onyirimba et al. 2003; Krishnan et al. 2004; Burkhart and Rayens 2005). While some non-adherence is unintentional (forgetting medications), much non-adherence is volitional and based on patient- or parent-reasoned and purposeful decision making, decisions based on the ecology of their asthma "community" including their interactions with health professionals (Adams et al. 2003; Bender et al. 2003; Osterberg and Blaschke 2005). The two types of non-adherence (intentional and non-intentional) both result from the person's asthma ecology (physical, cultural, economic and personal environment). However result from different interactions and therefore require different solutions. Tables 5.1 and 5.2 are summaries of the published literature on barriers and solutions to several ecological factors affecting asthma management. Table 5.1 addresses issues that are often unique to children and adolescents; issues common to adults with asthma are summarized in Table 5.2.

Table 5.1 Barriers to adherence: children and adolescents

Barriers to adherence: children and adolescents	Potential solutions
(1) Steroid fear (Yawn 2003a, b; Muntner et al. 2001)	
(2) Improper inhaler technique (Scarfone et al. 2002)	Nurse teaching (Hung et al. 2002; Rydman et al. 1999; O'Donnell et al. 1997)
(3) Side effects of drugs (Leickly et al. 1998; Bender and Bender 2005; Yawn 2003a, b; Muntner et al. 2001)	Better adherence with education and written action plan vs. usual care (Levy et al. 2000; Lindberg et al. 1999; Lindberg et al. 1999; Gibson et al. 2002)
(4) Parent unsure about effectiveness of medications (Leickly et al. 1998; Bender and Bender 2005; Yawn 2003a, b; Muntner et al. 2001)	Negative studies (Cowie et al. 2004; Colland et al. 2004)
(5) Child refuses meds (Leickly et al. 1998; Yawn 2003a, b)	
(6) Forgets meds (Leickly et al. 1998)	
(7) Can't avoid cigarette smoke and other triggers (Leickly et al. 1998)	Smoking cessation can be successfully provided at all ages. (Ryckman et al. 2006)
(8) Belief that disease is not severe (Bender and Bender 2005; Muntner et al. 2001)	
(9) Concerns about dependency on drugs and need to tough it out (Bender and Bender 2005; Yawn 2003a, b, Muntner et al. 2001)	
(10) Variable diagnoses of clinicians (Yawn 2003a, b)	
(11) Misunderstanding of use and role of medications.(Farber et al. 2003; Peterson-Sweeney et al. 2003)	
(12) Cost of medications (Bender and Bender 2005; Yawn 2003a, b)	
(13) Multiple caregivers (Rand 2005)	

Table 5.2 Barriers to adherence: adults

Barriers to adherence: adults	Potential solutions
(1) Fear of systemic steroids (Yawn 2003a, b; Janson et al. 2003)	
(2) Disruption of life activities (Bender and Bender 2005; Bender et al. 1998; Janson and Roberts 2003)	
(3) Minimization of symptoms (Janson and Roberts 2003)	(3) Use of Peak Flow Meters for poor perceivers (Gibson et al. 2002)
(4) Uncertainty regarding what to do (Bender and Bender 2005; Janson and Roberts 2003)	(4) Written asthma action plan that allows modification of doses (Gibson et al. 2002)
(5) Lack of understanding or belief in value of controllers (Farber et al. 2003; Butz et al. 2001)	(5) Self management education and nurse based case management (Adams et al. 2003; Gibson et al. 2002; Janson et al. 2003; Powell and Gibson 2006) Better explanations, regular appointments and written action plan (Adams et al 2003) Physicians who answer more questions, do more tests. (DiMatteo et al. 2000)
(6) Previous experiences (Yawn 2003a, b)	(6) Continuity of Care (Love et al. 2000)
(7) Need to "tough it out" (Yawn 2003a, b; Janson et al. 2003)	
(8) Costs (Bender and Bender 2005)	

Unintentional or intentional non-adherence may be caused by a stressed or chaotic lifestyle and be sporadic or consistent (Bender et al. 1998; DiMatteo 2004). Non-adherence based on intent is associated with a myriad of reasons and may vary with age, social economic status, gender, knowledge base, health-related beliefs, perceived symptom burden and risk of morbidity and mortality, co-morbid conditions, and cultural context (Apter 2003; Leickly et al. 1998; Rand 2005; Bender et al. 1998; DiMatteo 2004; DiMatteo et al. 2000; Bender and Bender 2005; Yawn 2003a, b; Janson and Becker 1998; Farber et al. 2003; Butz et al. 2001; Muntner et al. 2001; Peterson-Sweeney et al. 2003). The solutions for many of the barriers have been tested in limited populations making generalization to diverse ecological situations difficult, if not impossible. Other barriers require solutions that rely on culturally competent "common sense" and are seldom evaluated or shared in the medical literature. This area of inquiry remains wide open for research and quality improvement programs.

The Everyday Necessities and Ecology of Asthma

Every person requires food, water, and shelter to sustain life. Each of these necessities can interact with the systems that contribute to the biological and physiological basis of asthma. Literature is replete with information on the hygiene hypothesis of asthma, and the Allergic March (Klinnert et al. 2002; Annenberg Center, YR). These are usually presented in the context of childhood asthma, often dealing with the onset of asthma. In this section, a slightly different approach is taken.

In allergic asthma, the person's nutritional environment is generally approached as the source of triggers or allergens. Beginning with early exposure to sustenance other than breast milk, foods are seen as an exposure that may hasten a person along the allergy trajectory (Fig. 5.2). Even in-utero exposures have been mentioned as potential allergy triggers (Klinnert et al. 2002). However, little research have explored the social and psychological implications of foods as dangerous or "pathological" substances. One obvious consequence might be stigmatization of the child who cannot consume any food containing whey or peanuts. Imagine always having to think before you eat a cookie from a friend's lunch or have breakfast or dinner at a neighbor's house or even enjoy Valentine or Halloween candy. Little has been published on the social and psychological impact of having to "fear" something so closely associated with a happy childhood as a peanut butter and jelly sandwich, or milk and cookies. From the ecology perspective, issues can arise from the interactions among asthma, food, friends, social gatherings, and even self-image.

Food is not the only issue that can set the child or adult with asthma apart and set them up for exclusion or stigmatization by family, friends, and classmates

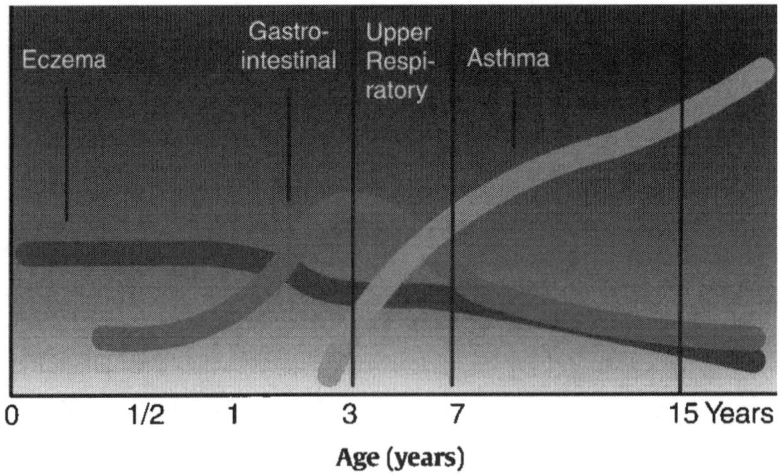

Fig. 5.2 The Allergic March. From: Anonymous 2000

(Yawn 2003a, b). Parents report not being able to work due to a child's asthma or a school's inability to manage asthma exacerbations and symptom variability. Adults must select occupations based on potential exposures to irritants and allergens. Families have to consider where they can live, where they can play or where they can vacation, whether or not they can have furry pets or friends with pets. Assessing and selecting acceptable physical environments can drive many life decisions for the family with asthma.

From the Parent Perspective

Parents of children with asthma report several concerns in their life with asthma. The medical aspects of properly identifying, and managing symptoms and inflammation are important and often difficult. However, there are many other concerns related to the child's ability to safely attend school as well as the stress that asthma places on every member of the family, including siblings of the child with asthma. Stress is a constant companion in any family with a child who has frequent symptoms or who has ever had an exacerbation leading to a visit to the emergency department or to a hospitalization. In the child with frequent symptoms, the mother may find working difficult since she is often called by day care, school, or after school care workers who are not always prepared to handle asthma flare-ups. The financial burden of asthma can be very large even with health insurance. And most important is the constant fear expressed by every parent regardless of the severity of their child's asthma (Yawn 2003a, b).

During a series of seven focus groups from around the US, parents of several races and ethnicities and from high, middle, and low socio-economic status developed consensus on a group of five major domains in their life with asthma. These domains describe a large part of the ecology of their asthma world: (1) Parents have many unmet asthma-related expectations, including being sure they have the proper diagnosis, and access to high quality care from professionals who can explain asthma, and its management in terms they understand. (2) The impact of asthma on daily life is pervasive. (3) Asthma can result in significant emotional burdens for those with asthma and for parents of children with asthma. (4) Financial concerns related to both asthma and asthma care are overwhelming for many families. (5) Parents of children with asthma often feel helpless and lack a sense of control over the disease and their lives.

From the Healthcare Perspective

Asthma ecology from the health care perspective is less well developed than it is from the patient and environmental perspective. In fact, only one paper could be found that included asthma, ecology, and health care, in the same title. That study attempted to move from the health care utilization study based in one setting, such as the office or emergency department, or one population, such as that of a large managed care organization (American Lung Association 2001; Donahue et al. 2000; Christakis et al. 2001; Department of Health and Human Services 2000; Persky et al. 1998; Yawn et al. 2004; Nelson et al. 1997; Rand et al. 2000; Legorreta et al. 2000) to a representative sample of the US population (Green 2001). The ecology model forces examination of the total context of health care, and it therefore provides useful additional information describing the patterns of contact in all health care settings giving the clinician, administrator, or policy maker the necessary foundation for interpreting the data. The point is to understand how people with asthma interface with the current health care system. Such information might help identify areas for capacity building, group empowerment, community relations enchancement, and culture challenges between the health care relations establishment and patients and families experiencing asthma.

In 1999, on average children with asthma were more likely to make contact with the health care system compared to children without any chronic illnesses: 1.3 times more likely to have at least one office visit; 2.2 times more likely to seek care in an emergency department (ED); and 3.2 times more likely to be hospitalized. For adults with asthma the impact was similar: they were 1.6 times more likely to make at least one office visit in 1 year; 2.9 times more likely to visit the ED; and 2.9 times more likely to be hospitalized compared to adults aged 18 to 45 without other chronic illnesses (Yawn et al. 2005).

But viewing asthma care through a patient centered ecology lens shows a different view of health care service use and variations in the patterns of use of

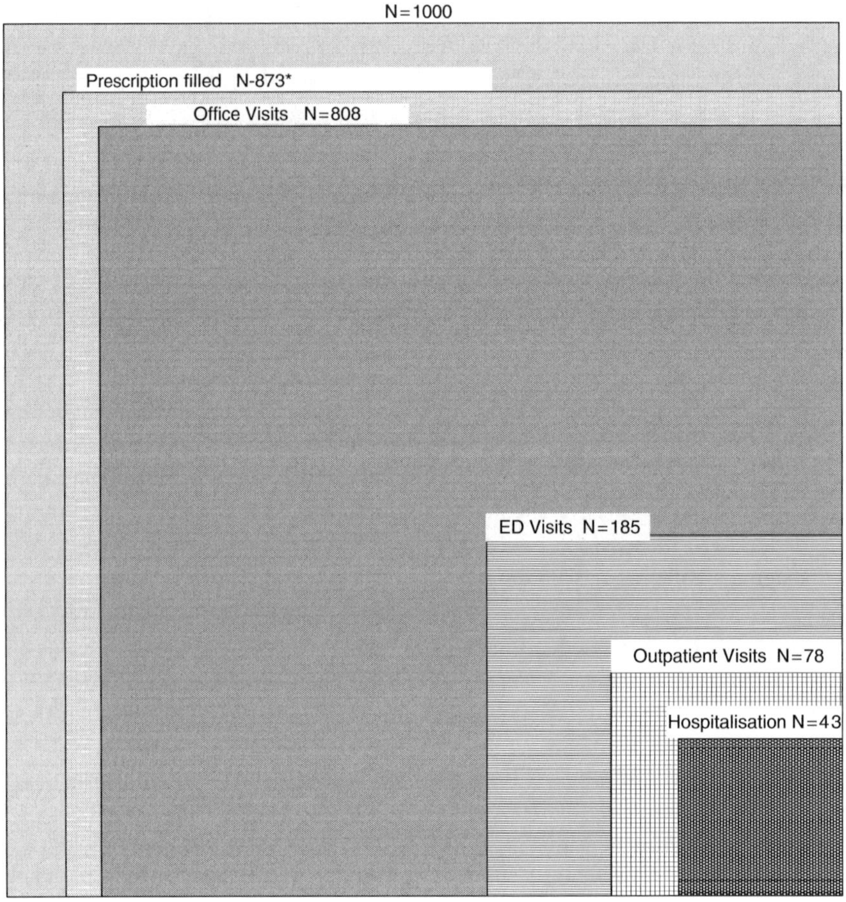

Fig. 5.3 Ecology of medical care for children with asthma

different types of services (Figs. 5.3 and 5.4). For example, data from the Medical Expenditure Panel Survey that completed in-depth interviews with a nationally representative sample of adults and the parents of children (Yawn et al. 2005; Green et al. 2001) reported that 13.6% of the parents of children with asthma reported that their child had asthma symptoms but no health care contact during 1999; 10.9% of adults with asthma symptoms made no health care visits. Overall these children and adults had the same average income, and racial distribution but were more likely to be uninsured ($p<0.01$) than those who had symptoms but made at least one ambulatory visit. In addition, 5.2% of children and 3.6% of young adults with asthma visited the ED or were hospitalized, but reported no ambulatory care visits during 1999. The children and adults with asthma who made ED or hospital visits but no ambulatory visits were more likely to be uninsured, to have no usual source of care, and to live in a metropolitan area, compared to adults and children with ED or hospital asthma visits plus ambulatory asthma visits during 1999 ($p<0.05$ for each characteristic). The adults with only ED or hospital asthma care visits also had a lower self-reported health status than adults with asthma having ambulatory visits as well as ED or hospital visits.

The ecology model of health professional asthma care not only serves to identify groups of patients with apparent gaps in care, but also serves to help reassess hypotheses related to patient characteristics and receipt and site of care. For example, the greater reliance on emergency department and hospital care for patients with asthma compared to those without asthma is not affected by the presence of insurance, contrary to the predictions of some researchers and policy makers (Department of Health and Human Services 2000; Nelson et al. 1997; Suissa and Ernst 2001). If it is contact with health care that leads to the diagnosis of asthma,

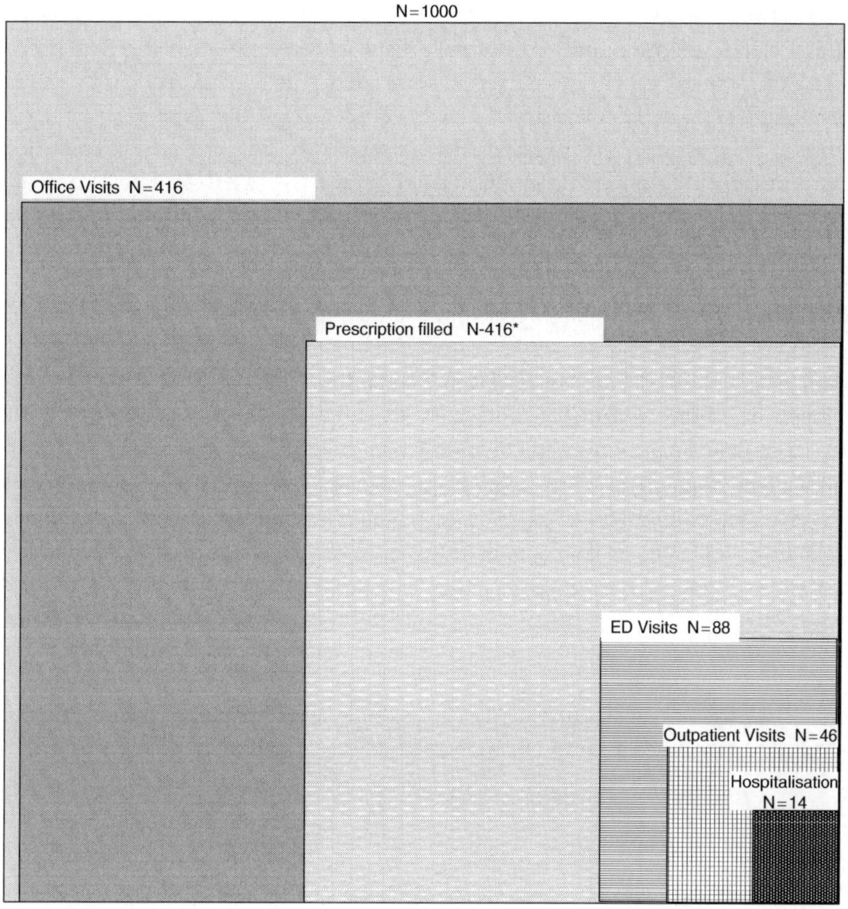

Fig. 5.4 Ecology of Medical Care for children with no chronic conditions. From: Yawn et al. 2005

using the recognition of asthma as a prerequisite for services may simply exacerbate the disparities related to undiagnosed (and therefore untreated) asthma for the estimated 75 million Americans without consistent health insurance (Olesen et al. 2001). The uninsured are often the people whose social, demographic and economic profiles are associated with an increased risk of having or developing asthma, thus amplifying the impact of current disparities.

How to Use Ecology Studies to Improve the Lives of People with Asthma

Social ecology has been suggested as a framework for transforming the impact of disease and health on people's lives (Stokols 1996). Maton suggests a need for a multi-disciplinary, multilevel approach that provides capacity-building, group empowerment, relational community-building and culture sensitivity (Maton 2000). Such a community effort requires several steps beginning with the recognition that much of health and disease is not a result of health care or the lack of it (The World Health Report 2006). Accepting this broader ecological model of health and disease often means that many community organizations and individuals will need to move outside the comfortable bounds where they usually provide care, education, services, or support. Attempts to lessen the burden of asthma must become the community and societal goals, not simply the responsibility of patients and health professionals. Many cities, counties, and even states have begun that transformation by moving smoking exposure to the center of our social consciousness and banning smoking in public places such as restaurants, near schools, at sporting events, and even in bars. This can be the first step to a "community of caring" for people with asthma.

Smoking bans require policy or even legislative change accomplished by people in many disciplines and professions working together (Maton 2000). In the 1990s, several groups moved single disease coalitions to a new level, forming asthma coalitions. Community coalitions are one well-recognized community organization model for impacting social ecology (Wandersman et al. 1996). Although the focus is on the community in these efforts, information from programs developed for other chronic conditions show that the impact must be on the family and include the eco-cultural features that affect their everyday routines. The effectiveness of programs developed by community asthma coalitions will be judged as positive or negative based on the relevance for individual family's ecology models.

Several groups of community asthma coalitions have taken on this challenge and succeeded to varying degrees (Clark et al. 2006a, b; Peterson et al. 2006; Lara et al. 2006; Nicholas et al. 2006; Rosenthal et al. 2006; Butterfoss et al. 2006; Kelly et al. 2006). The *Allies Against Asthma* is one of the largest and oldest of the collaborations of community asthma coalitions to develop integrated models of care by bringing together partners who can address the multiple factors influencing asthma (Clark et al. 2006a). Among these coalitions the term "care" is broadly defined to include all of the aspects of ecology that others have studied in asthma: medical care, indoor and outdoor environmental concerns, interpersonal support, financial burdens, psycho-social barriers to improved health and education matched to community members needs, and understanding (Clark et al. 2006a). The coalitions work because they bring together diverse groups to address issues of mutual concern, widen

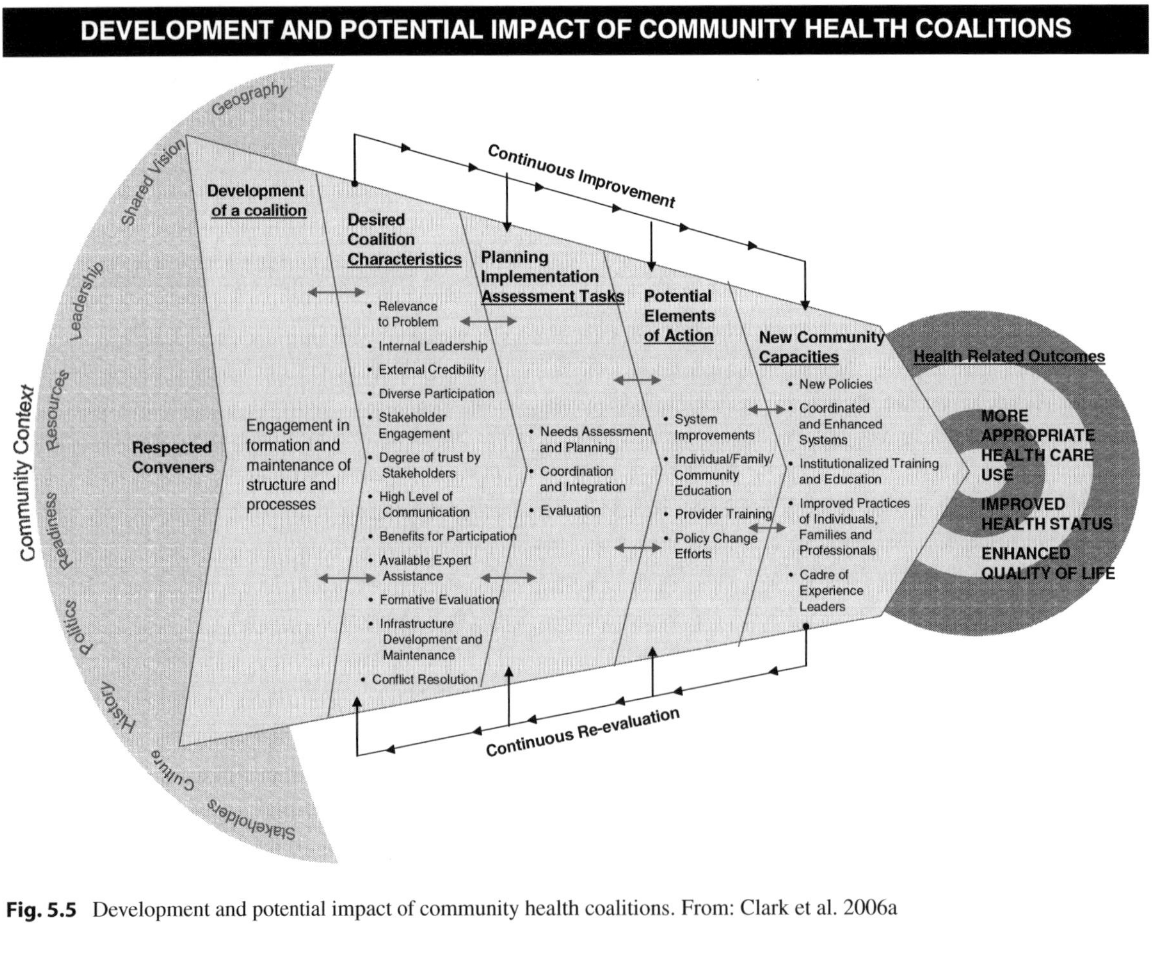

Fig. 5.5 Development and potential impact of community health coalitions. From: Clark et al. 2006a

people's spheres of influence, facilitate interaction to enhance creativity and innovation, and pool resources to address system-wide issues (www.AlliesAgainst-Asthma.org). The success of community coalitions is often based on the skills of individual leaders and facilitators and the persistence of the core group and needs that stimulated the programs. These community coalitions require many elements but primarily key leaders willing to accept the challenge and continue to work through the many layers of community change. The coalitions must use leverage points and linkages if they are to succeed (Grzywacz and Fuqua 2000). Sustainability is paramount to these coalition activities (Gallimore et al. 1989). Additional variations of the coalition model need to be developed and health professionals taught how to work effectively and collaboratively within a coalition model.

The ecology of asthma needs to be pulled together into a conceptual framework that will allow researchers, community activists, people with asthma and professionals in many fields to uncover common goals and action plans. The model presented by Clark and her colleagues drawn from the experiences of the *Allies Against Asthma* is a potential starting point for this framework (Fig. 5.5). Embedded in the context of the community (culture, history, politics, readiness, resources, etc.) and moving through the formation, planning, implementation, and evaluation to the birth of new community capacities and capabilities, this model can be expanded to incorporate the full spectrum of the ecology of asthma and serve as a road map to guide using ecology to change community and patient outcomes.

Summary

Like most chronic human conditions, asthma is the result of many environmental factors interacting with the human organism. The environmental factors must be considered in the broadest ecological sense including: the physical environment such as air quality, housing quality, and personal safety; a social environment that avoids stigmatization, supports diversity of beliefs, and personal resources; and a health care environment that minimizes barriers to access whether financial, geographic, ethnic, or informational as well as the corporal environment that maximizes use of current personal and physiological resources. The ecology models used by many disciplines appear to allow this broad approach to asthma prevention, and management. Until this ecological approach is embraced, it is likely that asthma will continue to be a major concern throughout the world and disparities in local, regional and national asthma burden will continue.

References

Adams RJ, Weiss ST, Fuhlbrigge A (2003) How and by whom care is delivered influences anti-inflammatory use in asthma: results of a national population survey. J Allergy Clin Immunol 112(2):445–450

Adams RJ, Wilson DH, Taylor AW, Daly A, Tursan d'Espaignet E, Dal Grande E, Ruffin RE (2004) Psychological factors and asthma quality of life: A population based study. Thorax 59(11):930–935

American Lung Association (2005) Epidemiology and statistics unit, best practice and program services. Trends in Asthma Morbidity and Mortality. http://www.lungusa.org/atf/cf/%7B7A8D42C2-FCCA-4604-8ADE-7F5D5E762256%7D/ASTHMA1.pdf

Anonymous (2000) Atopic factors in upper respiratory disease: Diagnosing and managing nasal symptoms. Sponsored by Annenberg Center for Health Sciences at Eisenhower

Apter AJ (2003) Clinical advances in adult asthma. J Allergy Clin Immunol 111(Suppl 3):S780–S784

Baker DW, Parker RM, Williams MV, Coates WC, Pitkin K (1996) Use and effectiveness of interpreters in an emergency department. JAMA 275(10):783–788

Bearison DJ, Minian N, Granowetter L (2002) Medical management of asthma and folk medicine in a Hispanic community. J Pediatr Psychol 27(4):385–392

Becker MH, Radius SM, Rosenstock IM (1978) Compliance with a medical regimen for asthma: a test of the health belief model. Public Health Rep 93:268–277

Bender BG (2006) Risk taking, depression, adherence, and symptoms control in adolescents and young adults with asthma. Am J Respir Crit Care Med 173(9):953–957

Bender BG, Bender SE (2005) Patient-identified barriers to asthma treatment adherence: Responses to interviews, focus groups, and questionnaires. Immunol Allergy Clin North Am 25(1):107–130

Bender B, Milgrom H, Rand C, Ackerson L (1998) Psychological factors associated with medication nonadherence in asthmatic children. J Asthma 35(4):347–353

Bender B, Milgrom H, Apter A (2003) Adherence intervention research: what have we learned and what do we do next? J Allergy Clin Immunol 112(3):489–494

Bousquet J, Bousquet PJ, Godard P, Daures JP (2005) The public health implications of asthma. Bull World Health Organ 83(7):548–554

Burkhart PV, Rayens MK (2005) Self-concept and health locus of control: factors related to children's adherence to recommended asthma regimen. Pediatr Nurs 31(5):404–409

Butterfoss FD, Lachance LL, Orians CE (2006) Building allies coalitions: Why formation matters. Health Promot Pract 7(Suppl 2):23S–33S

Butz AM, Eggleston P, Huss K, Kolodner K, Vargas P, Rand C (2001) Children with asthma and nebulizer use: Parental asthma self-care practices and beliefs. J Asthma 38(7):565–573

Cabana MD, Bruckman D, Meister K, Bradley JF, Clark N (2003) Documentation of asthma severity in pediatric outpatient clinics. Clin Pediatr 42(2):121–125

Children and Asthma in America (1997–2006) GlaxoSmithKline website http://www.asthmainamerica.com/children_index.html

Christakis DA, Mell L, Koepsell RD, Zimmerman FJ, Connell FA (2001) Association of lower continuity of care with greater risk of emergency department use and hospitalization of children. Pediatrics 107(3):524–529

Clark NM, Doctor LJ, Friedman AR, Lachance LL, Houle CR, Geng X, Grisso JA (2006a) Community coalitions to control chronic disease: Allies against asthma as a model and case study. Health Promot Pract 7(Suppl 2):14S–22S

Clark NM, Friedman AR, Lachance LL (2006b) Summing it up: Collective lessons from the experience of seven coalitions. Health Promot Pract 7(Suppl 2):149S–152S

Colland VT, van Essen-Zandvliet LE, Lans C, Denteneer A, Westers P, Brackel HJ (2004) Poor adherence to self-medication instructions in children with asthma and their parents. Patient Educ Couns 55(3):416–421

Couturaud F, Proust A, Frachon I, Dewitte JD, Oger E, Quiot JJ, Leroyer (2002) Education and self-management: A one-year randomized trial in stable adult asthmatic patients. J Asthma 39(6):493–500

Cowie RL, Underwood MF, Little CB, Mitchell I, Spier S, Fort GT (2002) Asthma in adolescents: a randomized, controlled trial of an asthma program for adolescents and young adults with severe asthma. Can Respir J 9(4):253–259

Cowie RL, Underwood MF, Field SK (2004) Inhaled corticosteroid therapy does not control asthma. Can Respir J 11(8):555–558

Department of Health and Human Services (2000) Actions Against Asthma. US Department of Health and Human Services. Washington DC

DiMatteo MR (2004) Social support and patient adherence to medical treatment: a meta-analysis. Health Psychol 23(2):207–218

DiMatteo MR, Lepper HS, Croghan TW (2000) Depression is a risk factor for noncompliance with medical treatment: meta-analysis of the effects of anxiety and depression on patient adherence. Arch Intern Med 160(14):2101–2107

Doak LG, Doak CC, Meade CD (1996) Strategies to improve cancer education materials. Oncol Nurs Form 23(8):1305–1312

Donahue JG, Fuhlbrigge AL, Finkelstein JA, Fagan J, Livingston JM, Lozano P, Platt R, Weiss ST, Weiss KB (2000) Asthma pharmacotherapy and utilization by children in 3 managed care organizations. The Pediatric Asthma Care Patient Outcomes Research Team. J Allergy Clin Immunol 106(6):1108–1114

Earls F, Carlson M (2001) The social ecology of child health and well-being. Ann Rev Public Health 22:143–166

Farber HJ, Capra AM, Finkelstein JA, Lozano P, Quesenberry CP, Jensvold NG, Chi FW, Lieu TA (2003) Misunderstanding of asthma controller medications: association with nonadherence. J Asthma 40(1):17–25

Flores G (2000) Culture and the patient-physician relationship: achieving cultural competency in health care. J Pediatr 136(1): 14–23

Flores G (2004) Culture, ethnicity, and linguistic issues in pediatric care: urgent priorities and unanswered questions. Ambul Pediatr 4(4):276–282

Gallimore R, Weisner RS, Kaufman SZ, Bernheimer LP (1989) The social construction of ecocultural niches: family accommodation of developmentally delayed children. Am J Ment Retard 94(3):216–230

Gautrin D, Boulet LP, Boutet M, Dugas M, Bherer L, L'Archeveque J, Laviolette M, Cote J, Malo JL (1994a) Is reactive airways dysfunction syndrome a variant of occupational asthma? J Allergy Clin Immunol 93(1 Pt 1):12–22

Gautrin D, D'Aquino LC, Gagnon G, Malo JL, Cartier A (1994b) Comparison between peak expiratory flow rates (PEFR) and FEV_1 in the monitoring of asthmatic subjects at an outpatient clinic. Chest 105(5):1419–1426

George M, Freedman TG, Norfleet AL, Feldman HI, Apter AJ (2003) Qualitative research-enhanced understanding of patients' beliefs: results of focus groups with low-income, urban, African American adults with asthma. J Allergy Clin Immunol 111(5):967–973

Gibson PG, Powell H, Coughlan J, Wilson AJ, Abramson M, Haywood P, Bauman A, Hensley MJ, Walters EH (2002) Limited (information only) patient education programs for adults with asthma. Cochrane Database Syst Rev (2):CD001005

Gold DR, Wright R (2005) Population disparities in asthma. Ann Rev Public Health 26:89–113

Green LA, Fryer GE, Yawn BP, Lanier D, Dovey SM (2001) The ecology of medical care revisited. N Eng J Med 344:2021–2025

Grzywacz JG, Fuqua J (2000) The social ecology of health: leverage points and linkages. Behav Med 26(3):101–115

Halbert RJ, Isonaka S, Internal Primary Care Respiratory Group (IPCRG) (2006) Guidelines: Integrating diagnostic guidelines for managing chornic respiratory diseases in primary care. Prim Care Respir J 15(1):13–19

Halm EA, Mora P, Leventhal H (2006) No symptoms, no asthma: the acute episodic disease belief is associated with poor self-management among inner-city adults with persistent asthma. Chest 129(3):573–580

Halterman JS, Aligne CA, Auinger P, McBride JT, Szilagyi PG (2000) Inadequate therapy for asthma among children in the United States. Pediatrics 105(1 Pt 3):272–276

Harper J (2004) Breathless in Houston: A political ecology of health approach to understanding environmental health concerns. Med Anthropol 23:295–326

Hart BJ, Whitehead L (1990) Ecology of house dust mites in Oxfordshire. Clin Exp Allergy 20(2):203–209

Hendrika JM, Kristjanson L, Coleman M (2003) The parenting competency framework: Learning to be a parent of a child with asthma. Int J Nurs Pract 9(6):368–373

Hung CC, Chen YC, Mao HC, Chiang BL (2002) Effects of systematic nursing instruction of mothers on using medication and on health status of asthmatic children. J Nurs Res 10(1):22–32

Israel E (2005) Genetics and the variability of treatment response in asthma. J Allergy Clin Immunol 115(Suppl 4): S532–S538

Janson S, Becker G (1998) Reasons for delay in seeking treatment for acute asthma: The patient's perspective. J Asthma 35(5): 427–435

Janson SL, Fahy JV, Covington JK, Paul SM, Gold WM, Boushey HA (2003) Effects of individual self-management education on clinical, biological, and adherence outcomes in asthma. Am J Med 115(8):620–626

Jonasson G, Carlsen KH, Mowinckel P (2000) Asthma drug adherence in a long term clinical trial. Arch Dis Child 83(4): 330–333

Kean EM, Kelsay K, Wamboldt F, Wamboldt MZ (2006) Posttraumatic stress in adolescents with asthma and their parents. J Am Acad Child Adolesc Psychiatry 45(1):78–86

Kelly CS, Meurer JR, Lachance LL, Taylor-Fishwick JC, Geng X, Arabia C (2006) Engaging health care providers in coalition activities. Health Promot Pract 7(Suppl 2):66S–75S

Kelso TM, Abou-Shala N, Heilker GM, Arheart KL, Portner TS, Self TH (1996) Comprehensive long-term management program for asthma: Effect on outcomes in adult African-Americans. Am J Med Sci 311(6):272–280

Kirsch RE (1993) Clin Res. S Afr Med J 83(10):757–759

Kleinman A, Eisenberg L, Good G (1978) Culture, illness, and care: clinical lessons from anthropologic and cross-cultural research. Ann Intern Med 88:251–258

Klinnert MD, Price MR, Liu AH, Robinson JL (2002) Unraveling the ecology of risks for early childhood asthma amoung ethnically diverse families in the southwest. Am J Public Health 92(5):792–798

Krishnan JA, Diette GB, Skinner EA, Clark BD, Steinwachs D, Wu AW (2001) Race and sex differences in consistency of care with national asthma guidelines in managed care organizations. Arch Intern Med 161(13):1660–1668

Krishnan JA, Riekert KA, McCoy JV, Stewart DY, Schmidt S, Chanmugam A, Hill P, Rand CS (2004) Corticosteroid use after hospital discharge among high-risk adults with asthma. Am J Respir Crit Care Med 170(12):1281–1285

Lanphear BP, Aligne CA, Auinger P, Weitzman M, Byrd RS (2001) Residential exposures associated with asthma in US children. Pediatrics 107(3):505–511

Lara M, Cabana MD, Houle CR, Krieger JW, Lachance LL, Muerer JR, Rosenthal MP, Vega I (2006) Improving quality of care and promoting health care system change: The role of community-based coalitions. Health Promot Pract 7(Suppl 2):87S–95S

Legorreta AP, Liu X, Zaher CA, Jatulis DE (2000) Variation in managing asthma; Experience at the Medical Group Level in California. Am J Man Care 6(4):445–453

Leickly FE, Wade SL, Crain E, Fruszon-Moran D, Wright EC, Evans R III (1998) Self-reported adherence, management behavior, and barriers to care after an emergency department visit by inner city children with asthma. Pediatrics 101(5):E8

Levy ML, Robb M, Allen J, Doherty C, Bland JM, Winter RJ (2000) A randomized controlled evaluation of specialist nurse education following accident and emergency department attendance for acute asthma. Respir Med 94(9): 900–908

Lindberg M, Ahlner J, Moller M, Ekstrom T (1999) Asthma nurse practice – a resource-effective approach in asthma management. Respir Med 93(8):584–588

Love MM, Mainous AG III, Talbert JC, Hager GL (2000) Continuity of care and the physician-patient relationship: the importance of continuity for adult patients with asthma. J Fam Pract 49(11):998–1004

Mannino DM (2004) Measuring asthma, respiratory symptoms, and changes over time. Int J Tuberc Lung Dis 8(12):1395

Manson A (1988) Language concordance as a determinant of patient compliance and emergency room use in patients with asthma. Med Care 26(12):1119–1128

Mansour ME, Lanphear BP, DeWitt TG (2000) Barriers to asthma care in urban children: parent perspectives. Pediatrics 106(3):512–519

Maton KI (2000) Making a difference: the social ecology of social transformation. Am J Community Psychol 28(1):25–57

Milton B, Whitehead M, Holland P, Hamilton V (2004) The social and economic consequences of childhood asthma across the lifecourse: a systematic review. Child Care Health Dev 30(6):711–728

Muntner P, Sudre P, Uldry C, Rochat T, Courteheuse C, Naef AF, Perneger TV (2001) Predictors of participation and attendance in a new asthma patient self-management education program. Chest 120(3):778–784

National Heart, Lung, and Blood Institute (1997) National Asthma Education and Prevention Expert Panel report 2: guidelines for the diagnosis and management of asthma. Bethesda (MD): National Institutes of Health Publ No. 97-4051. Available from URL: www.nhlbi.nih.gov/guidelines/asthma/asthgdln.htm

Nelson DA, Johnson CC, Divine GW, Strauchman C, Joseph CL, Ownby DR (1997) Ethnic differences in the prevalence of asthma in middle class children. Ann Allergy Asthma Immunol 78(1):21–26

Nelson HA, Weiss ST, Bleecker ER, Yancy SW, Dorinsky PM (2006) The Salmeterol Multicenter Asthma Research Trail: a comparison of usual pharmacotherapy for asthma or usual pharmacotherapy plus salmeterol. Chest 129(1):15–26

Neri M, Migliori GB, Spanevello A, Berra D, Nicolin E, Landoni CV, Ballardini L, Sommaruga M, Zanon P (1996) Economic analysis of two structured treatment and teaching programs on asthma. Allergy 51(5):313–319

Neri M, Spanevello A, Ambrosetti M, Ferronato P, Cagna C, Zanon P (2001) Short and long-term evaluation of two structured self management programmes on asthma. Monaldi Arch Chest Dis 56(3):208–210

Nicholas EA, Dwyer M, Murphy A, Taylor-Fishwick JC, Cohn JH, Kelly CS, Gould C, Di Stefano D (2006) Coalition-Based Approaches for Addressing Environmental Issues in Childhood Asthma. Health Promot Pract 7(Suppl 2):108S–116S

O'Donnell J, Birkinshaw R, Burke V, Driscoll PA (1997) The ability of A and E personnel to demonstrate inhaler technique. J Accid Emerg Med 14(3):163–164

Olesen C, Thrane N, Nielsen GL, Sorensen HT, Olsen J, EuroMAP Group (2001) A population based prescription study of asthma drugs during pregnancy: Changing the intensity of asthma therapy and perinatal outcomes. Respiration 68(3):256–261

Onyirimba F, Apter A, Reisine S, Litt M, McCusker C, Connors M, ZuWallack R (2003) Direct clinician-to-patient feedback discussion of inhaled steroid use: its effect on adherence. Ann Allergy Asthma Immunol 90(4):411–415

Osterberg L, Blaschke T (2005) Adherence to medication. N Engl J Med 353(5):487–497

Paasche-Orlow MK, Riekert KA, Bilderback A, Chanmugam A, Hill P, Rand CS, Brancati FL, Krishnan JA (2005) Tailored education may reduce health literacy disparities in asthma self-management. Am J Respir Crit Care Med 172(8): 980–986

Pachter LM, Weller SC (1993) Acculturation and compliance with medical therapy. J Dev Behav Pediatr 14(3):163–168
Pachter LM, Weller SC, Baer RD, de Alba Garcia JE, Trotter RT II, Glazer M, Klein R (2002) Variation in asthma beliefs and practices among mainland Puerto Ricans, Mexican-Americans, Mexicans, and Guatemalans. J Asthma 39(2):119–134
Parkes M, Panelli R, Weinstein P (2003) Converging paradigms for environmental health theory and practice. Environ Health Perspect 111(5):669–675
Patel R, Potter SJ (2004) Ten puffs to many. Arch Dis Child 89(12):1129
Pearlman DN, Zierler S, Meersman S, Kim HK, Viner-Brown SI, Caron C (2006) Race disparities in childhood asthma: Does where you live matter? J Natl Med Assoc 98(2):239–247
Persky VW, Slezak J, Contreras A, Becker L, Hernandez E, Ramakrishnan V, Piorkowski J (1998) Relationships of race and socioeconomic status with prevalence, severity, and symptoms of asthma in Chicago school children. Ann Allergy Asthma Immunol 81(3):266–271
Peterson JW, Lachance LL, Butterfoss FD, Houle CR, Nicholas EA, Gilmore LA, Lara M, Friedman AR (2006) Engaging the community in coalition efforts to address childhood asthma. Health Promot Pract 7(Suppl 2):56S–65S
Peterson-Sweeney K, McMullen A, Yoos HL, Kitzman H (2003) Parental perceptions of their child's asthma: management and medication use. J Pediatr Health Care 17(3): 118–125
Powell H, Gibson PG (2006) Options for self-management education for adults with asthma. The Cochrane Database of Systematic Reviews 2006 Issue 4. Copyright © 2006 The Cochrane Collaboration. Published by John Wiley and Sons, Ltd
Rand CS (2005) Non-adherence with asthma therapy: more than just forgetting. J Pediatr 146(2):157–159
Rand CS, Butz AM, Kolodner K, Huss K, Eggleston P, Malveaux F (2000) Emergency department visits by urban African American children with asthma. J Allergy Clin Immunol 105(1 Pt 1):83–90
Rastogi D, Shetty A, Neugebauer R, Harijith A (2006) National Heart, Lung, and Blook Institute guidelines and asthma management practices among inner-city pediatric primary care providers. Chest 129(3):619–623
Redd SC (2002) Asthma in the United States: burden and current theories. Environ Health Perspect 110(Suppl 4):557–560
Riekert KA, Butz AM, Eggleston PA, Huss K, Winkelstein M, Rand CS (2003) Caregiver-physician medication concordance and undertreatment of asthma among inner-city children. Pediatrics 111(3):e214–e220
Risser AL, Mazur LJ (1995) Use of fold remedies in a Hispanic population. Arch Pediatr Adolesc Med 149:978–981
Rosenthal MP, Butterfoss FD, Doctor LJ, Gilmore LA, Krieger JW, Meurer JR, Vega I (2006) The coalition process at work: Building care coordination models to control chronic disease. Health Promot Pract 7(Suppl 2):117S–126S
Ryckman KA, Bercaw DM, Ellis MR, Wolf DG, Elgert S (2006) Clinical inquires. What predicts a successful smoking cessation attempt? J Fam Pract 55(9):816–819
Rydman RJ, Sonenthal K, Tadimeti L, Butki N, McDermott MF (1999) Evaluating the outcome of two teaching methods of breath actuated inhaler in an inner city asthma clinic. J Med Syst 23(5):349–356
Rydstrom I, Dalheim-Englund AC, Segesten K, Rasmussen BH (2004) Relations governed by uncertainty: part of life of families of a child with asthma. J Pediatr Nurs 19(2):85–94
Scarfone RJ, Capraro GA, Zorc JJ, Zhao H (2002) Demonstrated use of metered-dose inhalers and peak flow meters by children and adolescents with acute asthma exacerbations. Arch Pediatr Adolesc Med 156(4):378–383
Shanawani H (2006) Health disparities and differences in asthma: concepts and controversies. Clin Chest Med 27(1):17–28
Stokols D (1996) Translating social ecological theory into guidelines for community health promotion. Am J Health Promot 10(4):282–298
Stoloff S (2000) Current asthma management: The performance gap and economic consequences. Am J Manag Care 6(Suppl 17):S918–S925 discussion S925–S929
Stoloff SW, Boushey HA (2006) Severity, control, and responsiveness in asthma. J Allergy Clin Immunol 117(3):544–548
Suissa S, Ernst P (2001) Inhaled corticosteroids: Impact on asthma morbidity and mortality. J Allergy Clin Immunol 107(6):937–944
Suissa S, Ernst P, Benayoun S, Baltzan M, Cai B (2000) Low-dose inhaled corticosteroids and the prevention of death from asthma. N Engl J Med 343(5):332–336
The World Health Report 2006 – working together for health. Geneva Switzerland. Available from URL www.who.int/whr/en/
Van Sickle D, Wright AL (2001) Navajo perceptions of asthma and asthma medications: clinical implications. Pediatrics 108(1):E11
Wandersman A, Valois R, Ochs L, de la Cruz DS, Adkins E, Goodman RM (1996) Toward a social ecology of community coalitions. Am J Health Promot 10(4):299–307
Weinberger M, Murray MD, Marrero DG, Brewer N, Lykens M, Harris LE, Seshadri R, Caffrey H, Roesner JF, Smith F, Newell AJ, Collins JC, McDonald CJ, Tierney WM (2002) Effectiveness of pharmacist care for patients with reactive airways disease: a randomized controlled trial. JAMA 288(13):1594–1602
Weinstein AG (2005) Should patients with persistent severe asthma be monitored for medication adherence? Ann Allergy Asthma Immunol 94(2):251–257
Williams MV, Baker DW, Honig EG, Lee TM, Nowlan A (1998) Inadequate literacy is a barrier to asthma knowledge and self-care. Chest 114(4):1008–1015
Williams LK, Pladevall M, Xi H, Peterson EL, Joseph C, Lafata JE, Ownby DR, Johnson CC (2004) Relationship between adherence to inhaled corticosteroids and poor outcomes among adults with asthma. J Allergy Clin Immunol 114(6):1288–1293
Woloshin S, Bickell NA, Schwartz LM, Gany F, Welch HG (1995) Language barriers in medicine in the United States. JAMA 273(9):724–728
Yawn BP (2003a) The impact of childhood asthma on daily life of the family. GPIAG 12(3):82–85
Yawn BP (2003b) The impact of childhood asthma on daily life of the family – a qualitative study using recurrent thematic analysis. Prim Care Respir J 12(3):82–85
Yawn BP (2004) Participatory research in rural primary care. Minn Med 87(9):52–54
Yawn BP, Bushy A, Yawn RA (eds) (1993) Exploring rural medicine: Issues and concepts, Publications, Inc., Thousand Oaks, CA

Yawn BP, Yunginger JW, Wollan PC, Reed CE, Silverstein MD, Harris AG (1999) Allergic rhinitis in Rochester, Minnesota residents with asthma: frequency and impact on health care charges. J Allergy Clin Immunol 103(1 Pt 1):54–59

Yawn BP, Wollan P, Kurland MJ, Scanlon P (2002) A longitudinal study of asthma prevalence in a community population of school age children. J Pediatr 140(5):576–581

Yawn BP, Mainous AG III, Love MM, Hueston W (2001) Do rural and urban children receive similar therapy for asthma? J Rural Health 17(1):32–39

Yawn BP, Fryer GE, Phillips RL, Dovey SM, Lanier D, Green LA (2005) Using the ecology model to describe the impact of asthma on patterns of health care. BMC Pulm Med 5:1–7

Part II
Managing Asthma

Chapter 6
Medical Management of Asthma

Andrej Petrov and Sally E. Wenzel

Introduction

Asthma is a chronic inflammatory disorder of the airways characterized by bronchial hyperresponsiveness (BHR) to a variety of stimuli and widespread but variable airflow obstruction that is often reversible either spontaneously or with treatment. Patients with asthma frequently have symptoms which can lead to limitations of daily activities, interrupted sleep, hospitalizations, and emergency department (ED) visits, and in small but significant group of patients, asthma can cause death.

The goal of asthma treatment is to enable patients with asthma to lead a normal life with minimal or no symptoms or exacerbations. Asthma has been traditionally classified based on frequency of symptoms and degree of airway obstruction into the following categories: mild intermittent, mildpersistent, moderate persistent and severe persistent (Table 6.1) (Global Initiative for Asthma (GINA) 2006). However, this classification has been recently modified and emphasis has moved away from severity classification toward classifying asthma by level of control. According to a new classification, patients with asthma should be categorized as controlled, partly controlled or uncontrolled (Table 6.2). This new concept recognizes that asthma is a disease with variable presentation where an individual's asthma symptoms may change over months or years. While severity reflects the chronic, underlying state of the disease, asthma control better reflects the variable day-to-day pattern of asthma. Therefore, the emphasis is placed on the periodic assessment of a patient's symptoms and the responsiveness to treatment. Studies suggest that the close monitoring of patients in this manner may lead to better treatment and prevention of asthma symptoms (Bateman et al. 2004).

Various therapeutic regimens have previously been proposed for different asthma severity categories. The most updated set of guidelines for asthma management have been released by Global Initiative for Asthma (GINA) in November of 2006 (Global Initiative for Asthma (GINA) 2006). In this chapter, we will discuss the new guidelines for asthma management, including the properties, efficacy and safety of the most common asthma medications, as well as recommendations for their use. The medications will be divided as they are in the various guidelines, into short-term reliever medications and controller medications. It must be noted that not all controller medications are additionally anti-inflammatory.

Medications: Short-Term Relievers

Short Acting Beta-2 Agonists

Pharmacology

Short acting beta-2 agonists (SABA) relax bronchial smooth muscle by binding to beta-2 agonist receptors on a smooth muscle cell. This leads to increases in cyclic AMP (cAMP) and subsequent relaxation of a smooth muscle cell. Additionally, relaxation of airway smooth muscle by β agonists may also involve the opening of potassium channels, without the involvement of cAMP

A. Petrov (✉)
Division of Pulmonary, Allergy and Critical Care Medicine, University of Pittsburgh School of Medicine,
UPMC Montefiore NW628, 3459 5th Avenue, Pittsburgh, PA, 15213, USA
e-mail: petrovaa@upmc.edu

A. Harver and H. Kotses (eds.), *Asthma, Health and Society: A Public Health Perspective*,
DOI 10.1007/978-0-387-78285-0_6, © Springer Science+Business Media, LLC 2010

Table 6.1 Classification of asthma severity by clinical features before treatment (From the Global Strategy for Asthma Management and Prevention, Global Initiative for Asthma (2006). Available at http://www.ginasthma.org/)

Intermittent
Symptoms less than once a week Brief exacerbations Nocturnal symptoms not more than twice a month • FEV_1 or PEF ≥ 80% predicted • PEF or FEV_1 variability < 20%
Mild Persistent
Symptoms more than once a week but less than once a day Exacerbations may affect activity and sleep Nocturnal symptoms more than twice a month • FEV_1 or PEF ≥ 80% predicted • PEF or FEV_1 variability < 20 – 30%
Moderate Persistent
Symptoms daily Exacerbations may affect activity and sleep Nocturnal symptoms more than once a week Daily use of inhaled short-acting β_2-agonist • FEV_1 or PEF 60-80% predicted • PEF or FEV_1 variability > 30%
Severe Persistent
Symptoms daily Frequent exacerbations Frequent nocturnal asthma symptoms Limitation of physical activities • FEV_1 or PEF ≤ 60% predicted • PEF or FEV_1 variability > 30%

(Giembycz and Newton 2006). Other important activation pathways have been described as well, which are beyond the scope of this chapter. Finally, beta-2 agonists may also exert nonbrononchodilator, anti-inflammatory actions, which have been suggested from some studies (Giembycz and Newton 2006). Beta-2 agonist receptors can be found on many pro-inflammatory cells and immune cells, including mast cells, macrophages, neutrophils, lymphocytes, and eosinophils. However, the clinical significance of these anti-inflammatory actions remains to be fully determined.

Efficacy

SABAs are the bronchodilators of choice in asthma and response to these agents (12% or greater improvement in FEV1) is a key element in the diagnosis of asthma. They are the most potent bronchodilators and should be used as rescue or reliever medications following the onset of bronchoconstriction for any number of reasons. In addition, they can be used prophylactically for the prevention of exercise-induced bronchospasm, being the most efficacious therapy for this condition.

General Usage

Most SABAs come as aerosol inhalers (metered dose inhalers (MDI)). The inhaled SABAs generally act within 10 min and have a duration of action of 4–5 h. A typical dose for the prevention and or treatment of acute episodes of bronchospasm is two inhalations as needed every 4–6 h. The majority of SABAs come in racemic form, 50:50 mixture of the left-sided (inert form) and right-sided (active form) enantiomers. Levalbuterol (Xopenex) is a right-sided Albuterol enantiomer and is typically dosed three times daily as needed. The drugs in this class are generally equally effective when used in comparable doses. These medications should not be dosed on a regular schedule, but rather as needed (Drazen et al. 1996).

Table 6.2 Levels of asthma control (From the Global Strategy for Asthma Management and Prevention, Global Initiative for Asthma (2006). Available at http://www.ginasthma.org/)

Characteristic	Controlled (All of the following)	Partly Controlled (Any measure present in any week)	Uncontrolled
Daytime symptoms	None (twice or less/week)	More than twice/week	Three or more features of partly controlled asthma present in any week
Limitations of activities	None	Any	
Nocturnal symptoms/awakening	None	Any	
Need for reliever/ rescue treatment	None (twice or less/week)	More than twice/week	
Lung function (PEF or FEV_1)‡	Normal	< 80% predicted or personal best (if known)	
Exacerbations	None	One or more/year*	One in any week†

* *Any exacerbation should prompt review of maintenance treatment to ensure that it is adequate.*
† *By definition, an exacerbation in any week makes that an uncontrolled asthma week.*
‡ *Lung function is not a reliable test for children 5 years and younger.*

The frequency of use of SABAs can also be used as a surrogate marker for asthma control, with an increase in use indicative of poor asthma control. Use of two or more canisters per month is associated with an increased risk of a severe, life-threatening asthma attack (Suissa et al. 1994).

Safety

The common side effects of SABAs are tachycardia, skeletal muscle tremor, headache, and irritability. The selectivity of these agents for the beta-2 receptor limits the cardiotoxicity of these drugs, which would occur through activation of the beta-1 receptor. However, at high doses, activation of the beta-1 receptor does occur. Hyperglycemia has been described, especially in children, with an overdose of SABAs. Hypokalemia has been noted in patients using high doses of albuterol, if they are already at risk for hypokalemia (e.g., diuretic use). These metabolic side effects are usually not seen with standard therapeutic doses of beta-2 agonists. Several recent studies have suggested that regular use of albuterol may lead to lower peak expiratory flow rates in patients homozygous for the arginine allele at codon 16 of beta agonist receptor (Israel et al. 2004).

Anticholinergics

Pharmacology

Acetylcholine, the most important neurotransmitter of the vagal nerve and parasympathetic pathway, plays a critical role in maintaining normal airway tone. In addition, it increases bronchial constriction by binding to muscarinic (M) receptors M3 on smooth muscle cells in bronchi and trachea. An additional important M receptor is the M2 receptor, which inhibits the release of acetylcholine from parasympathetic nerve endings in the airway. In contrast to antagonism of the M3 receptor, if the M2 receptor is blocked or downregulated, it may lead to increases in vagally induced bronchial constriction (Bowerfind et al. 2003).

Anticholinergic agents inhibit bronchial smooth muscle contraction by binding to M3 receptors and hence blocking the effects of acetylcholine. Ipratropium binds to M2 and M3 receptors with equal affinity, suggesting that its clinical efficacy may be limited by binding to the M2 receptor leading to increased release of acetylcholine and augmented bronchial constriction (Maclagan and Barnes 1989). Tiotropium is more selective for M3 receptors. Though it binds M2 and M3 receptors with equal affinity, it dissociates from the M2 receptor nearly ten times faster than from the M3 receptor (Disse et al. 1993). However, the clinical consequences for this remain difficult to discern.

Efficacy

Ipratropium has a slower onset of action (30–60 min to maximum effect) and is less potent than short acting beta-2 agonists in the majority of asthma patients. In acute severe asthma, the concomitant use of an anticholinergic has been shown to more rapidly and effectively improve FEV1 than beta agonists alone, although the absolute increase is small. In addition, there is some indication that their use may reduce the need for hospitalization (Rodrigo et al. 1999). Tiotropium has a long duration of action and is dosed one inhalation daily. It may have a small bronchodilatory response in asthma and decrease bronchial hyperresponsiveness (O'Connor et al. 1996). However, tiotropium is not indicated for use in asthma and its role in asthma therapy remains to be determined.

General Usage

Ipratropium bromide is typically dosed two to four inhalations every 4–6 h as needed. It is rarely used as first line bronchodilator therapy, but can be used as an adjunct to beta-2 agonist therapy, particularly in acute severe asthma. In chronic asthma, ipratropium can be used as a rescue inhaler in patients with intolerance to beta-2 agonists. Neither ipratropium nor tiotropium are approved for use in asthma. Of note, ipratropium is also available in combination with albuterol. There are no data to support efficacy of the combination in chronic asthma.

Safety

Common side effects include minimal mouth dryness or bad taste in the mouth.

Medications: Controllers

Glucocorticosteroids

Pharmacology

Glucocorticosteroids (GCs) suppress inflammation by inhibiting many steps in the inflammatory process. GCs produce anti-inflammatory effects by binding to glucocorticoid receptors (GRs), which are localized in the cytoplasm of target cells. The activated GR then translocates into the nucleus where it binds to the specific DNA sequences suppressing some genes while increasing others (Bodwell et al. 1998). In addition, GC bound to its receptor appears to inhibit binding of proinflammatory factors to DNA, inhibiting activation of inflammatory genes. The end effect is modification of behavior of target cells. The degree of histone acetylation may also be an important mechanism of controlling inflammatory gene expression and ineffective histone acetylation may contribute to lower steroid responses (Ito et al. 2000). There is strong evidence that GCs limit expression of multiple inflammatory cytokines and adhesion molecules, which in return decreases influx of inflammatory cells into the airway (Schleimer et al. 1997). They decrease numbers of osinophils, dendritic cells, mast cells, and T lymphocytes. The effect of GCs on B lymphocytes is modest and immunoglobulin levels may only be slightly decreased. Interestingly, GCs do not prevent mast cell degranulation (Otsuka et al. 1986) and they do not affect neutrophils, perhaps even augmenting neutrophil survival (Meagher et al. 1996). They decrease inflammation in the epithelial wall and marginally inhibit mucus secretion. Over time, they reduce BHR though rarely eliminate it (Kraan et al. 1988; Djukanovic et al. 1992a). GCs also inhibit nitric oxide (NO) production by inhibiting the enzyme inducible nitric oxide synthase. Recent studies suggest that measurement of sputum eosinophils, or perhaps exhaled NO to adjust inhaled GC therapy may improve control of asthma and/or lead to decreased medication use (Smith et al. 2005; Green et al. 2002).

Efficacy

GC inhalers have become the primary anti-inflammatory treatment for adults and children with asthma (Suissa et al. 2000; Djukanovic et al. 1992b; Barnes et al. 1998). GCs have a significant long-term impact on both FEV1 and BHR. The improvement in FEV1 takes days to weeks, while the effect on BHR takes several months. They are also efficacious in the treatment of asthma exacerbations, usually in a systemic form, leading to their occasional categorization as reliever medications. However, not all patients respond equally to GCs, with most studies suggesting about 70% response rates. Variability of response is believed to be dependent on genetic predisposition, asthma phenotype, as well as adherence to therapy (Szefler et al. 2002). Dose response curves for efficacy have been very difficult to generate in most studies of mild-moderate asthma. However, a clear dose response exists for safety parameters (see next section).

General Usage

GCs come as inhaled, oral, and intravenous preparations. Inhaled GCs (IGCs) are also called 'controller' medications since they prevent asthma symptoms and exacerbations. They should be used on a regular basis once or twice a day but can also be used for acute exacerbations. However, all IGCs are not equal. Fluticasone and mometasone are the most potent IGCs, while flunisolide is the least potent (Martin et al. 2002). In addition, the IGCs are all dosed differently. FP is sold in three dose strengths, mometasone in one (220 μg/puff) and budesonide in one (200 μg/puff). Some are available as dry powder inhalers, while others are metered dose inhalers, now primarily with hydrofluoroalkane (HFA) as the excipient. HFA beclomethasone is formulated as a solution leading to a smaller particle size and the greatest lung delivery of the available GCs (Verbanck et al. 2006). The implications of this greater delivery are still not clear. Inhaled fluticasone is most commonly used as a combination inhaler with the long-acting beta agonist (salmeterol) and a similar combination of budesonide with the long-acting beta agonist formoterol has recently been approved for use in the United States. Dry powder inhalers do not require a spacer device. However, MDI formulations should still be dosed with a spacer. In all cases, rinsing the mouth after use is recommended to prevent oral candidiasis.

Safety

IGCs are preferred over the systemic glucocorticosteroids because of the lower level of systemic side effects as compared to systemic GCs. However, all of the known side effects of systemic GCs have also been described with IGCs, but usually only at high doses (>600 μg of fluticasone) (Brus 1999). The common side effects of IGCs include oropharyngeal candidiasis and dysphonia. At higher doses, skin thinning and easy bruising, osteopenia/osteoporosis, cataracts, and glaucoma have all been reported. Hypothalamic-pituitary-adrenal axis suppression with use of IGCs does occur with higher doses, but the clinical significance in adults remains to be established. Fluticasone, budesonide, beclomethasone dipropionate, mometasone, and triamcinolone have all been shown to suppress the HPA axis (Brus 1999).

The side effects of long-term oral GC use include hypothalamic-pituitary-adrenal axis suppression, diabetes, osteoporosis, hypertension, obesity, skin thinning, muscle weakness, psychiatric disturbances, including mania and depression, cataracts and glaucoma. The rare but significant side effect of both short- and long-term use of systemic GCs is avascular necrosis of bone.

Cromones

Pharmacology

Cromones have been suggested to inhibit IgE mediated degranulation of the mast cells. They marginally reduce products of the early phase of mast cell activation, which include histamine, prostaglandin D2 as well as tryptase. They decrease eosinophils in the sputum and the airway (Calhoun et al. 1996; Manolitsas et al. 1995). However, the chief mechanism by which cromones are efficacious is not yet known.

Efficacy

Sodium cromoglycate and nedocromil sodium are representatives of this class of asthma medications. They inhibit both early and late asthmatic responses to inhaled allergens and they reduce airways reactivity resulting from exposure to a range of inhaled irritants, such as sulfur dioxide and cold air (Oseid et al. 1995; Koenig et al. 1988). They have no effect on BHR. They have no effect on chronic cough in children (The Cochrane Database of Systematic Reviews 2006).

General Usage

Cromones are less effective than IGCs (The Childhood Asthma Management Program Research Group 2000). Their current clinical role is mostly in patients with exercise-induced bronchospasm or in patients with mild persistent asthma who do not tolerate IGCs.

Safety

Cromones produce minimal side effects, such as occasional coughing upon inhalation of the powder formulation. Unpleasant taste is occasionally a side effect of nedocromil sodium.

Long Acting Beta-2 Agonists

Pharmacology

Long acting beta-2 agonists (LABA) relax airway smooth muscle and provide long-term bronchodilation for up to 12 h (probably less in severe asthma). Their general pharmacology is similar to short acting beta-2 agonists, but unlike SABAs, they have a longer duration of activation of the receptor. They include two inhaler preparations: salmeterol and formoterol. Salmeterol, a partial agonist of the beta-2 receptor, has an onset of action within 30 min, while formoterol, a full agonist has a more rapid onset of action. Like SABAs, they exert primarily a bronchodilator effect, with some in vitro studies to suggest they have anti-inflammatory effects. However, the clinical effect of LABAs has been insufficient to replace IGCs as primary therapy for asthma (Lazarus et al. 2001) and studies suggest that they should never be used alone. Nevertheless, LABAs and IGCs may have a synergistic effect. LABAs may augment the anti-inflammatory response of IGCs by increasing translocation of the glucocorticoid receptor into the nucleus of cells, which may contribute to an improved effect on inflammation (Eickelberg et al. 1999).

Efficacy

LABAs relax airway smooth muscle and provide long-term bronchodilation for up to 12 h. They are the preferred add-on medication to IGCs in patients inadequately controlled on IGCs alone, being more efficacious than doubling the dose of the IGC (Lemanske et al. 2001). Addition of LABAs to IGCs improves asthma symptoms, decreases asthma exacerbations and improves lung function (Pauwels et al. 1997; Bateman et al. 2004). Although they are effective bronchodilators when used alone, several studies suggest that using LABAs as single agents has an unacceptable safety profile and may lead to increased risks of fatal and near-fatal asthma exacerbations (Nelson et al. 2006).They reduce BHR for 24 h and demonstrate 12-h protection against exercise challenge. However, there is loss in bronchoprotection with exercise challenge at later time points after chronic treatment with LABAs (Edelman et al. 2000a). Another concern has been the possibility that LABAs may blunt the response to short acting beta-2 agonists. However, most studies suggest this does not occur (Korosec et al. 1999).

General Usage

Long acting beta-2 agonists are dosed via the inhaled route twice daily. In the United States, these medications are approved for use as a maintenance therapy for asthma. They should be used if a patient's symptoms are not adequately controlled with low to medium dose IGCs or if severity of disease requires two controller medications. In asthma, LABAs should only be used in combination with IGCs, never alone. Salmeterol is marketed in combination with fluticasone in a single dry powder disk device or metered dose inhaler. Formoterol has just recently been approved in the United States for use in combination with budesonide in an MDI. In Europe, formoterol (alone or in combination with the GC budesonide) has been also used a rescue medication in addition to its maintenance role, but use in this manner has not yet been approved in the United States. Salmeterol and formoterol are also approved for the prevention of exercise induced bronchospasm.

Safety

The common side effects of LABAs include tachycardia, skeletal muscle tremor and hypokalemia. β2-agonists have produced myocardial ischemia in susceptible individuals. All β2-adrenergic agonists can increase the QT_c interval. Recently, LABAs received a black box warning after publication of the Salmeterol Multicenter Asthma Research Trial (SMART) (Nelson et al. 2006). In this particular, trial there was a significant increase in asthma-related deaths in patients receiving salmeterol versus placebo. In Caucasians, the addition of IGCs prevented any increased risk, while a similar protective effect was not observed in African Americans. The mechanism for these safety concerns is not clear. Although focus has been on the effect of genetic polymorphisms, future large-scale studies are needed before the effect can be confirmed.

Methylxanthines

Pharmacology

Methylxanthines have many possible mechanisms of action. Their bronchodilatory effect derives from inhibition of phosphodiesterase and subsequent increase in intracellular cyclic 3(,5(-adenosine monophosphate (cAMP) and cyclic 3(,5(-guanosine monophosphate (cGMP) concentrations. However, this effect is not fully seen at therapeutic concentrations of methylxanthines (Rabe et al. 1995). Additionally, they may exert anti-inflammatory properties by preventing the translocation of the proinflammatory transcription factor nuclear factor kappa B (NF κB) into the nucleus and by increasing the activity of histone deacetylase during the transcription process (Ito et al. 2002). Theophylline has also been shown to have immunomodulatory effects on T lymphocytes. It is noteworthy that the anti-inflammatory effects may be exerted at lower plasma concentrations.

Efficacy

Theophylline should be used as an add-on therapy to IGCs in asthma. However, LABAs have been proven to be more effective and safer as an add-on therapy to IGCs than theophylline (Wilson et al. 2000). Therefore, theophylline should be used in selected patients with severe persistent asthma or nocturnal asthma as an add-on therapy to IGCs in patients who did not tolerate LABAs. Of note, theophylline does not have a significant effect on BHR.

General Usage

Methylxanthines come as oral and IV preparations. IV aminophylline was used extensively in the past for treatment of acute asthma exacerbations. However, aminophylline has fallen out of favor since it is less effective than nebulized beta-2 agonists and it may have significant side effects. Theophylline is an oral preparation, which should be administered only as a sustained release preparation.

When theophylline is used, levels should be kept below 10 mg/ml. Little data suggests that higher concentrations are more effective, but higher concentrations are associated with greater risk of toxicity.

Safety

At higher doses (10 mg/kg body weight/day or more), theophylline has the potential for significant adverse effects. Gastrointestinal symptoms, nausea, and vomiting are the early symptoms of theophylline intoxication. More serious side effects of theophylline intoxication include tachycardia, arrhythmias as well as seizures and death. Generally, serious toxic effects do not occur at serum concentrations below 15 μg/ml. Monitoring of serum concentrations is advised when high-dose theophylline therapy is started and at occasional intervals thereafter. However, certain conditions or concomitant medications can alter theophylline metabolism. For example, febrile illness, pregnancy, and antituberculosis medications reduce blood levels while liver disease, congestive heart failure and use of certain drugs including cimetidine, certain quinolones, and macrolides increase the risk of toxicity. Lower doses of theophylline are associated with less frequent side effects, and there is less need for measurement of plasma levels in patients on low-dose therapy.

Leukotriene Modifiers

Pharmacology

Leukotrienes (LTs) are important mediators of inflammation in asthma. Cysteinyl LTs (LTC4, LTD4 and LTE4) are produced by eosinophils, mast cells and basophils and long recognized as important contributors to allergic responses. LTB4 is produced by neutrophils and macrophages and its role in asthma is less clear. Cysteinyl LTs are important bronchoconstrictors and potent chemoattractants for neutrophils and eosinophils.

Leukotriene modifiers (LMs) act by blocking the cysteinyl leukotriene receptor (cysLR) 1 (Montelukast, Zafirlukast) or by preventing all leukotriene production through inhibition of the 5 lipoxygenase enzyme (Zileuton). Differences in efficacy of the two subclasses has never been confirmed. CysLR1 antagonists have a small effect on BHR following allergen challenge (Hui et al. 1991) and have been shown to modestly decrease inflammatory cell influx after allergen challenge (Kane et al. 1996; Calhoun et al. 1998). LMs decrease sputum, tissue and blood eosinophils (Pizzichini et al. 1999; Nakamura et al. 1998). They have a small effect on exhaled NO levels (Bisgaard et al. 1999; Wilson et al. 2001).

Efficacy

LMs are administered orally. They improve lung function, decrease asthma symptoms, and decrease asthma exacerbations (Reiss et al. 1998; Suissa et al. 1997). They inhibit exercise-induced bronchospasms and aspirin-related reactions in patients with sensitivity to nonsteroidal anti-inflammatories (Dahlen et al. 1998; Villaran et al. 1999; Edelman et al. 2000b). Patients' response to LMs is variable and it seems to be greatest in a subset of asthmatics in whom LTs are a major contributory factor to the asthma (Hasday et al. 2000). It appears that 30–50% of asthmatics respond to these medications (Malmstrom et al. 1999). As a general rule, LMs are less effective as controller asthma medications than IGCs, perhaps on the basis of the lesser overall percentage of responders.

LMs can be used as single therapy in mild persistent asthma (as a "nonpreferred" alternative to inhaled GCs) and in exercise-induced asthma. LABAs are generally more effective than LMs when added to IGCs in improving asthma control and decreasing exacerbations (Nelson et al. 2000; Fish et al. 2001). Although commonly used in conjunction with IGCs and LABAs in more severe asthma, there are no objective data to support that therapy with these three controller medications is an effective option.

General Usage

Montelukast is dosed once a day, Zileuton four times a day and Zafirlukast is dosed twice a day. LMs are indicated for use as controllers in persistent asthma. LMs can be used as single therapy in mild persistent asthma (as a "nonpreferred" alternative to IGCs) and in exercise-induced asthma. They can also be used as add-on therapy to IGCs as opposed to doubling the dose of IGCs (Price et al. 2003). Montelukast was also approved for treatment of allergic rhinitis. Interestingly, two studies have suggested that LMs are effective in the treatment of acute asthma in adults (Camargo et al. 2003; Silverman et al. 1999).

Safety

Zileuton and Zafirlukast may cause elevation of liver enzymes. Reversible hepatitis has been reported with Zileuton (Liu et al. 1996). This generally occurs in the first 3 months of therapy and can be monitored for by monthly checks of AST and ALT. The reaction to Zafirlukast is less predictable and can occur at any time (Reinus et al. 2000). No liver enzyme abnormalities have been reported with Montelukast. LMs have been linked to emergence of Churg-Strauss vasculitis in patients with asthma. However, most experts believe that appearance of Churg-Strauss vasculitis is caused by reducing steroid dose and not ongoing treatment with LMs (Wechsler et al. 2000).

Anti-IgE Therapy

Pharmacology

The cross-linking of IgE bound to mast cells is well recognized as a critical contributor to Type I acute hypersensitivity reactions linked to allergic responses. The cross-linking of the IgE causes immediate activation of mast cells/basophils to release histamine, proteases and produce a variety of lipid mediators, including leukotrienes and prostaglandins. In addition, more recent studies suggest that IgE may play a role in chronic asthma as well.

Omalizumab is a humanized monoclonal anti-IgE antibody, which binds free serum IgE to prevent binding of the IgE to mast cells and thereby inhibit activation. The effect lasts for 2–4 weeks, dependent on the starting IgE level and the weight of the patient. The secondary effect of decreased IgE level is down-regulation of IgE receptors on the surface of mast cells and basophils (MacGlashan et al. 1997; Beck et al. 2004). Additionally, omalizumab decreases sputum, airway tissue, and blood eosinophils, as well as surface IL-4 level (Djukanovic et al. 2004).

Efficacy

Omalizumab has been shown to inhibit both the early and late phases of allergic reactions. In large-scale clinical trials, omalizumab decreases the rate of exacerbations and improves asthma symptoms in patients whose asthma is not controlled on IGCs alone (Busse et al. 2001; Soler et al. 2001). While there are data to support efficacy when added to IGCs + LABA, the effect is less strong than in milder asthma (Humbert et al. 2005). Omalizumab does not cause a clinically significant improvement in FEV1 nor a decrease in BHR. Omalizumab has not been shown to improve asthma symptoms acutely and should not be used for treatment of acute asthma exacerbations.

General Usage

Omalizumab is dosed subcutaneously one to two times per month. The dose is determined by the serum IgE level and the weight of the patient. It is indicated for the treatment of moderate to severe allergic asthma, as defined by an IgE >30 IU/ml and documented specific IgE (either through skin testing or RAST). Omalizumab is a very expensive medication (>$10,000/year) and patients treated with this medication should have failed more standard therapy before preceding to this medication.

Safety

The most common side effects of omalizumab include local injection site reactions. Both early and delayed anaphylactic reactions are rarely observed in individuals receiving omalizumab therapy (less than 0.1%) and patients should be monitored for 2 h after injection. Patients should also have an epinephrine auto-injector (epipen) and be informed how to recognize and treat delayed anaphylaxis when it occurs. Omalizumab therapy has also been associated with increased incidence of neoplasms. Malignant neoplasms were observed in 0.5% of omalizumab-treated patients and in 0 .2% of control patients. There is presently an ongoing long-term clinical trial to evaluate whether there is causality between omalizumab and neoplasms.

Treatment of Asthma

Medication Administration Routes

Asthma medications can be administered via inhaled, oral, or parenteral routes. Inhalers are the preferred method of delivery for most asthma medications because of direct deposition of medication to the airways and few systemic side effects. On the other hand, the newer biological therapies in asthma (e.g., omalizumab) and LMs are all dosed systemically, either parenterally or orally.

Inhaler drug therapy requires that patients learn specific inhalation techniques for each of the available types of inhaler device. A less than optimal technique can result in decreased drug delivery and potentially reduced efficacy. There are several different types of inhaler devices and each type has its own advantages and disadvantages. Nebulizer/compressor systems require minimal patient cooperation and coordination, but are cumbersome and time-consuming to use. Metered dose inhalers (MDIs) are quicker to use and highly portable, but require the most patient training to ensure coordination for proper use. Up to 70% of patients fail to use them properly. The improper timing of MDI actuation with breath initiation is a common problem. The addition of a spacer/holding chamber allowed the aerosol delivered by the MDI to be contained in the spacer for a finite period of time, thereby circumventing the need for the coordinated actuation of the MDI with inhalation. This system of delivery of aerosolized medications also reduces oropharyngeal deposition (Brown et al. 1993). In the case of IGCs, this can diminish the incidence of oral candidiasis, and in many cases, improve lower airway deposition. Dry powder inhalers (DPIs) are easier to use than MDIs because they are breath-actuated, but require a relatively rapid rate of inhalation in order to provide the energy necessary for drug aerosolization. According to the American College of Chest Physicians and American College of Allergy and Immunology guidelines, there are no differences in pulmonary function response or symptom scores when the same dose of the same GC is used as a DPI or as an MDI with spacer/holding chamber (Dolovich et al. 2005). Delivery of SABAs via different delivery systems has been also studied in different clinical settings. In the ED or inpatient setting, administration of SABAs by nebulizers or MDIs with a spacer/holding chamber is equally effective for improving pulmonary function and reducing symptoms of acute asthma in both adults and pediatric patients (Cates et al. 2002).

Achieving Asthma Control

Periodic monitoring and assessment of patient with asthma through history, physical exam, and measurement of lung function are crucial in optimal asthma care. The physician should determine both the severity and the level of asthma control in relation to current medical treatment in each new or established asthma patient. If the patient is not on any maintenance medications, the severity of asthma is determined by frequency and intensity of symptoms and the level of functional impairment as well as obstruction of lung function measured by spirometry. However, the majority of patients are already on therapy when they present to specialist's office and in these patients the emphasis is changed to assessment of asthma control. This approach presumes that the severity of asthma is related to its responsiveness to treatment (Global Initiative for Asthma (GINA) 2006). Once the level of asthma control is determined, treatment should be adjusted accordingly (Fig. 6.1). If the patient's asthma is not controlled, treatment should be stepped up until full or maximal control is achieved. If asthma has been well controlled for at least 3 months, treatment can be stepped down.

The indicators of full asthma control include no daytime or nighttime symptoms, no asthma exacerbations, no rescue inhaler use, normal lung function, and normal activity levels. Asthma is considered partly

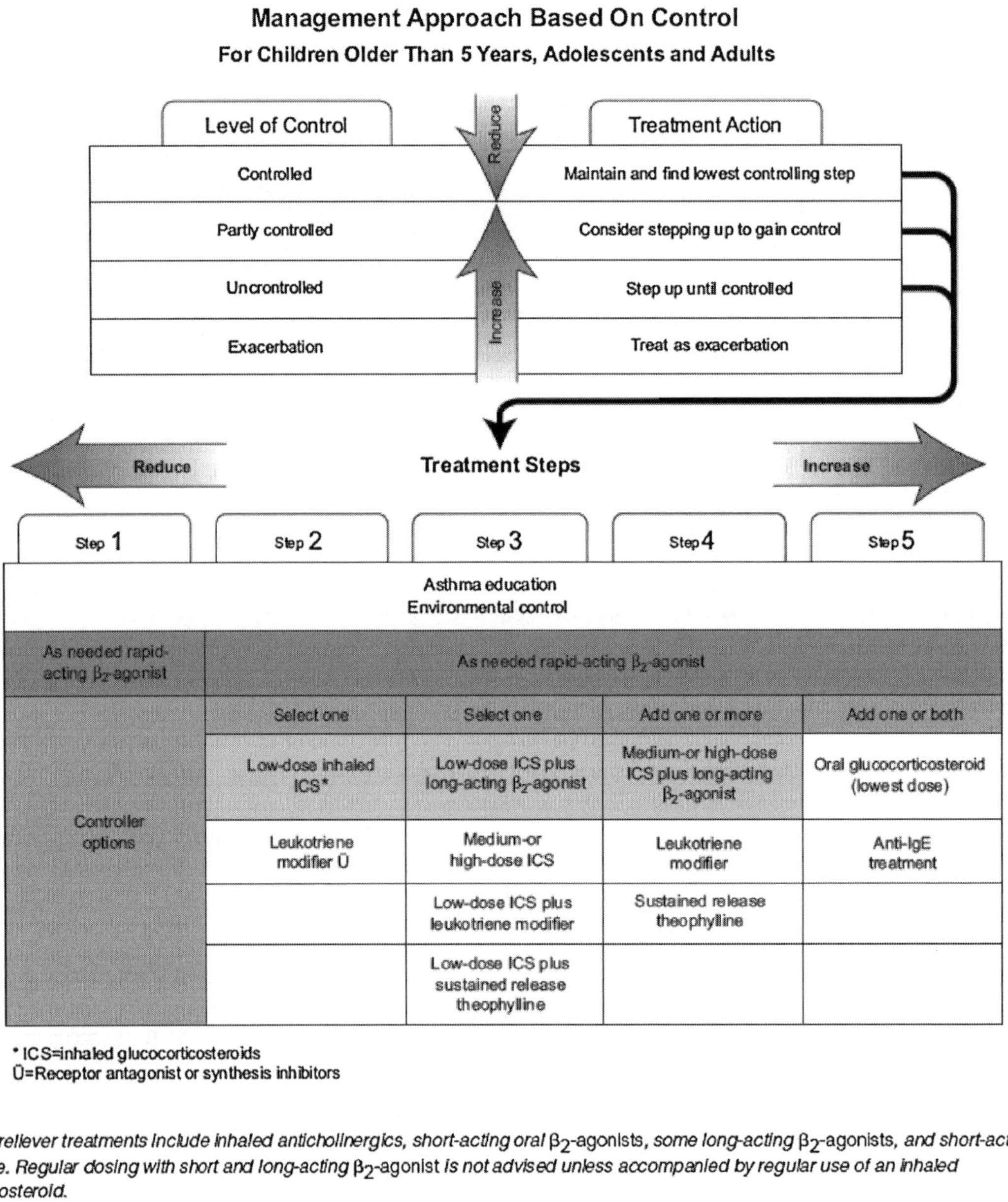

Fig. 6.1 Management approach based on control. From the Global Strategy for Asthma Management and Prevention, Global Initiative for Asthma (2006). Available at http://www.ginasthma.org/

controlled if one to two of the indicators of asthma control are not met. Asthma is uncontrolled if three or more indicators of asthma control are not reached.

The approach outlined in the 2006 GINA guidelines recommends a management approach based on control (Table 6.2). This new approach to managing asthma symptoms involves five treatment steps for achieving control of asthma.

STEP 1 treatment is reserved for patients with very mild symptoms that occur less than twice a week and have no exacerbations. These patients should be managed with as needed short acting beta-2 agonists only.

STEP 2 treatment involves adding a single controller therapy to rescue medication. The recommended controller is a low-dose IGC. An alternative approach is to use an LM. Studies of mild asthma treated with IGC or IGC plus LABA did not demonstrate any added benefit to the combination treatment with an inhaled GC alone (O'Byrne et al. 2001). Once the patient is committed to controller they should be well controlled for at least a year before a decision is made to discontinue controller therapy (Global Initiative for Asthma (GINA) 2006).

At *STEP 3*, the recommended treatment is to add a LABA to low-dose IGC. The alternative approach is to add a LM to low-dose IGC or increase IGC to medium to high dose.

At *STEP 4*, the preferred treatment is to increase the dose of IGC to medium to high dose IGC in combination with LABA. However, data from the GOAL study suggest that this approach further improves only a small percentage of patients (Bateman et al. 2004). If patients reach *STEP 5*, they have likely failed standard therapies. At this point other treatment modalities should be introduced. These include anti-IgE therapy and oral steroids. Difficult to control asthma will be discussed in more detail later.

Special Considerations

In every patient with asthma, the diagnosis of asthma should be confirmed with a compatible history, physical examination, and spirometric testing, generally pre- and post-SABA. Once the diagnosis is confirmed, one should look for potential triggers of asthma. The most common triggers include upper respiratory tract infections, environmental allergens with concomitant allergic rhinitis, gastroesophageal reflux disease, chronic rhinosinusitis, work-related triggers in occupational asthma, aspirin, and beta blockers. These triggers, if eliminated, can improve asthma control and decrease the dose of IGCs needed to maintain control of asthma symptoms (Platts-Mills 2004; Sandrini 2003; Adams 2002; Szczeklik et al. 2001; Covar et al. 2005; Harding et al. 2000; Patterson and Harding 1999).

Seasonal and perennial allergens are significant triggers of asthma symptoms. The indoor allergens are especially targeted as a potentially correctable cause of asthma exacerbations. However, it is very difficult to reduce an allergen load to the level where a significant clinical benefit will be noted (Luczynska et al. 2003; Woodcock et al. 2003; Wood et al. 1989). No large-scale studies have been able to show a sustained effect.

Allergen immunotherapy is based on the principle of inducing tolerance to environmental proteins. It has been used for decades for treatment of allergic asthma as well as for treatment of allergic rhinitis and stinging insect hypersensitivity. The inhaled allergens that trigger patient's asthma are usually identified with history and allergen skin testing.

The efficacy of allergen immunotherapy in allergic rhinitis and stinging insect hypersensitivity has been well established. However, the role of allergic immunotherapy in asthma has been controversial. A Cochrane review that examined 54 randomized trials suggested that allergen immunotherapy is effective in asthma, reducing asthma symptoms, and bronchial hyperresponsiveness (Abramson et al. 2003). Allergy immunotherapy should be reserved for patients with relatively mild allergic asthma, especially those whose triggers can be identified by clinical history and the presence of specific IgE (seasonal and/or perennial allergies). It is administered with subcutaneous injections of allergen vaccines, at weekly to monthly intervals. Due to potential for severe allergic reactions, allergen immunotherapy is contraindicated if the patient's FEV1 is below 70%. It is our opinion that allergen immunotherapy should not be used in moderate and severe persistent asthma because the risk of inducing severe asthma exacerbations outweighs the potential benefit of allergen immunotherapy. Allergen immunotherapy should not replace controller asthma medications and it should be used in addition to patient's maintenance medications.

Another important trigger of asthma symptoms is gastroesophageal reflux disease. Despite the lack of definitive studies to support the link between GERD and asthma symptoms, it is routinely recommended to aggressively treat any patient with GERD and asthma with dietary modifications, proton pump inhibitors or H-2 blockers and surgery for severely symptomatic patients. However, improvement in asthma control is inconsistently observed with this approach (Gibson et al. 2000) and, in fact, GERD may be consequence of poorly controlled asthma, as well as a cause of it. GERD may also contribute to vocal cord dysfunction which may be mistaken for asthma (Powell et al. 2000; Bahrainwala and Simon 2001).

Respiratory tract infections represent the most frequent triggers of asthma exacerbations (Martin 2006).

They enhance underlying airway inflammation and their effect may persist for weeks. Viral infections, such as rhinoviruses, are the most common triggers of asthma exacerbations in children and perhaps adults (Johnston et al. 1995; Nicholson et al. 1993). All patients with asthma should receive annual influenza vaccinations and probably pneumococcal vaccine as well. Supporting this approach, a recent study suggested that the diagnosis of asthma increased the risk for pneumonia (Talbot et al. 2005). Another potentially important cause of asthma worsening could be a chronic infection with *Mycoplasma pneumoniae* and *Chlamydia pneumoniae*. However, it is still uncertain whether infection with these bacteria plays a significant role in asthma pathogenesis (Martin 2006).

Exercise-induced asthma is a unique category of asthma since these patients have symptoms only with exercise. Effective strategies for treating exercise-induced asthma should be employed in the following order: two inhalations of SABA 15–20 min prior to exercise. If that fails, one may consider using a LM or a LABA 1–2 h prior to exercise (Edelman et al. 2000b). When exercise-induced symptoms occur more than twice a week, addition of IGC is recommended. Additionally, one may use inhaled cromones prior to exercise (Spooner et al. 2000). It is very important that patients with exercise-induced asthma immediately consult their physician if they develop asthma symptoms unrelated to exercise. In patients where the diagnosis is unclear, spirometry or peak flows pre- and postexercise should be ordered.

Anaphylaxis can be an important cause of asthma exacerbation. It is usually seen in the setting of a known trigger in a patient with underlying asthma. Examples of common anaphylactic triggers include foods, insect stings, latex, allergen immunotherapy injections, drugs, etc. The treatment of choice for these patients is intramuscular (IM) epinephrine followed by intravenous (IV) antihistamines and steroids.

Aspirin-induced asthma (AIA), also known as aspirin exacerbated respiratory disease, can affect up to 10% of adults with asthma (Nelson et al. 2003). Upon ingestion of aspirin and other NSAIDs, susceptible individuals will develop bronchoconstriction which may progress to full respiratory arrest. AIA is especially common in patients with nasal polyps and chronic sinusitis (Samter's triad), and it is frequently seen in more severe asthmatics. Aspirin-sensitive patients have an increased production of cysteinyl LTs at baseline and after aspirin challenge. While these patients should be instructed to avoid ASA and other nonsteroidal anti-inflammatory drugs (NSAIDs), the syndrome can persist and remain severe despite the absence of exposure to these medications. These patients can benefit greatly from LMs (Dahlen et al. 1998; 2002), although this is not true in every case. Some aspirin-sensitive patients benefit from aspirin desensitization (Pleskow et al. 1982). This can be particularly important if ASA or other NSAIDs are required for treatment of other conditions. However, the therapeutic effect was more convincing with upper airway disease than with lower airway disease.

Difficult to Treat Asthma

Patients with difficult to treat asthma do not achieve control with standard inhaler therapy. Their asthma can also be referred to as severe or refractory asthma. They appear to represent a minority of the asthma population (20–30%). They are characterized by frequent day and night-time symptoms, an FEV1 below 60% despite daily high doses of IGCs and frequently systemic GCs. While they often have a low FEV1, the ATS workshop definition of refractory asthma does not require the FEV1 to be persistently low, supporting the concept that asthma is a variable disease with different phenotypic presentations (Wenzel et al. 2000).

In all asthmatics, but particularly severe asthmatics, it is important to identify and treat potential triggers and co-morbidities. One should always review carefully the list of medications that the patient is taking for those which could potentially worsen underlying asthma, such as aspirin/NSAIDs and beta blockers. Additionally, the presence of GERD, chronic rhinosinusitis, bronchiectasis, obstructive sleep apnea, pulmonary hypertension, and other conditions should be determined and aggressive therapy instituted as needed. Asthma mimickers should be recognized since they can present as severe asthma and cause unnecessary treatments with steroids. Paradoxical vocal cord dysfunction is a common asthma mimicker, which is treated by addressing exacerbating factors, such as GERD, sinusitis, anxiety, and retraining breathing techniques (Bahrainwala and Simon 2001). Eosinophilic conditions can complicate severe asthma. The most common conditions are

Churg-Strauss vasculitis, allergic bronchopulmonary aspergillosis and chronic eosinophilic pneumonia.

Initial recommended treatment for patients with severe persistent asthma are high dose IGC plus LABA. However, nearly 40% of patients severe enough to require this combination of medications will not achieve adequate control of their asthma symptoms on this regimen and will continue to have frequent breakthrough asthma exacerbations (Bateman et al. 2004). Additional therapy should be offered to these patients, but there are very little data to support these additions. Adding LMs, specifically Zileuton, may be of some benefit when an aspirin-sensitive component is present (Dahlen et al. 1998). The monoclonal anti-IgE antibody omalizumab can be effective in patients with moderate to severe persistent asthma on combination therapy with high dose IGC and LABA, who have elevated total IgE and documented year-round environmental allergies (Humbert et al. 2005). When these approaches fail, consideration should be given to daily systemic GC. Once asthma control is established with systemic GCs, the dose should be reduced to the lowest dose at which asthma symptoms remain controlled. Unfortunately, some patients on higher doses of systemic steroids remain symptomatic and difficult to control. Because these patients are often complicated and difficult to treat, patients with severe persistent asthma often benefit from referral to an asthma specialist for further management.

Acute Asthma

Asthma exacerbations represent the most feared complication of this chronic disease. They can range from mild to severe and the patients can present acutely to the emergency room or their lung function can worsen gradually over time. Prompt treatment usually leads to full recovery. It is critical to identify individuals who are at high risk for asthma-related death since these patients will require more aggressive treatment and closer monitoring (Table 6.3). Finally, the poor perception of symptoms can delay care and patients need to be educated on how to recognize the beginning of asthma exacerbations and seek prompt medical care.

The treatment of asthma exacerbations begins by determining the severity of the exacerbation. Mild asthma exacerbations usually can be treated at home.

Table 6.3 Patients at high risk of asthma-related death

- History of near-fatal asthma requiring intubation and mechanical ventilation
- History of hospitalization or emergency care visit for asthma in the past year
- Current or recent use of oral glucocorticosteroids
- Patients are not currently using inhaled glucocorticosteroids
- Patients who are overdependent on rapid-acting inhaled beta-2 agonists, especially those who use more than one canister of salbutamol (or equivalent) monthly
- History of psychiatric disease or psychosocial problems, including the use of sedatives
- History of noncompliance with an asthma medication plan

Patients are frequently prescribed written action plans, which include identification of worsening asthma by symptoms, beta agonist use, and peak flows. These plans include instructions on how to manage their exacerbation. Regardless of whether the action plain is written or not, patients should be educated on how to recognize and treat an asthma exacerbation (Gibson et al. 2002). Of note, doubling the dose of IGC has not been shown to be effective in preventing an acute asthma exacerbation, although a fourfold higher dose may diminish the severity of an exacerbation (Harrison et al. 2004; FitzGerald et al. 2004; Foresi et al. 2000). Moderate to severe exacerbations often require treatment in the hospital or emergency room under close supervision. Early administration of systemic steroids has been show to decrease hospital admissions (Rowe et al. 2001a). Studies have demonstrated that intravenous and oral GC have similar efficacy supporting the dosing of steroids before arrival in the emergency room (Ratto et al. 1988; Harrison et al. 1986). It is still appropriate to administer IV steroid to the patient with severe asthma exacerbation, especially when nausea and vomiting are a concern. All asthma exacerbations should be treated with increasing doses of SABAs. In many cases, these may be the only class of medications required. As previously mentioned, delivery of SABAs in the ED setting by nebulizers or MDIs with holding chambers is equally effective for improving pulmonary function and reducing symptoms of acute asthma in asthma patients (Cates et al. 2002). Additionally, in the inpatient setting, the available evidence suggests that there is no difference in the pulmonary function response between using a nebulizer and using an MDI with a spacer/holding chamber for administering short-acting beta-2 agonist therapy (Dolovich et al. 2005). Continuous nebulization may be used in patients with severe asthma and may be better than intermittent in children with severe asthma exacerbations (Gibbs et al. 2000). Adding ipratropium to nebulized short acting beta agonist may reduce airway obstruction and hospital admissions, especially in patients with severe asthma (Rodrigo and Castro-Rodriguez 2005). Intravenous magnesium is not recommended for routine use, but it may be helpful in severe exacerbations (Rowe et al. 2001b). Patients who receive GCs in the ED should also receive GCs on discharge, preferably both as an oral GC burst and as an inhaled medication (Rowe et al. 1999).

Conclusion

Asthma is a treatable disease that affects millions of people, irrespective of their age. Patients who suffer from asthma are not identical and each individual patient presents to a physician's office with a unique combination of symptoms. The current guidelines for diagnosis and management of asthma are helpful for a busy physician because they summarize the latest evidence-based recommendations for treatment of asthma. However, the guidelines only represent an ancillary tool designed to foster better care. They are not designed to replace the art of practicing medicine, which still requires learning the "particulars" of every patient's story to devise a specific therapeutic plan for each patient. We are hopeful that this review of current medications and treatment approaches in asthma facilitates the process of determining the most appropriate therapy for patients with asthma.

References

(2000) Long-term effects of budesonide or nedocromil in children with asthma: The Childhood Asthma Management Program Research Group. N Engl J Med 343:1054.

Abramson MJ, Puy RM, Weiner JM (2003) Allergen immunotherapy for asthma. Cochrane Database Syst Rev (4):CD001186

Adams R (2002) Intranasal steroids and the risk of emergency department visits for asthma. J Allergy Clin Immunol 109(4):636–642

Bahrainwala AH, Simon MR (2001) Wheezing and vocal cord dysfunction mimicking asthma. Current Opin Pulm Med 7(1):8–13 Review [53 refs]

Barnes PJ, Pedersen S, Busse WW (1998) Efficacy and safety of inhaled corticosteroids. New developments. Am J Respir Crit Care Med 157:S1–S53

Bateman ED, Boushey HA, Bousquet J, Busse WW, Clark TJH, Pauwels RA, Pedersen SE, the GOAL Investigators Group (2004) Can guideline defined asthma control be achieved? Am J Respir Crit Care Med 170:836–844

Beck LA et al (2004) Omalizumab reduces skin mast cell IgE receptors and function. J Allergy Clin Immunol 114(3):464

Bisgaard H, Loland L, Anhoj J (1999) NO in exhaled air of asthmatic children is reduced by the leukotriene receptor antagonist montelukast. Am J Respir Crit Care Med 160:1227

Bodwell JE, Webster JC, Jewell CM et al (1998) Glucocorticoid receptor phosphorylation: overview, function and cell cycle-dependence. J Steroid Biochem Mol Biol 65:91

Bowerfind WML, Jacoby DB, Fryer AD (2003) Cholinergic mechanisms and anticholinergic therapy in respiratory diseases adkinson: Middleton's allergy: principles and practice, 6th ed. Mosby, Philadelphia, PA

Brown PH, Greening AP, Crompton GK (1993) Large volume spacer devices and the influence of high dose beclomethasone dipropionate on hypothalamo-pituitary-adrenal axis function. Thorax 48(3):233–238

Brus R (1999) Effects of high doses of inhaled corticosteroids on plasma cortisol concentrations in healthy adults. Arch Int Med 159:1903–1908

Busse W et al (2001) Omalizumab, anti-IgE recombinant humanized monoclonal antibody, for the treatment of severe allergic asthma. J Allergy Clin Immunol 108:184–190

Calhoun WJ, Jarjour NN, Gleich GJ et al (1996) Effect of nedocromil sodium pretreatment on the immediate and late responses of the airway to segmental antigen challenge. J Allergy Clin Immunol 98:S46

Calhoun WJ, Lavins BJ, Minkwitz MC et al (1998) Effect of zafirlukast (Accolate) on cellular mediators of inflammation. Am J Respir Crit Care Med 157:1381

Camargo CA Jr, Smithline HA, Malice MP, Green SA, Reiss TF (2003) A randomized controlled trial of intravenous montelukast in acute asthma. Am J Respir Crit Care Med 167(4):528–533

Cates CJ, Rowe BH, Bara A (2002) Holding chambers versus nebulizers for beta-agonist treatment of acute asthma. Cochrane Database Syst Rev (2):CD000052

Covar RA, Macomber BA, Szefler SJ (2005) Medications as asthma triggers. Immunol Allergy Clin North Am 25(1): 169–190

Dahlen B, Nizankowska E, Szczeklik A et al (1998) Benefits from adding the 5-lipoxygenase inhibitor zileuton to conventional therapy in aspirin-intolerant asthmatics. Am J Respir Crit Care Med 157:1187

Dahlen SE, Malmstrom K, Nizankowska E, Dahlen B, Kuna P, Kowalski M et al (2002) Improvement of aspirin-intolerant asthma by montelukast, a leukotriene antagonist: a randomized, doubleblind, placebo-controlled trial. Am J Respir Crit Care Med 165(1):9–14

Disse B, Reichl R, Speck G et al (1993) Ba 679 BR, a novel long-acting anticholinergic bronchodilator. Life Sci 52:537–544

Djukanovic R, Wilson JW, Britten KM et al (1992a) Effect of an inhaled corticosteroid on airway inflammation and symptoms in asthma. Am Rev Respir Dis 145:669

Djukanovic R, Wilson JW, Britten KM, Wilson SJ, Walls AF, Roche WR et al (1992b) Effect of an inhaled corticosteroid on airway inflammation and symptoms in asthma. Am Rev Respir Dis 145:669–674

Djukanovic R, Wilson SJ, Kraft M, Jarjour NN, Steel M, Chung KF, Bao W, Fowler-Taylor A, Matthews J, Busse WW, Holgate ST, Fahy JV (2004) Effects of treatment with anti-immunoglobulin E antibody omalizumab on airway inflammation in allergic asthma. Am J Respir Crit Care Med 170:583–593

Dolovich MB, Ahrens RC, Hess DR, Anderson P, Dhand R, Rau JL, Smaldone GC, Guyatt G (2005) Device selection and outcomes of aerosol therapy: evidence-based guidelines American College of Chest Physicians/American College of Asthma, Allergy, and Immunology. Chest 127:335–371

Drazen JM, Israel E, Boushey HA, Chinchilli VM, Fahy JV, Fish JE, Lazarus SC, Lemanske RF, Martin RJ, Peters SP, Sorkness C, Szefler SJ, the National Heart, Lung, and Blood Institute's Asthma Clinical Research Network (1996) Comparison of regularly scheduled with as-needed use of albuterol in mild asthma. N Engl J Med 335:841–847

Edelman JM, Turin JA, Bronsky EA et al (2000a) Oral montelukast compared with inhaled salmeterol to prevent exercise-induced bronchoconstriction. Ann Intern Med 132:97

Edelman JM, Turpin JA, Bronsky EA et al (2000b) Oral montelukast compared with inhaled salmeterol to prevent exercise-induced bronchoconstriction: a randomized, double-blind trial. Exercise Study Group. Ann Intern Med 132:97

Eickelberg O, Roth M, Lorx R et al (1999) Ligand-independent activation of the glucocorticoid receptor by β2-adrenergic receptor agonists in primary human lung fibroblasts and vascular smooth muscle cells. J Biol Chem 274:1005

Fish JE, Israel E, Murray JJ et al (2001) Salmeterol powder provides significantly better benefit than montelukast in asthmatic patients receiving concomitant inhaled corticosteroid therapy. Chest 120:423

FitzGerald JM, Becker A, Sears MR, Mink S, Chung K, Lee J, Canadian Asthma Exacerbation Study Group (2004) Doubling the dose of budesonide versus maintenance treatment in asthma exacerbations. Thorax 59(7):550–556

Foresi A, Morelli MC, Catena E (2000) Low-dose budesonide with the addition of an increased dose during exacerbations is effective in long-term asthma control. Chest 117:440–446

Gibbs MA, Camargo CA Jr, Rowe BH, Silverman RA (2000) State of the art: therapeutic controversies in severe acute asthma. Acad Emerg Med 7:800–815

Gibson PG, Henry RL, Coughlan JL (2000) Gastro-oesophageal reflux treatment for asthma in adults and children. Cochrane Database Syst Rev (2):CD001496.

Gibson PG, Powell H, Coughlan J, Wilson AJ, Abramson M, Haywood P, Bauman A, Hensley MJ, Walters EH (2002) Self-management education and regular practitioner review for adults with asthma. Cochrane Database Syst Rev (3):CD001117

Giembycz MA, Newton R (2006) Beyond the dogma: novel beta 2-adrenoceptor signaling in the airways. Eur Respir J 27:1286–1306

Global Initiative for Asthma (GINA) (2006) Global strategy for asthma management and prevention: NHLBI/WHO Workshop Report. National Institutes of Health, National Heart, Lung and Blood Institute, Bethesda

Green R, Brightling C, Wardlaw A, Pavord I (2002) Asthma exacerbations and sputum eosinophil counts. Lancet 361 (9365):1302–1303

Harding SM, Guzzo MR, Richter JE (2000) The prevalence of gastroesophageal reflux in asthma patients without reflux symptoms. Am J Respir Crit Care Med 162(1):34–39

Harrison BD, Stokes TC, Hart GJ, Vaughan DA, Ali NJ, Robinson AA (1986) Need for intravenous hydrocortisone in addition to oral prednisolone in patients admitted to hospital with severe asthma without ventilatory failure. Lancet 1(8474): 181–184

Harrison TW, Oborne J, Newton S, Tattersfield AE (2004) Doubling the dose of inhaled corticosteroid to prevent asthma exacerbations: randomized controlled trial. Lancet 363(9405): 271–275

Hasday JD, Meltzer SS, Moore WC et al (2000) Anti-inflammatory effects of zileuton in a subpopulation of allergic asthmatics. Am J Respir Crit Care Med 161:1229

Hui KP, Barnes NC, Hui KP, Barnes NC (1991) Lung function improvement in asthma with a cysteinyl-leukotriene receptor antagonist. Lancet 337:1062

Humbert M, Beasley R, Ayres J, Slavin R, Hébert J, Bousquet J, Beeh K-M, Ramos S, Canonica GW, Hedgecock S, Fox H, Blogg M, Surrey K (2005) Benefits of omalizumab as add-on therapy in patients with severe persistent asthma who are inadequately controlled despite best available therapy (GINA 2002 step 4 treatment): INNOVATE. Allergy 60(3):309–316

Israel E, Chinchilli VM, Ford JG, Boushey HA, Cherniack R, Craig TJ, Deykin A, Fagan JK, Fahy JV, Fish J, Kraft M, Kunselman SJ, Lazarus SC, Lemanske RF Jr, Liggett SB, Martin RJ, Mitra N, Peters SP, Silverman E, Sorkness CA, Szefler SJ, Wechsler ME, Weiss ST, Drazen JM, for the National Heart, Lung, and Blood Institute's Asthma Clinical Research Network (2004) Use of regularly scheduled albuterol treatment in asthma: genotype-stratified, randomised, placebo-controlled cross-over trial. Lancet 364:1505–1512

Ito K, Barnes PJ, Adcock IM (2000) Glucocorticoid receptor recruitment of histone deacetylase 2 inhibits interleukin-1beta-induced histone H4 acetylation on lysines 8 and 12. Mol Cell Biol 20:6891

Ito K, Lim S, Caramori G et al (2002) A molecular mechanism of action of theophylline: induction of histone deacetylase activity to decrease inflammatory gene expression. Proc Natl Acad Sci USA 99:8921

Johnston SL et al (1995) Community study of role of viral infections in exacerbations of asthma in 9-11 year old children. BMJ 310:1225–1229

Kane GC, Pollice M, Kim C-J et al (1996) A controlled trial of the effect of the 5-lipoxygenase inhibitor, zileuton, on lung inflammation produced by segmental antigen challenge in human beings. J Allergy Clin Immunol 97:646

Koenig JQ, Marshall SG, van Belle G et al (1988) Therapeutic range cromolyn dose-response inhibition and complete obliteration of SO_2-induced bronchoconstriction in atopic adolescents. J Allergy Clin Immunol 81:897

Korosec M, Novak RD, Myers E et al (1999) Salmeterol does not compromise the bronchodilator response to albuterol during acute episodes of asthma. Am J Med 107:209

Kraan J, Koeter GH, van der Mark TW et al (1988) Dosage and time effects of inhaled budesonide on bronchial hyperreactivity. Am Rev Respir Dis 137:44

Lazarus S, Boushey H, Fahy J, Chinchilli V, Lemanske R, Sorkness C, Kraft M, Fish J, Peters S, Craig T, Drazen J, Ford J, Israel E, Martin R, Mauger E, Nachman S, Spahn J, Szefler S, and the Asthma Clinical Research Network (2001) Long-acting ß2-agonist monotherapy vs continued therapy with inhaled corticosteroids in patients with persistent asthma: a randomized controlled trial. JAMA 285(20):2583–2593

Lemanske J, Sorkness C, Mauger E, Lazarus S, Boushey H, Fahy J, Drazen J, Chinchilli V, Craig T, Fish J, Ford J, Israel E, Kraft M, Martin R, Nachman S, Peters S, Spahn J, Szefler S, the Asthma Clinical Research Network (2001) Inhaled corticosteroid reduction and elimination in patients with persistent asthma receiving salmeterol: a randomized controlled trial. JAMA 285(20):2594–2603

Liu MC, Dube LM, Lancaster J et al (1996) Acute and chronic effects of a 5-lipoxygenase inhibitor in asthma: a 6-month randomized multicenter trial. J Allergy Clin Immunol 98:859

Luczynska C, Tredwell E, Smeeton N, Burney P (2003) A randomized controlled trial of mite allergen-impermeable bed covers in adult mite-sensitized asthmatics. Clin Exp Allergy 33(12):1648–1653

MacGlashan D Jr, Bochner B, Adelman D, Jardieu PM, Togias A, McKenzie-White J, Sterbinsky SA, Hamilton RG, Lichtenstein LM (1997) Down-regulation of FcεRI expression on human basophils during in vivo treatment of atopic patients with anti-IgE antibody. J Clin Immunol 158: 1438–1445

Maclagan J, Barnes PJ (1989) Muscarinic pharmacology of the airways. Trends Pharmacol Sci 88–92.

Malmstrom K, Rodriguez-Gomez G, Guerra J et al (1999) Oral montelukast, inhaled beclomethasone, and placebo for chronic asthma. Ann Intern Med 130:487

Manolitsas ND, Wang J, Devalia JL et al (1995) Regular albuterol, nedocromil sodium, and bronchial inflammation in asthma. Am J Respir Crit Care Med 151:1925

Martin R (2006) Infections and asthma. Clin Chest Med 27:87–98

Martin RJ, Szefler SJ, Chinchilli VM, Kraft M, Dolovich M, Boushey HA, Cherniack RM, Craig TJ, Drazen JM, Fagan JK, Fahy JV, Fish JE, Ford JG, Israel E, Kunselman SJ, Lazarus SC, Lemanske RF Jr, Peters SP, Sorkness CA (2002) Systemic effect comparisons of six inhaled corticosteroid preparations. Am J Resp Crit Care Med 165:1377–1383

Meagher LC, Cousin JM, Seckl JR et al (1996) Opposing effects of glucocorticoids on the rate of apoptosis in neutrophilic and eosinophlic granulocytes. J Immunol 156:4422

Nakamura Y, Hoshino M, Sim JJ et al (1998) Effect of the leukotriene receptor antagonist pranlukast on cellular infiltration in the bronchial mucosa of patients with asthma. Thorax 53:835

Nelson HS, Busse WW, Kerwin E et al (2000) Fluticasone propionate/salmeterol combination provides more effective asthma control than low-dose inhaled corticosteroid plus montelukast. J Allergy Clin Immunol 106:1088

Nelson H, Szczeklik A, Stevenson D (2003) Aspirin-induced asthma: advances in pathogenesis, diagnosis, and management. J Allergy Clin Immunol 111(5):913–921

Nelson HS, Weiss ST, Bleecker ER, Yancey SW, Dorinsky PM (2006) The salmeterol multicenter asthma research trial. A comparison of usual pharmacotherapy for asthma or usual pharmacotherapy plus salmeterol. Chest 129:15–26

Nicholson KG, Kent J, Ireland DC (1993) Respiratory viruses and exacerbations of asthma in adults. BMJ 307:982–986

O'Connor BJ, Towse LJ, Barnes PJ (1996) Prolonged effect of tiotropium bromide on methacholine-induced bronchoconstriction in asthma. Am J Respir Crit Care Med 154 (4 Pt 1):876–880

O'Byrne PM, Barnes PJ, Rodriguez-Roisin R, Runnerstrom E, Sandstrom T, Svensson K, Tattersfield A (2001) Low dose inhaled budesonide and formoterol in mild persistent asthma. The OPTIMA Randomized Trial. Am J Respir Crit Care Med 164:1392–1397

Oseid S, Mellbye E, Hem E (1995) Effect of nedocromil sodium on exercise-induced bronchoconstriction exacerbated by inhalation of cold air. Scand J Med Sci Sports 5:88

Otsuka I, Denburg JA, Befus AD et al (1986) Effect of beclomethasone dipropionate on nasal metachromatic cell subpopulations. Clin Allergy 16:589

Patterson PE, Harding SM (1999) Gastroesophageal reflux disorders and asthma. Curr Opin Pulm Med 5(1):63–67

Pauwels RA, Lofdahl CG, Postma DS, Tattersfield AE, O'Byrne P, Barnes PJ, Ullman A (1997) Effect of inhaled formoterol and budesonide on exacerbations of asthma. Formoterol and Corticosteroids Establishing Therapy (FACET) International Study Group. N Engl J Med 337(20):1405–1411

Pizzichini E, Leff JA, Reiss TF et al (1999) Montelukast reduces airway eosinophilic inflammation in asthma: a randomized, controlled trial. Eur Respir J 14:12

Platts-Mills TA (2004) Allergen avoidance. J Allergy Clin Immunol 113(3):388–391

Pleskow WW, Stevenson DD, Mathison DA, Simon RA, Schatz M, Zeiger RS (1982) Aspirin desensitization in aspirin-sensitive asthmatic patients: clinical manifestations and characterization of the refractory period. J Allergy Clin Immunol 69(1 Pt 1):11–19

Powell DM, Karanfilov BI, Beechler KB et al (2000) Paradoxical vocal cord dysfunction in juveniles. Arch Otolaryngol Head Neck Surg 126:29–34

Price DB, Hernandez D, Magyar P, Fiterman J, Beeh KM, James IG, Konstantopoulos S, Rojas R, van Noord JA, Pons M, Gilles L, Leff JA (2003) Randomised controlled trial of montelukast plus inhaled budesonide versus double dose inhaled budesonide in adult patients with asthma. Thorax 58:211–216

Rabe KF, Magnussen H, Dent G (1995) Theophylline and selective PDE inhibitors as bronchodilators and smooth muscle relaxants. Eur Respir J 8:637

Ratto D, Alfaro C, Sipsey J, Glovsky MM, Sharma OP (1988) Are intravenous corticosteroids required in status asthmaticus? JAMA 260(4):527–529

Reinus JF, Persky S, Burkiewicz JS et al (2000) Severe liver injury after treatment with the leukotriene receptor antagonist zafirlukast. Ann Intern Med 133:964

Reiss TF, Chervinsky P, Dockhorn RJ et al (1998) Montelukast, a once-daily leukotriene receptor antagonist, in the treatment of chronic asthma. Arch Intern Med 158:1213

Rodrigo GJ, Castro-Rodriguez JA (2005) Anticholinergics in the treatment of children and adults with acute asthma: a systematic review with meta-analysis. Thorax 60:740–746

Rodrigo G, Rodrigo C, Burschtin O (1999) A meta-analysis of the effects of ipratropium bromide in adults with acute asthma. Am J Med 107(4):363–370

Rowe BH, Bota GW, Fabris L, Therrien SA, Milner RA, Jacono J (1999) Inhaled budesonide in addition to oral corticosteroids to prevent asthma relapse following discharge from the emergency department: a randomized controlled trial. JAMA 281(22):2119–2126

Rowe BH, et al (2001) Early emergency department treatment of acute asthma with systemic corticosteroids. Cochrane Database Syst Rev (1):CD002178

Rowe BH, Edmonds ML, Spooner CH, Camargo CA (2001b) Evidence-based treatments for acute asthma. Respir Care 46(12):1380–1390

Sandrini A (2003) Effect of nasal triamcinolone acetonide on lower airway inflammatory markers in patients with allergic rhinitis. J Allergy Clin Immunol 111(2):313–320

Schleimer RP, Beck L, Schwiebert L et al (1997) Inhibition of inflammatory cell recruitment by glucocorticoids: cytokines as primary targets. In: Schleimer RP, Busse WW, O'Byrne P (eds) Topical glucocorticoids in asthma: mechanisms and clinical actions. Marcel Dekker, New York, p 203

Silverman RA, Miller CJ, Chen Y et al (1999) Zafirlukast reduces relapses and treatment failures after an acute asthma episode. Chest 116:296S

Smith AD, Cowan JO, Brassett KP, Herbison GP, Taylor DR (2005) Use of exhaled nitric oxide measurements to guide treatment in chronic asthma. N Engl J Med 352:2163–2173

Soler M, Matz J, Townley R, Buhl R, O'Brien J, Fox H, Thirlwell J, Gupta N, Della Cioppa G (2001) The anti-IgE antibody omalizumab reduces exacerbations and steroid requirement in allergic asthmatics. Eur Respir J 18:254–261

Spooner CH, Saunders LD, Rowe BH (2000) Nedocromil sodium for preventing exercise-induced bronchoconstriction. Cochrane Database Syst Rev (2):CD001183

Suissa S, Blais L, Ernst P (1994) Patterns of increasing beta-agonist use and the risk of fatal or near-fatal asthma. Eur Respir J 7:1602–1609

Suissa S, Dennis R, Ernst P et al (1997) Effectiveness of the leukotriene receptor antagonist zafirlukast for mild-to-moderate asthma: a randomized, double-blind, placebo-controlled trial. Ann Intern Med 126:177

Suissa S, Ernst P, Benayoun S, Baltzan M, Cai B (2000) Low-dose inhaled corticosteroids and the prevention of death from asthma. N Engl J Med 343:332–336

Szczeklik A, Nizankowska E, Bochenek G, Nagraba K, Mejza F, Swierczynska M (2001) Safety of a specific COX-2 inhibitor in aspirin-induced asthma. Clin Exp Allergy 31(2):219–225

Szefler S, Martin R, King T, Boushey H, Cherniack R, Chinchilli V, Craig T, Dolovich M, Drazen J, Fagan J, Fahy J, Fish J, Ford J, Israel E, Kiley J, Kraft M, Lazarus S, Lemanske R, Mauger E, Peters S, Sorkness C, for the Asthma Clinical Research Network (2002) Significant variability in response to inhaled corticosteroids for persistent asthma. J Allergy Clin Immunol 109:410–418

Talbot TR, Hartert TV, Mitchel E, Halasa NB, Arbogast PG, Poehling KA, Schaffner W, Craig AS, Griffin MR (2005) Asthma as a Risk Factor for Invasive Pneumococcal Disease. N Engl J Med 352:2082–2090

The Cochrane Database of Systematic Reviews Volume (4), 2006

Verbanck S, Schuermans D, Paiva M, Vincken W (2006) The functional benefit of anti-inflammatory aerosols in the lung periphery. J Allergy Clin Immunol 118:340–346

Villaran C, O'Neill SJ, Helbling A et al (1999) Montelukast versus salmeterol in patients with asthma and exercise-induced bronchoconstriction. J Allergy Clin Immunol 104:547

Wechsler ME, Finn D, Gunawardena D et al (2000) Churg-Strauss syndrome in patients receiving montelukast as treatment for asthma. Chest 117:708

Wenzel SE et al (2000) ATS Workshop. Am J Respir Crit Care Med 162:2342

Wilson AJ, Gibson PG, Coughlan J (2000) Long acting beta-agonists versus theophylline for maintenance treatment of asthma. Cochrane Database Syst Rev CD001281

Wilson AM, Dempsey OJ, Sims EJ et al (2001) A comparison of topical budesonide and oral montelukast in seasonal allergic rhinitis and asthma. Clin Exp Allergy 31:616

Wood RA, Chapman MD, Adkinson NF Jr, Eggleston PA (1989) The effect of cat removal on allergen content in household-dust samples. J Allergy Clin Immunol 83(4): 730–734

Woodcock A, Forster L, Matthews E, Martin J, Letley L, Vickers M et al (2003) Control of exposure to mite allergen and allergenimpermeable bed covers for adults with asthma. N Engl J Med 349(3):225–236

Chapter 7
Impact of Medication Delivery Method on Patient Adherence

Bruce G. Bender, Vasilisa Sazonov, and Karl J. Krobot

Synopsis

In this chapter, we provide a systematic review of randomized controlled trials, meta-analysis, case-control, or cohort studies that compared patient adherence with, or preference for, oral or inhaled controller medication for asthma. Among 17 studies meeting inclusion criteria for our review, patients were more adherent to oral than inhaled medications. Where queried, patients or parents expressed preference for oral medications. These findings were consistent across study designs, using contrasting measures of adherence, over varied time periods and including many with 12-month follow-up, and with patients who knew they were being monitored as well as those included in an anonymous database. Indirect evidence indicates that patient's preference for oral medication is not related to dosing frequency.

Introduction

Many patients with asthma are not adherent with treatment. Despite more than a decade of evidence-based physician guidelines for the management of asthma, hospitalization and emergency department visits for asthma remain high. Large, multinational, community-based surveys of asthma have shown that the majority of asthma patients suffer from alarmingly high rates of symptoms and disruption of life from their disease (Adams et al. 2002; Lai et al. 2003; Rabe et al. 2004). The tools to control asthma and prevent hospitalization are in place. Daily controller medicine can effectively treat most asthma symptoms, reducing airway inflammation and health care utilization (Szefler et al. 2000; Masoli et al. 2004; Schatz et al. 2003; Bateman et al. 2004). However, even the most effective medications have little value if not taken as prescribed.

Adherence to inhaled corticosteroids (ICS) in real-world settings is poor in all patient groups and across countries (Cerveri et al. 1999; DiMatteo et al. 2002; Melnikow and Kiefe 1994). Estimates of adherence rates to therapeutic recommendations in long-term medical regimens range from 40 to 65% (Adherence to long-term therapies: Evidence for action 2003). Children with asthma frequently receive less than half of their prescribed ICS treatments (Walders et al. 2005; McQuaid et al. 2003; Gibson et al. 1995; Coutts et al. 1992; Creer and Bender 1993). Similar findings have been reported for adult patients (Beardon 1993; Barr et al. 2002; Rand and Wise 1996).

Poor adherence leads to poor asthma control. A recent study demonstrated that in a cohort of 405 adults with asthma from a large health maintenance organization, overall adherence to ICS was approximately 50%. Lower adherence to ICS was associated with increasing numbers of oral steroid fills, emergency department visits, and asthma-related hospitalizations (Williams et al. 2004). Patients with a visit to the emergency department for exacerbation of asthma increased their medication adherence only temporarily before quickly returning to baseline rates (Stempel et al. 2004). Similarly, less than half of corticosteroid prescriptions were filled after children were hospitalized for asthma (Cooper and Hickson 2001). Under-utilization of ICS has been repeatedly linked to poor asthma control, reflected in increased symptoms, hospitalization, and asthma-related death (Suissa et al. 2000; Donahue et al. 1997; Williams et al. 2004).

B.G. Bender (✉)
Pediatric Behavioral Health, National Jewish Medical and Research Center, 1400 Jackson St, Denver, CO, 80206, USA
e-mail: benderb@njc.org

A. Harver and H. Kotses (eds.), *Asthma, Health and Society: A Public Health Perspective*,
DOI 10.1007/978-0-387-78285-0_7, © Springer Science+Business Media, LLC 2010

Multiple, complex factors influence patient adherence. Understanding of the illness, socioeconomic status, race, lifestyle, physician behavior, symptoms, medication cost, patient mental health, and side-effect potential have all been identified as variables that affect adherence (Rand 2005; Winnick et al. 2005; Apter et al. 1998, 2003). Patients' perception of their illness and treatment also clearly account for variability in adherence behavior. In one conceptualization, patients weigh their assessment of a medication's *necessity* against their *concerns* about it; adherence improves with the degree that the former exceeds the latter (Horne and Weinman 1999). Regardless of physician instructions, patients' beliefs about their illness and their requirement for medication are strongly correlated with their adherence motivation (Bender and Bender 2005).

Treatment characteristics can also influence adherence. Treatments that are easier to take and are better accepted by patients, and thus invite improved adherence. As treatment regimens call for more than two medication doses daily, adherence declines. A dramatic drop in adherence was observed at higher dosing frequencies in a study that randomized epileptic patients receiving the same oral tablet anti-seizure medication into four daily dosing groups – qd, bid, tid, and qid. Adherence decreased to 87, 81, 77, and 39%, respectively, with dramatically decreased adherence when dosing requirements reached four times daily (Cramer et al. 1989).

There is evidence that asthma patients prefer oral to inhaled medications, and that this preference may result in greater adherence with oral medication. In the current review, we sought to assess the collective evidence regarding patient preference for, and adherence to, oral medications in contrast to inhaled medications for asthma. We therefore searched for all randomized controlled trials, meta-analyses, case-control, and cohort studies in which asthma medication adherence or preference were measured and contrasted between these two classes of medications.

Approach

Criteria for studies to be included in this systematic review were as follows:

1. Address adherence/compliance/persistence with any leukotriene antagonist, theophylline, ICS, or oral corticosteroids.
2. Contrast adherence/compliance/persistence with multiple controller medications, including oral and inhaled medication.
3. Include a measure of adherence/compliance/persistence or satisfaction.
4. Include data from a pharmacy database, RCT, meta-analysis, case-control, cohort, or observational study.

The following databases and Boolian search strategies were used to find articles related to asthma-therapy-adherence and drug-delivery-methods: MEDLINE (1966 to July Week 3 2005); HealthSTAR (1966 to June 2005); and Cumulative Index to Nursing & Allied Health Literature (CINAHL, 1982 to July Week 4 2005). Citations were identified using the following National Library of Medicine's "Medical Subject Headings" and truncated text-words, located in the title and/or abstract of the article ("exp" in front of a Medical Subject Heading retrieves its narrower terms):

> (attitude to health/OR health knowledge, attitudes, practice/ OR patient acceptance of health care/OR patient compliance/OR patient participation/OR patient satisfaction/OR treatment refusal/OR sick role/OR patient dropouts/OR health behavior/OR patient education/) OR [(patient$) 2-word adjacency (prefer$ OR adher$ OR complian$)] OR (non-adher$ OR non-complia$) AND (exp dosage forms/OR exp drug delivery systems/OR exp drug administration routes/OR exp pharmaceutical preparations/OR prescriptions, drug/OR drug administration schedule/OR exp aerosols/OR exp "nebulizers and vaporizers"/OR self administration/OR self medication/)OR [(dose$ OR dosing OR dosages$ OR medications$ OR drug$) 2-word adjacency (characteristic$ OR frequenc$ OR form$)] OR (inhal$ OR nebuliz$ OR spray$) OR (drug delivery) AND exp asthma/(as a major topic) AND English AND human.

The following additional databases were also employed to identify articles related to asthma-therapy-adherence and drug-delivery-methods: Cochrane Database of Systematic Reviews (third Quarter 2005); ACP Journal Club (1991 to May/June 2005); Database of Abstracts of Reviews of Effects (second Quarter 2005); Cochrane Central Register of Controlled Trials (third Quarter 2005); Allied and Complementary Medicine (AMED, 1985 to July 2005); International Pharmaceutical Abstracts (1970 to July 2005); and PsycINFO (2000 to July Week 4 2005).

Citations were identified using the following search strategy:

(comply or complian$ or adher$ or refus$ or dropout$ or non-adher$ or non-compl$) AND asthma$.

Reference lists in each obtained article were searched for additional relevant articles not identified through the database search. The following information was abstracted from articles meeting inclusion criteria: study population, number of subjects, study design, study duration, outcome measures, and results. Additionally, the scientific quality of each article was rated using the criteria of Harbour and Miller (2001).

Although "adherence" and "compliance" are used interchangeably in the published literature, the term adherence has been adopted here. Adherence is generally defined as the amount of medication divided by the amount prescribed. Some of the identified studies provided this information expressed as percent adherence whether the amount of medication used was measured through electronic device (Krishnan et al. 2004) or self report (Bukstein et al. 2003b) in prospective studies, or as days or doses of medication filled in pharmacy claims studies (Dorais et al. 2005; Sherman et al. 2001). Other studies measured adherence as the percent of adherent patients (Balkrishnan et al. 2005) or mean number of refill obtained over 12 months (Bukstein et al. 2003a).

Results

Utilizing the search strategy described above and after de-duplication, 2,104 published articles were identified.

Titles from each article were reviewed. Those that clearly did not meet inclusion criteria were omitted. When criteria for exclusion for the remaining articles could not be cleanly identified in the abstracts, articles were included for full review. Following this procedure, the texts of 29 articles qualified for full review. These consisted of articles that examined adherence with, or preference for, oral or inhaled controller medication in a pharmacy database, RCT, meta-analysis, case-control, cohort, or observational study.

Twelve of the 29 articles were omitted from the final analysis because upon full review they did not meet inclusion criteria. Of these, nine included only one medication and hence allowed for no comparison between medications. Three included no measure of adherence.

Of the final 17 articles meeting inclusion criteria, 8 were pharmacy claims studies, 5 were RCTs, 2 were cohort studies, and 1 each were health maintenance organization claims or questionnaire studies (Table 7.1). All included comparisons between medications delivered orally or by inhalation. The oral medications included leukotriene antagonists (LTRA) in 12 studies, theophylline in three studies (one also including oxatomide and ketotifen), and oral corticosteroid in one study, with "tablet medication" included in a survey of medication delivery preference (Tuggey et al. 2001). Inhaled corticosteroid (ICS) medications were evaluated in 14 studies. Cromolyn sodium was included in four studies, two of which also included ICS, and "inhaler treatment" in a survey of medication delivery preference (Tuggey et al. 2001).

Regardless of study design, medication category, or method of measurement, patients expressed a preference for or used oral medications more often than inhaled medications. This difference occurred in both adult and pediatric asthma populations. In the one pharmacy claims study where mean obtained doses of montelukast did not significantly exceed ICS refills, the proportion of montelukast-adherent patients (51%) was still significantly greater than the proportion adherent with ICS (41%) (Carter and Ananthakrishnan 2003). Preference for oral medication over ICS was consistent despite considerable differences in the characteristics of theophylline, montelukast, or oral steroid. One exception to this finding documented higher self-reported adherence to oxatomide and ketotifen, but not theophylline, over ICS (Alessandro et al. 1994). Additionally, the only study examining adherence to oral and inhaled steroids found that, while mean oral adherence was higher, over time differences between the two disappeared (Krishnan et al. 2004).

Discussion

Patients appear more willing to take oral over inhaled medication for asthma. The 17 studies included in this systematic review produced a consistent picture of superior adherence with oral medication despite markedly different research designs that included RCT, cohort, retrospective pharmacy claims, and questionnaire studies. In most cases, differences were large, with some studies reporting oral medication adherence

[AU1]

Table 7.1 Adherence related to oral versus Inhaled medication for asthma

References	Population	Design	Duration	Outcomes measured	Key findings (with 95% CI, SD, or SEM if reported)	Scientific quality	Comment
Alessandro et al. (1994)	288 children with asthma	Prospective cohort study	30–45 days	Self-reported adherence	% fully adherent patients: Oral medications (theophylline, oxatomide, ketotifen) = 71.1% Inhaled Medications (cromolyn, beclomethasone) = 59.0%	2–	Only patient-reported data were included
Balkrishnan et al. (2005)	710 asthma patients, 2–64 years	Retrospective Medicaid claims study	12 months	Refills	% adherent patients: Montelukast = 18% Fluticasone = 9%	2–	No mean adherence data provided
Bukstein et al. (2003a)	343 asthma patients, 3–83 years	Retrospective pharmacy claims study	12 months	Refills, healthcare utilization	Means refills in 1 year: Montelukast = 5.1 Fluticasone = 3.1 No group difference in health outcomes	2+	
Bukstein et al. (2003b)	33 asthma patients, 6–11 years	RCT, open label, crossover	10 weeks	Parental self-reported adherence and preference	Mean % days of adherence: Montelukast = 96.3% Cromolyn = 79.7% Reported preference: Montelukast = 87% Cromolyn = 12%	1–	Only parent-reported data were provided;
Carter and Ananthakrishnan (2003)	141 asthma patients, 3–18	Retrospective pharmacy claims study; diagnosis confirmed by chart review	6 months	Refill adherence	Mean adherence (doses filled/ prescribed): Montelukast = 71% (CI=65–77) ICS=67% (CI=61–73) % adherent patients: Montelukast = 51% Fluticasone = 41%	2+	Includes pharmacy claims data only
Dorais et al. (2005)	2,529 asthma patients, 15–45 years	Retrospective pharmacy claims study	12 months	Refills	Mean adherence (days of medication obtained divided by 365) LTRA = 38 ICS = 19	2+	Includes pharmacy claims data only
Jones et al. (2003)	23,225 asthma patients, 6–55 years	Retrospective pharmacy claims study	12 months	Refills	Mean adherence (doses filled/ prescribed): LTRA = 67.7%, ICS = 33.8%, LABA = 40.0%	2+	Includes pharmacy claims data only

Kelloway et al. (1994)	276 asthma patients, 12–65 years	Retrospective pharmacy claims study; diagnosis confirmed by chart review	12 months	Refills	Mean (±SD) adherence (doses filled/prescribed): Theophylline = 79 ± 34% ICS = 54 ± 43% Cromolyn = 44 ± 34%	2+	Includes pharmacy claims data only
Krishnan et al. (2004)	Adults recently discharged from asthma hospitalization	Prospective cohort study	2 weeks	Electronic measurement of inhaled and oral corticosteroid use	Mean (±SEM) adherence (doses used/prescribed) ICS = 56.5 ± 4.6% Oral steroid = 68.6 ± 4.2% Patients discontinued OCS more quickly than ICS	2+	Relatively short follow-up period
Maspero et al. (2001)	124 asthma patients, 6–11 years	RCT, open label	6 months	PEFR, self-reported adherence, symptoms, health care utilization	Reported adherence: Montelukast = 97.6% Beclomethasone = 93.0% Parents preferred montelukast No differences in PEFR, symptoms, health care utilization	1–	Only self report adherence data were used
Sherman et al. (2000)	116 children with asthma	Retrospective Medicaid pharmacy claims study	12 months	Refills	Mean adherence (doses filled/ prescribed): Theophylline = 71.5% (CI=66–77) ICS = 61.4% (CI=54–74) Cromolyn = 37.6% (CI=23–53)	2–	Includes pharmacy claims data only
Sherman et al. (2001)	140 asthma patients, 1–21 years	Retrospective pharmacy claims study; diagnosis confirmed by chart review	3–12 months	Refills	Median adherence (doses filled/ prescribed): Montelukast = 59%(CI=48–65) Fluticasone = 44%(CI=35–50)	2+	Includes pharmacy claims data only
Stoloff et al. (2004)	2,511 asthma patients	Retrospective pharmacy claims study	12 months	Refills	Mean adherence (doses filled/ prescribed): Montelukast = 151 (CI=141–161) Fluticasone = 64 (CI=54–74) Fluticasone+salmeterol = 55 (CI=45–65) Fluticasone+montelukast = 46 (CI=36–55)	2+	Includes pharmacy claims data only

(continued)

Table 7.1 (continued)

References	Population	Design	Duration	Outcomes measured	Key findings (with 95% CI, SD, or SEM if reported)	Scientific quality	Comment
Tuggey et al. (2001)	715 asthma patients, less than 60 years	Mail questionnaire		Medication preferences surveyed	58% of respondents preferred tablets over inhaled medications	2–	Since only half of those surveyed responded, results are likely to be biased
Volovitz et al. (2000)	254 asthma patients, 6–11 years	RCT, open label	4 weeks	Medication preference and adherence, measured by parent self-report	% Preference: Montelukast = 88% Cromolyn = 12% Mean days of full adherence: Montelukast = 98% Cromolyn = 78% Beta-agonist use was lower in the Montelukast group	2–	Only self report adherence data were used; relatively short follow-up period
Weinberg and Naya (2000)	132 asthma patients, 12–17 years	RCT, open label	4 weeks	Preference measured by questionnaire	% preference: Zafirlukast = 79% Beclomethasone = 27%	2+	No behavior or disease outcome measured

Scientific quality (based upon Harbour and Miller 2001)

1–: Meta-analyses, systematic reviews or RCTs, or RCTs with a high risk of bias

2+: High quality systematic reviews of case-control or cohort studies or high quality case-control or cohort studies with a very low risk of confounding, bias, or chance and a high probability that the relationship is causal

PEFR peak expiratory flow rate, *SD* standard deviation, *SEM* standard error of the mean

2–: Case control or cohort studies with a high risk of confounding, bias, or chance, and a significant risk that the relationship is not causal.

twice that of inhaled medication (Table 7.1). While RCTs are generally held in higher regard than cohort studies when comparing drug properties, the assessment of adherence in RCTs has distinct disadvantages. Patients in RCTs are carefully selected, instructed, paid, and monitored. Their behavior, which can include medication "dumping" to create a false presentation of adherence (Simmons et al. 2000), may be markedly different from that seen in the "real world" of patient care. In this way, pharmacy claims studies have the advantage of surveying refill persistence in large groups of patients receiving routine medical care, although these studies cannot fully control other variables that may influence adherence. Prospective cohort studies can provide more accuracy in adherence assessment than pharmacy claims studies, but share with RCTs the limitations present when attempting to generalize about the larger population of asthma patients based on the behavior of a few who are willing to participate in a clinical study. It is the collective evidence across these research designs, each with particular strengths and weaknesses, that provide convincing evidence of greater adherence to oral medications.

Scientific quality of the 17 reports was variable. A total of eight retrospective studies and one RCT were rated in the category of highest qualify reflecting minimal risk of bias or confounding (Table 7.1). Areas of weakness in others included methods of data reporting, absence of a measure of variability, short follow-up period, or incomplete survey response. The single greatest limiting factor for the validity of any adherence study is frequently the method chosen to measure adherence. A large body of evidence clearly indicates that objective data are more accurate than self-reported adherence data. For example, in the study by Krishnan and colleagues (2004) patients reported an average of 85.6% adherence, while microchip-equipped metered-dose inhalers (MDIs) recorded actual adherence at 51.1%. A pediatric study similarly found about 50% adherence measured by another electronic device, while parents reported having administered more than 90% of the medicine to their children (Bender et al. 2000). Another strategy is to measure adherence by weighing the MDI canister before and after study visits and calculating number of doses emptied from the canister during the ensuing interval. This approach, which is somewhat less accurate than attaching an electronic device to a MDI (Krishnan et al. 2004; Bender et al. 2000), is nonetheless more objective and accurate than patient self-report, and is likely similar to pharmacy claims data in that both provide a gross measure of the amount of medication used but cannot discriminate doses accidentally discharged or lost in test puffs. No electronic measure can be introduced into a study without recruitment, informed consent, and study visits; hence, pharmacy refill claims remain the single most accurate method of measuring adherence in a large population of patients. Three of the reviewed studies used patient self report exclusively as the measure of adherence, which likely accounts for reports beyond the 95% adherence level (Bukstein et al. 2003a; Maspero et al. 2001; Volovitz et al. 2000). Given the likelihood that patient over-reporting of adherence was equally applied to oral and inhaled medication, the evidence of relative greater adherence to oral medications found in these studies is probably accurate even though the absolute levels of adherence are not.

Preference for oral medication in pharmacy claims and cohort studies may be confounded with dosing frequency. Specifically, oral medications are typically administered once daily and inhaled medications twice daily. Hence, it remains possible that greater adherence with oral medications reflects increased willingness to take a once-a-day (QD) medication over a twice-daily (BID) medication. However, most evidence indicates that within each medication category, there is little if any difference between QD and BID dosing for oral or inhaled medication. A comprehensive review of tablet adherence studies found similar mean adherence at once-daily (74%) and twice-daily (70%) medication, but both were dramatically higher than three (53%) or four (42%) doses per day (Greenberg 1984). Two studies of inhaled medications reported greater adherence when dosing was reduced from four to two doses (Coutts et al. 1992; Mann et al. 1992; Malo et al. 1995), but others found no dosing-related adherence difference (Gibson et al. 1995; Purucker et al. 2003; Bosley et al. 1994) and none have demonstrated clearly better adherence at QD over BID dosing. Thus, most evidence suggests that preference for oral over inhaled medications is not based on dosing frequency.

Summary

Adherence to oral medications is greater than adherence to inhaled controller medications in both adults and children with asthma. This finding was consistent across study designs using contrasting measures of adherence, over varied time periods, but including many with 12-month follow-up, and with patients who knew they were being monitored as well as those included in an anonymous database. When directly surveyed, patients expressed preference for oral over inhaled medication. Indirect evidence suggests that patient's preference for oral medication is not related to dosing frequency.

References

Adherence to Long-Term Therapies: Evidence for Action. World Health Organization, 2003

Adams RJ, Fuhlbrigge A, Guilbert T, Lozano P, Martinez F (2002) Inadequate use of asthma mediation in the United States: results of the asthma in America national population survey. J Allergy Clin Immunol 110:58–64

Alessandro G, Vincenzo Z, Marco S, Marcello G, Enrica R (1994) Compliance with pharmacologic prophylaxis and therapy in bronchial asthma. Ann Allergy 73:135–140

Apter A, Reisine S, Affleck G, Barrows E, ZuWallack R (1998) Adherence with twice-daily dosing of inhaled steroids. Am J Respir Crit Care Med 157:1810–1817

Apter A, Boston R, George M et al (2003) Modifiable barriers to adherence to inhaled steroids among adults with asthma: it's not just black and white. J Allergy Clin Immunol 111:1219–1226

Balkrishnan R, Nelsen LM, Kulkarni AS, Pleasants RA, Whitmire JT, Schechter MS (2005) Outcomes associated with initiation of different controller therapies in a Medicaid asthmatic population: a retrospective data analysis. J Asthma 42(1):35–40

Barr R, Somers S, Speizer F, Camargo CJ (2002) Patient factors and medication guideline adherence among older women with asthma. Arch Intern Med 162:1761–1768

Bateman ED, Boushey HA, Bousquet J et al (2004) Can guideline-defined asthma control be achieved? The gaining optimal asthma control study. Am J Respir Crit Care Med 170:836–844

Beardon PH (1993) Primary non-compliance with prescribed medication in primary care. Br Med J 307:846–848

Bender BG, Bender SE (2005) Patient-identified barriers to asthma treatment adherence: responses to interview, focus groups, and questionnaires. Immunol Allergy Clin North Am 25:107–130

Bender B, Wamboldt F, O'Connor S et al (2000) Measurement of children's asthma medication adherence by self report, mother report, canister weight, and Doser CT. Ann Allergy Asthma Immunol 85:416–421

Bosley CM, Parry DT, Cochrane GM (1994) Patient compliance with inhaled medication: does combining beta-agonists with corticosteroids improve compliance? Eur Respir J 7(3): 504–509

Bukstein D, Luskin AT, Bernstein BA (2003a) "Real-world" effectiveness of daily controller medicine in children with mild persistent asthma. Ann Allergy Asthma Immunol 90: 543–549

Bukstein DA, Bratton DL, Firriolo KM et al (2003b) Evaluation of parental preference for the treatment of asthmatic children aged 6 to 11 years with oral montelukast or inhaled cromolyn: a randomized, open-label, crossover study. J Asthma 40(5): 475–485

Carter ER, Ananthakrishnan M (2003) Adherence to montelukast versus inhaled corticosteriods in children with asthma. Pediatr Pulmonol 36:301–304

Cerveri I, Locatelli F, Zoia MC, Corsico A, Accordini S (1999) International variations in asthma treatment compliance: the results of the European Community Respiratory Health Survey (ECRHS). Eur Respir J 14:288–294

Cooper WO, Hickson GB (2001) Corticosteroid presciption filling for children covered by Medicaid following an emergency department visit or a hospitalization for asthma. Arch Pediatr Adolesc Med 155:1111–1115

Coutts JA, Gibson NA, Paton JY (1992) Measuring compliance with inhaled medication in asthma. Arch Dis Child 67:332–333

Cramer J, Mattson R, Prevey M, Scheyer R, Oullette V (1989) How often is medication taken as prescribed? A novel assessment technique. JAMA 261:3273–3277

Creer G, Bender G (1993) Psychophysiological Disorders Research and Clinical Applications. In: Gotchel R, Blanchard E (eds) Asthma. American Psychological Association, Washington, DC, pp 151–208

DiMatteo MR, Giordani PJ, Lepper HS, Croghan TW (2002) Patient adherence and medical treatment outcomes: a meta-analysis. Med Care 40:794–811

Donahue JG, Weiss ST, Livingston JM, Goetsch MA, Greineder DK, Platt R (1997) Inhaled steroids and the risk of hospitalization for asthma. JAMA 277:887–891

Dorais M, Glais L, Chabot I, LeLorier J (2005) Treatment persistence with leukotriene receptor antagonists and inhaled corticosteriods. J Asthma 42:385–393

Gibson N, Ferguson A, Aitchison T, Paton J (1995) Compliance with inhaled asthma medication in preschool children. Thorax 50:1274–1279

Greenberg RN (1984) Overview of patient compliance with medication dosing: a literature review. Clin Ther 6(5):592–598

Harbour R, Miller JA (2001) A new system for grading recommendations in evidence based guidelines. BMJ 323:334–336

Horne R, Weinman J (1999) Patients' beliefs about prescribed medicines and their role in adherence to treatment in chronic physical illness. J Psychosom Res 47(6):555–567

Jones C, Santanello NC, Boccuzzi SJ, Wogen J, Strub P, Nelsen LM (2003) Adherence to prescribed treatment for asthma: evidence from pharmacy benefits data. J Asthma 40(1):93–101

Kelloway JS, Wyatt RA, Adlis SA (1994) Comparison of patients' compliance with prescribed oral and inhaled asthma medications. Arch Intern Med 154:1349–1352

Krishnan JA, Riekert KA, McCoy JV et al (2004) Corticosteriod use after hospital discharge among high-risk adults with asthma. Am J Respir and Crit Care Med 170:1281–1285

Lai CK, DeGuia TS, Kim YY, Asthma insights and reality in Asia-Pacific Steering Committee et al (2003) Asthma control in the Asia-Pacific region: the asthma insights and reality in Asia-Pacific Study. J Allergy Clin Immunol 111:263–268

Malo JL, Cartier A, Ghezzo H, Trudeau C, Morris J, Jennings B (1995) Comparison of four-times-a-day and twice-a-day

dosing regimens in subjects requiring 1200 *ug* or less of budesonide to control mild to moderate asthma. Respir Med 89:537–543
Mann M, Eliasson O, Patel K, ZuWallack L (1992) A comparison of the effects of bid and qid dosing on compliance with inhaled flunisolide. Chest 101(2):496–499
Masoli M, Weatherall M, Holt S, Beasley R (2004) Systematic review of the dose-response relation of inhaled fluticasone propionate. Arch Dis Child 89:902–907
Maspero JF, Duenas-Meza E, Volovitz B et al (2001) Oral montelukast versus inhaled beclomethasone in 6 to 11 year old children with asthma: results of an open-label extension study evaluating long-term safety satisfaction, and adherence with therapy. Curr Med Res Opin 17(2):96–104
McQuaid E, Kopel S, Klein R, Fritz G (2003) Medication adherence in pediatric asthma: reasoning, responsibility, and behavior. J Pediatr Psychol 28:323–333
Melnikow J, Kiefe C (1994) Patient compliance and medical research: issues in methodology. J Gen Intern Med 9:96–105
Purucker ME, Rosebraugh CJ, Zhou F, Meyer RJ (2003) Inhaled fluticasone propionate by diskus in the treatment of asthma. Chest 124:1584–1593
Rabe KF, Adachi M, Lai CK et al (2004) Worldwide severity and control of asthma in children and adults: the global asthma insights and reality surveys. J Allergy Clin Immunol 114:40–47
Rand C (2005) Non-adherence with asthma therapy: more than just forgetting. J Pediatr 146:157–159
Rand CS, Wise R (1996) Adherence with asthma therapy in the management of asthma: review and clinical guidelines. In: Szefler SJ, Leung DYM (eds) Severe asthma: pathogenesis and clinical management. Marcel Dekker, New York, pp 436–464
Schatz M, Cook EF, Nakahiro R, Petitti D (2003) Inhaled corticosteriods and allergy speciality care reduce emergency hospital use for asthma. J Allergy Clin Immunol 111:503–508
Sherman J, Hutson A, Baumstein S, Hendeles L (2000) Telephoning the patient's pharmacy to assess adherence with asthma medications by measuring refill rate for prescriptions. J Pediatr 136(4):532–535
Sherman J, Patel P, Hutson A, Chesrown S, Hendeles L (2001) Adherence to oral montelukast and inhaled fluticasone in children with persistent asthma. Pharmacotherapy 21(12): 1464–1467
Simmons MS, Nides M, Rand C (2000) Unpredictability of deception in compliance with physician-prescribed bronchodilator inhaler use in clinical trial. Chest 118:290–295
Stempel DA, Roberts CS, Stanford RH (2004) Treatment patterns in the months prior to and after asthma-related emergency department visit. Chest 126:75–80
Stoloff SW, Stempel DA, Meyer J, Stnaford RH, Rosenzweig JR (2004) Improved refill persistence with fluticasone propionate and salmeterol in a single inhaler compared with other controller therapies. J Allergy Clin Immunol 113(2): 245–251
Suissa S, Ernst P, Benayoun S, Baltzan M, Cai B (2000) Low-dose inhaled corticosteroids and the prevention of death from asthma. N Engl J Med 343:332–336
Szefler S, Weiss SR, Tonascia J, Childhood Asthma Management Program Group (2000) Long-term effects of budesonide or nedocromil in children with asthma. N Engl J Med 15: 1054–1063
Tuggey J, Hosker HS, Chetcuti P, Brownlee K, Taylor J, MacGowan C (2001) Choice of add-on therapy in asthma – another inhaler or a tablet/syrup? A survey of 1415 UK asthmatics. Prim Care Respir J 10(1):27–30
Volovitz B, Duenas-Meza E, Chmielewska-Szewczyk DA et al (2000) Comparison of oral montelukast and inhaled cromolyn with respect to preference, satisfaction, and adherence: a multicenter, randomized, open-label, crossover study in children with mild to moderate persistent asthma. Curr Ther Res 61(7):490–506
Walders N, Kopel SJ, Koinis-Mitchell D, McQuaid EL (2005) Patterns of quick-relief and long-term controller medication use in pediatric asthma. J Pediatr 146:177–182
Weinberg EG, Naya I (2000) Treatment preferences of adolescent patients with asthma. Pediatr Allergy Immunol 11:49–55
Williams LK, Pladevall M, Xi H et al (2004) Relationship between adherence to inhaled corticosteriods and poor outcomes among adults with asthma. J Allergy Clin Immunol 114:1288–1293
Winnick S, Luca D, Hartment AL, Toll D (2005) How do you improve compliance? Pediatrics 115:718–724

Chapter 8
Asthma Self-Management

Harry Kotses and Thomas L. Creer

Asthma self-management represents a systematic way of educating patients to control the disease by avoiding it when possible and reducing it when necessary. In its present form, it has been practiced for little more than 30 years. It was encouraged initially by the National Institute of Health (NIH) through support of extramural asthma self-management research, and subsequently, by its inclusion in the first NIH asthma diagnosis and treatment guidelines (NIH 1991). The seminal programs (Clark et al. 1980; Creer et al. 1988; McNabb et al. 1985) developed with the help of NIH were concerned with control of pediatric asthma. Subsequent work has expanded to cover a variety of other populations, both pediatric and adult, as well as individualized programs. This chapter represents an overview of existing self-management programs as well as an evaluation of their effectiveness.

The term 'self-management' is not to be confused with 'self-care.' While the goal of self-care is to reduce the role of the physician in the treatment of disease, self-management recognizes the importance of the physician and encourages the patient to partner with the physician in the management of the disease. The partnering relationship implies that the physician's effectiveness in managing asthma increases in direct proportion to the quality of asthma information provided by the patient. To be successful, asthma self-management requires the patient to understand the essential features of asthma including: the physical changes underlying difficult breathing, asthma triggers and symptoms, how to evaluate asthma severity, and how to prevent asthma and reduce its exacerbation. These facets of asthma constitute a blueprint for the development of asthma self-management programs, and represent the elements of effective, chronic disease management.

The Elements of Asthma Self-Management Programs

Most asthma self-management programs have two objectives: increasing asthma knowledge; and promoting asthma control (Kotses et al. 1990). Asthma knowledge refers to information about the disease whereas asthma control refers to techniques that effectively limit the disease. There is evidence that patients who simply increase their knowledge of asthma without a systematic effort to control the disease do not necessarily improve their management of asthma (Gibson et al. 2002). The same may be said of patients who attempt control of asthma in the absence of knowledge of the disease (Kotses et al. 2006). Asthma knowledge and asthma control appear to be requisites of successful asthma self-management programs; each must be used in conjunction with the other for effective management of the disease.

Asthma knowledge is associated with such things as the physical changes, causes, and symptoms of asthma. It includes information about the variety and purposes of asthma medications, and about special problems that could be encountered in specific circumstances. Asthma control, on the other hand, is concerned both with the prevention and the reduction of asthma. There is considerable overlap between the two, particularly in providing information about asthma and its treatment. Some procedures, such as techniques for improvement of medication compliance

H. Kotses (✉)
Emeritus Professor of Psychology, Ohio University, Athens, OH, 45701, USA
e-mail: kotses@comcast.net

A. Harver and H. Kotses (eds.), *Asthma, Health and Society: A Public Health Perspective*,
DOI 10.1007/978-0-387-78285-0_8, © Springer Science+Business Media, LLC 2010

or avoiding triggers may be thought of primarily as preventative measures, whereas others such as using variations in severity to prompt corrective action are more closely related to asthma reduction. In self-management programs, both prevention and the reduction procedures are commonly executed within the context of a strategy to control asthma in accordance with a series of escalating symptoms. The strategy can include an action plan, a set of instructions that outline adjustments as dictated by variations in either symptom or pulmonary function measures. It is important to note that action plan adjustments may consist of either behavioral (i.e., avoiding known triggers, rest and relaxation, and ingesting fluids) or pharmacological procedures for controlling asthma. Apart from elements concerned strictly with asthma knowledge and control, several less common elements relating to relaxation training and social skills training sometimes are included in self-management programs. An outline of the elements of asthma self-management is provided in Table 8.1.

Asthma self-management programs are both numerous and varied. They differ from one another in the instructional model around which they are organized, in their format, and in their method of delivery. No single standard defines the form of asthma self-management programs; no body of knowledge is uniformly taught, and no form or method of instruction is universally employed. The only guidelines that have reached a broad audience are those offered by NIH (1991). They are broad enough to encompass programs that differ substantially in instructional model, in format, and in method of delivery. These qualities are described below.

Instructional Model

Asthma self-management programs adhere to one of three basic instructional models: group training (e.g., Creer et al. 1988; Kotses et al. 1995), tailored training (e.g., Kotses et al. 1996; Wilson et al. 1993), and self-administered training (Rubin et al. 1986). Group training programs are those in which training is given simultaneously to a number of patients. The programs are written with an eye toward suitability for a wide range of asthma patients. In most cases, a group consists of no more than 10–12 patients, as larger groups might tend to erode the mutual support that patients can develop for one another. Self-administered training is similar to group training in that the same program is offered to many individuals, but different in that the training is applied one patient at a time. Tailored training, on the other hand, takes into consideration the special circumstances of each patient. This form of training implies a somewhat different program for each patient depending upon the patient's special needs. There are advantages and drawbacks to each instructional model. Group and self-administered programs are desirable because, once developed, they may be offered at a low cost and present few

Table 8.1 Components of asthma self-management: informational elements are shown on left and training elements are on right. Overlapping elements are presented on the same line. Less common elements shown in lower box

Asthma Education (Informational)	Asthma Control (Training)
Physical changes caused by asthma	
The causes of asthma	Identify patient's triggers
Signs and symptoms of asthma	Symptom definition and quantification; identify patient's symptoms
Asthma medications	Distinguish between patient's rescue and control medications
	Proper use of medication. Improve medication compliance.
	Asthma monitoring (use of asthma diary and peak flow meter)
	Action plan: pair diary information with control measures (behavior and /or adjustment)
Self-management outside the home (school, work, travel)	Identify and eliminate or reduce patient's triggers at school or work (e.g., reduce effects of physical activity; eliminate environmental irritants; insure availability of medication)
Relaxation training	Progressive relaxation training; systematic desensitization; breathing exercises; biofeedback
Social skills training	Decision making; self reliance; assertiveness and communication training

organizational problems. However, because they are directed to asthma patients in general, they compel most patients to deal with at least some material that may not be relevant to their disease. From a patient's point of view, tailored programs are preferable to either group or self-administered programs because they can be organized exclusively around those aspects of self-management that are useful to the patient. Material that is irrelevant for a particular patient may be safely dropped. Unfortunately, relatively few programs are tailored, an acknowledgement, no doubt, of both the difficulty and the cost associated with developing a unique program for each patient.

Program Setting

The settings in which programs are conducted vary widely. A program may be given in a hospital (e.g., Chiang et al. 2005), a clinic (e.g., Hilton et al. 1986), a home (e.g., Butz et al. 2005; Brown et al. 2002), or a school (e.g., Bruzzese et al. 2008; Horner and Fouladi 2008; Velsor-Freidrich et al. 2004; Christiansen et al. 1997); and some programs are community-based (e.g., Bryant-Stevens and Li 2004). However, other venues also may be used, including pharmacies (e.g., Smith et al. 2007; Barbanel et al. 2003; Diamond and Chapman 2001) and churches (Ford et al. 1996). The unique qualities of each setting may demand that either a group or an individual approach be used, but some settings may accommodate either. Hospital and clinic staff, for example, may find individual programs more convenient to implement than group programs, but community-based programs may be impractical if they do not adhere to a group format. At the present time, no particular advantage in terms of effectiveness may be attributed to any format and setting combination.

Method of Delivery

Asthma self-management education may be conducted by presentation, by written materials (i.e., Behera et al. 2005), or electronically by computer or related electronic devices. Each method has its strengths. A presentation insures that patients receive program material, and often affords them an opportunity for interaction with health care providers during which they may clarify questions or receive further guidance about asthma control. On the other hand, written instruction, in the form of pamphlets or books, allows unlimited review of a program, a benefit not to be taken lightly. In most programs, patients are given presentations in addition to written material so as to capitalize on the strengths of both (Clark et al. 1980; Creer et al. 1988). The vast majority of asthma self-management programs have made use of either presentational or written methods of delivery or a combination of the two. However, a newer method of delivery, electronic delivery, combines elements of both and offers unique advantages. Electronic delivery is now in its early stages but has been embraced enthusiastically. It encompasses a wide range of strategies, including innovative computer programs for teaching asthma self-management to children (Rubin et al. 1986) and their parents (Fall et al. 1998), teleconsultation (Ostojic et al. 2005), and even daily adjustment of medication schedules based on transmission of peak flow information from patients to health care providers (Pinnock et al. 2007; Ryan et al. 2005). Although the promise of electronic programs is great, their development is hindered by the enormous investment of time and equipment they require. A positive aspect of these programs, however, is that once they are developed, their subsequent application may prove to be both inexpensive and convenient.

The combinations and permutations of program content, instructional format, and method of presentation have given rise to a large number of asthma self-management programs. Their variety suggests that self-management is adaptable to a wide range of conditions, a positive quality. On the other hand, the multiplicity of programs demonstrates that the essential elements of asthma self-management are not well understood, a failure that precludes clear guidance as to the contents of programs. To say that this has complicated evaluation of asthma self-management effectiveness is an understatement. Because programs vary so much, the demonstrated effectiveness of one asthma self-management program is not predictive either of the effectiveness or the degree of effectiveness of another. This needs to be taken into consideration when interpreting the results of research. It may be the case that inconsistent findings are related to differences between programs in what, where, and how they teach asthma self-management. Additionally, programs cannot always be classified with precision, and they may be organized without much forethought. As a result, programs are often not clearly described. Group programs, for example, that include some meetings with individual patients may or may not include a tailored training component, and programs employing more than one method of instruction rarely, if ever, clarify the interactions between methods or to tease out the contribution of each asthma control. These departures from the best experimental design practices make it difficult to paint a portrait of the effectiveness of asthma self-management with anything other than the broadest strokes. Experimental refinement may come, however, as more is learned about how the individual elements of self-management contribute to its overall effectiveness. After a brief excursion into the asthma self-management theory, the following sections outline the use and effectiveness of asthma self-management programs in pediatric and adult populations, and deal with the problems of tailoring self-management to individuals.

Asthma Self-Management Theory: Basic Considerations

The self-management theory has not received a great deal of attention, and no single formulation has dominated self-management research. Two competing theories, both concerned with how behavior is controlled have been advocated in efforts to organize self-management findings, and to formulate questions for further research: one has to do strictly with environmental control of behavior, and the other emphasizes control of behavior through its interaction with private events such as cognitions and emotions (Kotses et al. 1990). Both approaches may be described as behavioral, but in the former, the elements controlling behavior are features of the environment, and in the latter, they may additionally reside in the individual.

Environmental theory, most clearly articulated by operant conditioning theory (Skinner 1953), makes extensive use of the concept of reinforcement, defined as any event that increases the frequency or probability of occurrence of some behavior. Essential in this formulation is the temporal relationship between the target behavior and the reinforcing event: reinforcement must follow the behavior. As it applies to asthma self-management, the reinforcement increases the frequency of behaviors capable of controlling asthma. In general terms, reinforcement consists both of events or outcomes that patients ordinarily avoid (i. e., the symptoms and consequences of the disease) and of events that patients seek (i. e., the benefits of good health). The likelihood of avoiding or seeking specific outcomes is facilitated by use of symptom monitoring and asthma attack management, procedures introduced by self-management training. Monitoring provides the patient a series of benchmarks for initiation of behavior intended to avoid asthma, and attack management consists of guidelines to reduce the severity of an attack. Both monitoring and attack management may consist of a series of graded steps that provide explicit behavioral recommendations depending on asthma severity. In this way, the stages of asthma severity serve as cues, discriminative stimuli in technical parlance, for progressively ramping up behavior whose goal is asthma control. Mild symptoms, for example, cue for minimal interventions, whereas more severe symptoms are cues for potent control measures. Successful management of individual asthma episodes for a period of time insures that larger systems of reinforcement come into play, including lowered treatment costs, fewer disruptions of daily activities due to asthma, and positive regard from others for successful control of asthma. Asthma self-management, viewed from this perspective, represents a series of control measures taken in response to specific environmental cues related to the severity of asthma. A chief benefit of the approach is that both the cues that signal the occurrence of asthma and behaviors that reduce asthma are objective, a quality that ensures patients can be given clear and specific guidance as to how the disease may be controlled. Among those with philosophical leanings toward environmental control of behavior, progress in asthma self-management might involve increasing the number or the saliency of environmental cues built into training programs so as to facilitate or improve control of the disease. Critics of environmental theory have argued that the approach is mechanistic and cannot adequately account for the complexity of human behavior. In addition, environmental theory makes no provision for inclusion of important human qualities such as mood, emotion, and thinking. The failure to consider these qualities contributes to resistance to the theory.

Behavior control that includes the influence of private events represents an alternative to environmental control. Formulations within this tradition are known generally as social learning theory. As a group, they posit an additional level of explanation mediating between environmental stimuli and reactions to them. Various terms have been used to describe the mediators, but mostly they may be considered cognitive factors. In asthma self-management, the most influential of this group of theories is social cognitive theory (Bandura 1986). Consistent with operant theory, it places an emphasis on reinforcement, but in addition, social cognitive theory takes into account the interactions between the person and both the environment and behavior. It is the addition of the person to the mix that gives this and other similar theories their distinctiveness (e.g., Creer 2008). Thinking, for example, a concept that has no place in a strictly behavioral approach, both influences and is influenced by behavior according to the social cognitive theory.

Self-management in the social cognitive theory relies on a form of internal control, rather than exclusively on reinforcement. It is greatly affected by observational learning, meaning learning without behavior, and by self-efficacy (Lavoi et al. 2008), referring to the belief that one can achieve some standard of performance (Bandura 1991a, b). In self-management, observational learning allows for a rapid determination of appropriate control behavior, while self-efficacy provides the motivation to perform appropriately. These abilities and beliefs guide behavior relevant to the control of disease while influencing and being influenced by the environment. Developing a self-management program along these lines might involve increasing opportunities for observational learning and seeking ways to improve self-efficacy. A benefit of this approach is the antithesis of a problem that plagues environmental theory: the acknowledgment that humans are capable of complex behavior in the absence of reinforcement and the recognition that human qualities such as thinking and emotion play a role in controlling behavior. In addition, theories of this sort are compatible with efforts in behavioral neuroscience to identify physiological elements related to cognition. Criticism of the approach often focuses on the use of unobservable quantities. It is important to note that all elements of asthma self-management may be conceptualized in terms of either operant or social cognitive theory, and that reliance on one theory or another is a matter of preference.

Pediatric Asthma Self-Management Programs

By any measure, childhood asthma is a serious disease. It is the most common of the chronic childhood diseases, affecting 4.8 million of those aged 0–18 years (Adams and Marano 1995). Information from 2003 showed that 3.1 million children experienced an asthma episode during the previous 12 months (American Lung Association 2005). These attacks, no doubt, accounted for a major portion of the 14.7 million school days missed in 2002 (Centers for Disease Control and Prevention [CDC], 2004). Unfortunately, not all attacks can be successfully reduced either at home or by a visit to the doctor. Among those 15 years and younger, asthma is the third-ranking reason for hospitalization (Popovic 2001). And some attacks simply cannot be reduced. Although the asthma death rate among the young is not large, 3,850 deaths of individuals up to 24 years of age were reported between 1980 and 1993 (CDC 1996). This level of morbidity and mortality consumes a significant portion of our heath care budget. An estimated $3.2 billion is spent annually treating asthma in those younger than 18 (Weiss et al. 2000). There is little doubt that the early encouragement and support of pediatric self-management by NIH was well considered.

At the outset, and at the risk of stating the obvious, asthma self-management programs for children are not solely for children; they are for children and their families. This is the chief distinction between programs for children and those for adults. The reason that families must be included in pediatric programs is twofold. First, many children do not have the skills needed to conduct the program on their own. The practice of asthma self-management is not especially complex, but it does require symptom monitoring often assisted by use of a peak flow meter, record keeping, data interpretation, decision-making, and discipline to conduct these activities on a regular basis. Each of these skills may be developed with practice, but they are beyond the ability of younger patients and they must be supported, in large measure, by parents until children are capable of dealing with the program demands on their own. Second, a child's asthma cannot help but be affected by the actions of members of the child's family. Parental responsibilities such as controlling allergens and irritants within the home, insuring the availability of medication, mediating conflicts related to a child's asthma between and among family members, communicating with health care providers, and intervening with school and community officials to neutralize potential asthma hazards must be included in a comprehensive disease management program. These considerations should not be taken to suggest that the families of adult asthma patients are unimportant in asthma self-management, but only to emphasize that in pediatric asthma self-management, cooperation between all members of a child's family is essential for success.

The decade of the 1980s witnessed the rapid development of asthma self-management programs for children; by 1990, several dozen programs had been produced (Wigal et al. 1990). Each of these early programs may be considered a pioneering effort, and each resulted in asthma morbidity improvement. Unfortu nately, a number of the studies evaluating the programs were plagued by procedural problems (Creer et al. 1990). In subsequent years, more attention had been paid to research procedure, but problems remained. A meta-analytic review of pediatric asthma self-management studies (Wolf et al. 2003) detected a number of these. Of the 32 programs reviewed, group assignment was biased potentially in 20, confounding was evident in 6, and differential withdrawal was noted in 8. A similar review that included 25 randomized control trials in children (Smith et al. 2005) echoed these concerns. Of the trials, randomization was based on a unit or group rather than the individual in 4; was restricted by matching in 5, by stratification in 4; and was based on inadequate methods in 3. Smith and her colleagues (2005) also reported that only 10 of the 25 programs were blinded in some fashion, that only 9 were free of the potential for selective reporting, that only 7 reported power calculations, and that only 15 featured adequate reporting. Some of these problems could be related to the difficulty of conducting research in pediatric self-management, but that doesn't excuse them. Research difficulty merely underscores the importance of knowledge of common research pitfalls.

In spite of the complexity inherent in pediatric asthma self-management research, the effectiveness of self-management was confirmed by meta-analysis. In their systematic review, Wolf and his colleagues (2003) concluded that self-management programs were associated with improvement in airflow, school absenteeism, restricted activity days, and emergency room visits. A similar review (Coffman et al. 2008) documented an association between asthma education and improvement both in hospital admissions and emergency visits, and a review that included adult as well as pediatric studies (Smith et al. 2005) concluded that self-management positively affected hospital admission and asthma symptoms in children. Descriptive as these summary statements are, they fail to communicate a flavor of the breadth of self-management effects. Broadly speaking, dependent variables of interest in pediatric self-management studies may be grouped into eight categories: (a) physical condition, (b) activity restriction, (c) cognitive factors, (d) quality-of-life, (e) asthma self-management behavior, (f) use of health care facilities, (g) school attendance, and (h) health care cost. We consider each of these in the following sections.

Physical Condition

Aspects of physical condition may be the most commonly recorded indices of asthma in self-management studies. They include the common asthma symptoms: wheeze, cough, chest tightness, and dyspnea. Because of vast differences both within and between patients in expression of symptoms, it is difficult to detect reliable change in any one symptom. Therefore, symptoms are often measured in the aggregate, as asthma exacerbations or attacks. They may be measured either as occurrences of asthma, as days on which unspecified asthma symptoms occurred, or as ratings of symptoms on some scale of severity. Extreme exacerbations of symptoms are termed asthma attacks or episodes and are frequently compiled independently of symptom episodes; they differ from the occurrence of symptoms only in degree. Symptoms that occur at night have been expressed either as a measure of severity or frequency and are sometimes measured separately from those that occur during the day. They can include awakenings as a separate category. In addition, the category of physical condition includes pulmonary variables, most notably peak flow, but other quantities derived from the forced expiratory volume maneuver also have been studied.

1. *Symptoms*. Two aspects of quantifying asthma symptoms may result in confusion. First, the various ways of measuring asthma symptoms: occurrences,

symptom days, and ratings, are not necessarily consistent with one another. More than one symptom occurrence, for example, may take place on a single day, thereby giving rise to a discrepancy between the number of occurrences and the number of symptom days. And ratings, clearly based on a property other than frequency, may or may not coincide either with the number of symptom occurrences or with the number of symptom days. This is no small matter. When measurement method is not taken into consideration, its implications for findings and conclusions can go unrecognized. It is entirely possible to reach different conclusions from the same data depending on how symptom scores were computed. Second, quantification of asthma attacks is subject to interpretation by the patient. The same degree of symptom exacerbation may be classified as an attack by a patient on one day but not on another, or classified differently by different patients. Efforts to circumvent this are made by specifying objective criteria for identification of asthma attacks, but ultimately, the judgment is made subjectively and is subject to within- as well as between-patient variability.

These cautionary considerations on scoring procedures notwithstanding, improvement in asthma symptoms frequently is associated with self-management. Children who were given self-management training experienced fewer symptom days (Clark et al. 2004; Evans et al. 1987) or more symptom-free days (Brown et al. 2002) than children who were not. Improvement not only in symptom days but also in symptom ratings occurs with administration of asthma self-management. In a study of a home-based education program for low-income families (Brown et al. 2002), caregivers of children aged 1–3, given self-management training assigned lower severity ratings on the symptom subscale of the Paediatric Asthma Quality of Life Questionnaire (Juniper et al. 1996a, b) than did caregivers of children not given training. Consistent with these findings were results reported for hospitalized children who were given training in an effort to reduce readmission (Madge et al. 1997). The improved symptom severity ratings obtained with the Usherwood index (Usherwood et al. 1990) applied to all ages (2–14) and extended to night symptoms, in addition to those noted in the day. Even a 5-item questionnaire consisting of questions relating to symptoms and activity restriction was sensitive to asthma education (Christiansen et al. 1997). Six months after the start of the study, children who received education had lower symptom ratings than control children. Other measures of asthma symptoms that improved by their association with self-management included: number of children experiencing night symptoms (Deaves 1993); frequency of awakening due to asthma (Colland 1993); and parental reports of symptom frequency (Colland 1993). An indirect measure of symptoms, use of reliever medication, also improved in children taught self-management (Dahl et al. 1990; Glasgow et al. 2003). As for findings concerning specific symptoms, few reports exist, but one (Glasgow et al. 2003) detailed a reduction of speech-limiting wheeze in children who had undergone brief self-management training given by general practitioners.

Reduction of asthma attacks has also been reported in studies of asthma self-management. Both the number of asthma attacks (Creer et al. 1988; Evans et al. 1987; Fireman et al. 1981), and the duration of attacks decreased (Evans et al. 1987) when children were given self-management training. Fireman and his colleagues (1981) compared asthma attacks in self-managed and control patients during their study, whereas the others based their comparisons on improvement from a baseline taken prior to the study. In no case, however, was a standard criterion for asthma given to children, leaving open the possibility that the meaning of an asthma attack varied among studies.

2. *Pulmonary measures*. Peak expiratory flow, another aspect of physical condition, was initially thought to be capable of supplanting reliance on symptoms for the purpose of gauging the severity of asthma. This has not happened, as the relationship between peak flow and symptoms was found to be only moderate and complex (e.g., Apter et al. 1997). Detracting from the relationship are factors that affect the measurement both of peak flow and of symptoms. Peak flow is effort-dependent, and for that reason some of the variability it exhibits is not due to physical condition but other factors under the control of the patient. And a portion of symptom score variability, as noted previously, is due to patient interpretation and independent of physical condition.

Much like asthma symptoms, peak flow may be expressed in a number of different ways. It may be presented as the recorded value, but this is a risky practice as peak flow is affected by the height, age, and sex of the patient. If adjustment is not made for these factors, the peak flow value may be misleading. Despite this, unadjusted peak flow in one study improved in a self-management group relative to a control group (Weingarten et al. 1985). The averaged peak flow scores observed in the study did not differ between the groups at baseline, but differed after intervention. A more common practice is to express peak flow relative to some standard such as the predicted values for a specific child. Using percent of predicted values, Creer and his colleagues (1988) observed that children in a self-management group were breathing below their predicted values at the start of treatment, but reached their predicted values at follow-up, some 18 months after the beginning of the study. A similar finding was reported for trained children but not for controls in a study of the effects of asthma education provided by nurses in the homes of patients (Carswell et al. 1989). It is also possible to compare asthma patients on the frequency of peak flow scores occurring within a specific range of percent of predicted values. In one such comparison (Charlton et al. 1994), trained children had a lower frequency of peak flow scores below 30% of their predicted value than did untrained children. Pulmonary measures other than peak flow for evaluation of self-management are uncommon, but they are recorded occasionally. Of these, one-second forced expiratory volume (FEV_1) has been used more than others. In a community-based asthma self-management program, higher FEV_1 values were observed in children who received the program as compared with those who did not (Toelle et al. 1993). The program included education and treatment for children and involved parents, doctors, nurses, pharmacists, and teachers.

Activity Restriction

Restriction of activity may be considered a consequence of asthma, placing it in the same category as school attendance, doctor visits, and other variables. Nevertheless, it is useful to consider restriction of activity independently of other consequences because it represents a salient patient complaint. As with any chronic condition, asthma patients complain that they cannot engage in many activities. Activity restriction has been quantified by tabulating asthma diary entries, by interview, and by questionnaire.

A number of investigators have reported evidence of changes in activity restriction as a function of asthma self-management. In a single group study (Hindi-Alexander and Cropp 1984), activity restrictions based on diary entries declined over the course of the study. Activity restrictions referred to such things as participation in Little League, newspaper delivery, and participation in intramural gymnastics. Diary entries also confirmed a differential decline in activity restriction between children given an asthma self-management program and those who were not (Charlton et al. 1994). The change favored the trained group. Information gleaned from interviews has supplemented data from asthma diary entries in support of beneficial self-management effects on activity restriction. In a study of a school-based, general program of asthma self-management (Cicutto et al. 2005), interviews guided by the activities scale of Paediatric Quality of Life Questionnaire (Juniper et al. 1996a, b) revealed that children who received the intervention had higher levels of activity than did control children at 2-month follow-up. The difference in activity level held up a year later when the measurement was taken on a questionnaire that the authors called a tracking sheet. A modified version of an adult asthma quality of life scale (Juniper et al. 1993) also was sensitive to differences in activity level between children who received a teacher-led asthma education program and those that did not (Henry et al. 2004).

Cognitive Factors

Among the most commonly studied variables in asthma self-management research, cognitive factors include measures of knowledge, attitude, and emotion. They represent an important dimension of asthma that is not addressed by traditional morbidity measures. They are important in another way: they interact with traditional measures of morbidity and can thereby influence them.

1. *Knowledge*. Asthma knowledge represents familiarity with materials presented in education sessions of self-management programs. It consists of information about the nature of asthma, its symptoms, and ways to control the disease. It has been evaluated with positive results over a dozen times. Both children (e.g., Holzheimer et al. 1998) and parents

(e.g., Deaves 1993; Parcel et al. 1980) have been tested. Instruments used to evaluate knowledge have included true false items (e.g., Parcel et al. 1980; Christiansen et al. 1997), multiple choice items (e.g. Talabere 1993), and pictorial multiple-choice items (Holzheimer et al. 1998). Knowledge has also been evaluated by interview (Deaves 1993). All efforts to evaluate the effect of asthma education on asthma knowledge have consistently shown that education improves knowledge.

2. *Attitude*. Self-management requires that the patient shoulder much of the burden for control of disease. Accordingly patient attitudes relating to such things as factors responsible for disease, and patient ability to control disease have a bearing on the success of asthma self-management. One concept that captures the essence of these concerns is locus of control, a measure of beliefs or attitudes about the source of control of matters affecting one's life. A patient may believe he or she either can control an asthma attack or cannot control it because it is under the control by factors independent of the patient. A scale that measures the tendency of patients to assign control of health matters either to themselves or to other factors was developed years ago and is known as Health Locus of Control (HLOC) scale (Parcel and Meyer 1978). As might be expected, self-management training is associated with changes in locus of control away from external control and toward internal control. This has been confirmed by changes in locus of control of children undergoing asthma self-management training a number of times (Hindi-Alexander and Cropp 1984; Henry et al. 2004; Kubly and McClellan 1984; Parcel et al. 1980; Robinson 1985; Taggart et al. 1987), and at, least once, in their parents (Hindi-Alexander and Cropp 1984). In related work, children's attitudes toward themselves and their ability to manage asthma changed positively, as documented by the Children's Asthma Attitude Scale in an early program (Creer et al. 1988).

Self-efficacy is a concept that bears some similarity to locus of control. While locus of control is concerned solely with beliefs about the source of control, self-efficacy, as noted previously in the section on theory, is concerned with the degree to which patients are confident they can control important disease factors. This concept has not been used much in pediatric asthma self-management studies, but it promises to have an impact. In one study (Cicutto et al. 2005), self-efficacy measured from baseline to post-intervention was greater in elementary school children who received an asthma education program than it was in their controls. The children who received the program experienced gains in their confidence to use an inhalation device, control asthma, manage triggers, and prevent asthma from getting worse.

One other attitudinal measure that has been used with some frequency, but with mixed results in evaluations of asthma self-management programs for children, is the Piers-Harris Self-Concept Inventory. The inventory measures how children feel about themselves. Positive increases in self-concept following self-management training have been reported on two occasions (Creer et al. 1988; Weiss and Hermalin 1987), but in two other studies (Parcel et al. 1980; Rubin et al. 1986), changes in self-concept were not observed.

3. *Emotion*. A connection between asthma and emotion has been recognized for over a hundred years. Some of the evidence is drawn from observations of innocuous objects causing asthma. MacKenzie (1886) noted that a paper rose elicited chest tightness and dyspnea in a patient who was being treated for a variety of allergic and asthma-like symptoms that occurred annually between spring and fall. And Dekker and Groen (1956) described patients whose asthma was brought on by picture of a horse, in one case, and a toy goldfish in a bowl in another. In each of these cases, a seemingly harmless stimulus apparently triggered an arousal of emotion, a condition that has the effect of narrowing airways caliber. This consequence of emotion is fairly well known. In healthy individuals, respiratory resistance is increased under conditions of emotion or stress (Kotses et al. 1987a; b; Wigal et al. 1988), an effect most likely due to an elevation in bronchomotor tone. The underlying mechanism, of course, is not related to asthma, but its action in asthma patients may affect breathing and may, at times, combine with inflammation to produce a serious asthma exacerbation. This is recognized in many asthma self-management programs by inclusion of instructions to rest and relax in the face of an attack. An even more effective way of nullifying the deleterious effects of emotion in asthma is by training patients to relax. It is for this reason that relaxation training of one form or another sometimes is included in asthma self-management programs.

Progressive muscle relaxation, a form of relaxation training that involves teaching a patient to distinguish between tension and relaxation by alternately tensing and relaxing each of the major muscle groups of the body while attending to the accompanying sensations has been shown to affect pulmonary function. In two experiments, Alexander and his colleagues (Alexander et al. 1972; Alexander 1972), provided evidence that progressive relaxation training resulted in an increase in the peak flow scores of children with asthma. Biofeedback relaxation, a form of training in which electronic feedback is used to assist the patient to relax specific muscles also is associated with pulmonary improvement in children with asthma (Kotses et al. 1991a, 1978, 1976), and with improvement in attitudes toward asthma and chronic anxiety (Kotses et al. 1991a). Apart from relaxation-induced asthma improvement, there is some evidence that self-management training alone may be responsible for a decrease in anxiety. In particular, self-management resulted in a decrease in trait anxiety for all patients, and asthma-specific anxiety in a subgroup of children who had a high level of asthma anxiety (Colland 1993). In addition, self-management children exhibited more favorable scores than controls on the emotion domain of a quality-of-life index (Cicutto et al. 2005; Henry et al. 2004).

Asthma self-management appears to reduce anxiety in children, even without the inclusion of relaxation training procedures. The case is much stronger, however, when specialized training in relaxation is given. Unfortunately, the time it takes to train children in progressive relaxation or biofeedback is often considered too great for the return it provides. Consequently, few programs today include much training in relaxation.

Quality-Of-Life

Asthma quality-of-life combines measures of asthma symptoms, activity restriction, and emotion (Juniper 1998). It is assessed most frequently with the Paediatric Asthma Quality of Life Questionnaire (Juniper et al. 1996a), an instrument that may be administered in about 10 min. As we described earlier, individual subscales of the questionnaire have been used to document symptoms and activity restriction. The scale has also been used in its entirety in asthma self-management research to obtain a global measure of quality-of-life. In a school-based program of self-management conducted by asthma educators, quality-of-life scores increased from baseline to post-intervention for children who received the training, but evidenced no change for children who did not (Cicutto et al. 2005). Closer examination revealed that the changes were limited to emotion and activity domains. Similar results for both total and domain scores were reported in another school-based study, this one led by teachers (Henry et al. 2004). Not only is quality-of-life improved by self-management in children with asthma, but benefits of training accrue even to caretakers. A caretaker quality-of-life scale developed by Juniper and her colleagues (Juniper et al. 1996b) was sensitive to caretaker improvement both at 3 months and at a year after children received the intervention. The improvement was limited to caretakers of children who themselves improved after self-management.

Thus far, quality-of-life indices have not been used extensively to evaluate self-management programs, but their potential is great because they ferret out information of several types that may negatively affect asthma patients. They also represent a convenient and economical way of obtaining a great deal of information for a small investment in time. In addition, these instruments may be put to use in diagnostic applications.

Asthma Self-Management Behavior

Changing the way patients respond to asthma is a primary goal of asthma self-management; therefore, determining whether behavior changed as a result of self-management is a key concern. An increase in the ability of self-management children to cope with an asthma exacerbation has been documented a number of times (Charlton et al. 1994; Colland 1993; Evans et al. 1987; Holzheimer et al. 1998; Hughes et al. 1991; Lewis et al. 1984; Rakos et al. 1985; Rubin et al. 1986; Whitman et al. 1985; Wilson-Pessano and McNabb 1985). Usually, the determination is made by questionnaire, but other procedures, including interviews, analyses of diary entries, tabulation of responses to a single item, and observation of targeted skills have been used. Adherence to medication recommendations, an important self-management behavior, also has been found to increase in children given self-management training (Holzheimer et al. 1998; Lewis et al. 1984).

Use of Health Care Facilities

Examination of two variables, emergency treatment and hospital admission frequency, make up the bulk of research on how health care facility use is affected by self-management. Typically, researchers tabulated frequencies in treatment and control groups of patients during lengthy periods of observation before and after the intervention. The before and after measures are needed so as to control for individual variation, especially when the number of patients studied is small. The observation periods are often a year in length so as to control for seasonal variation. Analyses of the frequency of emergency treatment in self-management and control patients for a year before and a year after the intervention have favored self-management (Alexander et al. 1988; Greineder et al. 1999; Lewis et al. 1984; McNabb et al. 1985). Findings consistent with these were reported when observation periods shorter than a year (but still a year apart) were used (Colland 1993), when patients were used as their own controls (Hindi-Alexander and Cropp 1984), and when self-management and control groups were compared only after the intervention was delivered (Fireman et al. 1981).

Evidence indicates that self-management training also improves hospital admission for asthma, but the case is not as strong as it is for emergency visits. The strongest evidence comes from only one study in which improvements in hospital admission were measured from before to after the intervention for a self-management group and a control group (Greineder et al. 1991). In several other studies (Fireman et al. 1981; Madge et al. 1997), hospital admissions were tabulated only during a post-intervention period and may have been subject to individual variation. In addition, frequencies were small, in one case (Fireman et al. 1981), and observations were limited to patients that had been hospitalized for asthma, in another case (Madge et al. 1997).

Two additional variables relating to health care facility use that could be examined for self-management effects: scheduled physician visits and number of hospital days may not be reliable measures for that purpose. Scheduled physician visits are as likely to increase as they are to decrease following self-management training, and therefore, a consistent prediction as to the effects of self-management cannot be made. Hospital days, on the other hand, may be affected by factors other than asthma condition, including insurance plan provisions and availability of hospital facilities. In addition, hospital rates may be affected by the practices and beliefs of individual physicians who treat asthma. A series of articles a decade or so ago suggested that these were due, in part, to whether or not patients were treated by asthma specialists (e.g., Bartter and Pratter 1996; Mahr and Evans 1993). The consensus was that specialists were significantly better at treating asthma than general practice physicians. More recently, there has been concern as to whether the rate of hospital referrals was due to whether or not physicians followed national and international guidelines for the treatment of asthma (e.g., Vermeire et al. 2002). This debate is ongoing. However, it should be emphasized that there is a spectrum of physician views in deciding whether to refer asthma patients to a hospital. At one end, there are the physicians and medical personal who see the need to refer a patient to a hospital for asthma as unnecessary. At the other end of the continuum, there are physicians and medical personal who actively encourage their patients to seek hospital services in the event of an attack. This breadth of practices makes hospital use a highly problematic outcome variable in comparing data gathered across studies.

School Attendance

School attendance is a difficult variable to measure because it takes a long time to evaluate. Additionally, school records often do not distinguish absences by cause; so missing a day of school for asthma is recorded in the same way as missing a day for some other reason. To the extent possible, investigators have tried to collect school attendance data not only for periods of active self-management investigation, but also for periods prior to the start of the study. Weiss and Hermalin (1987) recorded school attendance for 2 years prior to and for 1 year after introduction of Superstuff, a self-administered asthma self-management program. School attendance in their treatment and control groups before the intervention was not different, but after the intervention the treatment group attended about five more days of school. on average, than did the control group. The difference was statistically reliable. Similar findings for observation periods of only 1 month (Colland 1993; Dahl et al. 1990), for within-patient comparisons of pre- and post-intervention performance (Creer et al. 1988; Hindi-Alexander and Cropp 1984), and for post-intervention only comparisons of intervention and control group (Cicutto et al. 2005; Clark et al. 2004; Fireman et al. 1981) also have been reported. In addition, the academic grades of self-management patients but not of control patients increased after the intervention was introduced (Clark et al. 2004; Evans et al. 1987). The assumption was that school attendance influences academic performance.

Cost of Healthcare

It is difficult to estimate the cost of treating a child with asthma and easy to understand why. For most families, insurance of one type or another or public assistance keeps the cost of treatment stable from month to month and independent of the condition of the child. Only in a few families does the cost of asthma care accurately reflect the need for medical services. In families such as these, the percentage of net family income devoted to the treatment of the child was 1.79 after self-management training, a drop from 2.71 prior to training (Creer et al. 1988). These data were based on only nine families and may not be representative of asthma costs in a larger segment of the population. A partial measure of asthma care cost, the amount a family spent on the use of facilities not covered by their health care plan, also went down following self-management training (Greineder et al. 1999). The average cost after training was $471 per family as compared to $2692 prior to training. The analogous figures in a control condition were $1638 and $2266, respectively. The difference between the drop in the trained group and that in the control group was statistically reliable. In one other comparison, the combined hospitalization and emergency treatment costs over the course of a year were estimated at $35 for 13 patients in self-management group, and $2955 for 13 patients in a control group (Fireman et al. 1981). Admittedly, a conclusion about the effect of self-management on health care cost is difficult to reach based on these few observations. However, it is not unreasonable to expect self-management to decrease health care costs owing to the reduction it brings about in the need for some medical services.

Adult Asthma Self-Management

Asthma self-management for adults was a natural outgrowth of pediatric programs. The programs began to appear in numbers in the decade of the 1990s. As a group, they are similar to children's programs with the following exceptions. First, and most obviously, adult programs do not require extensive participation of all members of the patient's family. Unlike pediatric programs, adult programs can be restricted to the patient, although this probably does not represent the ideal circumstance. Second, because a certain level of comprehension may be assumed with most adult patients, adult self-management programs may be more complex than those designed only for children. This has promoted use of procedures such as action plans that permit patient adjustment of medication in adult programs as compared with those for children. Finally, developmental considerations may be less a problem with adult than with children's programs. Children at different stages of development may require the use of somewhat different educational and behavioral control procedures, a problem not encountered in adult population. Perhaps partially for these reasons, the effects of adult programs appear to be more robust than those of children's programs. A systematic review of adult programs (Gibson et al. 2002) concluded that use of self-management in adults is correlated with clinically significant reductions in hospital admission, emergency treatment, days lost from work, nocturnal asthma episodes, and costs; and in improved quality-of-life.

As we did in our review of pediatric programs, we grouped outcome variables of adult programs into the following eight categories: (a) physical condition, (b) activity limitation, (c) cognitive factors, (d) quality-of-life, (e) self-management behavior, (f) use of health care facilities, (g) work absenteeism, and (h) cost. We consider only those studies that examined the effects of a comprehensive self-management program, one that included both an education and an asthma control component. We tolerated wide latitude of asthma control procedures including: those in which either symptoms or peak flow was monitored, either with or without a formal action plan; and both those that provided and those that did not provide for medication adjustment. In the studies we examined, self-management training usually was compared with customary care. This is by far the most common form of comparison, even though it is not entirely trouble-free. We shall return to this point in a subsequent section. To avoid redundancy, we omit extended discussion of outcome variables in studies of adults. Interested readers may refer to analogous coverage of outcome variables in children's programs.

Physical Condition

Self-management is associated with a reduction in either the number or the severity of asthma exacerbations in adult patients. The effect of self-management on exacerbation has been confirmed by both direct and indirect means. In some cases, self-management reduced the frequency of exacerbations (Bailey et al. 1990; Kotses et al. 1995; Snyder et al. 1987); in others, it increased the number of symptom-free days (Cote et al. 2000; Wilson et al. 1993); and in still others, it improved scores on symptom severity scales based either on self-reports of patients (de Oliveira et al. 1999; Levy et al. 2000; Put et al. 2003) or on questionnaires of patient experience that were completed by others (Wilson et al. 1993; Yilmaz and Akkaya 2002). In addition, the symptom dimension of quality-of-life scales indicated improvement following self-management in several studies (Cote et al. 2001; de Oliveira et al. 1999; Put et al. 2003). Other aspects of physical condition that improved with self-management training included peak expiratory flow (Ghosh et al. 1998; Ignacio-Garcia and Gonzalez-Santos 1995; Kotses et al. 1995; Levy et al. 2000; Put et al. 2003), and airway responsiveness to methacholine (Cote et al. 2000). Additionally, a decrease in eosinophils, a biological marker of airway inflammation, was reported in sputum samples (Janson et al. 2003) of patients who received self-management training as compared with patients who did not. In general, findings regarding the effects of self-management on physical condition in adults were consistent with those observed in children. The evidence makes a strong case that self-management training improves physical condition.

Activity Restriction

In contrast to studies of children, there is relatively little support showing that self-management affects activity level in adults, but some evidence exists. Information about activity limitation was gathered in a multi-site study of 323 adult patients who were given either group or individual self-management training and followed for a year after training (Wilson et al. 1993). A trained nurse administered questionnaires that sampled information about activity limitation at 5 months and at 1 year after the intervention. One year after the intervention, patients who had received group training reported less activity limitation than either patients who received individual training or patients in control groups. A somewhat similar result was reported in a study of patients given self-management training after they had been hospitalized with acute asthma (Osman et al. 2002). One year after the intervention, more patients in the intervention group than in the control group, 60% vs. 52% respectively, reported experiencing no activity limitation. Perhaps the strongest evidence of the effects of self-management on activity restriction comes not from activity reports but from quality-of-life measures. On more than one occasion, the activity domain of quality-of-life indicated improvement following self-management (Cote et al. 2001; de Oliveira et al. 1999; Put et al. 2003). In each case, activity questions on the scale had been individualized according to interests of the patient. It is possible that changes in activity restriction effected by self-management are less apparent in adults than in children because overall level of activity is lower in older patients. A lower level of activity is likely to be associated with lower variability making changes in activity restriction more difficult to demonstrate.

Cognitive Factors

1. *Knowledge.* Ample evidence shows that asthma self-management training improves asthma knowledge in adults. Improvement of knowledge has been reported in a number of controlled studies that included baseline and post-intervention measures (Allen et al. 1995; Cote et al. 1997, 2001; Kotses et al. 1995; Put et al. 2003; Snyder et al. 1987). In each case, knowledge was assessed by questionnaire. The inclusion of a baseline measure is important for control of pre-existing knowledge differences. Studies in which knowledge questionnaires were administered only after the intervention also documented knowledge differences in favor of

the self-management group (Abdulwadud et al. 1999; Brewin and Hughes 1995; Yilmaz and Akkaya 2002; Yoon et al. 1993). In one study (de Oliveira et al. 1999), the dependent variable on which knowledge was evaluated consisted, not of questionnaire score, but of the percentage of patients in self-management and control groups correctly answering questions related to knowledge. Here too, as in all other studies, the comparison favored the self-management group. Considered as a group, these studies strongly support the assertion that self-management increases knowledge of asthma in adult patients.

2. *Attitude.* Work concerning attitudes in studies of adult asthma self-management is largely limited to asthma control, self-efficacy, and asthma health beliefs. The research suggests that self-management training leads to an improvement in: willingness to work within the framework of self-management toward greater asthma control, confidence to manage asthma, and beliefs about asthma drugs. Positive changes in willingness to control asthma (Put et al. 2003) and self-efficacy (Kotses et al. 1995) were observed in adult patients given self-management training but not in waiting-list controls. And beliefs concerning whether asthma drugs are addictive or lose effectiveness with time shifted in an appropriate direction in self-management but not control patients (Yoon et al. 1993). Beliefs concerning asthma drugs, however, were based on responses to only five statements.
3. *Emotion.* Emotional changes associated with self-management in adults have been registered on the Negative Emotionality Scale (NEM) (Tellegen et al. 1988), on the emotion dimension of the McMaster Asthma Quality-of-Life Questionnaire (AQLQ) (Juniper et al. 1992), and on the Beck Depression Inventory (BDI) (Beck 1967). The NEM measures such things as irritability, instability, and nervousness, the AQLQ is a general quality-of-life questionnaire for adult patients, and the BDI is a widely employed test of depression useful for identifying severe depression requiring intervention. Improvement in both in negative emotionality and in emotion measured by a quality-of-life scale was observed in self-management patients throughout a period of 6 months after training, but not in control patients (Put et al. 2003). Similar findings were reported for depression (Kotses et al. 1995), but the depression scores of both trained and untrained patients were entirely within the normal range of values before and after the intervention. That suggested that depression is not prominent in the majority of patients with asthma. On the other hand, the findings for negative emotionality and emotion measured as a part of quality-of-life are of interest and deserve further study.

Quality-Of-Life

The quality of life of adult asthma patients has been measured by the AQOL (Juniper et al. 1992), and the St. George Respiratory Questionnaire (SGRQ) (Jones et al. 1992). The AQOL has four domains (symptoms, emotions, exposure to environmental stimuli, and activity limitation), and the SGRQ has three (symptoms, activity, and impacts of daily life). Of the two, the AQOL seems to have greater responsiveness (Juniper 1998) and has become the instrument of choice. Following self-management, improvement has been observed in total AQOL score (Cote et al. 2000; Put et al. 2003; Yilmaz and Akkaya 2002), in total SGRQ score (Lahdensuo et al. 1996), and in a total measure that combined aspects of the AQOL and SGRQ (de Oliveira et al. 1999). Positive change in the individual domains of quality-of-life also has been reported for exposure to environmental stimuli (Put et al. 2003), and as noted in earlier sections above, for the domains of symptoms, physical activity, and emotion.

Asthma Self-Management Behavior

As expected, the frequency with which patients practice asthma self-management behavior increases as a result of self-management training. Confirmation of the expectation has come in the form of both: an overall measure of self-management behavior frequency and measurement of specific behavior frequency. Patients who had undergone self-management training reported a higher frequency of self-management behavior than patients in a control group (Kotses et al. 1995). The comparison was made on the basis of the number of self-management behaviors endorsed on the Report of Episode/Attack of Asthma (Creer 1992), a checklist of behaviors useful for reducing an exacerbation. Specific behaviors reported to have increased after self-management training included improvement in the control of both house dust mites (Cote et al. 2000) and of the bedroom environment (Wilson et al. 1993). The latter referred to such things as elimination of allergenic bedroom furnishings, dust control, and cleaning practices. An improvement in the frequency with which peak flow was checked also has been reported (Knoell et al. 1998), as well as an increase in keeping follow-up appointments after training in self-management (George et al. 1999).

Adherence to medication recommendations has attracted more interest than any other self-management behavior. Taking medication as prescribed can be a problem for asthma patients as many think they have no need for medication during symptom-free periods. Self-management helps the problem. Adherence to inhaled steroid medication, measured in a variety of ways, improved in conjunction with self-management (Berg et al. 1997; Cote et al. 1997; Janson et al. 2003; Levy et al. 2000), as did both self-report measures of medication adherence (Bailey et al. 1990; Put et al. 2003) and rated medication adherence (Bailey et al. 1990). Ability to properly operate a metered dose inhaler also improved with self-management training (Bailey et al. 1990; de Oliveira et al. 1999; Wilson et al. 1993). Assessment of the inhaler technique was made in each case following a standardized procedure (Manzilla et al. 1989).

Use of Health Care Facilities

Self-management reduced unscheduled visits of adult asthma patients to medical facilities. Most studies were concerned with emergency room use. Supporting evidence derived from contrasts of: the number of emergency room visits in self-management and control groups (Cowie et al. 1997); the number of emergency room visits in self-management and control groups before and after the intervention (Cote et al. 2001; George et al. 1999; Ghosh et al. 1998; Yoon et al. 1993); the average number of emergency room visits per patient in the self-management and control groups (Ignacio-Garcia and Gonzalez-Santos 1995); and the percentage of patients making emergency room visits in the self-management and control groups (Gallefoss and Bakke 2000; Lahdensuo et al. 1996). Although these estimates of emergency room use do not necessarily yield identical results, the conclusions in the studies cited were consistent. Similar findings also were reported for a closely related variable: number of unscheduled physician consultations (Moudgil et al. 2000).

Hospital admission rate research has targeted high-risk patients, those who have experienced hospitalization for asthma in the past. Typically, hospitalized individuals are given self-management and their rate of hospital admission is compared with controls for periods before and after training.

Hospital admission rates follow a pattern much like that of emergency room visits. And dependent variables used to measure admission rates are similar to those used to measure emergency visits. These include: hospital admission frequency (George et al. 1999; Yoon et al. 1993); admissions per patient (Mayo et al. 1990); and percentage of patients admitted (Castro et al. 2003; Osman et al. 2002). In each study, a lower rate of hospital admission was associated with self-management training.

Number of hospital days is another variable of health care facility use. As noted previously, it is a difficult quantity to work with because factors other than patient health can affect the length of time one spends is a hospital. Despite this, the number of days spent in the hospital declined for patients who had self-management training. The findings were expressed either as number of hospital days (Ghosh et al. 1998) or as hospital days per patient (Mayo et al. 1990). It is of interest to note that effects of self-management on number of hospital days are limited to these two reports. This may be an indication of influence of other factors on this variable.

Absenteeism

The findings regarding absenteeism in adults are consistent with the results of research on school absenteeism due to asthma in children, but our information regarding the former is less extensive than that of the latter. Comparisons of self-management and control group for a period of a year after training revealed lower rates of absenteeism for self-management patients (Ghosh et al. 1998; Lahdensuo et al. 1996). In each case, absenteeism of patients in the self-management group was about half that of patients in the control group. A more thorough comparison included information about absenteeism not only after training but also for a period prior to training (Ignacio-Garcia and Gonzalez-Santos 1995). Work days lost were roughly equivalent between groups during a 6-month period before training but dropped sharply in self-management patients during the 6 months after training, a change that did not occur in control patients. Although these outcomes seem straightforward, it should be noted that factors other than asthma severity could contribute to days lost from work. These factors include type of work performed and manner of remuneration.

Cost of Healthcare

Like some other self-management outcome variables, cost of healthcare is difficult to pin down precisely because health care costs in parts of the world and at different times vary greatly. As noted earlier, even within a region, differences between patients in medical insurance coverage adds further variability to costs. These factors make it difficult to compare cost figures between studies, and sometimes even cost figures between individuals within the same study. However, changes in health care costs in self-management training may be examined if these considerations are kept in mind.

Determining changes in the cost of health care for adult patients who receive self-management training has been studied in two ways: by between-group cost comparisons, and by cost-benefit analyses. Average cost estimates per patient for asthma care in India in the early 1990s were $210.52 and $270.24 in self-management and control groups, respectively, for a period of a year after training (Ghosh et al. 1998). By contrast, the per patient costs for total health care in St. Louis in the late 1990s were $5,726.00 and $12,188.00, respectively, in self-management and control groups (Castro et al. 2003). Both direct and indirect costs were included in each study. Indirect costs were especially difficult to estimate accurately because they included the cost of lost workdays, a figure greatly affected by the patient's rate of pay. A technique that gets around some of the problems of comparability is cost-benefit analysis. It is concerned not so much with a comparison of cost between those who have had self-management training and those who have not, but the degree to which healthcare cost changes for an individual who is given training. Cost-benefit analyses take into consideration cost of self-management training as well as the cost of asthma care. A cost-benefit analysis of an adult asthma self-management program revealed that self-management reduced asthma care cost by an average of $475.29 per patient as compared to cost of care prior to training (Taitel et al. 1995). The greatest savings occurred in hospitalization cost and in income lost as a result of lost workdays due to asthma. Comparability between studies remains a problem in cost-benefit studies, but it may be reduced if the savings were expressed as a percentage of asthma care costs.

Tailored Asthma Self-Management

Tailoring of treatment and management recommendations is customary in medicine, but not in asthma self-management. Enthusiasm for it has been hindered by the complexity of asthma self-management programs and by variability between patients in their need for asthma control. The main stumbling block to widespread use of tailoring is the lack of a clear and convenient way to assess a patient's need for a large number of practices that potentially can control asthma. But for the lack of such an assessment, a unique program could be developed for each patient, one that would include only those practices effective for the patient. Asthma self-management has far to go before this ideal is achieved, but some preliminary work has been done.

Tailoring in asthma self-management has proceeded along two lines: tailoring individual elements of self-management, and tailoring entire self-management programs. One other practice, a form of tailoring intended for specific populations rather than for individuals also has received attention, but will not be considered in this section because such programs are directed to groups, not to individual patients. For the interested reader, examples of asthma self-management programs for specific populations include those for inner city children (e.g., Butz et al. 2005; Velsor-Freidrich et al. 2004), preschool children (Mesters et al. 1994 Wilson et al. 1996), and college students (Tehan et al. 1989), to name a few.

Tailoring Elements of Asthma Self-Management

The most readily tailored element of asthma self-management is medication requirement. An early example of this consisted of a children's computer game whose program could be altered for each child to include the child's medication (Rubin et al. 1986). A different approach was used in a study of adult patients who received booklets at monthly intervals that were tailored for medication requirement and for information either requested by the patient or deemed valuable to the patient (Osman et al. 1994). These programs yielded positive results, but the tailored aspects of the programs were not independently evaluated.

A common form of limited tailoring consists of combining medication need with an action plan that includes recommendations for medication use and for seeking assistance. The intent is to establish a series of progressively aggressive measures for controlling asthma. Recommendations for increasing medication use or for initiating other measures to control asthma may be based on the status of asthma as indicated by symptoms or by peak expiratory flow level. Perhaps the first study of this sort of tailoring was conducted in a Maori community, where individuals were given a card that outlined procedures for asthma assessment and intervention based on information about peak expiratory flow, and provided specific instruction for when to seek emergency assistance (D'Souza et al. 1984). Unfortunately, the program could not be evaluated because of the design of the study. More recently, research related to limited tailoring has been done within the context of evaluating home monitoring of asthma. Specifically, action plans that include medication adjustments have been studied. Although a great deal of attention has been focused on this area, the contribution of a tailored action plan to a comprehensive asthma self-management program remains unclear. The reason for this resides in the experimental designs of most studies. What is needed to determine the incremental value of an action plan to self-management is a study of programs with and without an action plan. In studies of home monitoring, the converse has been done: action plans with and without self-management have been compared with traditional medical management. In addition, various action plans have been compared with one another. None of this work addresses the value of tailoring in self-management, and for that reason will not be reviewed here. These studies, however, are the subject of several reviews (Kotses et al. 2006; Toelle and Ram 2004), and additionally, are discussed in a separate chapter in this volume.

Tailoring Asthma Self-Management Programs

At least two approaches to tailoring of self-management programs have been attempted. They differ in how information for tailoring is collected. Ultimately, all tailoring is based on patient experience. But in some studies, tailoring decisions are made by asking patients about their asthma, and in others, by analyzing data collected by patients. Asking patients about their asthma is the simpler of the two. It has been used on several occasions to tailor self-management programs (e.g., Bailey et al. 1990; Dahl et al. 1990; Fireman et al. 1981; Sockrider et al. 2006; Thoonen et al. 2002; Wilson et al. 1993). Improvements were reported in each study, but tailoring was evaluated independently only in one (Wilson et al. 1993). In the latter study, the effectiveness of tailored self-management programs was compared with that of a small group program. The tailored programs were assembled, on the basis of an interview, from a pool of 18 instructional modules that represented the entire content of the small group self-management program. Patients in both conditions improved in comparison to controls, but the improvement favored the group-trained participants to a slight degree. The investigators also pointed out that group participants benefited from peer support and that group programs were cheaper to conduct than tailored programs.

Tailoring that relies on data collected by patients also has produced positive outcomes. In two studies (Creer et al. 1988; Kotses et al. 1995), patients participating in a group self-management program completed a questionnaire relating to both triggers and control practices for each asthma episode they experienced. Patients reviewed the reports periodically for evidence of consistency in either their triggers or effective controls. The intent of this was to help each patient understand the causes and countermeasures of his or her asthma. These tailoring procedures were not evaluated independently of the self-management programs. But a closely related procedure (Kotses et al. 1991 b, 1996) was evaluated independently and produced evidence of effective asthma control for tailored programs. Patients were asked to collect information regarding the date and time of their asthma attacks, their daily peak flow scores, and their contact with a number of asthma triggers. The information the patients gathered was analyzed statistically for the relationship of asthma attacks both to triggers and to peak flow. On the basis of these analyses, a unique program was designed for each patient that took into consideration the patient's triggers. Patients who were given these programs did at least as well as patients given a group self-management program.

These studies make it clear that tailored self-management programs can be effective. A major benefit of tailoring is a practical one: tailoring is consistent with medical practice. As in customary medical practice, tailoring concerns the individual, not the group. By contrast, group self-management is more closely associated with education than it is with medicine. It requires teaching competencies and facilities that may not be readily available in some medical settings: complex scheduling arrangements, classroom space, teaching equipment, and supplies. Tailored asthma self-management, therefore, might be feasible where group training is impractical. The benefit is, however, offset by its high cost. Even if the costs for development of the two self-management formats were equivalent, the difference between them in the cost of staff time needed for administration would be greater for tailored than for group programs, a problem that could preclude widespread use of tailored programs. But even this barrier may be surmounted by research, possibly by developing tailored programs that can be self-administered, at least to some extent. This and other challenges of tailoring wait to be taken up.

Asthma Self-Management in Hindsight

Our review of asthma self-management focused almost exclusively on outcome. With the exception of our mention of a few methodological problems, we did not consider procedures. But procedures matter, and some of the results we described may not withstand close scrutiny. One serious problem that plagues asthma self-management research concerns its most common control procedure: usual care. While usual care may appear to fulfill the requirements for control adequately, there is reason to believe that it does not. All research requires that a control condition be identical to the experimental condition in all relevant ways except for the treatment variable: the intervention, in the case of self-management. The requirement includes amount of time spent with patients, a hard thing to balance between groups, as self-management training almost always involves more time spent with the patient than usual care. If both self-management training and time spent with patients differ between groups, research outcomes cannot be fully attributed to self-management.

The argument is underscored by research showing that subtle factors can affect research outcome. In self-management research, the outcome of training may be affected by both demand characteristics and experimenter bias. The former refers to the tendency of patients to behave in ways expected of them and the latter to the expectations of the experimenter. These influences have not been fully explored for asthma-related variables, but related findings have been reported. Evidence of the influence of demand, consisting of air volume and flow variation resulting from the change of single word in forced expiatory maneuver instructions (Harm et al. 1984, 1985), has been reported in healthy individuals. Research has also shown that the expectancy of the experimenter affects respiratory resistance in healthy subjects despite a total lack of awareness on the part of the experimenter that an expectation was communicated (Wigal et al. 1997). The sensitivity of individuals to experimental conditions, as documented in these studies, suggests the likelihood that interactions with self-management patients during periods of extended contact may give rise to influences that affect outcome independently of training. Failure to control such influences could lead to misleading conclusions.

The possibility of this sort of contamination suggests that some of our conclusions regarding the effects of self-management may be overly optimistic. That we have reached this uneasy understanding after much effort researching self-management is not surprising. Conducting research in a naturalistic setting is a tall order. In the case of asthma self-management, the best medical and research practices are often in conflict, a hurdle that limits research effectiveness. Additionally, neither patients nor their health care providers necessarily play the roles we ask of them in self-management research, and their interactions may be affected by variables of which we know relatively little. Even our best experimental designs may falter against these obstacles. We are encouraged, however, by volume of evidence of self-management effectiveness, even as we recognize that only more research will resolve questions of its efficacy once and for all.

Some Trends in Asthma Self-Management Research

A recent survey of asthma self-management practice in Canada (Tsuyuki et al. 2005) noted that the records of more than half of the asthma patients contained no evidence that they received any type of self-management training, and that only 2% had been given an action plan. The fact that so many asthma patients do not receive self-management training suggests the presence of significant barriers to training. These may include cost, time and money, and possibly the failure of self-management programs to accommodate the needs of some patients. Fortunately, trends in research suggest remedies for these problems are on the way. Recently, an increasing amount of asthma self-management research has been devoted to special populations and to special settings. Both inner-city populations, in which prevalence of the disease is especially high, and school settings, where children may be reached conveniently and at modest cost, have been studied extensively. These investigations may bring access to self-management to a greater number of people. Augmenting these trends is an increase in short forms of asthma self-management. The length of the early self-management programs was six to eight sessions, but more recently programs requiring a little as a single session have been developed. Short programs increase access to training by reducing both the time needed to complete a program and the financial cost of the program. Additional improvement may result from tailoring programs for individual patients. Among new approaches to tailoring, the use of biomarkers may eventually play a role in developing asthma treatment and management programs for individuals (Szefler 2008) Tailored programs provide the ultimate degree of flexibility and efficiency for asthma self-management. If they could be conducted inexpensively, they would extend the benefits of asthma self-management to every patient who needs it.

References

Abdulwadud O, Abramson M, Forbes A, James A, Walters EH (1999) Evaluation of a randomized controlled trial of adult asthma education in a hospital setting. Thorax 54:493–500

Adams PF, Marano MA (1995) Current estimates from the National Health Interview Survey, 1994. Vital Health Stat 10(193 Pt 1):1–260

Alexander AB (1972) Systematic relaxation and flow rates in asthmatic children: relationship to emotional precipitants and anxiety. J Psychosom Res 16:405–410

Alexander AB, Miklich DR, Hershkoff H (1972) The immediate effects of systematic relaxation training on peak expiratory flow rates in asthmatic children. Psychosom Med 34:388–394

Alexander JS, Younger RE, Cohen RM, Crawford LV (1988) Effectiveness of a nurse-managed program for children with chronic asthma. J Pediatr Nurs 3:312–317

Allen RM, Jones MP, Oldenburg B (1995) Randomized trial of an asthma self-management programme for adults. Thorax 50:731–738

American Lung Association, Epidemiology and Statistics Unit, Research and Program Services (2005). Trends in asthma morbidity and mortality. Retrieved 26 May, 2006 from http://www.lungusa.org/atf/cf

Apter AJ, Affleck G, Reisine ST, Tennen HA, Barrows E, Wells M et al (1997) Perception of airway obstruction in asthma: sequential daily analyses of symptoms, peak expiratory flow rate, and mood. J Allergy Clin Immunol 99:605–612

Bailey WC, Richards JM, Brooks M, Soong S, Windsor RA, Manzella BA (1990) A randomized trial to improve self-management practices in adults with asthma. Arch Intern Med 150:1664–1668

Bandura A (1991a) Self-efficacy mechanism in physiological activation and health promoting behavior. In: Madden J IV (ed) Neurobiology of learning, emotion and affect. Raven, New York, pp 229–270

Bandura A (1991b) Self-regulation of motivation through anticipatory and self-regulatory mechanisms. In: Dienstbier RA (ed) Perspectives on motivation: Nebraska symposium on motivation 38. University of Nebraska Press, Lincoln, pp 69–164

Bandura A (1986) Social foundation of thought and action: a social cognitive theory. Prentice-Hall, Englewood Cliffs NJ

Barbanel D, Eldridge S, Griffiths C (2003) Can a self-management programme delivered by a community pharmacist improve asthma control? A randomized trial. Thorax 58:851–854

Bartter T, Pratter MR (1996) Asthma: better outcome at lower cost? The role of the expert in the care system. Chest 110:1589–1596

Beck AT (1967) Depression: clinical, experimental, and theoretical aspects. Harper & Row, New York

Berg J, Dunbar-Jacob J, Sereika SM (1997) An evaluation of a self-management program for adults with asthma. Clin Nurs Res 6:225–238

Behera D, Kaur S, Gupta D, Verma SK (2005) Evaluation of self-care manual in bronchial asthma. Indian J Chest Dis Allied Sci 48:43–48

Brown JV, Bakeman R, Celano MP, Demi AS, Kokbrynski L, Wilson SR (2002) Home-based asthma education for you low-income children and their families. J Pediatr Psychol 27:677–688

Brewin AM, Hughes JA (1995) Effects of patient education on asthma management. Br J Nurs 4:81–101

Bruzzese JM, Unikel L, Gallagher R, Evans D, Colland V (2008) Feasibility of a school-based intervention for families of urbanized adolescents with asthma: results from a randomized pilot trial. Fam Process 47:95–113

Bryant-Stevens T, Li Y (2004) Community asthma education program for parents of urban asthmatic children. J Natl Med Assoc 9:954–960

Butz AM, Syron L, Johnson B, Spaudling J, Walker M, Bollinger ME (2005) Home-based asthma self-management education for inner city children. Public Health Nurs 22:189–199

Carswell F, Robinson EJ, Hek G, Shenton T (1989) A Bristol experience: benefits and cost of an 'asthma nurse' visiting the homes of asthmatic children. Bristol Med Chir J 104:11–12

Castro M, Zimmermann NA, Crocker S, Bradley J, Leven C, Schechtman KB (2003) Asthma intervention program prevents readmissions in high healthcare users. Am J Respir Crit Care Med 168:1095–1098

Centers for Disease Control and Prevention (1996) Asthma mortality and hospitalization among children and young adults – United States, 1980–1993. Morb Mort Wkly Rep 45:350–353

Centers for Disease Control and Prevention (2004) Asthma prevalence, health care use and mortality, 2002. National Center for Health Statistics, Hyattsville, Maryland

Charlton I, Antoniou AG, Atkinson J, Campbell MJ, Chapman E, Mackintosh T et al (1994) Asthma at the interface: bridging the gap between general practice and a district general hospital. Arch Dis Child 70:313–318

Chiang L, Huang J, Chao S (2005) A comparison by quantitative and qualitative methods, between the self-management behaviors of parents with asthmatic children in two hospitals. J Nurs Res 13:85–95

Chaucer G (Ca. 1387-1400). The Canterbury tales; the monk's tale, Line 2139. Retrieved 1 May, 2006 from http://etext.lib.virginia.edu/etcbin/toccerold?id=Cha2Can&images=images/modeng&data=/lv1/Archive/mideng-parsed&tag=public&part=42&division=div1

Christiansen SC, Martin SB, Schleilcher NC, Koxiol JA, Mathers KP, Zuraw BL (1997) Evaluation of a school-based asthma education program for inner-city children. J Allergy Clin Immunol 10:613–617

Cicutto L, Murphy S, Coutts D, O'Rourke J, Lang G, Chapman C et al (2005) Evaluating an asthma center's efforts to provide education to children with asthma in schools. Chest 128:1928–1935

Clark NM, Brown R, Joseph CLM, Anderson EW, Liu M, Valerio MA (2004) Effects of a comprehensive school-based asthma program on symptoms, parental management, grades, and absenteeism. Chest 125:1674–1679

Clark NM, Feldman CH, Freudenberg N, Millman EJ, Wasilewski Y, Valle I (1980) Developing education for children with asthma through study of self-management behavior. Health Educ Q 7:278–297

Coffman JM, Cabana MD, Halpin HA, Yelin EH (2008) Effects of asthma education on children's use of acute care services: a meta-analysis. Pediatrics 121:575–586

Colland VT (1993) Learning to cope with asthma: a behavioural self-management program for children. Patient Educ Couns 22:141–152

Cote J, Bowie DM, Robichaud P, Parent J, Battisti L, Boulet L (2001) Evaluation of two different educational interventions for adult patients consulting with an acute asthma exacerbation. Am J Respir Crit Care Med 163:1415–1419

Cote J, Cartier A, Robichaud P, Boutin H, Malo J, Rouleau M et al (2000) Influence of asthma education on severity, quality of life and environmental control. Can Respir J 7:395–400

Cote J, Cartier A, Robichaud P, Boutin H, Malo J, Rouleau M et al (1997) Influence on asthma morbidity of asthma education programs based on self-management plans following treatment optimization. Am J Respir Crit Care Med 155:1509–1514

Cowie RL, Revitt SG, Underwood MF, Field SK (1997) The effect of peak flow action plans in the prevention of exacerbations of asthma. Chest 112:1534–1538

Creer TL (2008) Behavioral and cognitive processes in the self-management of asthma. J Asthma 45:81–94

Creer TL (1992) Psychological and behavioral assessment of childhood asthma. Part II: behavioral approaches. Pediatr Asthma Allergy Immunol 6:21–34

Creer TL, Backial M, Burns KL, Leung P, Marion RJ, Micklich DR et al (1988) Living with asthma I. Genesis and development of a self-management program for childhood asthma. J Asthma 25:335–362

Creer TL, Wigal JK, Kotses H, Lewis P (1990) A critique of 19 self-management programs for childhood asthma: part II. Comment regarding the scientific merits of the programs. Pediatr Asthma Allergy Immunol 4:41–55

Dahl J, Gustafsson D, Melin L (1990) Effects of a behavioral treatment program on children with asthma. J Asthma 27:41–46

Deaves DM (1993) An assessment of the value of health education in the prevention of childhood asthma. J Adv Nurs 18:354–363

Dekker E, Groen J (1956) Reproducible psychogenic attacks of asthma. J Psychosom Res 1:58–67

de Oliveira MA, Faresin SM, Bruno VF, de Bittencourt AR, Fernandes ALG (1999) Evaluation of an educational programme for socially deprived asthma patients. Eur Respir J 14:908–914

Diamond SA, Chapman KR. (2001). The impact of a nationally-coordinated pharmacy-based asthma education intervention. Can Respir J 8:261–265.

D'Souza W, Crane J, Burgess H, Te Karu H, Fox C, Harper M et al (1984) Community-based asthma care: trial of a "credit card" asthma self-management plan. Eur Respir J 7:1260–1265

Evans D, Clark NM, Feldman CH, Rips J, Kaplan D, Levison MJ et al (1987) A school health education program for children with asthma aged 8–11 years. Health Educ Q 14:267–279

Fall AJ, Henry RL, Hazell T (1998) The use of an interactive computer program for the education of parents of asthmatic children. J Pediatr Child Health 34:127–130

Fireman P, Friday GA, Gira C, Virthaler WA, Michaels L (1981) Teaching self-management skills to asthmatic children and their parents in an ambulatory care setting. Pediatrics 68:341–348

Ford ME, Edwards G, Rodriguez JL, Gibson RC, Tilley BC (1996) An empowerment-centered, church-based asthma education program for African-American adults. Health Soc Work 21:70–75

Gallefoss F, Bakke PS (2000) Impact of patient education and self-management on morbidity in asthmatics and patients with chronic obstructive pulmonary disease. Respir Med 94:279–287

George MR, O'Dowd LC, Martin I, Lindell KO, Whitney F, Jones M et al (1999) A comprehensive educational program improves clinical outcome measures in inner-city patients with asthma. Arch Intern Med 159:1710–1716

Ghosh CS, Ravindran P, Joshi M, Stearns SC (1998) Reductions in hospital use from self-management training for chronic asthmatics. Soc Sci Med 46:1087–1093

Gibson PG, Powell H, Coughlan J, Wilson AJ, Hensley MJ, Abramson, et al. (2002). Limited (information only) patient education programs for adults with asthma. The Cochrane Database of Systematic Reviews, Issue 1. Art. No.: CD001005

Glasgow NJ, Ponsonby A, Yates R, Beilby J, Dugdale P (2003) Proactive asthma care in childhood: general practice based randomized control trial. Br J Med 327:659–665

Greineder DK, Loane KC, Parks P (1999) A randomized control trial of a pediatric asthma outreach program. J Allergy Clin Immunol 103:436–440

Harm DL, Marion RJ, Creer TL, Kotses H (1985) Effects of instructions on pulmonary function values. J Asthma 22:289–294

Harm DL, Marion RJ, Kotses H, Creer TL (1984) Effects of subject effort on pulmonary function measures: a preliminary investigation. J Asthma 21:295–298

Henry RL, Gibson PG, Vimpani GV, Francis JL, Hazell J (2004) Randomized controlled trial of a teacher-led asthma education program. Pediatr Pulmonol 38:434–442

Hilton S, Sibbald B, Anderson HR, Freeling P (1986) Controlled evaluation of the effects of patient education on asthma morbidity in general practice. Lancet 1:26–29

Hindi-Alexander M, Cropp GJ (1984) Evaluation of a family asthma program. J Allergy Clin Immunol 46:143–148

Holzheimer L, Mohay H, Master IB (1998) Educating young children about asthma: comparing the effectiveness of a developmentally appropriate asthma education video tape and picture book. Child Care Health Dev 24:85–99

Horner SD, Fouladi RT (2008) Improvement of rural children's asthma self-management by lay health educators. J Sch Health 78:506–513

Hughes DM, McLeod M, Garner B, Goldbloom RB (1991) Controlled trail of a home and ambulatory program for asthmatic children. Pediatrics 87:54–61

Ignacio-Garcia JM, Gonzalez-Santos P (1995) Asthma self-management education program by home monitoring of peak expiratory flow. Am J Respir Crit Care Med 151: 353–359

Janson JL, Fahy JV, Covington JK, Paul SM, Gold WM, Boushey HA (2003) Effects of individual self-management education on clinical, biological, and adherence outcomes in asthma. Am J Med 115:620–626

Jones PW, Quirk FH, Baveystock CM, Littlejohns (1992) A complete measure of health status of chronic airflow limitation. The St. George's Respiratory Questionnaire. Am Rev Respir Dis 145(6):1321–1327

Juniper EF (1998) Quality-of-life measures. In: Kotses H, Harver A (eds) Self-management of asthma. Marcel Dekker, New York, pp 91–115

Juniper EF, Guyett GH, Epstein RS, Ferrie PJ, Jaeschke R, Hiller TK (1992) Evaluation of impairment of health-related quality of life in asthma: development of a questionnaire for use in clinical trails. Thorax 47:76–83

Juniper EF, Guyett GH, Feeny DH, Ferrie PJ, Griffith LE, Townsend M (1996a) Measuring quality of life in children with asthma. Qual Life Res 5:27–34

Juniper EF, Guyett GH, Feeny DH, Ferrie PJ, Griffith LE, Townsend M (1996b) Measuring quality of life in parents of children with asthma. Qual Life Res 5:35–46

Juniper EF, Guyett GH, Ferrie PJ, Griffith LE (1993) Measuring quality of life in asthma. Am Rev Respir Dis 147:832–838

Knoell DL, Pierson JF, Marsh CB, Allen JN, Pathak DS (1998) Measurement of outcomes in adults receiving pharmaceutical care in a comprehensive outcome clinic. Pharmacotherapy 18:1365–1374

Kotses H, Bernstein IL, Bernstein DI, Korbee L, Wigal JK, Ganson E, Stout C, Creer TL (1995) A self-management program for adults with asthma. Part I: development and evaluation. J Allergy Clin Immunol 95:529–540

Kotses H, Glaus KD, Bricel SK, Edwards JE, Crawford PC (1978) Operant muscular relaxation and peak expiratory flow rate in children. J Psychosom Res 22:17–23

Kotses H, Glaus KD, Crawford PC, Edwards JE, Sherr MS (1976) Operant reduction of frontalis EMG activity in the treatment of asthma in children. J Psychosom Res 20:453–459

Kotses H, Harver A, Humphries CT (2006) Home monitoring in asthma self-management. J Asthma 43:649–655

Kotses H, Harver A, Segretto J, Glaus KD, Creer TL, Young GA (1991a) Long-term effects of biofeedback-induced facial relaxation on measures of asthma severity in children. Biofeedback Self Regul 16:1–21

Kotses H, Rawson JC, Wigal JK, Creer TL (1987a) Respiratory airway changes in response to suggestion in normal individuals. Psychosom Med 49:536–541

Kotses H, Lewis P, Creer TL (1990) Environmental control of asthma self-management. J Asthma 27:357–384

Kotses H, Stout C, McGonnaughy K, Winder JA, Creer TL (1996) Evaluation in individualized asthma self-management programs. J Asthma 33:113–118

Kotses H, Stout C, Wigal JK, Carlson B, Creer TL, Lewis P (1991b) Individualized asthma self-management: a beginning. J Asthma 28:287–289

Kotses H, Westlund R, Creer TL (1987b) Performing mental arithmetic increases total respiratory resistance in individuals with normal respiration. Psychophysiology 24:678–682

Lahdensuo A, Haahtela T, Herrala J, Kava T, Kiviranta K, Kuusisto P et al (1996) Randomized comparison of guided self-management and traditional treatment of asthma over one year. Br Med J 312:748–752

Lavoi KL, Bouchard A, Joseph M, Campbell TS, Favreau H, Bacon SL (2008) Association of self-efficacy to asthma control and quality of life. Ann Behav Med 36:100–106

Levy ML, Robb M, Allen J, Doherty JM, Winter RJD (2000) A randomized controlled evaluation of specialist nurse education following accident and emergency department attendance for acute asthma. Respir Med 94:900–908

Lewis CE, Rachelefsky G, Lewis MA, de la Sota A, Kaplan M (1984) A randomized trial of A. C. T. (Asthma Care Training) for kids. Pediatrics 74:478–486

Kubly LS, McClellan MS (1984) Effects of self-care instruction on asthmatic children. Issues Compr Pediatr Nurs 7:121–130

MacKenzie JN (1886) The production of so called "rose cold" by means of an artificial rose. Am J Med Sci 91:45–57

Madge P, McColl J, Paton J (1997) Impact of a nurse-led management training programme in children admitted to hospital with acute asthma: a randomized control study. Thorax 52:223–228

Mahr TA, Evans R 3rd (1993) Allergist influence in asthma care. Ann Allergy 71:115–120

Manzilla BA, Brooks CM, Richards JM, Windsor RA, Soong S, Bailey WC (1989) Assessing the use of metered dose inhalers by adults with asthma. J Asthma 26:223–230

Mesters I, Meertens R, Kok G, Parcel GS (1994) Effectiveness of a multidisciplinary education protocol in children with asthma. J Asthma 33:347–359

Mayo PH, Richman J, Harris HW (1990) Results of a program to reduce admissions for adult asthma. Ann Intern Med 112:864–871

McNabb WL, Wilson-Pessano SR, Hughes GW, Scamagas P (1985) Self-management education of children with asthma: AIR WISE. Am J Public Health 75:1219–1220

Moudgil H, Marshall T, Honeybourne D (2000) Asthma education and quality of life in the community: a randomized control study to evaluate the impact on white European and Indian subcontinent ethnic groups from socioeconomically deprived areas of Birmingham, UK. Thorax 55:177–183

National Institute of Health (1991) Guidelines for the diagnosis and management of asthma. Expert Panel Report. J Allergy Clin Immunol 88(3(Pt. 2)):425–534

Osman LM, Abdalla MI, Beattie JAG, Ross SJ, Russell IT, Friend JA et al (1994) Reducing hospital admissions through computer supported education for asthma patients. Br Med J 308:568–571

Osman LM, Calder C, Godden DJ, Friend JAR, Mckenzie L, Legge JS, Douglas JG (2002) A randomised trial of self-management planning for adult patients admitted to hospital with acute asthma. Thorax 57:869–874

Ostojic B, Cvoriscec B, Ostojic SB, Reznikiff D, Stipic-Markovic A, Tudjman Z (2005) Improving asthma control through telemedicine: a study of short-message service. Telemed J E Health 11:28–35

Parcel GS, Meyer MP (1978) Development of an instrument to measure children's health locus of control. Health Educ Monogr 6:149–159

Parcel GS, Nader PR, Tiernan K (1980) A health education program for children with asthma. Dev Behav Pediatr 1:128–132

Pinnock H, Slack R, Pagliari C, Price D, Sheikh A (2007) Understanding the potential role of mobile phone-based monitoring on asthma self-management: qualitative study. Clin Exp Allergy 37:794–802

Popovic JC (2001) 1999 National hospital discharge survey: annual summary with detailed diagnosis and procedure data. National Center for Health Statistics. Vital Health Stat 13(151):21 Table 10

Put C, van den Bergh O, Lemaigre V, Demedts M, Vereden G (2003) Evaluation of an individualised asthma programme directed at behavioural change. Eur Respir J 21:109–115

Rakos RF, Grodek MV, Mack KK (1985) The impact of a self-administered behavioral intervention program on pediatric asthma. J Psychosom Res 29:101–108

Robinson LD (1985) Evaluation of an asthma summer camp program. Chest 87:105S–107S

Rubin DH, Leventhal JM, Sadock RT, Letovsky E, Schottland P, Clemente I et al (1986) Educational intervention by computer in childhood asthma: a randomized clinical trial testing the use of a new teaching intervention in childhood asthma. Pediatrics 11:1–77

Ryan D, Cobern W, Wheeler J, Price D, Tarassenko L (2005) Mobil phone technology in the management of asthma. J Telemed Telecare 11(Suppl 1):43–46

Skinner BF (1953) Science and human behavior. New York: Macmillan

Smith L, Bosnic-Anticevich SZ, Mitchell B, Saini B, Kress I, Armour C (2007) Treating asthma with a self-management model of illness behaviour in an Australian community pharmacy setting. Soc Sci Med 64:1501–1511

Smith JH, Mugford M, Holland R, Candy B, Noble J, Harrison BWD et al (2005) A systematic review to examine the impact of psycho-educational interventions on health outcomes and cost in adults and children with difficult asthma. Health Technol Assess 9:23

Snyder SE, Winder JA, Creer TL (1987) Development and evaluation of an adult asthma self-management program: Wheezers Anonymous. J Asthma 24:153–158

Sockrider MM, Abramson S, Brooks E, Caviness AC, Pliney S, Koerner C et al (2006) Delivering tailored family asthma family education in a pediatric emergency department: a pilot study. Pediatrics 117:S135–S144

Szefler SJ (2008) Individualizing asthma therapy: application of biomarkers. J Asthma 45(S1):29–31

Taggart VS, Zuckerman A, Lucas C, Acty-Lindsey A, Bellanti JA (1987) Adapting a self-management education program for asthma for use in an outpatient clinic. Ann Allergy 58:173–178

Taitel MS, Kotses H, Bernstein IL, Bernstein DI, Creer TL (1995) A self-management program for adult asthma, Part II: cost-benefit analysis. J Allergy Clin Immunol 95:672–676

Talabere LR (1993) The effects of an asthma education program on selected health behaviors in school-aged children with asthma. In: Funk SG (ed) Key aspects of caring for the chronically ill: hospital and home. Springer, New York, pp 319–330

Tehan N, Sloan BC, Walsh-Robert N, Chamberlain MD (1989) Impact of asthma self-management education on the health behavior of young adults. J Adolesc Health Care 10:513–519

Tellegen A, Lykken DT, Bouchard TJ, Wilcox KJ, Segal NL, Rich S (1988) Personality similarity in twins reared apart and together. J Pers Soc Psychol 54:1031–1039

Thoonen BPA, Schermer TJR, Jansen M, Smeele I, Jacobs AJE, Grol R et al (2002) Asthma education tailored to individual patient needs can optimise partnerships in asthma self-management. Patient Educ Couns 47:355–360

Toelle BG, Peat JK, Salome CM, Mellis CM, Bauman AE, Woolcock AJ (1993) Evaluation of a community-based asthma management program in a population sample of school children. Med J Aust 158:742–746

Toelle BG, Ram FSF (2004) Written individualized management plans for children and adults. Cochrane Database Syst RevIssue1,Art.No.CD002171.pub2.DOI:10.1002/14651858. CD002171. pub2.

Tsuyuki RT, Sin DD, Sharpe HM, Cowie RL, Nilsson C, Man P (2005) Management of asthma among community-based primary care physicians. J Asthma 42:163-167

Usherwood TP, Scrimgeour A, Barber JH (1990) Questionnaire to measure perceived symptoms and disability in asthma. Arch Dis Child 87:376–379

Velsor-Freidrich B, Pigott TD, Louloudes A (2004) The effects of a school-based intervention on the self-care and health of African-American inner-city children. J Pediatr Nurs 19:247–256

Vermeire PA, Rabe KF, Sorian JB, Maier WC (2002) Asthma control and differences in management practices across seven European countries. Respir Med 96:142–149

Weingarten MA, Goldberg BM, Teperberg Y, Harrison N, Oded BA (1985) A pilot study of the multidisciplinary management of childhood asthma in a family practice. J Asthma 22:261–265

Weiss JH, Hermalin JA (1987) The effectiveness of a self-teaching asthma self-management training program for school age children and their families. Prev Health 5:57–78

Weiss KB, Sullivan SD, Lytle CS (2000) Trends in the cost of illness for asthma in the United States, 1985–1994. J Allergy Clin Immunol 106:493–499

Whitman N, West D, Brough FK, Welch M (1985) A study of a self-care rehabilitation program in pediatric asthma. Health Educ Q 12:333–342

Wigal JK, Creer TL, Kotses H, Lewis P (1990) A critique of 19 self-management programs for childhood asthma: part I. Development and evaluation of the programs. Pediatr Asthma Allergy Immunol 4:17–39

Wigal JK, Kotses H, Rawson JC, Creer TL (1988) The effects of suggestion on total respiration resistance in healthy female subjects. J Psychosom Res 32:409–416

Wigal J, Stout C, Kotses H, Creer T, Fogle K, Gayhart L et al (1997) Experimenter expectancy in resistance to respiratory air flow. Psychosom Med 59:318–322

Wilson-Pessano SR, McNabb WL (1985) The role of patient education in the management of childhood asthma. Prev Med 14:670–687

Wilson SR, Scamagas P, German dF, Hughes GW, Lulla S, Coss S et al (1993) A controlled trial of two forms of self-management education for adults with asthma. Am J Med 94:564–576

Wilson SR, Latini D, Starr NJ, Fish L, Loes LM, Page A et al (1996) Education of parents of infants and very young children with asthma: a developmental evaluation of the Wee Wheezers Program. J Asthma 33:239–254

Wolf FM, Guevara JP, Grum CM, Clark NM, Cates CJ (2003) Educational interventions for asthma in children (Cochrane Review). In: The Cochrane Library (1). Oxford: Update Software http://www.update-software.com/abstracts/ab000326.htm

Yilmaz A, Akkaya E (2002) Evaluation of long-term efficacy of an asthma education programme in an out-patient clinic. Respir Med 96:519–524

Yoon R, McKenzie DK, Bauman A, Miles DA (1993) Controlled trial evaluation of an asthma education programme for adults. Thorax 48:1110–1116

Chapter 9
Home Monitoring of Asthma: Symptoms and Peak Flow

Andrew Harver, Maeve O'Connor, Sam Walford, and Harry Kotses

Monitoring is an established component of asthma control. Its purpose is to provide the patient an ongoing evaluation of the severity of the disease. The importance of such an evaluation cannot be overestimated as it guides corrective measures needed to keep asthma under control. All asthma patients monitor severity at some level, but only some do it systematically. The term 'home monitoring' implies the latter. It has been a part of asthma self-management programs since their inception. And while no one questions the necessity of monitoring for asthma control, its contribution to asthma self-management is not fully understood.

Two forms of home monitoring have emerged: symptom monitoring and peak flow monitoring. Symptoms monitored include both subjective elements of an asthma exacerbation (i.e., dyspnea, chest tightness, cough, wheeze, and congestion), and objective indices of asthma severity such as activity limitation and nighttime awakenings. Respiratory indices monitored can include any of the several lung functions but only peak expiratory flow rate (PEFR) has been used widely. It is not uncommon for symptom and peak flow monitoring to be practiced together for asthma self-management. Despite the accepted value of monitoring, a great deal of interest has been devoted to examining the relative effectiveness of the two in asthma control.

In this chapter, we describe common home monitoring practices and validation procedures, outline developments with potential to improve accuracy of symptom and PEFR indices, and review research on effectiveness of home monitoring in asthma self-management.

A. Harver (✉)
Department of Public Health Sciences, The University of North Carolina at Charlotte, 9201 University City Blvd, Charlotte, NC, 28223-0001, USA
e-mail: arharver@uncc.edu

Home Monitoring Practice

Symptom Monitoring

Monitoring of symptoms includes practices that differ in terms of the demands they place on patients. In the simplest case, symptom monitoring is not considered an intervention but conducted to gain information about variability of symptoms that might be useful in the interpretation of findings (Charlton et al. 1994; Ignacio-Garcia and Gonzalez-Santos 1995). Although patient reactions to monitoring are not of primary interest in this procedure, the act of observing and recording symptoms may affect the way in which some patients deal with their asthma. A somewhat more demanding procedure involves providing the patient with general guidelines for reacting to symptoms. These may involve instruction in tracking the severity of asthma with symptoms, in using symptoms to identify triggers of asthma, and in corrective action required when symptoms occur (e.g., Creer et al. 1988; Kotses et al. 1995). Symptom monitoring may be made even more demanding when combined with an action plan, a formal set of recommendations for control of asthma at different levels of severity. One such plan, for example, specified symptom benchmarks that cued administration of an increasing amount of a bronchodilator and initiation of steroid administration (Turner et al. 1998). The National Institute of Health (NIH) recommends use of a formal action plan (NIH 2007).

Symptoms such as cough, wheeze, and others may be recorded individually (e.g., Santanello et al. 1997) or in the aggregate by expressing the effect of all symptoms in a single asthma severity score (e.g., Fritz et al. 1990). The two forms of monitoring yield different information. Recording symptoms individually has the

A. Harver and H. Kotses (eds.), *Asthma, Health and Society: A Public Health Perspective*,
DOI 10.1007/978-0-387-78285-0_9, © Springer Science+Business Media, LLC 2010

advantage of preserving the response characteristics of patients and the disadvantage of complicating the interpretation of symptoms. Symptoms monitored in the aggregate resolve the interpretation problem but mask unique symptom patterns that may be potentially important. There is no compelling reason for preferring one form of symptom assessment consistently over the other.

PEFR Monitoring

The PEFR is the fastest rate of exhalation that can be maintained for 10 ms (Wright and McKerrow 1959). Patients can measure it at home with an inexpensive meter. The measurement requires the patient to exhale forcefully through the meter and to record the value indicated. Introduction of a meter, even one as simple as that used by most patients, necessitates patients be trained in its use. As consistency of patient recording procedures is desirable, a commonly used set of training guidelines is recommended.

Several issues must be dealt with before the patient can use the meter effectively. First, it is essential that the meter be kept clean, in good working condition, and recalibrated periodically. The latter is important because some meters lose calibration after a few hundred tests (Shapiro et al. 1991). Second, the PEFR is effort-dependent. To get a good reading, exhalation into the meter must be as forceful as possible. Inevitably, the effort-dependency of PEFR recording leads to error, as it is difficult to achieve maximum expiratory effort consistently (Gannon et al. 1999). Additional error is introduced because effort-dependent pulmonary functions can be influenced by subtle factors (Harm et al. 1984). To compensate for these errors, the best of three PEFR readings taken a minute apart is considered as the best estimate of PEFR (NIH 2007). Third, the PEFR is subject to diurnal variation; it is usually lower in the morning than it is in the evening. If daily range is of interest, two scores a day, one in the morning and one in the evening, must be taken. If daily variation is not of interest, or if two recordings per day are judged to place too heavy a burden on the patient, one recording will suffice. When PEFR is recorded but once a day, it is important that the reading be made at the same time each day. Fourth, the procedure for recording the PEFR is standardized. NIH recommends specific steps (i.e., stand up, take a deep breath, etc.) be followed in testing PEFR (NIH 2007).

A single PEFR score is meaningless to the individual and useless for managing asthma. To be informative, the score must be compared to a standard. Any one of a number of standards may be used, but the benchmark recommended by NIH (2007) is the "personal best" score. It is the highest score the patient can achieve during regular testing throughout a 2-week period. Asthma severity is measured by PEFR expressed as the percentage of personal best score. NIH (2007) recommends the distribution of percentage scores be subdivided into severity ranges representing little or no asthma (80–100% personal best–green zone), worsening asthma (50–79% personal best–yellow zone), and dangerous asthma (below 50% personal best–red zone). Each zone is associated with specific recommendations for asthma management.

Like its symptoms counterpart, PEFR monitoring has been used in asthma self-management programs that feature different levels of patient demand including: solely for data collection (e.g., Ignacio-Garcia and Gonzalez-Santos 1995), in moderately structured self-management (e.g., Creer et al. 1988), and in self-management that includes a formal action plan. (e.g., Turner et al. 1998). Recent recommendations from the National Asthma Education and Prevention Program Expert Panel Report-3 (NIH 2007) include peak flow monitoring in patients who: have moderate or severe persistent asthma; have a history of severe exacerbations; poorly perceive airflow obstruction and worsening asthma; or prefer this monitoring method. The latter two recommendations were based more on panel consensus judgment than on sufficient clinical literature that would provide stronger, evidence-based conclusions.

Considerations of usage and attitudes bear on peak flow monitoring preferences. First, the percentage of patients who use a meter regularly is low, reportedly 10% in one study (Kendrick et al. 1993) and 16% in another (Garrett et al. 1994). Second, patients who described a scenario of a slowly evolving asthma attack mentioned a peak flow meter only 25% of the time (Garrett et al. 1994). Third, only 20% of the parents of pediatric patients described a peak flow meter as useful for detecting of respiratory problems when the child was not exhibiting signs of respiratory distress (Lloyd and Ali 1992). Clearly, peak flow monitoring has not been highly endorsed by patients, but the question of monitoring preference has not been answered directly.

Several investigations have confirmed low levels of patient compliance with regular peak flow monitoring (e.g., Cote et al. 1998; Kamps and Brand 2001). If patients do not see benefits to monitoring adherence is likely to be poor (Clark et al. 1992), routine monitoring of peak flow may be difficult; it requires the availability of both a meter and a suitable place in which to execute an expiratory maneuver, and it may interfere with other activities. Aspects of peak flow monitoring may be inconvenient or distracting for both pediatric and adult patients and place demands on patients that make the practice of peak flow monitoring challenging (McMullen et al. 2002). Finally, it is inconclusive whether peak flow monitoring interventions are cost-effective (Willems et al. 2006).

Validating Measures Used in Home Monitoring

Symptoms

Objective measures of lung function have long been considered the most suitable criteria for validating most categories of asthma symptoms. Therefore, correlations between symptom scores and respiratory indices represent the key estimates of validity. The correlations indicate how closely symptoms mirror aspects of respiration but they do not address the question of symptom-monitoring effectiveness. Nevertheless, evidence that symptoms represent a reliable, subjective index of airflow obstruction is important if they are to provide useful information about asthma. Unfortunately, validation studies of asthma symptoms have painted something less than a clear picture.

A summary of findings from a score of studies may be stated briefly: the relationship between asthma symptoms and lung function varies considerably between patients and, on average, is characterized by a correlation in the low-to-moderate range. Some patients exhibit a strong relationship between symptoms and lung function, but others do not. Patients who exhibit perceptual error demonstrate a significant difference between objective levels of airflow obstruction and subjective measures of perceived asthma severity. In a study of 37 children with asthma, for example, Fritz et al. (1990) reported correlations between symptom severity and PEFR that ranged from 0.16 to –0.86. Similar findings were reported by Brouwer et al. (2006); in a study of 36 children with asthma, correlations between asthma severity scores and corresponding FEV_1 values in individual patients ranged from 0.51 to –0.28. Individuals in the low portion of the distribution of correlations may be said to exhibit perceptual error. Perceptual error also has been reported in studies of: (a) changes in bronchomoter tone induced by drugs (Burden et al. 1982; McFadden et al. 1973; Orehek et al. 1982; Rubinfeld and Pain 1976), (b) naturally occurring pulmonary variation (Bye et al. 1992; Ferguson 1988; Nguyen et al. 1996), (c) asthma symptoms recorded either in the aggregate (Fonseca et al. 2006; Fritz et al. 1990; Higgs et al. 1986; Kendrick et al. 1993; Peiffer et al. 1989), and (d) or individually (Apter et al. 1997; Apter et al. 1994; Cabral et al. 2002; Atherton et al. 1996; Pauli et al. 1985; Reeder et al. 1990; Santanello et al. 1997; Shingo et al. 2001). A recent review (Kotses et al. 2006) described these studies and others in detail.

The reasons for perceptual error in the interpretation of asthma symptoms are not altogether clear, but several factors may be involved. One factor may be adaptation or tolerance to obstruction. Perceptual error is greater in patients who either have become accustomed to a high level of obstruction (Rietveld and Everaerd 2000) or exhibit low values of either FEV_1 (Burden et al. 1982; Bijl-Hofland et al. 1999) or $FEF_{25–75\%}$ (Apter et al. 1997) compared to other patients. It is greater in patients with life-threatening asthma than in others (Julius et al. 2002), and it is more likely to occur during asthma exacerbation (Yoos et al. 2003) than at other times. Each of these findings suggests that asthma severity in one form of another interferes with symptom perception, but evidence to the contrary also has been reported (Cabral et al. 2002; Fritz et al. 1990; Rietveld et al. 2001).

Psychological factors that interact with environmental variables may contribute to perceptual error. They are invoked when changes in breathlessness are reported in the absence of concomitant changes in lung function, and other antecedent conditions cannot be identified. Asthma patients reported more symptoms in the absence of pulmonary change either when listening to wheezing sounds (Rietveld et al. 1997) or during conditioning of asthma symptoms (De Peuter et al. 2005). Similarly, imagery was associated with increased perceptual error in patients (Rietveld et al.

1999), as was watching affective film clips (von Leupoldt et al. 2006). These changes have been attributed to the effects of emotional or cognitive factors.

Psychological factors considered as traits also have been linked to perceptual error. In general, psychological trait relationships are hard to evaluate, as often closely related measures of the same construct do not agree. Consistency can also be a problem, especially when relationships are weak. Anxiety in children as measured by the Revised Children's Manifest Anxiety Scale, for example, has been reported to be both related (Chen et al. 2006) and unrelated (Fritz et al. 1996a, b) to symptom perception. Another personality trait, repressive defensive style, was associated with heightened symptom perception in adult asthma patients (Steiner et al. 1987), but not in children with asthma (Fritz et al. 1996a, b).

An additional set of factors comes from the field of sensory psychophysics and turns on appreciation of the separate and independent forces of *perceptual sensitivity* and *response bias* on judgments of the presence or absence of airflow obstruction (Harver and Mahler 1990, 1998). The first of these, sensitivity, represents the patient's capability for making discrimination about the presence or absence of acute airflow obstruction; how well a patient is able to make correct judgments and avoid incorrect ones. The second, response bias, provides an index of the patient's criterion for acting on information arising from the discrimination and refers to the non-sensory factors that affect judgments of symptom severity; how risky a patient might be in acting on the perceived discrimination (Baird 1998).

Demographic factors such as age, gender, and race represent yet another category of perceptual error inquiry. For these variables, the results have been mostly negative (e.g., Cabral et al. 2002; Fritz et al. 1990; Fritz et al. 1996a, b). Intelligence was related to perceptual accuracy in children (Fritz et al. 1996a, b), but the relationship was not strong. Overall, demographic variables do not appear to have a major impact on symptom perception of asthma.

Peak Expiratory Flow Rate

The PEFR is used in asthma monitoring because it is an indirect index of airway tone, an all-important quantity associated with asthma symptomatology. In home monitoring, there is no particular reason for preferring PEFR to other airflow measures except that it was the first measure used for that purpose (Wright 1978), and, as a result, continues to be the standard. Both mechanical testing and testing in patients have been conducted to determine whether PEFR describes airway status adequately.

Mechanical testing of accuracy and reliability of a number of PEFR meters was conducted by subjecting them to airflow patterns generated by a computer-controlled syringe (Gardner et al. 1992). Each meter was tested with a number of different airflow patterns all of which adhered to the testing recommendations of the American Thoracic Society (Gardner et al. 1987). Overall, the response of the meters was judged to be acceptable. The meters tended to overestimate mid-range PEFRs, but not by very much. All of them appeared to be capable of tracking airflow variation as required in asthma self-management.

The accuracy of PEFR measured mechanically is far different from that measured by patients during home monitoring. The latter has been studied most notably by comparing PEFR recordings both to measures of airflow derived from a forced expiratory volume maneuver and to measures of airflow resistance. Such studies have shown that PEFR is related to other pulmonary responses, but not strongly, a conclusion consistent between studies with widely dissimilar methodologies. In half of over 6,000 adult patients, percent-of-predicted PEFR differed from percent-of-predicted FEV_1 by more than 10% (Aggarwal et al. 2006). In 18% of 91 children with asthma, PEFR was in the normal severity zone but FEV_1 was not, and concordance between PEFR and $FEF_{25-75\%}$ was low (Klein et al. 1995). In twenty-four asthma patients who exhibited an FEV_1 drop large enough to place the patient in a lower zone of severity, the associated PEFR drop did not affect severity zone status (Gautrin et al. 1994). In 102 patients, intra-subject variability was greater in PEFR than it was in FEV_1 (Vaughan et al. 1989). And in healthy individuals, the correlation between PEFR and total respiratory resistance was, on an average, only −0.41 (Westlund et al. 1987).

Error in PEFR recordings may be introduced by any one of the several factors. Of these, the most important may be the effort-dependency of PEFR. As noted earlier, an accurate PEFR requires the patient to apply maximal effort during the expiratory volume maneuver. If the patient does not, the reading will underestimate the patient's airflow capability. Related to effort dependency of the PEFR is the quality of its expiratory maneuver. A less than maximal effort may result in reduction of maneuver quality, a quantity that may be evaluated by examination of the flow-volume curve. Maneuver quality is affected by age and by anti-inflammatory medication usage (Thompson et al. 2006). Therefore, it is possible that these variables affect PEFR accuracy. Air trapping, a result of airway closure caused by inflammation, also can affect the PEFR accuracy. In a study of 669 patients with asthma and 85 healthy individuals, air trapping was accompanied by normal PEFR but reduced FEV_1 and $FEF_{25-75\%}$, and a concomitant decrease of the ability of PEFR to predict the other measures (Eid et al. 2000).

Improving Effectiveness of Home Monitoring

Symptom Perception

The lack of agreement between objective and subjective measures of asthma severity is a vexing problem for many patients. As noted earlier, most patients use symptoms as guides in asthma control, but the practice is helpful only to some. Others, those in whom the link between symptoms and asthma severity functions imperfectly or not at all, may often be left feeling overwhelmed by the enormity of efforts needed to control asthma, and constantly surprised by the seriousness of the condition when it demands their attention. Such patients require techniques that have the potential to reduce the difference between objective and subjective measures of asthma severity and improve understanding of the physiological basis of asthma symptoms (Banzett et al. 2000; Stahl 2000). Unfortunately, the available candidates for such a role are few, but several approaches have been examined.

1. *Peak expiratory flow rate training*. In efforts to improve the accuracy of subjective respiratory sensations, patients estimated PEFR daily and compared their estimates with actual PEFR and respiratory sensations. It was assumed that improvement in the accuracy of PEFR estimates would generalize to recognition of asthma symptoms. This is a plausible idea, and studies were successful in showing PEFR estimation with feedback resulted in more accurate estimates of PEFR (Silverman et al. 1990; Silverman et al. 1987). The early studies were confirmed by recent work that included better controls. Children with asthma who estimated PEFR for at least 15 days under conditions of accurate feedback exhibited less error in their estimates than children who received no feedback (Kotses et al. 2008). The potential usefulness of all PEFR training studies was limited, however, by the restricted range of PEFR values to which the children were exposed.
2. *Detection of added resistive loads*. To overcome the restricted range problem, researchers have turned to added resistive load detection. Combining added loads with feedback can provide training conveniently in the recognition of respiratory resistance throughout a wide range of values. Briefly, the technique consists of inserting screens that obstruct airflow, to varying degrees, into the patient's breathing circuit, and recording the patient's sensitivity to them. Feedback of accuracy of the patient's perception of added loads has the effect of improving the patient's sensitivity to them (Harver 1994; Harver et al. 2008; Stout et al. 1997). Because asthma symptoms involve a large measure of respiratory resistance decreases, improvement in recognition of respiratory loads could generalize to improvement both in recognition of asthma symptoms and in asthma; but empirical tests of this hypothesis have only begun.
3. *Error grid analysis*. This procedure combines a graphic representation of clinically meaningful asthma severity zones (e.g., the NIH green, yellow and red zones) with a scatter diagram of actual versus estimated PEFR scores both expressed as a percent of personal best (Feldman et al. 2007; Fritz and Wamboldt 1998; Fritz et al. 1996a, b; Klein et al. 2004). Points representing the divergence between estimated and actual PEFR fall into safe or dangerous areas as defined by asthma severity zones. Examination of the scatter diagram of estimated versus actual PEFR values may reveal characteristic patterns of over- or underestimation of PEFR and thereby provide guidance for improved accuracy. Scatter diagrams may be based either on estimates made by a sample of patients or on numerous estimates made by a single patient. The error grid analysis has yet to be applied systematically in clinical settings.

Pulmonary Monitoring

Widespread PEFR home monitoring did not begin until after the introduction of the mini-Wright meter (Wright 1979), a low-cost device that patients could keep at home. That meter and a number of similar meters developed shortly thereafter were limited to measurement of a single quantity, the PEFR. Subsequent development in technology produced meters that measured multiple pulmonary functions and included storage capability. Such meters provided additional possibilities for monitoring asthma severity and maintained records conveniently. It is likely that the next stage of meter development will include devices with the ability to derive functions based on one or more measures that can improve both evaluation of asthma severity and prediction of asthma exacerbation. Potential improvements in the usefulness of pulmonary monitoring described below suggest such a possibility.

1. *Conditional probability.* Conditional probability, as the term is applied to asthma, represents the probability of an asthma attack given the occurrence of a critical PEFR value. The critical PEFR value, determined empirically, is the PEFR score at which prediction of an asthma attack is maximized. The difference between the likelihood of an attack when PEFR is above or below the critical value represents the increase in predictability afforded by the computation of conditional probabilities. Using this procedure, Taplin and Creer (1978) documented a threefold increase in predictability of asthma in two patients. Additional improvements in the procedure led to a nearly fivefold increase in asthma predictability (Harm et al. 1985). There is no doubt that improved prediction of attacks based on PEFR would be useful for patients. But it is equally apparent that computation of conditional probabilities is beyond the capabilities of many patients. Incorporating computation of conditional probabilities into a meter that also has the ability to record and store PEFR values as well as record asthma attacks may benefit asthma management.
2. *Identifying periods of ineffective pulmonary monitoring.* Air trapping is characteristic of individuals with severe asthma (Sorkness et al. 2008), a group representing 5–10% of asthma cases. Patients with severe asthma exhibit a great deal of asthma morbidity and utilize health care facilities to a disproportionate degree. As noted earlier, they also fail to benefit from PEFR monitoring, as increases in air trapping result in dissociation between PEFR and other pulmonary functions (Eid et al. 2000). Other patients may be subject to air trapping, but for only some of the time. Air trapping episodes may identify periods during which the pulmonary monitoring yields unusual results or is ineffective. The simultaneous monitoring and comparison of several pulmonary functions may help identify these periods.
3. *Other possibilities.* There is no end to the potential improvement for control of asthma that more comprehensive monitoring may bring (Reddel 2006). Some patients, for example, may be more likely to benefit from monitoring an index other than PEFR. Others may require a complex derivative function to adequately describe their asthma condition. Whatever the need, it is likely to be met in future versions of pulmonary meters for home use.

Effectiveness of Home Monitoring in Asthma Self-Management

We start this section with two conclusions: (a) the contribution of home monitoring to asthma control is not clear; and (b) the relative effectiveness of symptom and PEFR monitoring has not been determined. These conclusions are bewildering, in view of the amount of research conducted on asthma self-management including enthusiasm for the role of peak flow monitoring in asthma management that has persisted for decades (e.g., Cross and Nelson 1991; Jain et al. 1998), and the degree of effort devoted to ferreting out the most efficient form of monitoring. But a look at the details of self-management research quickly reveals the source of the confusion. Asthma self-management is not just one intervention; it is a group of loosely related interventions. Within this somewhat unstructured universe, self-management programs differ from one another in their content, in their method of instruction, and in the setting in which they are applied. Interactions between the various elements of self-management may produce outcomes that cannot always be duplicated by any of the components. It is one thing, for example, to be taught the use of a PEFR meter by a nurse and another to learn the skill by reading a pamphlet, just as it is different to learn the proper use of asthma medication at a group meeting or in a conference with one's physician. And appreciating the distinction between control and quick-relief medications may be difficult unless one has some understanding of the nature of asthma. Returning to questions of home monitoring, it is possible that both the effectiveness of home monitoring and the relative superiority of either symptom or PEFR monitoring vary between self-management programs that differ in their composition. It is also possible that the relative advantage of one method over the other is contingent on patient variables such as illness severity, sociodemographics, and race (Yoos et al. 2002).

In this section, we review research on home monitoring in asthma self-management. We discuss controlled studies in which home monitoring was an independent variable as well as studies that focused on formal peak flow action plans. The studies fall into two categories as determined by their experimental designs: peak flow monitoring versus medical management, and peak flow monitoring versus symptom monitoring. Designs vary somewhat within the categories.

Peak Flow Monitoring Versus Medical Management

Evaluating peak flow monitoring is not straightforward. Because, it is a technique that is usually a part of an asthma self-management program, it makes sense to evaluate it within that context. But this is not the only possibility. Peak flow monitoring may be evaluated simply as an independent treatment. This was done in three studies (Ayers and Campbell 1996; Drummond et al. 1994; Jones et al. 1995) that featured individualized peak flow plans for adult asthma patients in which two thresholds were identified: one signaling either a start or an increase in steroid use, and a second indicating a need to seek medical assistance. Except for two additional independent variables in one study (Drummond et al. 1994), one of which consisted of enhanced education, other interventions relating to asthma self-management were not included. Controls used in the studies also were similar. They involved medication adjustments made by physicians. Investigators in the threes studies examined a variety of dependent variables including pulmonary scores, medication use, symptoms, health-care usage, and psychological factors. At the end of the study periods, which varied between roughly 6 (Ayers and Campbell 1996) and 12 (Drummond et al. 1994) months, differences between the patient-adjusted and the physician-adjusted medication groups were not observed.

PEFR action plans also have been evaluated as a part of a more comprehensive asthma self-management program. In this case, they have been compared to a control condition approximating medical management. Programs for adults (Gallefoss and Bakke 2000; Ignacio-Garcia and Gonzalez-Santos 1995; Lahdensuo et al. 1996) and for children with asthma (Charlton et al. 1994) have been tested. Most frequently, the action plans have been paired with educational programs that covered, at the very least, aspects of medication and basic asthma physiology, but in some studies, education was extensive. Patients in studies were followed for periods ranging from 6 to 12 months. In each study, improvements accrued to the PEFR group. The types of improvements that were observed included reductions in symptoms, work or school absenteeism, clinic visits, medication use, and improvement in quality of life. Additionally, a complex action plan that included a combination of both PEFR and symptom monitoring yielded benefits in comparison to a medical management group, but the number of patients studied was small (Woolcock et al. 1988).

Peak Flow Versus Symptom Monitoring

Comparisons of PEFR and symptom monitoring plans also have yielded inconsistent findings. Just as in comparisons between PEFR plans and medical management, the inconsistencies may be related to the inclusion of other interventions. In general, when other interventions were kept at a minimum, differences between PEFR and symptom monitoring plans did not emerge (Adams et al. 2001; Buist et al. 2006; Charlton et al. 1990; Malo et al. 1990; Wensley and Silverman 2004). Patients in these studies were both adults (Adams et al. 2001; Buist et al. 2006; Charlton et al. 1990; Malo et al. 1990) and children (Charlton et al. 1990; Wensley and Silverman 2004) who were tested on a variety of dependent variables throughout periods ranging from 3 to 12 months, or longer. In some studies, information about asthma was provided to patients either in the form of leaflets and pamphlets (Adams et al. 2000) or in informal discussions (Charlton et al. 1990), but it did not seem significant, as it was far less than that included in a comprehensive asthma education program.

In some investigations, however, peak flow monitoring proved to be more useful than symptom monitoring, at least for some patients (Bheekie et al. 2001; Yoos et al. 2002). Additionally, when patients were given extensive asthma education in addition to the action plans, PEFR monitoring usually was superior to symptom monitoring (Cowie et al. 1997; Lopez-Vina and del Castillo-Arevalo 2000; Turner et al. 1998). Those who monitored asthma severity with PEFR had either fewer emergency visits (Cowie et al. 1997) or unscheduled physician visits (Turner et al. 1998) than those who monitored symptoms. Patients using PEFR action plans also exhibited better treatment adherence and had slightly higher percent of predicted FVC scores than those using symptom plans (Lopez-Vina and del Castillo-Arevalo 2000). These observations lead to an obvious conclusion, but one that may be misleading. The findings represent only a few of the variables tested. The vast majority of variables were not sensitive to the type of action plan employed.

A consistent observation, not only in comparisons between symptom and PEFR plans but also in evaluations of PEFR plans against medical management is the association between PEFR plan benefits and education. The effects of PEFR plans appear to be potentiated by education (McGrath et al. 2001). But this conclusion may be overstated. It is contradicted by one study in which educated patients with a PEFR plan did not differ from those either with a symptom plan or with no plan (Cote et al. 1997). The authors attributed the failure, in part, to sustained care, a benefit enjoyed by all patients in the study. But it is possible that sustained care confers benefits that in some way are similar to those afforded by comprehensive asthma education.

In a recent review, Brouwer and Brand (2008) concluded that monitoring lung function adds little, if anything, to symptom monitoring in tracking asthma severity. Their conclusion is reasonable, despite some evidence to the contrary in the form of studies attesting to PEFR benefits. However, PEFR monitoring should not be written off. As we noted in our discussion of technical progress, its potential is great. But more importantly, a number of basic questions about the effects of PEFR monitoring have not been answered completely. These include concerns both about the training and the conduct of PEFR monitoring, and the wide variability consistently evident among patients between objective and subjective assessment of asthma severity. Once such questions are resolved, strong recommendations about the best ways to monitor asthma severity will emerge.

References

Adams RJ, Boath K, Homan S, Campbell DA, Ruffin RE (2001) A randomized trial of peak-flow and symptom-based action plans in adults with moderate-to-severe asthma. Respirology 6:297–304

Aggarwal AN, Gupta D, Jindal SK (2006) The relationship between FEV_1 and peak expiratory flow in patients with airways obstruction is poor. Chest 130:1454–1461

Apter AJ, ZuWallack RL, Clive J (1994) Common measures of asthma severity lack association for describing its clinical course. J Allergy Clin Immunol 94:732–737

Apter AJ, Affleck G, Reisine ST, Tennen HA, Barrows E, Wells M, Willard A, ZuWallack RL (1997) Perception of airway obstruction in asthma: sequential daily analyses of symptoms, peak expiratory flow rate, and mood. J Allergy Clin Immunol 99:605–612

Atherton HA, White PT, Hewett G, Howells K (1996) Relationship of daytime asthma symptom frequency to morning peak expiratory flow. Eur Respir J 9:232–236

Ayers JG, Campbell RMA (1996) A controlled assessment of an asthma self-management plan involving a budesonide dose regimen. Eur Respir J 9:886–892

Baird JC (1998) Sensory psychophysics. In: Kotses H, Harver A (eds) Self-management of asthma. Marcel-Dekker, New York

Banzett RB, Dempsey JA, O'Donnell DE, Wamboldt MZ (2000) Symptom perception and respiratory sensation in asthma. Am J Respir Crit Care Med 162:1178–1182

Bheekie A, Syce JA, Weinberg EG (2001) Peak expiratory flow rate and symptom self-monitoring of asthma initiated from community pharmacies. J Clin Pharm Ther 26:287–296

Bijl-Hofland ID, Cloosterman SGM, Folgering HTM, Akkermans RP, van Schayck CP (1999) Relationship between the perception of airway obstruction to the severity of asthma. Thorax 54:15–19

Brouwer AF, Brand PL (2008) Asthma education and monitoring: what has been shown to work. Pediatr Respir Rev 9:193–199

Brouwer AF, Roorda RJ, Brand PLP (2006) Home spirometry and asthma severity in children. Eur Respir J 28:1131–1137

Buist AS, Wollmer WM, Wilson SR, Frazier EA, Hayward AD (2006) A randomized clinical trial of peak flow versus symptom monitoring in older adults with asthma. Am J Respir Crit Care Med 174:1077–1087

Burden JG, Juniper EF, Killian KJ, Hargreave FE, Campbell EJ (1982) The perception of breathlessness in asthma. Am Rev Respir Dis 126:825–828

Bye MR, Kerstein D, Barsh E (1992) The importance of spirometry in the assessment of childhood asthma. Am J Dis Child 146:977–978

Cabral ALB, Conceicao GM, Saldiva PHN, Martins MA (2002) Effect of asthma severity on symptom perception in childhood asthma. Braz J Med Biol Res 35:319–327

Charlton I, Charlton G, Broomfield J, Mullee MA (1990) Evaluation of peak flow and symptoms only self-management plans for control of asthma in general practice. Br Med J 301:1355–1359

Charlton I, Antoniou AG, Atkinson J, Campbell MJ, Chapman E, Mackintosh T et al (1994) Asthma at the interface: bridging the gap between general practice and a district general hospital. Arch Dis Child 70:313–318

Chen E, Hermann C, Rodgers D, Oliver-Welker T, Strunk RC (2006) Symptom perception in childhood asthma: the role of anxiety and asthma severity. Health Psychol 25:389–395

Clark NM, Evans D, Mellins RB (1992) Patient use of peak flow monitoring. Am Rev Respir Dis 145:722–725

Cote J, Cartier A, Robichaud P, Boutin H, Malo J, Rouleau M et al (1997) Influence on asthma morbidity of asthma education programs based on self-management plans following treatment optimization. Am J Respir Crit Care Med 155:1509–1514

Cote J, Cartier A, Malo JL, Rouleau M, Boulet LP (1998) Compliance with peak expiratory flow monitoring in home management of asthma. Chest 113:968–972

Cowie RL, Revitt SG, Underwood MF, Field SK (1997) The effect of peak flow action plans in the prevention of exacerbations of asthma. Chest 112:1534–1538

Creer TL, Backial M, Burns KL, Leung P, Marion RJ, Micklich DR et al (1988) Living with asthma. I. Genesis and development of a self-management program for childhood asthma. J Asthma 25:335–362

Cross D, Nelson HS (1991) The role of peak flow meter in the diagnosis and management of asthma. J Allergy Clin Immunol 8:120–128

De Peuter S, Van Diest I, Lemaigre V, Li W, Verleden G, Demedts M, Van den Bergh O (2005) Can subjective asthma symptoms be learned? Psychosom Med 67:454–461

Drummond N, Abdalla M, Beattie JAG, Buckingham JK, Lindsay T, Osman LM et al (1994) Effectiveness of routine self-monitoring of peak flow in patients with asthma. Br Med J 308:1355–1359

Eid N, Yandell B, Howell L, Eddy M, Sheikh S (2000) Can peak expiratory flow predict airflow obstruction in children with asthma. Pediatrics 105:354–358

Feldman JM, McQuaid EL, Klein RB, Kopel SJ, Nassau JH, Mitchell DK, Wamboldt MZ, Fritz GK (2007) Symptom perception and functional morbidity across a 1-year follow-up in pediatric asthma. Pediatr Pulmonol 42:339–347

Ferguson AC (1988) Persisting airway obstruction in asymptomatic children with asthma with normal peak expiratory rates. J Allergy Clin Immunol 82:19–22

Fishwick D, Beasley R (1996) Use of peak flow-based self-management plans by adult asthmatic patients. Eur Respir J 9:861–865

Fonseca ACCF, Fonseca MTM, Rodrigues MESM, Lasmar LMLBF, Camargos PAM (2006) Peak expiratory flow monitoring in asthmatic children. J Pediatr 82:465–469

Fritz GK, Wamboldt MZ (1998) Psychosomatic interactions and symptom perception. In: Kotses H, Harver A (eds) Self-management of asthma. Marcel-Dekker, New York

Fritz GK, Klien RB, Overholzer JC (1990) Accuracy of symptom perception in childhood asthma. J Dev Behav Pediatr 11:69–72

Fritz GK, McQuaid EL, Spirito A, Klien RB (1996a) Symptom perception in pediatric asthma. J Am Acad Child Adolesc Psychiatry 35:1033–1041

Fritz GK, Yeung A, Wamboldt MZ, Spirito A, McQuaid EL, Klein R et al (1996b) Conceptual and methodological issues in quantifying perceptual accuracy in childhood asthma. J Pediatr Psychol 21:153–173

Gallefoss F, Bakke PS (2000) Impact of patient education and self-management on morbidity in asthmatics and patients with chronic obstructive pulmonary disease. Respir Med 94:279–287

Gannon PFG, Belcher J, Pantin CFA, Burge PS (1999) The effect of patient technique and training on the accuracy of self-recorded peak expiratory flow. Eur Respir J 14:28–31

Gardner RM, Hankinson JL, Clausen JL, Crapo RO, Johnson RL, Epler GR (1987) ATS statement of standardization of spirometry–1987 update. Am Rev Respir Dis 136: 1285–1298

Gardner RM, Crappo RO, Jackson BR, Jensen RL (1992) Evaluation of accuracy and reproducibility of peak flowmeters at 1400 m. Chest 101:948–952

Garrett J, Fenwick JM, Taylor G, Mitchell E, Rea H (1994) Peak expiratory flow meters (PEFMs) – who uses them and how and does education affect the patter of utilisation? Aust N Z J Med 24:521–528

Gautrin D, D'Aquino LC, Gagnon G, Malo JL, Cartier A (1994) Comparison between peak expiratory flow rates (PEFR) and FEV_1 in the monitoring of asthmatic subjects at an outpatient clinic. Chest 106:1419–1426

Harm DL, Marion RJ, Kotses H, Creer TL (1984) Effect of subject effort on pulmonary function measures: a preliminary investigation. J Asthma 21:295–298

Harm DL, Kotses H, Creer TL (1985) Improving the ability of peak expiratory flow rates to predict asthma. J Allergy Clin Immunol 76:688–694

Harver A (1994) Effects of feedback on the ability of asthmatic subjects to detect increases in the flow-resistive component to breathing. Health Psychol 13:52–62

Harver A, Mahler DA (1990) The symptom of dyspnea. In: Mahler DA (ed) Dyspnea. Futura Publishing Co., Inc., Mount Kisco, New York, pp 1–53

Harver A, Mahler DA (1998) Perception of increased resistance to breathing. In: Kotses H, Harver A (eds) Self-management of asthma. Marcel Dekker, New York, pp 147–193

Harver A, Ersek J, Humphries CT, O'Connor M, Kotses H (2008) Effects of feedback on the detection of inspiratory resistive loads in children with persistent asthma: an ROC approach. Annual meeting of the International Society for the Advancement of Respiratory Psychophysiology, Ann Arbor

Higgs CMB, Richardson RB, Lea DA, Lewis GTR, Laszlo G (1986) Influence of knowledge of peak flow on self-assessment of asthma: studies with a coded peak flow meter. Thorax 41:671–675

Ignacio-Garcia JM, Gonzalez-Santos P (1995) Asthma self-management education program by home monitoring of peak expiratory flow. Am J Respir Crit Care Med 151:353–359

Jain P, Kavuru MS, Emerman CL, Ahmad M (1998) Utility of peak expiratory flow monitoring. Chest 114:861–876

Jones KP, Mullee AM, Middelton M, Chapman E, Holgate ST (1995) Peak flow based asthma self-management: a randomized control study in general practice. Thorax 50:851–857

Julius SM, Davenport LL, Davenport PW (2002) Perception of intrinsic and extrinsic respiratory loads in children with life-threatening asthma. Pediatric Pulmonol 34:425–433

Kamps AWA, Brand PLP (2001) Education, self-management and home peak flow monitoring in childhood asthma. Paediatr Respir Rev 2:165–169

Kendrick AH, Higgs CMB, Whitfield MJ, Laszlo G (1993) Accuracy of perception of severity of asthma: patients treated in general practice. Br Med J 307:422–424

Klein RB, Fritz GK, Yeung A, McQuaid EL, Mansell A (1995) Spirometric patterns in childhood asthma: peak flow compared with other indices. Pediatr Pulmonol 20:372–379

Klein RB, Walders N, McQuaid EL, Adams S, Yaros D, Fritz GK (2004) The asthma risk grid: clinical interpretation of symptom perception. Allergy Asthma Proc 25:1–6

Kotses H, Bernstein IL, Bernstein DI, Korbee L, Wigal JK, Ganson E et al (1995) A self-management program for adults with asthma. Part I: development and evaluation. J Allergy Clin Immunol 95:529–540

Kotses H, Harver A, Humphries CT (2006) Home monitoring in asthma self-management. J Asthma 43:649–655

Kotses H, Hyseni, H, Harver A, Walford S, Hardy SJ (2008) Effects of feedback on the correspondence between estimated and actual PEFR in children with persistent asthma. Paper presented at the annual meeting of the International Society for the Advancement of Respiratory Psychophysiology, Ann Arbor, MI

Lahdensuo A, Haahtela T, Herrala J, Kava T, Kiviranta K, Kuusisto P et al (1996) Randomized comparison of guided self-management and traditional treatment of asthma over one year. Br Med J 312:748–752

Lloyd BW, Ali MH (1992) How useful do parents find home peak flow monitoring for children with asthma? Br Med J 30:1128–1129

Lopez-Vina A, del Castillo-Arevalo F (2000) Influence of peak expiratory flow monitoring on an asthma self-management education programme. Respir Med 94:760–766

Malo JL, L'Archeveque JL, Trudeau C, d'Aquino C, Cartier A (1990) Should we monitor peak expiratory flow rates or record symptoms with a simple diary in the management of asthma. J Allergy Clin Immunol 91:702–709

McFadden ER Jr, Kiser R, DeGroot WJ (1973) Acute bronchial asthma: Relationships between clinical and physiologic manifestations. N Engl J Med 288:221–225

McGrath AM, Gardner DM, McCormack J (2001) Is home peak expiratory flow monitoring effective for controlling asthma symptoms? J Clin Pharm Ther 26:311–317

McMullen AH, Yoos HL, Kitzman H (2002) Peak flow meters in childhood asthma: parent report of use and perceived usefulness. J Pediatr Health Care 16:67–72

National Institute of Health (2007) Guidelines for the diagnosis and management of asthma. Expert Panel Report 3 (NIH Publication No. 07-4051). Department of Health and Human Services, Washington, DC

Nguyen BP, Wilson SR, German DF (1996) Patients' perception compared with objective ratings of asthma severity. Ann Allergy Asthma Immunol 77:209–215

Orehek J, Beaupre P, Badier M, Nicoli MM, Delpierre S (1982) Perception of airway tone by asthmatic patients. Bulletin European de Physiopathologie Respiratoire 18:601–607

Pauli G, Biggot H, Peletier A, Kopferschmitt-Kubler MC, Roegel E (1985) A study of the criteria used for clinical evaluation of prophylactic treatment of bronchial asthma. Eur J Respir Dis 67:369–377

Peiffer C, Marsac J, Lockhart A (1989) Chronobiological study of the relationship between dyspnoea and airway obstruction in symptomatic asthmatic subject. Clin Sci 77:237–244

Reddel HK (2006) Peak flow monitoring in clinical practice and clinical asthma trials. Curr Opin Pulm Med 12:75–81

Reeder KP, Dolce JJ, Dule L, Raczynski JM, Bailey WC (1990) Peak flow meters: are they monitoring tools or training devices. J Asthma 27:219–227

Rietveld S, Everaerd W (2000) Perception of asthma by adolescents at home. Chest 117:433–439

Rietveld S, Kolk AM, Prins PJM, Colland VT (1997) The influence of respiratory sounds on breathlessness in children with asthma: a symptom-perception approach. Health Psychol 16:547–553

Rietveld S, Everaerd E, van Beest I (2000) Excessive breathlessness through emotional imagery in asthma. Behav Res Ther 38:1005–1014

Rietveld S, Prins PJM, Colland VT (2001) Accuracy of symptom perception in asthma and illness severity. Children Health Care 301:27–41

Rubinfeld AR, Pain MCF (1976) Perception of asthma. Lancet 93:883–884

Santanello NC, Barber BL, Reiss TF, Friedman BS, Juniper EF, Zhang J (1997) Measurement characteristics of two asthma symptom diary scales for use in clinical trials. Eur Respir J 10:646–651

Shapiro SM, Hendler JM, Ogirala Rg, Aldrich TK, Shapiro MB (1991) An evaluation of the accuracy of assess and mini-Wright peak flow meters. Chest 99:358–362

Shingo S, Zhang J, Reiss TF (2001) Correlation of airway obstruction and patient-reported endpoints in clinical studies. Eur Respir J 17:220–224

Silverman BT, Mayer D, Sabinsky R, Williams-Akita A, Feldman J, Schneider AT, Chiaramonte LT (1987) Training perception of air flow obstruction in asthmatics. Ann Allergy 59:350–354

Silverman B, Cassilda J, Misra S, Schneider AT, Chiaramonte LT (1990) Training perception of acute airflow obstruction. Ann Allergy 64:373–375

Sorkness RL, Bleecker ER, Busse WW, Calhoun WJ, Castro M, Chung KF et al (2008) J Appl Physiol 104:394–403

Stahl E (2000) Correlation between objective measures of airway caliber and clinical symptoms in asthma: a systematic review of clinical studies. Respir Med 94:735–741

Steiner H, Higgs C, Fritz GK, Laszlo G, Harvey JE (1987) Defense style and perception of asthma. Psychosom Med 49:35–44

Stout C, Kotses H, Creer TL (1997) Improving perception of air flow obstruction in asthma patients. Psychosom Med 59:201–206

Taplin PS, Creer TL (1978) A procedure for using peak expiratory flow rate data to increase the predictability of asthma episodes. J Asthma Res 16:15–19

Thompson R, Delfino RJ, Tjoa T, Nussbaum E, Cooper D (2006) Evaluation of daily home spirometry for school children with asthma: new insights. Pediatr Pulmonol 41:819–828

Turner MO, Taylor D, Bennett R, Fitzgerald JM (1998) A randomized trial comparing peak expiratory flow with symptom self-management plans for patients with asthma attending a primary care clinic. Am J Respir Crit Care Med 157:540–546

Uwyyed K, Springer C, Avital A, Bar-Yishay E, Godfrey S (1996) Home recording of PEF in young asthmatics: does it contribute to management. Eur Respir J 9:872–879

Vaughan T, Weber RW, Tipton WR, Nelson HS (1989) Comparison of PEFR and FEV1 in patients with varying degrees if airway obstruction: effects of modest altitude. Chest 95:558–562

von Leupoldt A, Riedel F, Dahme B (2006) The impact of emotions on the perception of dyspnea in pediatric asthma. Psychophysiology 43:641–644

Wensley D, Silverman M (2004) Peak flow monitoring for guided self-management in childhood asthma: a randomized controlled trial. Am J Respir Crit Care Med 170: 606–612

Westlund RE, Theofanous AG, Wigal JK, Rawson JC, Kotses H, Creer TL, Harm DL (1987) Total respiratory resistance and spirometric measures: within-subject comparisons. J Asthma 24:5–8

Willems DCM, Joore MA, Hendriks JJE, Wouters EFM, Severens JL (2006) Cost-effectiveness of self-management in asthma: a systematic review of peak flow monitoring interventions. Int J Technol Assess Health Care 22:436–442

Woolcock AJ, Yan K, Salome CM (1988) Effect of therapy on bronchial hyperresponsiveness in the long-term management of asthma. Clin Allergy 18:165–176

Wright BM (1978) A miniature Wright peak-flow meter. Br Med J 2:1627–1628

Wright BM, McKerrow CB (1959) Maximum force expiratory flow rate as a measure of ventilatory capacity. Br Med J 2:1041–1047

Yoos HL, Kitzman H, McMullen A, Henderson C, Sidora K (2002) Symptom monitoring in childhood asthma: a randomized clinical trial comparing peak expiratory flow rate with symptom monitoring. Ann Allergy Asthma Immunol 88:283–291

Yoos HL, Kitzman H, McMullen A, Sidora K (2003) Symptom perception in childhood asthma: how accurate are children and parents? J Asthma 40:27–39

Chapter 10
Computer-Based Applications in the Management of Asthma

Ross Shegog and Marianna M. Sockrider

Introduction

Asthma has emerged as a significant chronic disease affecting an estimated 300 million people worldwide (Masoli et al. 2004), including over 20 million people in the United States. Poor asthma control results in significant morbidity including lost work days for adults and school days for children (11.8 million and 14.7 million, respectively, in 2002), preventable mortality (estimated at 4,261 deaths per year), and also contributes substantially to the burden of health-care expenditures (estimated at a total cost of $16.1 billion in 2004) (Schiller and Bernadel 2004; NHLBI 2004). Prevalence of childhood asthma, as estimated in the 2007 National Health Information Survey, remains at historically high levels with 9.1% of children (6.7 million) estimated to have asthma (Akinbami et al. 2009). Controlling asthma is a public health challenge. Complicating this are reported discrepancies in how asthma is managed by health-care providers and patients. These discrepancies include under-estimation of disease severity by patients (Worstell 2000), under-treatment of symptoms by health-care providers (Wolfenden et al. 2003), low rates of outpatient follow-up after emergency room visits and hospitalizations (Smith et al. 2004; Cabana et al. 2003), and under-utilization of preventive measures such as influenza vaccination (Figaro and Belue 2005).

Clinical guidelines can help to curtail these practice deficiencies by providing evidence-based and standardized approaches to the management of asthma (NHLBI 1991, 1995, 1997, 2002, 2007; British Thoracic Society 1990; Woolcock et al. 1989; Spector and Nicklas 1995; Creer et al. 1999; Jadad 2002; GINA 2006). These clinical practice guidelines have been widely disseminated to health-care providers and are freely accessible through the Internet. However, the success of guidelines is predicated on health-care providers adopting and implementing them. Although providers report a high awareness of the guidelines, specific practices such as prescribing anti-inflammatory controller medications, giving patients written action plans, and using objective measures of lung function have remained at low-to-moderate rates (NHLBI 1991, 2002; Grant et al. 1999; Gregson et al. 1995; Lieu et al. 1997; Dawson et al. 1995; Legorreta et al. 1998; Finkelstein et al. 2002). In the past 15 years since the publication of the first NAEPP guidelines, a slow but steady adoption of key guideline messages appears evident (Ruchi and Weiss 2009). Reasons for practice variances include cognitive and motivational factors such as lack of familiarity with specific guideline recommendations or skills to implement them; low efficacy or outcome expectations; clinical practice constraints, such as time and reimbursement for education; guideline-specific factors such as lack of clarity or inadequate evidence of effectiveness; and health system decision support (Cabana et al. 1999; Cabana et al. 2000; Cabana et al. 2001; Ruchi and Weiss 2009). Asthma guidelines are purportedly one of the more commonly adopted when compared to other chronic disease guidelines (Flores 2000). Despite this, application of asthma guidelines is a behavioral and organizational challenge.

Computer applications offer potential to enhance the application of asthma management guidelines. The refinement of clinical and behavioral asthma care practices and the evolution of computer-based technology

R. Shegog (✉)
Center for Health Promotion & Prevention Research, UT School of Public Health, 7000 Fannin, Suite 2668, Houston, TX 77030, USA
e-mail: ross.shegog@uth.tmc.edu

A. Harver and H. Kotses (eds.), *Asthma, Health and Society: A Public Health Perspective*,
DOI 10.1007/978-0-387-78285-0_10, © Springer Science+Business Media, LLC 2010

have led to a steady increase in studies evaluating the use of computers in asthma management. Computer-based applications have been described throughout the therapeutic stream of asthma management (Fig. 10.1). A recent review lists 64 publications devoted to informatics applications in asthma, but few of those have moved from the testing environment to widespread use in patient care (Sanders and Aronsky 2006). This chapter will briefly describe the emergence of computers in health-care and examine empirical research on using computer-based applications in the management of asthma. Research will be described in three operational domains: (1) in support of clinician practice and decision-making, (2) to educate patients and/or health-care professionals in asthma management and skills, and (3) to allow patients to monitor asthma self-management practices and control.

Emergence of Computer Applications in Health-Care

Computer-based applications for asthma management have evolved in tandem with the evolution of computer technology. The transition from the industrial age to the information age in the latter twentieth century ushered in dramatic computing advances in health-care from medical practice to education and research (Morris 1994; Sanders and Aronsky 2006). Early developments were focused on Health Information Systems (HIS), large computerized data bases used to store health and administrative information, communicate orders, and/or report results from pharmacies and laboratories (e.g., Technicon Medical Information Systems, Mountain View, CA.; the HELP system, Latter Day Saints Hospital, Salt Lake City, Utah; and the HIS at the National Institutes of Health Clinical Center, Bethesda, MD.) (Staggers et al. 2001). Support for clinical practice was limited in the 1970s and 1980s, with computerized billing functions often superseding care functions (Ozbolt et al. 1990). By the late 1980s, HIS vendors (e.g., Shared Medical Systems, HBOC, Center) began developing and marketing clinical applications. Early diagnostic and medical record data bases were the vanguard for applications that mirror the expanding demands of modern disease management. These include applications for maintaining patient records, clinical decision making (e.g., diagnostic systems, expert systems, decision support systems), management education (e.g., computer-assisted instruction programs), and information resources (e.g., Internet sites, electronic textbooks) (Hunt et al. 1998; Shiffman et al. 1999).

Medical Record Systems

A shift to managed care in the 1980s and 1990s brought a changing focus from the traditional physician-orientation to a payer-orientation that emphasized health promotion, disease prevention, and cost containment (Staggers et al. 2001). New information technology (IT) support developed to integrate health-care delivery networks from diverse types of healthcare settings. Computer-based patient records (CPRs) or electronic medical records (EMRs) emerged to track patient care within managed networks, enabling strategic goals to fuse business and clinical operations. These systems became

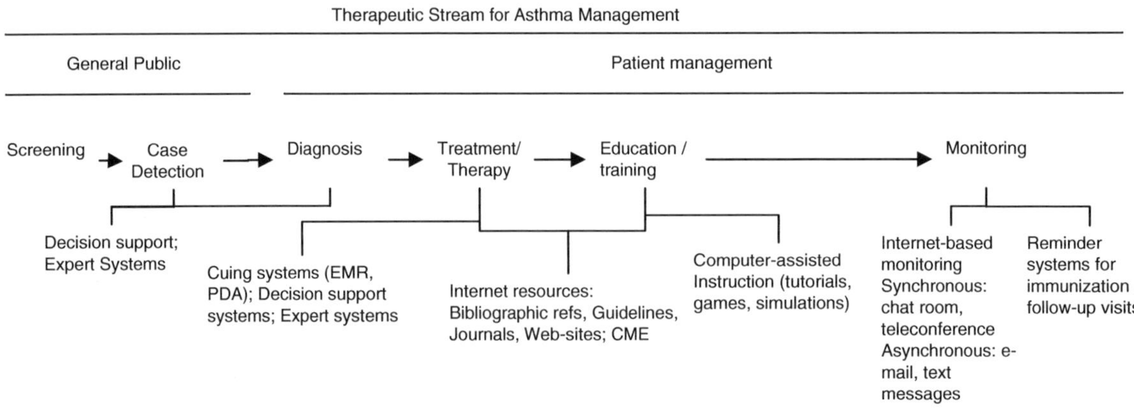

Fig. 10.1 Applications in the management of asthma

part of the Institute of Medicine's recommendations for improving patient records by managing clinical data through the lifespan and across interdisciplinary teams (Dick and Steen 1991). By providing data that is consistent, accurate, accessible, and with minimal redundancy, CPRs have been projected to save tens of billions of dollars in hospital care costs due to earlier clinical intervention and fewer patient visits. By the end of the 1980s, computing and communication technology had converged as telephone lines were superseded by coaxial cables and then fiberoptic lines. Open network architecture and interconnection protocols allowed compatibility of computers from different vendors (Morris 1994). Complimentary advances have included data standardization through groups such as the American National Standards Institute (ANSI), Healthcare Informatics Standards Board Vocabulary Working Group and the computer-based Patient Records Institute Working Group on Codes and Structure (Chute et al. 1998). The legal, privacy, and security issues in handling shared data are also being addressed through policy initiatives such as The Health Insurance Portability and Accountability Act (HIPAA) of 1996. This act calls for strict limits on disclosure and use of healthcare information and mandates individual health information protection (Christiansen 1999).

Expert Systems and Decision Support Systems

Computer-based expert systems are programs that are designed to mimic expert human performance in a narrow domain. An expert system comprises a knowledge base and an inference engine (Alessi and Trollip 1991; Giarrantano and Riley 1989). The knowledge base contains the content of the program, including decisions to be made based on the gathered clinical data, questions that provide required clinical data, and decision rules that operate upon that data. The inference engine is the program that uses the components of the knowledge base to provide conclusions to the user (Alessi et al. 1991; Giarrantano and Riley 1989).

Early clinical decision making applications developed in the 1950s focused on assisting in medical diagnosis (e.g., Iliad, DxExplain, Internist-I, MYCIN, and QMR) (Staggers et al. 2001). These applications provided broad-based support in diagnosing a range of diseases but lacked integration into existing CPRs causing providers to enter data into separate programs.

Computer-based tools that help to improve physician's evidence-based decision making (EBDM) can be categorized as *passive* tools that can be searched (including on-line guidelines, journals, texts) and *active* tools which continuously survey computer-physician interactions and are programmed to intervene under defined conditions (Schneider and Eisenberg 1998; Haug et al. 1999). Active tools can be broadly termed as decision support systems (DSSs). Functions of DSSs can include: (a) alerting the care provider to situations of concern, (b) critiquing previous decisions, (c) suggesting interventions at the direct request of the care provider, and (d) conducting retrospective quality assurance reviews, or combinations of these (Haug et al. 1999; Shiffman et al. 1999). The utility of DSSs in medical practice has been demonstrated in enhancing clinician adherence with practice guidelines including drug dosing (Johnston et al. 1994; Walton et al. 1999), diagnosis and referral of high-risk patients for respiratory assessment (Chase et al. 1983), and in acute medical care (Johnston et al. 1994; Hunt et al. 1998; Shiffman et al. 1999; Creer 1993). Cumulative evidence suggests that computerized medical DSSs can improve clinician compliance with practice guidelines and improve preventive and active care, especially when delivering patient-specific advice at the time and place of a consultation (Johnston et al. 1994; Grimshaw and Russell 1993; Tierney et al. 1986).

A systematic review of the functionality and effectiveness of computer-based decision support systems found that they improved guideline adherence and documentation and contributed to the improved process, delivery, and evaluation of medical care (Johnston et al. 1994; Hunt et al. 1998; Shiffman et al. 1999). Recommendations for future asthma care include the enlistment of health information technology (Ruchi and Weiss 2009). Despite this, development of these systems is still evolving slowly with relatively few being widely implemented into medical practice (Hunt et al. 1998; Johnston et al. 1994; Austin et al. 1996; Shiffman et al. 1999; Sanders and Aronsky 2006).

Computer-Assisted Instruction

In recent decades, computer-based applications have evolved for patient and family health education and behavior change in health promotion, disease prevention, and disease management (Skinner and Kreuter 1997; Brennan et al. 1991; Brown et al. 1997; Dijkstra et al. 1998; Rhodes et al. 1997; Bartholomew et al. 2001; Gustafson et al. 1987; Williams et al. 1995). Collectively, such programs have been shown to positively affect learner attention, motivation, memory, and comprehension, while also promoting active learning, attitude change, and increased transfer of learning (Alessi and Trollip 1985; Lieberman 1997; Rimal and Flora 1997; Niemiec and Walberg 1987; Skinner and Kreuter 1997; Clark et al. 2009).

Information Resources

Interactive health communication (IHC) has been broadly defined as "the interaction of an individual-consumer, patient, caregiver, or professional – with or through an electronic device or communication technology to access or transmit health information to or receive guidance and support on health-related issues" (Science Panel on Interactive Communication and Health 1999). Increased accessibility (through the World Wide Web (WWW), increased transmission speed, portable digital devices (PDAs), and wireless communication) is enabling greater use of the technology by providers and patients who are less constrained by location (hospital, clinic, home, and school). This technology is heralding a change in how providers and patients communicate about health-care issues. As the Internet emerges as a principal source of health information (Pew Internet American Life 2006), the role for health-care providers is changing from health information "providers" to health information "brokers" who may guide judicious selection of e-health-related information in websites and online chat rooms. The evolution of hardware has led to increasing use of integrated handheld technology (PDAs, cell phones, iPods™) which has barely gained attention in the evaluation literature to date (Chang et al. 2003).

Applications in Support of Clinician Practice in Asthma

National Heart Lung and Blood Institute (NHLBI) NAEPP guidelines delineate four essential elements of asthma management: diagnosis and monitoring using objective measures of lung function; control of inflammation and bronchospasm through pharmacotherapy; environmental trigger identification and avoidance; and patient education and collaboration in care (NHLBI 1991, 1995, 1997, 2002, 2007). Computer-based applications used by clinicians to achieve the following clinical guideline objectives are described in this section: diagnosis and case detection, objective monitoring of lung function, support in implementing therapeutic guidelines, and engendering the physician-patient collaborative partnership.

Diagnosis and Case Detection

Case detection and diagnosis of asthma are critical first steps in management (National Heart Lung and Blood Institute 1997). Sanders and Aronsky (2006) reviewed 18 evaluation studies (from a pool of 64 informatics studies in asthma) devoted to diagnosis and case detection. These include applications that analyze clinical data (e.g., using pulmonary function tests or peak flow values) to determine presence and severity of asthma; programs to identify asthma patients on the basis of administrative data (e.g., discharge summaries, billing codes); and computer-based surveys to screen for asthma or characterize disease severity and control (Sanders and Aronsky 2006). Historically, diagnostic functions have provided some of the earliest clinical decision making support in asthma as well as other chronic diseases.

Broad-based expert systems (e.g., Iliad, MYCIN) have provided input to physicians on diagnosis of varied diseases including asthma and more recently have been devoted to successfully detecting asthma or assessing its severity (Redier et al. 1995; Ray et al. 1995; Shegog et al. 2004). Examples of such systems include *AsthmaExpert*©, which has been favorably compared to 3 pre-existing severity-scoring systems (Gautier et al. 1996) and OASYS-2, a computer-assisted diagnostic aid for the visual analysis of peak expiratory flow plotted records, found feasible in confirming cases of occupational asthma (Gannon et al. 1996; Burge et al. 1999). Systems have also been reported that compare favorably with human examiners in detecting airway obstruction through the classification of breath sounds (Tinkelman et al. 1991; Rietveld et al. 1999) as well as differentiating tidal breathing patterns (van der Ent et al. 1996).

Automated systems can significantly reduce manual chart review burden while maintaining adequate levels of precision. Evaluations of chart review systems for health-care organizations have included a system to identify acute exacerbations in pediatric asthma (Aronow et al. 1995a, b), a natural language processing system to identify diagnostic, co-morbidity, and smoking status in discharge summaries for asthma patients (Zheng et al. 2006), and a system to identify the prevalence of asthma (Vollmer et al. 2004). Documentation from a *Computer-Assisted Triage System©* (CATS) was reported to compare satisfactorily to written records for all visit detail items and 9 out of 10 triage detail items and less favorably for nursing observations and medical details (Kabir et al. 1998). A study of EMR impact on delays of diagnosis of asthma in children did not show a significant difference in delays before the implementation of the EMR vs. delays subsequent to implementation, though a positive trend was indicated (Yoo and Molis 2007).

Electronic versions of data acquisition surveys such as the Pediatric Asthma Quality of Life Questionnaire and Pediatric Asthma Caregivers Quality of Life Questionnaire are becoming available and have the added value of immediate scoring and graphical feedback (Mussaffi et al. 2007). A validation study comparing electronic to written collection methods for the International Study of Asthma and Allergies in Childhood Questionniare indicated no appreciable difference in the quality of data collected in a sample of Dutch adolescents (Raat et al. 2007). Computer-based data acquisition of medication prescription information from patients has shown acceptable validity (Porter et al. 2006). Medication adherence, however, represents a greater challenge. In a study assessing the effect of interview mode on self-reported adherence to a corticosteroid regimen indicated that while all modes (audio computer-assisted self interviewing (ACASI), face-to-face interviews, and self-administered paper and pencil questionnaire) showed a discrepancy between self-report and objectively measured adherence, the ACASI condition showed the most discrepancy (Bender et al. 2007). At least in the domain of adherence, the advantages of ACASI were not demonstrated as they have been in other health domains (i.e., risky sexual behavior and illicit drug use).

Though beyond the scope of this chapter, asthma case detection systems have been used for both epidemiological research and community screening in the general population (Grassi et al. 2001; Hirsch et al. 2001); predicting at-risk children from outpatient populations (Lieu et al. 1998); predicting mortality risk in adult outpatients (Tierney et al. 1997); predicting chronic obstructive pulmonary disease (COPD) in asthma patients (Himes et al. 2009), and predicting emergency room utilization based on environmental data (Bibi et al. 2002). Other applications include genetic data bases for asthma phenotypes (Wjst and Immervoll 1998), electronic nose applications to discriminate between patients with asthma and controls through the analysis of volatile organic compounds in exhaled air (Dragonieri et al. 2007), and community-based approaches such as the application of geographic information systems (Rob 2003; Peled et al. 2005; Peled et al. 2006). Collectively, such systems appear to have public health utility, and demonstrate appropriate sensitivity and specificity.

Objective Monitoring of Lung Function

Objective measurement of lung function continues to be an essential element of the NHLBI NAEPP guidelines (NHLBI 2007). The measurement of lung function using spirometry provides a measure of disease severity and a means to track the disease's course and response to therapy (Miller et al. 2005; NHLBI 2007). Computer-based applications have been shown to successfully train patients to perform the spirometry technique, even in young children. An innovative computer-animated interactive system (*SpiroGame©*) was developed to teach and measure tidal breathing, encourage participation, and train preschool children to provide valid and reproducible spirometric test results (Vilozni et al. 2001). Children 3–6 years of age showed acceptable spirometry maneuvers through the use of the system which includes a game teaching tidal breathing technique before performing FVC maneuvers, an interactive visual interface, and a small, child friendly, ice cream cone-shaped pneumotachograph. Submission of digital video through the Internet has been demonstrated as a method of assessing peak flow meter technique in 7–16-year-old children (Chan et al. 2003; Chan et al. 2007). This asynchronous approach is described more fully under home monitoring later in this chapter.

Implementing Therapeutic Guidelines for Asthma

As the asthma guidelines have continued to be refined, so have computer-based applications designed to facilitate their use in clinical practice. In a review of informatics application for asthma management, Sanders and Aronsky (2006) report 20 publications (31% of publications reviewed) devoted to implementing or evaluating applications in support of clinical guidelines. These included systems in support of drug dosing, outpatient clinic practices, critiquing care plans, and vaccination reminder systems.

Prototypes have been described based on both the British Thoracic Society and NHLBI NAEPP guidelines (Austin et al. 1996; Shiffman et al. 2000). Studies in the United Kingdom have found mixed results in the application of DSSs for clinician decision making and patient outcomes. Epistemological and computational models for system design of a DSS under the aegis of the GAMES-II project was reported by Austin and colleagues though clinical outcomes have not been reported (Austin et al. 1996). A web-based, guideline-based DSS for acute asthma was assessed for its effect on clinician decisions using clinical scenario testing (Thomas et al. 1999). The DSS improved decision making across disciplines and modalities. Nonpulmonary nurses using the asthma DSS scored the same as experts (89% vs. 88%) and medical residents using the DSS scored significantly better than residents using a pen and paper application (92% vs. 84%). Also supportive was that patients whose physicians used a DSS in general practice clinics in the UK had fewer acute asthma exacerbations and initiated fewer practice consultations for asthma by 6 month follow-up than patients whose physician did not use a DSS (McCowan et al. 2001a, b). Less encouraging results using a DSS were found in a study of general practitioners and nurses in general practice clinics in N.E. England (Eccles et al. 2002). Measures taken 12 months before and 12 months following the introduction of the asthma DSS found no improvement in consultation rates, process of care measures, or reported patient outcomes. This study highlighted the importance of training and system design to avoid reported low levels of system adoption. A randomized controlled trial of 246 physicians, 20 outpatient pharmacists, and 706 of their patients with asthma and chronic COPD failed to show an effect of computer-generated care suggestions from clinical workstations to enhance physician and pharmacist adherence to evidence-based guidelines (Tierney et al. 2005). Conversely, computer clinic workstations have been an effective medium for delivery of interventions to effect physician ordering behaviour (Tierney et al. 1990) and to establish computerized physician order entry (CPOE) systems to help standardize order sets, reduce practice variation, and promote best practice (McAlearney et al. 2006).

Use of a handheld system based on the NHLBI NAEPP guidelines was associated with increased physician adherence to guideline recommendations including measures of lung function (peak flow and O_2 saturation) and pharmacotherapy (beta agonist use) though use of the system also resulted in prolonged and more costly visits with no demonstrated improvement in intermediate-term patient outcomes (Shiffman et al. 2000; Karras et al. 1999). The majority of users applied the system in real time concurrently with patient care and appreciated its cuing and reminder functions (Shiffman et al. 1999).

A traditional usability barrier to the computer-based support of guideline implementation has been that DSSs have not been integrated into EMRs causing providers to access different programs and duplicate data entry. In follow-on work, Shiffman and colleagues successfully translated the NHLBI guidelines into workflow decision support for the Logician™ EMR system. To date, the principles governing design activities and the steps to achieve integration into the existing workflow have been published (Shiffman et al. 2004). This work reflects a next generation of integrated decision support.

Descriptive and feasibility studies have also been conducted on another integrated system, "*Asthma Critic*," a "non-inquisitive" program designed to review or critique physician's diagnostic and treatment plans for asthma and chronic COPD using existing data already available in the EMR, hence requiring no additional data input from physicians (Kuilboer et al. 2002; Kuilboer et al. 2003). The system provides feedback of two types: critique as a patient specific comment based on the current clinical data, and transformed clinical measurement including calculation of measurement values (e.g., predicted peak flow based on gender, age, and height). A prospective feasibility study of over 100,000 electronic case records from primary care practices determined that the program was able to detect asthma and COPD records ($n = 8{,}784$) and produce patient specific feedback, mostly related to prescription type (for patients ≥12 years of age) and route (for patients ≤12 years). A randomized clinical trial of "AsthmaCritic" in 32 practices (40 Dutch general practitioners) compared the program with usual practice and determined that it changed the manner in which physicians monitored patients (i.e. increased FEV1 and PEF measures and ratio of coded measurements), conducted treatment (i.e. decreased cromoglycate prescriptions), and changed data-recording habits (Kuilboer et al. 2006).

Decision-support systems and EMR's can represent complex solutions to enhance the implementation of evidence-based clinical guidelines. Low-end solutions, while less complex, can provide elegant alternatives. Microsoft Access™ has been modified for the creation of asthma action plans using the "form entry" function, providing a database that can be queried to document best practices, is user-friendly, and networkable (Mangold and Salzman 2005).

Computer-based applications, EMRs, and DSSs have potential in influencing provider behavior and provide a likely candidate to address the call to develop and critically assess innovative interventions that encourage providers to adhere to guideline recommendations for inpatient as well as outpatient populations (Kattan 2008).

Physician-Patient Partnership, Collaboration and Communication

While acknowledging the importance of collaborative self-management, existing asthma management guidelines are less specific on how to establish an effective patient-provider partnership and how patients can overcome barriers to asthma self-care (NHLBI 1997, 2002; Shegog et al. 2004; NHLBI 2007). Theoretically-based tailored interventions have proven effective in influencing clinicians to train and motivate their patients to perform self-management (Clark 1989; Clark and Zimmerman 1990; Clark et al. 1995). While computer-based CD-ROMs have been used as a medium for an interdisciplinary training program in helping care providers understand overlapping roles in the clinical management of asthma (Rodehorst et al. 2005) the practical guidance in applying such models, as well as communication techniques that are effective with patients, have not been systematically addressed in an easily applicable form for providers and thus have been more slowly incorporated in DSS design (National Heart Lung and Blood Institute 2007; Glanz et al. 1997).

The *Stop Asthma Clinical System* (*SACS*) DSS provides support to the health-care provider in using tailored behavioral intervention strategies as a means of assessing and addressing problems of adherence to medication taking and environmental trigger control while also supporting asthma severity determination, pharmacotherapy, and action plan development. (Shegog et al. 2004; Shegog et al. 2006a, b). The decision rules in this DSS are based on inductive and deductive knowledge acquisition approaches, as well as Social Cognitive Theory and the Transtheoretical Stages of Change methods and strategies (Bandura 1991; Prochaska and Velicer 1997). While feasibility for the application has been established, the affects of *SACS* on physician behaviors and patient outcomes has yet to be determined (Shegog et al. 2006a, b). A modified version of the *SACS* (*AE-BACKER*) has been evaluated in a randomized controlled trial of a self-management intervention delivered in an emergency department setting for children aged 1–18 years of age (Sockrider et al. 2006). Asthma educators used *AE-BACKER* to tailor intervention messages and provide a customized asthma action plan and educational summary. Treatment subjects had higher confidence to prevent/treat asthma episodes 14 days after intervention; reported more well-asthma visits by 9 months after intervention; and had significantly fewer return emergency department visits. Although a greater proportion of subjects in the intervention group reported well-asthma visits than subjects in the control group, this return rate was still <50%. Despite computer-based decision support the ability to link children with emergency department visits back to primary care for well-asthma care remains a challenge, and even when follow-up occurs, the impact on subsequent asthma control remains uncertain (Sockrider et al. 2006).

In service of enhancing the patient-provider partnership, Hartman and colleagues have developed a website, *MyExpertDoctor.com*©, designed to raise patient awareness about what questions to ask their physicians prior to a clinic visit to increase the likelihood of receiving asthma care consistent with evidence-based guidelines (Hartmann et al. 2007). Results of qualitative evaluation indicate that patients had positive shifts in attitudes regarding interaction with their physician and became more involved in asthma care. Porter and colleagues report on two studies of the *Asthma Kiosk* ©, a DSS program, accessed during an emergency department visit, that collects child patient data from parents on symptoms of chronic severity, current medications, assessment of care needs, and environmental risk and provides output to clinicians that highlights level of chronic severity, symptom data supporting the severity rating, current controller medicines, mismatches between severity medicine and use of controllers, and asthma-specific needs regarding environmental risks, access to care and medicines, and educational topics (Porter et al. 2004; Porter et al. 2005; Porter et al. 2006). Patients rated the *Asthma Kiosk* © favorably as a good use of time and knowledge, easy to use, and not burdensome (Porter et al. 2004) and it was found to be a valid source of patient medication data (Porter et al. 2005). Parent satisfaction with care was measured by information-sharing by providers and by perceived involvement in their child's care during the ED visit. There was no change in information-sharing with patients reporting that they received as much information as they wanted at baseline and during the study. Satisfaction ratings worsened on the involvement rating from baseline to follow-up, possibly due to providers' inattention to concerns that were communicated via the kiosk (Porter et al. 2006). These results support the contention that to have an impact on patient outcomes, providers not only require salient patient information of the kind provided by programs such as *Asthma Kiosk*, but also they need to believe the correctness of the information they receive and take action to provide effective tailored recommendations using behavior change strategies to promote self-management as offered in programs like *SACS* or *AE-BACKER* (Clark et al. 1995).

Applications for Asthma Management Education

Patient and family education is essential for successful management of asthma as a chronic disease (NHLBI 1991, 1997, 2002, 2007; USDHHS 2003). Without adequate education, management recommendations on following a written action plan, correctly administering medications, and taking appropriate actions early in the event of an asthma exacerbation are rendered ineffective (Cabana and Tao 2005; Toelle and Ram 2004; Clark et al. 2009). The expansion of asthma educational programs has been driven, at least in part, by a growing acceptance that patients be actively involved in the management of their chronic disease and in treatment decisions (NHLBI 1991, 1997, 2007). The practical importance of teaching patients and their families self-management skills to lessen the impact of chronic illness has been well elucidated (Clark and Zimmerman 1990; Thoresen and Kirmil-Gray 1983; Bailey et al. 1992; Clark et al. 1993; Guevara et al. 2003). Such skills include adherence to medical regimens as well as the complex cognitive-behavioral tasks of self-monitoring, decision-making, and communicating about both symptoms and treatment regimens (Clark and Zimmerman 1990; Thoresen and Kirmil-Gray 1983; Bailey et al. 1992; Clark et al. 1993).

The benefits of asthma education programs include improved knowledge, feelings of competence, use of specific self-management behaviors, adherence to medical regimen, decreased emergency room and unscheduled doctor visits, reduced financial burden of asthma, enhanced partnerships with health-care providers, and quality of life (Evans 1992; Clark et al. 1986; Peterson et al. 2001; Klingelhofer and Gershwin 1988; Wigal et al. 1990). More recent systematic reviews have indicated improved objective measures of lung function, frequency of asthma symptoms, and health-care utilization (Velsor-Friedrich and Srof 2000a, b; Gibson et al. 2002; Wolf et al. 2002).

Recommendations for contemporary asthma education programs include that they (1) recognize the multiple factors that influence asthma and its control; (2) assess the individual's risk factors and needs in achieving control; (3) be individualized and tailored to the patient's asthma characteristics; (4) be more closely based on sound self-management and learning principles so that the patients and families can assume greater responsibility to self-manage their own asthma; (5) account for the importance of context and contextual variables (physical and social environments) on asthma management; (6) involve significant family members in intervention activities; (7) use venues where learning can be optimized (e.g., schools); and (8) be integrated into the provision of medical care in an efficient form to allow convenient implementation in the context of a clinic visit (Creer et al. 1990; Creer et al. 1992;

Kotses et al. 1990; Kotses et al. 1991; Velsor-Friedrich and Srof 2000a, b; McPherson et al. 2001, 2005; Clark et al. 2009). This section will describe evaluations of computer-assisted instruction programs that address these recommendations. Trends in professional training and the Internet as an information resource will also be briefly described.

Computer-Based Instruction for Asthma

The number of published empirical trials of asthma related computer-based instruction (CAI) is increasing. Reviews of computer-based interventions have listed as few as one study on asthma education in 2001 to as many as 13 in 2006 (Revere and Dunbar 2001; Osman et al. 1994; Sanders and Aronsky 2006; Bussey-Smith and Rossen 2007; Stinson et al. 2008). CAI now utilizes the full advantages of multimedia computing, providing interactive, tailored lesson content in engaging forms such as games, tutorials, quizzes, or simulations that are self-paced, more easily disseminated, and provide a range of visual (animation, graphics, video) and auditory (sound effects, music, voice over) strategies (Table 10.1).

Pediatric Asthma Education

Children with chronic conditions are playing a much more pivotal role in their management and treatment decisions, leading to an expansion of asthma education programs designed for their use. McPherson et al. (2005) describe two major computer-based educational approaches for children with asthma: stand-alone games and Internet-enabled programs. Gaming has long been considered a core educational strategy for computer applications and is currently enjoying an emergence with Serious Gaming and Gaming for Health initiatives (Serious Games Initiative 2006; Games for Health 2006). Early use of CAI gaming with children with asthma (7–12 years of age) was investigated using a computer game, *Asthma Command* © (Rubin et al. 1986; Rubin et al. 1989). The game content included symptom recognition, "aggravators," medicines, appropriate use of health providers, and encouragement to attend school. Children who played *Asthma Command*© for 40 min every 6 weeks for a period of 10 months in the outpatient clinic showed significantly improved knowledge and self-reported asthma management behaviors compared to children who did not have this exposure. A revised version of this program, *Asthma Control* ©, was created to reflect changes in the expert guidelines including the importance of preventive medication and expanded simulated environments and educational content (Homer et al. 2000). Children 3–12 years of age who used *Asthma Control*© in hospital, primary care or health clinic settings increased asthma knowledge and could report more environmental triggers than those children receiving usual care. They also showed improvement in a range of asthma management outcomes equivalent to children receiving usual care, which suggests the potential for computer-based applications to be a cost-effective educational approach in the long term (McPherson et al 2001).

A school-based program, *AirAcademy: The Quest for Airtopia* ™, was introduced as part of a 4th grade general health curriculum for students (9 and 10 years of age) (Yawn et al. 2000). It uses a science fiction theme to cover topics including anatomy of the lung, pathophysiology of asthma, environmental triggers, symptoms, therapeutic compliance and management, and goals of asthma management. Children using *AirAcademy*™ showed significant improvement in knowledge scores at 4-week follow-up compared to children not using the program.

These early studies reported change in knowledge about asthma and its management. As advances were being made in the theoretical and empirical underpinnings of self-management behavior, the design and evaluation of computer-based applications have moved from a focus on impacting knowledge to include other determinants of self-management behavior. *Bronki the Bronchiasaurus*™ is a Nintendo ™ psychomotor game where children guide a cartoon character to manage asthma including taking medicines, using an inhaler, recognizing and avoiding asthma triggers, monitoring peak flow, and using a sick day plan (Lieberman 1997, 2001). Multiple choice questions also cover an array of asthma management topics. Children, 6–16 years of age, who played the game for 40 min in an outpatient setting showed significant improvements in asthma knowledge, self-efficacy for asthma self-management, and self-efficacy for communicating with their parents about asthma. In another outpatient study, children

Table 10.1 Advantages and disadvantages of computer-based instruction and online resources

Advantages of CAI
• Convenient: Accessible at time and place convenient to user, and to geographically disparate populations
• Safe: Allows for safe exploration of concepts and applications
• Interactive: Often requires active input and response from users
• Flexible: Can be used as a stand-alone program, adaptable to changing data, can provide personalized and tailored instruction/information, operated at the users' own pace, search and personalized display capabilities
• Social: Can provide a sense of community through bulletin boards, e-mail, virtual worlds, can enhance communication with peers
• Motivational: Attractive to users, especially youth
• Attractive: Incorporates multimedia applications
• Accessible and egalitarian: Easily disseminated to underserved populations
Disadvantages of CAI
• Accessibility: May be dependant on cost and location causing disparities ("digital divide")
• Literacy: Depends on user's ability to read, many websites are in high-level English
• Interactivity: Often websites are simply "page turners"
• Turnover: Programs are often superseded in terms of sophistication and content
• Quality: Website content quality is variable and may be dated, a number of checklists to assess website quality exist but none are definitive, expert moderation is required in chat rooms and bulletin boards
• User demographics: It is still unclear who benefits most from using CAI and which factors are salient predictors of success (e.g., I.Q., disease severity, education level)
• Cost: Up-front costs are often high and development processes are long and detailed

Adapted from (Glasgow et al. 1999; Owen 2002; McPherson et al. 2001; D'Alessandro and Dosa 2001; Croft and Peterson 2002; Oermann et al. 2003)

using the program for 30 min showed significantly greater self-efficacy for asthma self-care activity than children watching a 30-min videotape about asthma self-care (Lieberman 2001).

STARBRIGHT World™ is an on-line virtual experience designed for hospitalized children that has generated research across health domains (Starlight Foundation 2009). In this application children can learn about asthma or other diseases and interact with other users online. Children, 8–18 years of age, many with asthma, who used STARBRIGHT World™ during their hospitalization showed increased knowledge about asthma compared to those experiencing traditional hospital educational and recreational activities (Hazzard et al. 2002). The experience of the on-line virtual community did not significantly increase perceived social support from peers or coping skills compared to the traditional hospital experience.

Recent evaluation studies have been reporting findings that promise greater impact on behavioral and clinical outcomes of asthma. Outpatient children 7–14 years of age who accessed a self-management computer program from home called *The Asthma Files©* had greater knowledge and locus of control at 1 month and were less likely to have required oral corticosteroid or time off school during a 6-month follow-up period when compared to children not accessing the computer program (McPherson et al. 2001). Other outcome parameters including FEV1, PEF, and unscheduled visits to the clinic or hospital were not significantly different. In two separate studies evaluating Internet-enabled applications for outpatient education Krishna et al. (2003) have shown promise in supplementing conventional asthma care with interactive multimedia education to improve knowledge and reduce the burden of childhood asthma. Children 7–17 years of age visiting a pediatric pulmonary clinic who received an Internet-enabled multimedia asthma education program in addition to face-to-face patient education significantly increased asthma knowledge, decreased asthma symptom days, and decreased number of ER visits compared to children receiving patient education alone (Krishna et al. 2003). These children were also using a significantly lower average daily dose of inhaled corticosteroid (beclomethasone equivalent) at 12 months follow-up. A subsequent version of this program entitled "*Interactive Multimedia Program for Asthma Control and Tracking*"© (*IMPACT*) comprised Internet-based scenarios, and exercises on causes, triggers, and treatment of asthma in 44 linear lessons that was supervised by health-care professionals (Krishna et al. 2006). Children 7–18 years of age and parents of children 0–6 years of age who used the program demonstrated significantly improved knowledge (child and parent), reduced days of asthma symptoms, emergency care, and school days missed, and reduced activity limitation compared to children and parents using verbal and printed information. Quality of life and lung function indices were not significantly improved.

Another Internet-based asthma education program was able to significantly impact quality of life and lung function, as well as missed school days and asthma-related emergencies (Runge et al. 2006). Four hundred and thirty eight youth (8–16 years of age) were assigned to either a standardized patient management program (SPMP) or to a SPMP with the adjunct Internet-based program and compared after 12 month follow-up. In addition to the previously mentioned outcomes, the combined SPMP/Internet programs also demonstrated positive cost-benefits.

By approximating real life situations, simulations offer great potential to increase transference of asthma management skills to real world behaviors. Findings from studies examining these types of programs are yielding mixed results. Hopper (2005) described an online simulation that used branching-logic in a frame-based application targeting skills training in inner city youth at Atlanta's *Zap Asthma*© headquarters. A sample of 12 inner city children 7–14 years of age provided initial formative evaluation on the application which simulates decision making regarding environmental triggers, medication use, and self-assessment. Field testing and usability testing indicated no significant comprehension or navigation problems but impact and outcome evaluation results have yet to be reported. In *Wee Willee Wheezie*©, asthma management is simulated in life-like settings with the goal to avoid the simulated consequences of exacerbations of asthma and trips to hospital (Huss et al. 2003). Children 7–12 years of age who accessed the program from home for 20 min showed no significant difference on knowledge, symptom, self-management, lung function, or quality of life variables when compared to children who used a non-asthma health related computer game.

A simulation game, *Watch, Discover, Think, and Act* (*WDTA*)©, was designed to include a self-regulation meta-cognitive framework as a central program theme in addition to asthma-specific skills training (Bartholomew et al. 2000a, b). Self-regulation can be described as a sequence of steps of goal setting, self-monitoring, problem identification (self-judgment), solution identification, action (self-reaction), and evaluation (Clark and Zimmerman 1990; Clark et al. 1981; Creer et al. 1992; Bandura 1991; Clark et al. 1984; Macro Int'l 1994). These cognitive skills have been identified as important in assessing and solving asthma related problems as well as more traditional academic problems (Clark et al. 1981, 1984; Creer et al. 1992; Hindi-Alexander and Cropp 1981; Fireman et al. 1981; Creer and Winder 1986; Schunk 1983, 1986; Zimmerman 1986, 1989; Zimmerman and Ringle 1981). Programs that teach self-management behavior in the context of a meta-cognitive framework of self-regulation have shown promise (Clark and Zimmerman 1990; Thoresen and Kirmil-Gray 1983; Creer et al. 1992; Kotses et al. 1990; Clark and Partridge 2002; Clark et al. 2007). The *WDTA* program was found to positively impact self-efficacy and attributions to asthma management in children 9–12 years of age in a laboratory-based impact evaluation (Shegog et al. 2001). Inner city children, 8–16 years of age, who used *WDTA* in outpatient settings rated the program as motivationally appealing and had fewer hospitalizations, better symptom scores, increased functional status, greater knowledge of asthma management, better self-reported self-management behavior, and greater clinic return rates than those receiving usual care only (Bartholomew et al. 2000a, b; Shegog et al. 2006a, b). In a subsequent school-based evaluation of multifaceted screening and educational intervention that included the *WDTA* program, children receiving the intervention demonstrated improved knowledge, self-efficacy, and self-reported self-management including reported trigger management, exercise pre-treatment, and self-management of episodes at home (Bartholomew et al. 2006). While feasible for school use, the multi-component nature of the school-based intervention made the particular effects of *WDTA* program, in comparison to other intervention components, difficult to determine.

Adult Asthma Education

Education programs for adult patients tend to take three primary forms: conventional instruction as tutorials; programs that assist in disease monitoring (described in the next section); and Internet resources offering a smorgasbord of information and materials for self-tailored use (described later in this section). Relatively few evaluation studies have been published on stand-alone applications for adult education, with most being in outpatient settings.

Computer-generated personalized booklets have been found to compare favorably to traditional face-to-face asthma education at outpatient or surgery visits in adult outpatients (Osman et al. 1994). The significant findings included 54% fewer hospital admissions than the control group and 80% reduction in sleep disturbance. While not a computer-based intervention in the strictest sense, this study provides an adjunctive use of data management to provide personalized and tailored printed interventions that include the drug regimen used by the patient. Another clinic-based program, *Breathe Smart*©, targeted parents of children with asthma (<12 years of age) and comprised a touch screen interface with photos and graphic media (Fall et al. 1998). Though the program was well received by parents, there was no significant knowledge increase at 1-month follow-up in parents who used the program in a single outpatient clinic visit.

Computer-based applications can be effective as stand-alone programs; however, their efficacy is often greatest when used as an adjunct with conventional education or face-to-face interaction with clinic personnel. A CAI drill and practice program was developed for adult outpatients to instruct them on asthma management and equipment techniques (i.e., peak flow) using a quiz format (Takabayashi et al. 1999). Although older patients (>65 years) required more time, most patients had no difficulty using the program and stated it was beneficial and validated their understanding of asthma. Clinical outcomes were mixed in the small study sample with 8 of 26 patients having decreased emergency visits while 2 patients had deteriorated control. Mixed results were also found for a combined 30-min computer program followed by a 30-min discussion with a specialized asthma nurse in a sample of young adults, 18–25 years of age (Sundberg et al. 2005). Those using the program had significantly increased FEV1, especially among atopic patients. No other benefits were observed in ER visits, symptoms, knowledge, lung function, or quality of life.

The efficacy of using supplementary CAI for environmental trigger control has also been assessed. At 12-week follow-up, patients with dust mite allergy who used a CAI program in addition to conventional instruction (physician verbal and written guidance) scored significantly higher on adherence to avoidance strategies and had lower house dust mite allergen levels in the bedroom compared to control subjects who had conventional instruction alone (Huss et al. 1991; Huss et al. 1992a, b).

Professional Asthma Education

Health-care providers require training programs in the clinical process and management of disease, and continuing medical education (CME) for accreditation purposes. Increasingly, training programs are relying on computer-based applications to provide learning opportunities. Peterson et al. (2001) surveyed hospital -based teaching programs to assess the interest and feasibility of using computer-based delivery for asthma education to train health-care professionals (Peterson et al. 2001). At the time of the survey, 69% of hospital training programs had computers available with 60% linked to the Internet. Eighty five percent of programs reported they could use a computer-based program if one was available though cost and time constraints remain the primary barriers. The development and evaluation of how CAI fits into medical school curricula has been suggested as a future focus of CAI (Adler and Johnson 2000).

With the focus of "just-in-time" learning opportunities for the health-care provider, the computer-based decision support systems offer the potential for "hands-on" training and education in real time. This raises the question as to the effectiveness of the current generation of computer-based education programs. Published evaluations of computer-assisted CME and training programs in asthma education are lagging behind their implementation though some web-based programs are being reported as suitable for delivering educational materials to primary care physicians locally and internationally (Sly et al. 2006).

The Internet provides a breadth of professional resources. Resources generally comprise, but are not limited to, professional associations, pulmonary and medical journals, asthma information sites, disease foundations, and general health information sites. Examples of these links for the pulmonary practitioner can be viewed at the University of Missouri health web page http://intmed.muhealth.org/pulm/pulm_links.html. Further, recent developments in Internet, multimedia, and wireless broadband can facilitate information access to databases devoted to providing support for EBDM including the Cochrane Library, Best Evidence, Clinical Evidence, and the National Guideline Clearinghouse (Jadad 2002; Bero et al. 1998). Relatively few published articles have devoted themselves to professional resources on the Internet and those that have are frequently dated due to the continually evolving offerings (Smith 1999a, b).

The Internet as an Asthma Management Resource

The Internet is also a resource for information on asthma pathophysiology and management for patients and families. Originated through the U.S. government's Advanced Research Projects Agency in 1969, the Internet was designed to be a sustainable network, allowing communication between computer users from one university to another, while allowing routing and rerouting in more than one direction in the event of parts of the network being inoperative (Staggers et al. 2001). It has since evolved into a diverse interaction of "virtual" communities that share information or human experience, mushrooming into a public, cooperative, and self-sustaining facility accessible to hundreds of millions of people worldwide (the World Wide Web).

While potentially beneficial, the Internet can also be a confusing information resource for patients to navigate. For example, when the word "asthma" was entered into three search engines resultant "hits" totalled 2,740,320 (Oermann et al. 2003). Further, the structure of decentralized control makes it difficult to enforce quality-control on sites raising concern about the potential harm caused by health-related Websites through misleading or incorrect information (Kiley 2002; Robinson et al. 1998). The criteria used by people with chronic disease (including asthma) and their caregivers to assess websites, as determined using qualitative survey methods, are information content, presentation, interactivity, and trustworthiness (Kerr et al. 2006). To ease confusion and provide formal criteria, organizations including the American Medical Association (AMA), British Healthcare Internet Association, Health on the Net (HON) Foundation, and the Health Summit Working group have each developed rating tools to objectively evaluate websites (Kim et al. 1999; Health Summit Working Group 1997; Chang et al. 2003). Broadly, these criteria are (1) credibility including sources or references, currency, relevance, site evaluation, (2) content including accuracy, disclaimers from authors or sponsors, completeness, (3) disclosure including purpose and profiling, (4) links including selection, architecture, content, and back linkages, (5) design including accessibility, logical organization, ease of use, and internal search capability, (6) interactivity including mechanisms for users to provide feedback, and (7) caveats including agendas that users need-to-know (Chang et al. 2003).

These criteria have been used to review asthma education on the WWW. The significant strides that have been made in disseminating resources on asthma to the general public have been published that categorize sites into those providing general information, multipurpose sites, and discussion lists (Higgenbottom and Smith 2002) as well as websites catering to adolescents (Chang et al. 2003). Cabana (2005) has echoed the overall results of these evaluation studies, stating that resources on the web vary in their quality and content, often fail to meet the information needs of patients and make little innovative use of technology. An assessment of 145 asthma websites from four major search engines determined that the mean number of HON principles met was 6.3 of 8 (only 14 sites conformed to all), and the mean number of asthma educational concepts was 4.9 of 8 (only 20 sites contained all of these) (Croft and Peterson 2002). The sites also scored low on accessibility. The reading level required to use the websites was greater than 10th grade and only 9 sites had multilingual asthma education content. Few websites used innovative or interactive components with many websites being little more than "electronic books." A subsequent study evaluated asthma websites for patient education using Yahoo™, Google™, and AOL™ search engines and found just ten websites meeting HON criteria and NHLBI content criteria and being recommended for patients and parents of children with asthma (Oermann et al. 2003). The authors also caution that these websites were not excluded on the basis of higher than recommended reading levels. Findings have been similar in international studies that cite highly variable information, and lack of core asthma educational concepts and justifiability (Berland et al. 2001; Heung-Woo et al. 2004).

The challenge of the WWW does not reside in content quality alone. Accessibility, in technical and communication terms, has also represented a challenge. While "adoption of the Internet as a health information resource continues to lag among vulnerable populations who could benefit the most, including patients of lower socioeconomic status and the elderly" (Murray et al. 2003), it is also true that more individuals are gaining access to this resource. "Historically, no communications technology (including the telephone) has been adopted as rapidly as the Internet" (Glasgow et al. 1999). While a segment of the population is becoming increasingly directive of their health-care, there is also a segment which is not "plugged in" and which is still operating in a pre-electronic mode requiring the health-care system to be flexible to handle both conditions (Murray et al. 2003).

An advantage of the Internet is the contact that can be provided for people across a wide geographic distribution to the health-care professional. As previously described, this can be through knowledge assessment and simple feedback (Krishna et al. 2001) or more complex approaches of transmitting detailed management information to ensure they are adhering to the asthma management plan (Chan et al. 2003).

Applications to Monitor Asthma Management and Control

Successful management of a dynamic chronic disorder such as asthma requires consistent monitoring to detect early signs and symptoms and initiate rescue plans, to control airway inflammation, to recognize and avoid environmental triggers, and to maintain collaborative care (NHLBI 1997; Wainright and Wootton 2003). Computer-based monitoring applications have been designed to assist patients in these self-management activities (Chang et al. 2003; Rasmussen et al. 2005). Computer-based monitoring applications comprise a monitoring component and a communication component (Chang et al. 2003). The monitoring component includes individual assessment with feedback that compares patient data such as current lung function (e.g., peak flow, spirometry) or medicine use with past values. Ideally feedback is based on established national guidelines and accounts for the individual patient's characteristics including goals, behaviors, environment, signs, and symptoms. The communication component comprises some form of telecommunications technology. This might be through the Internet or non-Internet-dependent telemedicine systems (Schneider and Eisenberg 1998a, b). Communication can be synchronous or asynchronous. Synchronous communication occurs in real time and includes chat-room modules or teleconferences for conversations between patients that can be monitored by health-care professionals. Synchronous or real-time connections have been described as inconvenient for patients and providers and too dependent on temperamental video connections (Chan et al. 2007). Asynchronous communication, also described as "store and forward" technology, allows patients to accrue data which can be forwarded to health-care providers for subsequent review. This can include e-mails or text messages that might contain a symptom diary-associating peak flow, environmental triggers, activity level, and feelings so that the health-care provider can understand the antecedents of asthma control. This can also include video exemplifying specific management techniques. Monitoring systems also usually encompass an educational component to reinforce information received from the health-care provider (Chang et al. 2003). Examples include commonly asked questions and answers, a library of education materials, video clips, brochures related to asthma, and website links.

Computer-based monitoring has the potential to facilitate the patient-provider communication, provide the opportunity for the patient to work with their own data in real time, to have ongoing management education, and reduce the chance of decay of knowledge and skills gained from previous management education (Finkelstein et al. 1998; Finkelstein et al. 2000; Finkelstein et al. 2001). The number of published evaluation studies is growing with Sanders and Aronsky (2006) reporting 13 papers (20% of their total reviewed pool) devoted to monitoring and prevention. Of these, 10 studies focused primarily on applications allowing patients to record the degree of symptom control, reminding patients to use prescribed medicines, or for tracking the use of rescue medicines. Applications for patient-centered, home-based monitoring of asthma management are described in this section.

Home Internet Monitoring (Management Monitoring Studies)

The rise of the Internet has increased the viability of home-based monitoring. Results to date are encouraging. An Internet-based asthma diary with a feedback system, integrated asthma action plan, and treatment decision support system for use by adult patients was assessed over a 6-month period and led to a significant reduction in symptoms and airway hyper-responsiveness, and improved quality of life and lung function when compared to clinical assessment by specialists or general practitioners (Rasmussen et al. 2005). The opportunity to continually register symptoms provided patients with a more accurate picture of disease severity. This, coupled with greater adherence to their asthma action plan and more efficient monitoring, helped the Internet subjects take the recommended dose of inhaled corticosteroid and maintain asthma control.

The feasibility of this store and forward technology had been established in a separate study where spirometry data (PEFR and FEV) from the Vitalgraph® 2110 home spirometer were uploaded into a PC for subsequent review and analysis and found to generate accurate and reliable data with 67.4% of morning and 71.7% evening recordings meeting acceptable criteria (Hamid et al. 1998). A more recent adherence study in children with persistent asthma used the AccuTrax™ Personal Diary Spirometer, which is a handheld device capable of measuring and recording PEF and FEV_1 values in conjunction with date and time (Burkhart et al. 2007). Daily telemonitoring of exhaled nitric oxide data (from a NIOX MINO™ airway inflammation monitor via PalmOne™ PDA) in children 6–18 years with mild-moderate asthma, though found to be feasible, was not found to provide an appreciable advantage from symptom telemonitoring alone (de Jongste et al. 2009).

Studies of the feasibility of Internet-based home monitoring for low income, inner city patients who have little or no prior computer experience have also been reported (Finkelstein et al. 1998; Finkelstein et al. 2000). A system comprising portable spirometers and pocket-sized palmtop computers for registering lung function and symptoms was evaluated over a 3-week period with a sample of 17 inner city adults with asthma (Finkelstein et al. 1998) and in another sample of 31 inner city adults (Finkelstein et al. 2000). Subjects felt that self-testing was important and uncomplicated, but the clinical impact of this system has yet to be reported (Finkelstein et al. 2001).

Monitoring systems have also been developed for children. The "*Health Buddy*"© (HB) telemonitoring program queries children on their asthma management and provides immediate feedback as well as transmitting trivia and asthma facts on a daily basis (Guendelman et al. 2002). Evaluation results at 6 and 12 week follow-up showed that children 8–16 years of age using HB had less limitation of activity, lower frequency of sub-optimal PEF, more unprompted controller medication use, and less urgent calls to the hospital than children using a conventional asthma diary. Another study compared use of an Internet based store and forward system for submission of digital video of peak flow meter use and symptom diaries to office-based (face-to-face) education in improving peak flow and inhaler technique (Chan et al. 2003). Children who were 7 years of age with persistent asthma showed significant improvement in inhaler technique and peak flow values equivalent to children having face-to-face training. However, the investigators noted that there was a significant decline in electronic submission of monitoring videos and diaries from children over time. Therefore, they suggested that intermittent monitoring be instituted mainly at times when the patient's clinical status or regimen is changing (Chan et al. 2003). Similar results were found in a subsequent study examining the long-term comparison of an Internet-based asynchronous case management and education program with traditional face-to-face, office-based case management (Chan et al. 2007). At 12 month follow-up both groups had achieved asthma control suggesting a role for Internet-based case management as a long-term and cost-effective option for ongoing management. Those using the web-based application demonstrated better metered-dose inhaler technique scores and were more adherent to diary submission than those in the traditional face-to-face condition, though adherence to submission of monitoring data was still inconsistent. A study of electronic monitoring of nebulizer medication in inner city children with asthma was found to be more precise than self-report on diary cards and feasible for this population (Butz et al. 2005).

The LinkMedica™ resource site represents a collaborative between AstraZeneca, academic, and patient groups. This is a web service for asthma patients and health-care providers that includes an asthma diary for monitoring and self-management (Jadad 2002; Anhoj and Nielsen 2004). Patient and caregiver use of the site was assessed using quantitative and qualitative evaluations which determined two main uses of the site, "outside-in" in which an asthma management problem arises and users seek answers in the site, and "inside-out" where users focus on the use of the diary feature with little browsing activity. Studies of adolescent's perceived uses, barriers and benefits of the Internet (as well as short message service) for asthma self-management have been conducted. Support is provided on the potential of this technology for long term monitoring, particularly by those adolescents with poor asthma control (van der Meer et al. 2007) and for younger adolescent's who, in one study, were found to have a greater interest in learning about asthma (Rhee et al. 2006). Outcomes from a randomized trial of a tailored web-based asthma management program for urban African-American high school students supports this contention (Joseph et al. 2007; Joseph 2000). In a trial with 314 15–19-year-old teens 21-month follow-up indicated that students using the website, *Puff City*©, reported fewer symptom days, symptom nights, school days missed, restricted activity days, and hospitalizations for asthma compared to control students. Asthma control (average PEF, symptom scores), adherence, quality of life, and asthma knowledge were also positively impacted in a randomized controlled trial of *Blue Angel for Asthma*, an Internet-based multimedia asthma education program with interactive asthma telemonitoring and retrieval analysis system (Jan et al. 2007). The system was evaluated with 164 children (6–12 years of age) with persistent asthma for a period of 12 months.

The National Asthma Education Program Panel (NAEPP) guidelines have been used as a criteria for analyzing ongoing (bi-monthly) asthma data (symptoms, health-care utilization, and medication use) that is then used to provide medication management recommendations (increase, decrease, no change) to the primary care physician via computerized letters (Kattan et al. 2006). Children who used this system had more follow-up care visits, increased asthma visits in which medications were stepped-up when clinically indicated, and had fewer emergency department visits.

Electronic peak flow monitoring has been associated with better patient adherence than with conventional paper recording of peak flow readings (Reddel et al. 1998; Bruderman and Abboud 1997; Lieu et al. 1997). However, the small sample sizes and short duration of published studies make it difficult to generalize or comment on sustainability and a common finding is that monitoring behavior is quickly extinguished or subject to mixed adherence (Finkelstein et al. 1998; Guendelman et al. 2002; Streel et al. 2002). The "Health Buddy©" (HB) system, for example, was well received by the children but there was also a reported decline in use of HB (and also the asthma diary) over the course of the study. In the Internet-monitoring studies by Finkelstein and colleagues, adherence was at issue with only 29.5% of subjects independently reviewing their results at home at least once a week. Despite favorable responses from patients and doctors regarding credibility and reliability, users of the LinkMedica™ site were unwilling to use the site for an extended calendar period and patients stopped using the diary function after a short time. This suggests that the most salient use of the system may be at critical times in care management (e.g., at the start of care for asthma or after an acute exacerbation, an ED visit, a hospitalization, or a step-up in severity class) (Guendelman et al. 2002). Internet-based telemonitoring systems tested in more recent studies have often included a bundling of an educational program and ongoing monitoring in one application. The impact of these programs indicate a positive trend toward greater efficacy in impacting self-management and related outcomes (Kattan et al. 2006; Joseph et al. 2007; Jan et al. 2007).

Computer-Based Reminder Systems

Computer-based reminder systems provide monitoring or tracking functions and cue health-care providers to remind patients to return for clinic visits for prevention services. These systems have positively effected immunization rates and asthma management behaviors (Barnett et al. 1983; McDowell et al. 1989; Rosser et al. 1992; Johnston et al. 1994; Martin 2006). A reminder system used to identify children with asthma and to send a reminder letter followed by an autodial telephone message (sent 6 weeks later) caused a significant increase in influenza vaccines for children from 5.4 to 32.1% (Gaglani et al. 2001). Similar results have been found in a study of children in four private medical practices in Denver where the influenza immunization rate for those receiving a staged reminder letter and postcard was 42% compared to 25% in control subjects (Daley et al. 2004). Reminded subjects were more likely to have an office visit and less likely to have a missed opportunity to immunize. A computer-based reminder system that targeted adult asthma patients was evaluated in outpatient clinics (Curtin et al. 1998). The system comprised an automatic reminder accompanied by a care plan focused on self-management.

Computer-generated point of service reminders and annual birthday card reminders mailed to patients improved self-management and reduced hospitalizations. Intervention patients had significantly greater number of peak flow meter readings and use of the clinical guideline management plan (Asthma Game Plan), as well as fewer hospital admissions and ED visits.

Conclusion

Research on the feasibility, efficacy, and effectiveness of computer-based applications has determined their potential to support guideline implementation throughout the therapeutic stream of asthma management (Fig. 10.1). Future possibilities for computers in the management of asthma are vast and will continue to be linked to two parallel developments, that of new and more sophisticated computer-based systems and communication methods, and the continual evolution of best practice methods (pharmaceutical, technological, behavioral) in asthma management. Success will ultimately by measured when the innovative prototypic applications migrate from the "lab bench" to the broad clinic application. To facilitate this transfer of applications from the realm of scientific investigation to mainstream use will require stringency on the part of researchers, developers, and clinicians to attend to rigorous evaluations of their effectiveness and diffusion.

To date, the effectiveness of computer-based systems in improving asthma management is encouraging but not conclusive. Ongoing work is required. A review of primary care computing from 1980 to 1997 was aptly titled "a descriptive feast but an evaluative famine" (Mitchell and Sullivan 2001) and other authors noted the dominance of demonstration articles over comparison studies with few appearing in "core" medical journals (Adler and Johnson 2000).

In 1994, Johnson and colleagues noted that system assessment occurred primarily at earlier developmental phases, such as measuring reliability, accuracy, and acceptability and called for studies to progress from the lab to the clinical population in a systematic way (Johnston et al. 1994). A decade later, little has changed with respect to scientific validation of computer-based applications for asthma management. Sanders and Aronsky (2006) determined that only a handful of studies demonstrated "maturity," marked by influence (how routinely applications are used in patient care) and by rigor of study design (Sanders and Aronsky 2006). Prospective randomized clinical controlled trials were represented in only 16 publications and were limited mainly to primary care clinics with relatively few in emergency room care and hospital care (Sanders and Aronsky 2006). A relative dearth of efficacy and effectiveness studies of home-based computer applications has also been noted (Clark et al. 2009). Prospective informatics studies have been particularly lacking in the asthma domains of detection, diagnosis, and monitoring (Sanders and Aronsky 2006).

Claims for effectiveness of computer-based applications need to be assessed with the same rigor as any other therapeutic innovation. This will require study designs that can suggest causality such as randomized controlled trials. While clinical controlled trials continue to be the gold standard in evaluation of systems, Harris et al. (2006) point out that quasi-experimental designs, used extensively in the social sciences, could be more utilized in informatics evaluations. Unlike pharmaceutical trials, the use of computer-based systems preclude blinding the health-care provider to condition and clinical settings often preclude complete separation of intervention and control groups (Harris et al. 2006). Studies of patient outcomes bring the added burden of large numbers of participants and substantial budgets. These quasi-experimental designs are often more amenable for use in the constraints of health-care settings. Progress of research in this field will need to confront the challenges presented by a heterogeneity of study designs and varied measures of clinical outcomes if meaningful cross-study comparisons are to be made (Mattke et al. 2009).

While the current state of the literature appears somewhat top heavy with respect to design descriptions and feasibility studies, it is necessary that researchers not throw the "baby out with the bath water" and continue to publish design innovations and prototype testing. A criticism of existing literature, not confined to informatics, is that often critical information about programs is missing and there is wide variation in methods and content, meaning that replication is difficult and that most effective components are difficult to identify (Sudre et al. 1999). Researchers will also need to find a balance between reporting on innovative applications with the risk of fuelling the criticism that asthma intervention research is often underwhelming with results that report short-term knowledge change but not behavioral effects (Clark et al. 2009).

A consistent challenge with rapidly moving technology is that dissemination of programs outstrips their evaluation. A paradox exists where corporate or foundation collaborations produce programs that are disseminated but have limited empirical data to indicate their effectiveness. An example is the computer-assisted instruction program entitled "*Quest for the Code*"® (Starlight Foundation 2009) that comprises a game-like strategy, uses well known entertainers, and sophisticated multimedia interface. This program is one of a suite of programs available online through the Starlight Foundation, offering appeal and the potential for efficacious asthma education but having yet to be evaluated for effectiveness in the peer-reviewed literature.

The continued evolution of decision support systems raises a broader question as why such systems are not more ubiquitous in general medical practice. Reasons proffered for this include the labor and cost investments, lack of universal vocabularies to allow for integrated systems, need for more effectiveness trials, the legal and ethical issues related to medical decision-making, and the clinical viability of such systems (Staggers et al. 2001; Lehmann 2004; Johnston et al. 1994; Rosenstein 1999) (Table 10.2). For optimal dissemination, innovative decision-support systems should satisfy the principles of successful diffusion of innovation and demonstrate cost-effectiveness, usability, and clinical integration, all critical predictors of successful adoption (Rogers 1995); Helitzer et al. 2003; Dixon and Dixon 1994; Davis 1989).

For a computer-based application to be successfully disseminated, it must be considered to be effective in facilitating asthma care and reducing costs. There is a general lack of cost-effectiveness studies for computer-based applications for asthma management (Johnston et al. 1994; Wainright and Wootton 2003; Rosenstein 1999; Chang et al. 2003) despite cost-effectiveness being a fundamental antecedent to institutionalization. A recent systematic review of interactive computer-based asthma patient education programs indicated that none of the studies under review fully addressed the cost-benefit ratio of developing and implementing these computer programs (Bussey-Smith and Rossen 2007). This may be rectified as studies mature toward more trials of effectiveness and determine the gains from the direct and indirect improvements in cost, quality, and patient-focused outcomes.

Table 10.2 Challenges for developing and deploying computer-based systems in support of asthma management

(1) Strategic planning that links decisions about clinical strategy, care delivery process requirements, and investment in technology
(2) Developing standard and effective data models that describe clinical activities, data definitions, and approaches for data integrity
(3) Defining common practice standards (i.e., nomenclature, clinical vocabulary, and protocols)
(4) Addressing efficient, economic, and effective clinical practice processes before automation
(5) Investing in "people-ware" (i.e., clinicians and other user groups), particularly in education and training
(6) Collaborating, educating, and self-assessing for quality improvement in an unequivocally interdisciplinary way; rewarding creativity and innovations
(7) Exploring risk-sharing and partnership opportunities with vendors
(8) Refining cost-effectiveness approaches to support better long-term decisions

Adapted from (Mathews and Newell 1999; Adler and Johnson 2000; Staggers et al. 2001)

Computer-based applications in the clinic setting often present an irony. Systems can reduce medical errors, improve the use of treatment guidelines, reduce redundant testing, and enhance delivery of both physician and patient education at the point of care. These enhancements often come at a cost of the increased time taken in using the systems. Time management, ironically, is one of the reasons for instituting computer-based systems in the first place. Time constraints have been frequently cited in past studies as a critical barrier to adoption of clinic-based applications (Shiffman et al. 2000; Gadd et al. 1998; Cabana 2005). This presents integration and design challenges. Design criteria that make computer systems usable and time effective within the context of the often hectic clinic begins at the front-end of development with end-user input to guide development and include: (1) Obtaining the end-user's perspective, (2) Developing information appropriate in level and quality, (3) Connecting via wireless technology, (4) Maintaining security and privacy, (5) Justifying cost (Chang et al. 2003). Tangible strategies to mitigate time taken to use a DSS include thorough training, consistent system use, integration of DSS functions into existing EMR workflow and a design that organizes information, provides process and decision models, and suggest courses of action as seamlessly as possible. Computer-based applications can also provide allied health professionals with the opportunity for more input in collecting and providing information, relieving the time and task burden from the physician.

Asthma care is a multidisciplinary pursuit that requires coordination and communication between patients and health-care providers in home, outpatient, and acute care settings. This requires computer systems such as EMRs to be integrated across locations and the need to examine computer-based applications in varied settings (Sanders and Aronsky 2006). The outpatient clinic is the most common study setting. Relatively few studies have been conducted in inpatient settings. Studies of CAI, for example, have indicated that it is a strategy best used as a component of a multi-faceted approach, and not as a replacement to other educational and clinical management approaches (Revere and Dunbar 2001; Bartholomew et al. 2000a, b; McPherson et al. 2001; Fall et al. 1998).

In addition to the challenge of integration is the need to individualize asthma management plans and revise therapy based on patient response. Replicating static care guidelines into a computer system is an inadequate solution. Effective systems will need to track patient outcomes over time and be able to generate personalized care plans for both acute and chronic asthma care (Sanders and Aronsky 2006). Coupled with this is the need for application of behavioral theory to guide specification of program objectives, health behaviors, cognitive determinants of behavior (such as knowledge, attitudes, social perceptions, and self-efficacy), change methods, and evaluation and measurement protocols (Skinner and Kreuter 1997; Lieberman 1997; Rhodes et al. 1997; Revere and Dunbar 2001). Systematic approaches have been described that assist developers in the application of theory in computer-based applications and simulations (Bartholomew et al. 2001; Shegog et al. 2006a, b). Further, novel approaches to asthma management include the application of a computer-based decision-making paradigm for multiple risk behaviors such as cigarette, alcohol, and marijuana use that might exacerbate adolescent asthma management (Rhee et al. 2008).

It cannot be said that computer-based programs thus far created offer a blueprint for clinical practice because evaluation results have generally not been replicated and few studies have followed subjects longer than 1 year (Peterson et al. 2001; Klingelhofer and Gershwin 1988). Future evaluation challenges for computer-based applications for the management of asthma will include diffusion studies that examine the integration of computers into the clinical and management repertoires of health-care providers, effectiveness trials of alternative and emerging technological modalities such as the Internet, PDAs, iPods™, cellular phones (Lee et al. 2005); and economic analyses regarding the cost and time benefits of computer applications in clinic and hospital settings (Adler and Johnson 2000; Street and Rimal 1997). We have only begun to realize the benefits of computer-based applications for asthma management. If history is an indicator, then a future of exciting innovation is assured.

References

Adler MD, Johnson KB (2000) Quantifying the literature of computer-aided instruction in medical education. Acad Med 75(10):1025–1028

Akinbami L, Moorman JE, Garbe PL, Sondik EJ (2009) Status of childhood asthma in the United States, 1980–2007. Pediatrics 123:S131–S145

Alessi SM, Trollip SR (1991) Computer-based instruction: Methods and development. Prentice-Hall, Englewood Cliffs

Anhoj J, Nielsen MA (2004) Quantitative and qualitative usage data of an Internet-based asthma monitoring tool. J Med Internet Res 6(3):e23

Aronow DB, Soderland S, Ponte JM, Feng F, Croft WB, Lehnert WG (1995a) Automated classification of encounter notes in a computer based medical record. Medinfo 8(Pt 1):8–12

Aronow DB, Cooley JR, Soderland S (1995b) Automated identification of episodes of asthma exacerbation for quality measurement in a computer-based medical record. Proc Annu Symp Comput Appl Med Care 309–313

Austin T, Iliffe S, Leaning M, Modell M (1996) A prototype computer decision support system for the management of asthma. J Med Syst 20(1):45–55

Bailey WC, Clark NM, Gotsch AR, Lemen RJ, O'Connor GT, Rosenstock IM (1992) Asthma prevention. Chest 102(3):216s–231s

Bandura A (1991) Social cognitive theory of self regulation. Special issue: Theories of cognitive self-regulation. Organ Behav Hum Decis Process 50:248–287

Barnett GO, Winickoff RN, Morgan MM, Zielstorff RD (1983) A computer-based monitoring system for follow-up of elevated blood pressure. Med Care 21(4):400–409

Bartholomew LK, Shegog R, Parcel GS, Gold R, Fernandez M, Czyzewski D, Sockrider MM, Berlin N (2000a) Watch, discover, think, and act. A model for patient education program development. J Patient Educ Couns 39:253–268

Bartholomew LK, Gold R, Parcel GS, Czyzewski DI, Sockrider MM, Fernandez M, Shegog R, Swank PR (2000b) Watch, discover, think then act: Evaluation of computer-assisted instruction to improve asthma self-management in inner-city children. J Patient Educ Couns 39:269–280

Bartholomew LK, Parcel GS, Kok G, Gottlieb N (2001) Intervention mapping: A process for designing theory-and evidence-based health promotion programs. Mayfield Publishing Co, California, p 515

Bartholomew LK, Tortolero S, Czyzewski DI, Sockrider MM, Abramson SL, Swank PR, Tyrell S, Markham C, Shegog R, Parcel GS (2006) Partners in school asthma management: Evaluation of a self-management program for children with asthma. J Sch Health 76(6):283–290

Bender BG, Bartlett SJ, Rand CS, Turner C, Wamboldt FS, Zhang L (2007) Impact of interview mode on accuracy of child and parent report of adherence with asthma-controller medication. Pediatrics 120:e471–e477

Berland GK, Elliott MN, Morales LS, Algazy JI, Kravitz RL, Broder MS, Kanouse DE, Muñoz JA, Puyol J-A, Lara M, Watkins KE, Yang H, McGlynn EA (2001) Health information on the Internet: Accessibility, quality, and readability in English and Spanish. JAMA 285(20):2612–2621

Bero LA, Grilli R, Grimshaw JM, Harvey E, Oxman AD, Thomson MA (1998) Closing the gap between research and practice: An overview of systematic reviews of interventions to promote the implementation of research findings. The Cochrane Effective Practice and Organization of Care Review Group. Brit Med J 317(7156):465–468

Bibi H, Nutman A, Shoseyov D, Shalom M, Peled R, Kivity S, Nutman J (2002) Prediction of emergency department visits for respiratory symptoms using an artificial neural network. Chest 122(5):1627–1632

Brennan P, Ripich S, Moore S (1991) The use of home-based computers to support persons living with AIDS/ARC. J Community Health Nurs 8(1):3–14

British Thoracic Society (1990) Statement by the British Thoracic Society, Research Unit of the Royal College of Physicians of London, King's Fund Centre, National Asthma Campaign: Guidelines for management of asthma in adults. I. Chronic persistent asthma. Br Med J 301:797–800

Brown SJ, Lieberman DA, Germeny BA, Fan YC, Wilson DM, Pasta DJ (1997) Education video game for juvenile diabetes self-care: Results of a controlled trial. Med Inform (Lond) 22(1):77–89

Bruderman I, Abboud S (1997) Telespirometry: Novel system for home monitoring of asthmatic patients. Telemed J 3(2):127–133

Burge PS, Pantin CFA, Newton DT, Gannon PFG, Bright P, Belcher J, McCoach J, Baldwin DR, Burge CBSG and the Midlands Thoracic Society Research Group (1999) Development of an expert system for the interpretation of serial peak expiratory flow measurements in the diagnosis of occupational asthma. Occup Environ Med 56:758–764

Burkhart PV, Rayens MK, Oakley MG, Abshire DA, Zhang M (2007) Testing an intervention to promote children's adherence to asthma self-management. J Nurs Sch 39(2):133–140

Bussey-Smith KL, Rossen RD (2007) A systematic review of randomized control trials evaluating the effectives of interactive computerized asthma patient education programs. Ann Allergy Asthma Immunol 98:507–516

Butz AM, Donithan M, Bollinger ME, Rand C, Thompson RE (2005) Monitoring nebulizer use in children: Comparison of electronic and asthma diary data. Ann Allergy Asthma Immunol 94(3):360–365

Cabana MD (2005) Tao TL challenges in asthma patient education. J Allergy Clin Immunol 115:1225–1227

Cabana MD, Rand CS, Powe NR, Wu AW, Wilson MH, Abboud PA et al (1999) Why don't physicians follow clinical practice guidelines? A framework for improvement. JAMA 282(15):1458–1465

Cabana MD, Ebel BE, Cooper-Patrick L, Powe NR, Rubin HR, Rand CS (2000) Barriers pediatricians face when using asthma practice guidelines. Arch Pediatr Adolesc Med 154(7):685–693

Cabana MD, Rand CS, Becher OJ, Rubin HR (2001) Reasons for pediatrician non-adherence to asthma guidelines. Arch Pediatr Adolesc Med 155(9):1057–1062

Cabana MD, Bruckman D, Bratton SL, Kemper AR, Clark NM (2003) Association between outpatient follow-up and pediatric emergency department visits. J Asthma 40(7):741–749

Chan DS, Callahan CW, Sheets SJ, Moreno CN, Malone FJ (2003) An Internet-based store-and-forward video home telehealth system for improving asthma outcomes in children. Am J Health Syst Pharm 60(19):1976–1981

Chan DS, Callahan CW, Hatch-Pigott VB, Lawless H, Proffitt L, Manning NE, Schweikert M, Malone FJ (2007) An Internet-based store-and-forward video home telehealth system for improving asthma outcomes in children. Pediatrics 119:569–578

Chang BL, Omery A, Mayo A (2003) Use of personal digital assistants by adolescents with severe asthma. Can they enhance patient outcomes? AACN Clin Issues 14(3):379–391

Chase CR, Vacek PM, Shinozaki T, Giard AM, Ashikaga T (1983) Medical information management: Improving the transfer of research results to pre-surgical evaluation. Med Care 21(4):410–424

Christiansen J (1999) Health IT and privacy: The legal perspective. MD Comput 16(4):15–16

Chute CG, Cohn SP, Campbell JR (1998) A framework for comprehensive health terminology systems in the United States: Development guidelines, criteria for selection, and public policy implications. JAMA 5:503–510

Clark NM (1989) Asthma self-management education research and implications for clinical practice. Chest 95(5):1110–1113

Clark NM, Partridge MR (2002) Strengthening asthma education to enhance disease control. Chest 121:1661–1669

Clark NM, Zimmerman BJ (1990) A social cognitive view of self-regulated learning about health. Health Educ Res 5(3):371–379

Clark NM, Feldman CH, Evans D, Millman EJ, Wasilewski Y, Valle I (1981) The effectiveness of education for family management of asthma in children: A preliminary report. Health Educ Quarterly 8(2):166–174

Clark NM, Feldman CH, Evans D, Wasilewski Y, Leveson MJ (1984) Changes in children's school performance as a result of education for family management of asthma. J Sch Health 54:143–145

Clark NM, Feldman CH, Evans D, Levison MJ, Wasilewski Y, Mellins RB (1986) The impact of health education on frequency and cost of health-care use by low income children with asthma. J Allergy Clin Immunol 78:108–115

Clark NM, Gotsch A, Rosenstock IR (1993) Patient, professional, and public education on behavioral aspects of asthma: A review of strategies for change and needed research. J Asthma 30(4):241–255

Clark NM, Nothwehr F, Gong M, Evans D, Maiman LA, Hurwitz ME, Roloff D, Mellins RB (1995) Physician-patient partnership in managing chronic illness. Acad Med 70(11):957–959

Clark NM, Gong ZM, Wang SJ, Lin X, Bria WF, Johnson TR (2007) A randomized trial of a self-regulation intervention for women with asthma. Chest 132:88–97

Clark NM, Mitchell HE, Rand CS (2009) Effectiveness of educational and behavioral asthma interventions. Pediatrics 123:S185–S192

Creer TL (1993) Medication compliance and childhood asthma. In: Krusnejer CA, Epstein L, Johnson SB, Yafti SJ (eds) Developmental aspects of health compliance behavior. Lawrence Erlbaum Associates, Hillsdale, NJ

Creer TL, Winder JA (1986) Asthma. In: Holroyd KA, Creer TL (eds) Self-management of chronic disease: Handbook of clinical interventions and research. Academic, New York, pp 269–303

Creer TL, Wigal JK, Kotses H, Lewis PA (1990) Critique of 19 self-management programs for childhood asthma: Part II. comments regarding the scientific merit of the programs. Pediatr Asthma Allergy Immunol 4(1):41–55

Creer TL, Kotses H, Wigal JK (1992) A second-generation model of asthma self-management. Pediatr Asthma Allergy Immunol 6(3):143–165

Creer TL, Winder JA, Tinkelman D (1999) Guidelines for the diagnosis and management of asthma: Accepting the challenge. J Asthma 36(5):391–407

Croft D, Peterson M (2002) An evaluation of the quality and contents of asthma education on the World Wide Web. Chest 121:1301–1307

Curtin K, Hayes BD, Holland CL, Katz LA (1998) Computer-generated intervention for asthma population care management. Eff Clin Pract 1(1):43–46

D'Alessandro D, Dosa NP (2001) Empowering children and families with information technology. Arch Pediatr Adol Med 155:1131–1136

Daley MF, Barrow J, Pearson K, Crane LA, Gao D, Stevenson JM et al (2004) Identification and recall of children with chronic medical conditions for influenza vaccination. Pediatrics 113(1 Pt 1):e26–e33

Davis FD (1989) Perceived usefulness, perceived ease of use, and user acceptance of information technology. MIS Quarterly 13:319–340

Dawson KP, Van Asperen P, Higgins C, Sharpe C, Davis A (1995) An evaluation of the action plans of children with asthma. J Paediatr Child Health 31(1):21–23

de Jongste JC, Carraro S, Hop WC, Baraldi E, CHARISM Group (2009) Daily telemonitoring of exhaled nitric oxide and symptoms in the treatment of childhood asthma. Am J Respir Crit Care Med 179:93–97

Dick R, Steen E (1991) The computer-based patient record: An essential technology for healthcare. Institute of Medicine & National Academy Press, Washington, DC

Dijkstra A, De Vries H, Roijackers J (1998) Long-term effectiveness of computer-generated tailored feedback in smoking cessation. Health Educ Res Theory Pract 13(2):207–214

Dixon DR, Dixon BJ (1994) Adoption of information technology enabled innovations by primary care physicians: Model and questionnaire development. SCAMC 631–635

Dragonieri S, Schot R, Mertens BJA, LeCessie S, Gauw SA, Spanevello A, Resta O, Willard NP, Vink TJ, Rabe KF, Bel EH, Sterk PJ (2007) An electronic nose in the discrimination of patients with asthma and controls. J Allergy Clin Immunol 120:856–862

Eccles M, McColl E, Steen N, Rousseau N, Grimshaw J, Parkin D et al (2002) Effect of computerised evidence based guidelines on management of asthma and angina in adults in primary care: Cluster randomised controlled trial. BMJ 325(7370):941

Evans R (1992) Asthma among minority children. A growing problem. Chest 101(6):368S–371S

Fall AJ, Henry RL, Hazell T (1998) The use of an interactive computer program for the education of parents of asthmatic children. J Paediatr Child Health 34(2):127–130

Figaro MK, Belue R (2005) Prevalence of influenza vaccination in a high-risk population: Impact of age and race. J Ambul Care Manage 28(1):24–29

Finkelstein J, Hripcsak G, Cabrera M (1998) Telematic system for monitoring of asthma severity in patient's homes. MEDINFO '98, 9th World Congress on Medical Informatics. IOS Press, Amsterdam, The Netherlands Pt 1, pp 272–276

Finkelstein J, Cabrera MR, Hripcsak G (2000) Internet-based home asthma telemonitoring: Can patients handle the technology? Chest 117(1):148–155

Finkelstein J, O'Connor G, Friedmann RH (2001) Development and implementation of the home asthma telemonitoring (HAT) system to facilitate asthma self-care. MedInfo 10(Pt 1):810–814

Finkelstein JA, Lozano P, Farber HJ, Miroshnik I, Lieu TA (2002) Underuse of controller medications among Medicaid-insured children with asthma. Arch Pediatr Adol Med 156(6):562–567

Fireman P, Friday GA, Gira C, Vieshaler WA, Michaels L (1981) Teaching self-management skills to asthmatic children and their parents in an ambulatory care setting. Pediatrics 68:341–348

Flores G (2000) Pediatrician's attitudes, beliefs, and practices regarding clinical practice guidelines: A national survey. Pediatrics 105(2 Pt 1):496–501

Gadd CS, Baskaran P, Lobach DF (1998) Identification of design features to enhance utilization and acceptance of systems for Internet-based decision support at the point of care. Proc AMIA Symp 91–95

Gaglani M, Riggs M, Kamenicky C, Glezen WP (2001) A computerized reminder strategy is effective for annual influenza immunization of children with asthma or reactive airway disease. Pediatr Infect Dis J 20(12):1155–1160

Games for Health (2006) Available at: http://www.gamesforhealth.org/index3.html. Accessed Dec 3rd, 2006

Gannon PFG, Newton DT, Belcher J, Pantin CFA, Burge PS (1996) The development of Oasys-2; a system for the analysis of serial measurement of peak expiratory flow in workers with suspected occupational asthma. Thorax 51:484–489

Gautier V, Rédier H, Pujol JL, Bousquet J, Proudhon H, Michel C, Daures JP, Michel FB, Godard P (1996) Comparison of an expert system with other clinical scores for the evaluation of severity of asthma. Eur Respir J 9(1):58–64

Giarrantano J, Riley G (1989) Expert systems: Principles and programming. PWS-KENT Publishing Company, Boston

Gibson PG, Powell H, Coughlan J, Wilson AJ, Abramson M, Haywood P, Bauman A, Hensley MJ, Walters EH, Roberts JJL (2002) Self-management education and regular practitioner review for adults with asthma. Cochrane Database Syst Rev CD001117

Glanz K, Lewis FM, Rimer BK (eds) (1997) Health behavior and health education. Theory, research, and practice, 2nd edn. Josey-Bass Publishers, San Francisco

Glasgow RE, McKay G, Boles SM, Vogt TM (1999) Interactive computer technology, behavioral science, and family practice. J Fam Pract 48(6):464–470

Global Initative for Asthma (2006) Pocket guide for asthma management and prevention. Rev Dec http://www.ginasthma.com/

GuidelinesResources.asp?l1 = 2&l2 = 0. Accessed February 11, 2007
Grant EN, Moy JN, Turner-Roan K, Daugherty SR, Weiss KB (1999) Asthma care practices, perceptions, and beliefs of Chicago-area primary-care physicians. Chicago Asthma Surveillance Initiative Project Team. Chest 116(4 Suppl 1): 145S–154S
Grassi M, Villani S, Marinoni A (2001) Classification methods for the identification of "case" in epidemiological diagnosis of asthma. Eur J Epidemiol 17(1):19–29
Gregson RK, Warner JO, Radford M (1995) Assessment of the continued supervision and asthma – management knowledge of patients possessing home nebulizers. Respir Med 89(7):487–493
Grimshaw JM, Russell IT (1993) Effect of clinical guidelines on medical practice: A systematic review of rigorous evaluations. Lancet 342(8883):1317–1322
Guendelman S, Meade K, Benson M, Chen YQ, Samuels S (2002) Improving asthma outcomes and self-management behaviors of inner-city children: A randomized trial of the Health Buddy interactive device and an asthma diary. Arch Pediatr Adolesc Med 156(2):114–120
Guevara JP, Wolf FM, Grum CM, Clark NM (2003) Effects of educational interventions for self-management of asthma in children and adolescents: Systematic review and meta-analysis. BMJ 326(7402):1308–1309
Gustafson DH, Bosworth K, Chewning B, Hawkins RP (1987) Computer-based health promotion: Combining technological advances with problem-solving techniques to effect successful health behavior changes. Annu Rev Public Health 8:387–415
Hamid S, Corden ZM, Ryan DP, Burnett I, Cochrane GM (1998) Evaluation of an electronic hand-held spirometer in patients with asthma. Respir Med 92:1177–1180
Harris A, McGregor JC, Perencevich EN, Furuno JP, Zhu J, Peterson DE, Finkelstein J (2006) The use and interpretation of quasi-experimental studies in medical informatics. J Am Med Inform Assoc 13:16–23
Hartmann CW, Sciamanna CN, Blanch DC, Mui S, Lawless H, Manocchia M, Rosen RK, Pietropaoli A (2007) Website to improve asthma care by suggesting patient questions for physicians: Qualitative analysis of user experiences. J Med Internet Res 9(1):e3
Haug P, Gardner R, Evans R (1999) Hospital-based decision support. In: Berner E (ed) Clinical decision support systems: Theory and practice. Springer, New York, pp 77–103
Hazzard A, Celano M, Collins M, Markoy Y (2002) Effects of STARBRIGHT World on knowledge, social support, and coping in hospitalized children with sickle cell disease and asthma. Child Health Care 31(1):69–86
Health Summit Working Group (1997) White paper: Criteria for consumers. Healthcare providers, and technical developers on evaluating healthcare websites. Mitretek Systems, McLean, Va, available at http://hitiWeb.mitretek.org/hswg/documents/default.asp. Accessed January 2007
Helitzer D, Heath D, Maltrud K, Sullivan E, Alverson D (2003) Assessing or predicting adoption of telehealth using the diffusion of innovations theory: A practical example from a rural program in New Mexico. Telemed E-Health J 9(2):179–187
Heung-Woo P, Min Kyung-Up, You-Young K, Sang-Heon C (2004) Assessing the quality and contents of asthma-related information on the Korean Internet as an educational material for patients. J Korean Med Sci 19:364–368
Higgenbottom PC, Smith JT (2002) Asthma: An annotated guide to resources on the World Wide Web. Health Care Internet 6(3):45–52
Himes BE, Dai Y, Kohane IS, Weiss ST, Ramoni MF (2009) Prediction of chronic obstructive pulmonary disease (COPD) in asthma patients using Electronic Medical Records. J Am Med Inform Assoc doi:10.1197/jamia.M2846
Hindi-Alexander M, Cropp GJ (1981) Community and family programs for children with asthma. Ann Allergy 46:143–148
Hirsch S, Shapiro JL, Turega MA, Frank TL, Niven RM, Frank PI (2001) Using a neural network to screen a population for asthma. Ann Epidemiol 11(6):369–376
Homer C, Susskind O, Alpert HR, Owusu M, Schneider L, Rappaport LA, Rubin DH (2000) An evaluation of an innovative multimedia educational software program for asthma management: Report of a randomized, controlled trial. Pediatrics 106(1 Pt 2):210–215
Hopper KB (2005) An online simulation in pediatric asthma management. In: Association for Educational Communications and Technology (AECT) 2004 Proceedings vol 2. Association for Educational Communications and Technology, Bloomington, IN, pp 252–265
Hunt DL, Haynes RB, Hanna SE, Smith K (1998) Effects of computer-based clinical decision support systems on physician performance and patient outcomes: A systematic review. J Am Med Assoc 280(15):1339–1346
Huss K, Salerno M, Huss RW (1991) Computer-assisted reinforcement of instruction: Effects on adherence in adult atopic asthmatics. Res Nurs Health 14(4):259–267
Huss K, Huss RW, Squire EN, Carpenter GB, Smith LJ, Salata K, Salerno M, Agostinelli D (1992a) Computer education for asthmatics: What effects? J Nurs Care Qual 6(3):57–66
Huss K, Squire EN Jr, Carpenter GB, Smith LJ, Huss RW, Salata K, Salerno M, Agostinelli D, Hershey J (1992b) Effective education of adults with asthma who are allergic to dust mites. J Allergy Clin Immunol 89(4):836–843
Huss K, Winkelstein M, Nanda J, Naumann PL, Sloand ED, Huss RW (2003) Computer game for inner-city children does not improve asthma outcomes. J Pediatr Health Care 17(2):72–78
Jadad AR (2002) Evidence-based decision making and asthma in the Internet age: The tools of the trade. Allergy 57(Suppl 74):15–22
Jan R, Wang J, Huang M, Tseng S, Su H, Lui L (2007) An Internet-based interactive telemonitoring system for improving childhood asthma outcomes in Taiwan. Telemed J E Health 13(3):257–268
Johnston ME, Langton KB, Haynes RB, Mathieu A (1994) Effects of computer-based clinical decision support systems on clinician performance and patient outcome. A critical appraisal of research. Ann Intern Med 120(2):135–142
Joseph C (2007) Tailored asthma management for urban teens. Available at http://ClinicalTrials.gov Identifier: NCT00201058. Accessed Feb. 2, 2007.
Joseph C, Peterson E, Havstad S, Johnson CC, Hoerauf S, Stringer S, Gibson-Scipio W, Ownby DR, Elston-Lafata J, Pallonen U, Strecher V (2007) A web-based, tailored asthma management program for urban African–American high school students. Am J Respir Crit Care Med 175(9):888–895
Kabir A, Hanson R, Mellis CM, van Asperen PP (1998) Is asthma documentation improved by computer-facilitated data entry? J Qual Clin Practice 18:187–193

Karras BT, Nath SD, Corb GJ, Engles-Horton L, Shiffman RN (1999) PalmAsthma: Design of a system for the implementation of asthma guidelines on handheld computers. Proceedings of AMIA, Orlando, FL. (no pub med)

Kattan M (2008) Quality of inpatient care for asthma: Challenges and opportunities. Pediatrics 122:1369–1370

Kattan M, Crain EF, Steinbach S, Visness CM, Walter M, Stout JW, Evans R, Smartt E, Gruchalla RS, Morgan WJ, O'Connor GT, Mitchell HE (2006) A randomized clinical trial of clinician feedback to improve quality of care for inner city children with asthma. Pediatrics 117:e1095–e1103

Kerr C, Murray E, Stevenson F, Gore C, Nazareth I (2006) Internet interventions for long-term conditions: Patient and caregiver quality criteria. J Med Internet Res 8(3):e13

Kiley R (2002) Does the Internet harm health? Some evidence exists that the Internet does harm health. BMJ 324(7331):238–239

Kim P, Eng TR, Deering MJ, Maxfield A (1999) Published criteria for evaluating health related Websites: Review. BMJ 318:647–649

Klingelhofer EL, Gershwin ME (1988) Asthma self-management programs: Remises, not promises. J Asthma 25(2):89–101

Kotses H, Lewis P, Creer TL (1990) Environmental control of asthma self-management. J Asthma 27(6):375–384

Kotses H, Stout MA, Wigal JK, Carlson B, Creer TL, Lewis P (1991) Individualized Asthma Self-management: A beginning. J Asthma 28(4):287–289

Krishna S, Francisco B, Balas E (2001) A randomized controlled trial to evaluate an interactive multimedia asthma education program. Third Triennial World Asthma Meeting, Chicago

Krishna S, Francisco BD, Balas A, Konig P, Graff G, Madsen RW (2003) Internet-enabled interactive multimedia asthma education program: A randomized trial. Pediatrics 111:503–510

Krishna S, Balas E, Francisco B, Konig P (2006) Effective and sustainable multimedia education for children with asthma: A randomized controlled trial. Child Health Care 35(1):75–90

Kuilboer MM, van Wijk MAM, Mosseveld M, van der Does E, Ponsioen BP, de Jongste JC, Overbeek SE, van der Lei J (2002) Feasibility of AsthmaCritic, a decision-support system for asthma and COPD which generates patient-specific feedback on routinely recorded data in general practice. Fam Pract 19(5):442–447

Kuilboer MM, van Wijk MAM, Mosseveld M, vander Lei J (2003) AsthmaCritic: Issues in designing a noninquisitive critiquing system for daily practice. J Am Med Inform Assoc 10(5):419–424

Kuilboer MM, van Wijk MAM, Mosseveld M, van der Does E, de Jongste JC, Overbeek SE, Ponsioen B, van der Lei J (2006) Computed critiquing integrated into daily clinical practice affects physicians' behaviour – A randomized clinical trial with AsthmaCritic. Methods Inf Med 45(4):447–454

Lee HR, Yoo SK, Jung SM, Kwon NY, Hong CS (2005) A web-based mobile asthma management system. J Telemed Telecare 11(Suppl 1):56–59

Legorreta AP, Christian-Herman J, O'Connor RD, Hasan MM, Evans R, Leung KM (1998) Compliance with national asthma management guidelines and specialty care: A health maintenance organization experience. Arch Intern Med 158(5):457–464

Lehmann ED (2004) Computerized decision-support tools in diabetes care: Hurdles to implementation. Diabetes Technol Ther 6(3):422–429

Lieberman DA (1997) Interactive video games for health promotion: Effects on knowledge, self-efficacy, social support, and health. In: Street R, Gold W, Manning T (eds) Health Promotion and interactive technology: Theoretical applications and future directions. Lawrence Erlbaum Associates, Mahwah

Lieberman DA (2001) Management of chronic pediatric diseases with interactive health games: Theory and research findings. J Ambul Care Manage 24(1):26–38

Lieu TA, Quesenberry CP Jr, Capra AM, Sorel ME, Martin KE, Mendoza GR (1997) Outpatient management practices associated with reduced risk of pediatric asthma hospitalization and emergency department visits. Pediatrics 100(3):334–341

Lieu TA, Quesenberry CP, Sorel ME, Mendoza GR, Leong AB (1998) Computer-based models to identify high-risk children with asthma. Am J Respir Crit Care Med 157:1173–1180

Macro International, Inc. (1994) Developing and implementing educational strategies and interventions for controlling asthma in inner city and high risk populations. First Technical Progress Report Contract No. N01-H0-39220

Mangold RA, Salzman GA (2005) Electronic asthma action plan database: Asthma action plan development using Microsoft Access. J Asthma 42(3):191–196

Martin E (2006) Improving influenza vaccination rates in a pediatric asthma management program by utilization of an electronic medical record system. Clin Pediatr 45:221

Masoli M, Fabian D, Holt S, Beasley R (2004) The global burden of asthma: Executive summary of the GINA Dissemination Committee report. Allergy 59(5):469–478

Mathews P, and Newell L (1999) Clinical information systems: Paving the way for clinical information management. Journal of Healthcare Information Management 13(3):97–111

Mattke S, Martorelli F, Sharma P, Malveaux F, Lurie N (2009) Quality of care for childhood asthma: Estimating impact and implications. Pediatrics 123:S199–S204

McAlearney AS, Chisolm D, Veneris S, Rich D, Kelleher K (2006) Utilization of evidence-based computerized order sets in paediatrics. Int J Med Inform 75:501–512

McCowan C, Neville RG, Ricketts IW, Warner FC, Hoskins G, Thomas GE (2001a) Lessons from a randomized controlled trial designed to evaluate computer decision support software to improve the management of asthma. Med Inform 26(3):191–201

McCowan C, Neville RG, Ricketts IW, Warner FC, Hoskins G, Thomas GE (2001b) Computer-assisted assessment and management of patients with asthma. Am J Resp Crit Care Med 163(5):A506

McDowell I, Newell C, Rosser W (1989) A randomized trial of computerized reminders for blood pressure screening in primary care. Med Care 27:297–305

McPherson A, Glazebrook C, Smyth A (2001) Double click for health: The role of multimedia in asthma education. Arch Dis Child 85(6):447–449

McPherson AC, Glazebrook C, Smyth AR (2005) Educational interventions – computers for delivering education to children with respiratory illness and to their parents. Pediatr Resp Rev 6:215–226

Miller MR, Hankinson J, Brusasco V, Burgos F, Casaburi R, Coates A, Crapo R, Enright P, van der Grinten CPM, Gustafsson P, Jensen R, Johnson DC, MacIntyre N, McKay R, Navajas D, Pedersen OF, Pellegrino R, Viegi G, Wanger J (2005) Standardization of spirometry. Eur Respir J 26:319–338

Mitchell E, Sullivan FA (2001) Descriptive feast but an evaluative famine: Systematic review of published articles on primary care computing during 1980–1997. BMJ 322:279–282

Morris C (1994) The origins of informatics. J Am Med Inform Assoc 1:91–107

Murray E, Lo B, Pollack L, Donelan K, Catania J, White M et al (2003) The impact of health information multimedia on the Internet on the physician-patient relationship. Arch Intern Med 163:1727–1734

Mussaffi H, Omar R, Prais D, Mel-Zahav M, Weiss-Kasirer T, Botzer Z, Blau H (2007) Computerized pediatric asthma quality of life questionnaires in routine care. Arch Dis Child 92(8):678–682

National Heart Lung and Blood Institute (1995) National Institutes of Health: Global strategy for asthma management and prevention. National Institutes of Health, Bethesda, MD

National Heart Lung and Blood Institute (1997) National Asthma Education and Prevention Program, Expert Panel 2: Guidelines for the diagnosis and management of asthma. National Institutes of Health, Bethesda, MD, Report #97-4051

National Heart Lung and Blood Institute (2007) National asthma education and prevention program, expert panel 3: Guidelines for the diagnosis and management of asthma. National Institutes of Health, Bethesda, MD

National Heart, Lung, and Blood Institute (1991) National Asthma Education Program Expert Panel Report. Guidelines for the diagnosis and management of asthma. National Institutes of Health, Bethesda, MD Report #91-3042

National Heart, Lung, and Blood Institute (2002) Guidelines for the diagnosis and management of asthma. Update on selected topics. NIH Publication, Bethesda, MD Report No. 02-5074

National Heart, Lung, and Blood Institute NHLBI (2004) Morbidity and mortality chart book on cardiovascular, lung, and blood diseases. National Institutes of Health, Bethesda, MD

Niemiec R, Walberg HJ (1987) Comparative effects of computer-assisted instruction: A synthesis of reviews. J Educ Comput Res 3(1):19–35

Oermann MH, Gerich J, Ostosh L, Zaleski S (2003) Evaluation of asthma websites for patient and parent education. J Pediatr Nurs 18(6):389–396

Osman LM, Abdalla MI, Beattie JA, Ross SJ, Russell IT, Friend JA, Legge JS, Douglas JG (1994) Reducing hospital admission through computer supported education for asthma patients Grampian Asthma Study of Integrated Care (GRASSIC). BMJ 308(6928):568–571

Owen N, Fotheringham MJ, Marcus BH (2002) Communication technology and health behavior change. In Glanz K, Rimer BK, Lewis FM (eds) Health Behavior and health Education. Theory, research, and Practice. 3rd ed. San Francisco, CA., Jossey-Bass, John Wiley & Sons, Inc.

Ozbolt J, Abraham I, Shultz S II (1990) Nursing information systems. In: Shortcliffe E, Perrealt L (eds) Medical informatics: Computer applications in healthcare. Addison-Wesley, Reading, MA, pp 244–272

Peled R, Tal A, Pliskin JS, Reuveni H (2005) A computerized surveillance system for the quality of care in childhood asthma. J Healthcare Quality 27(5):28–33

Peled R, Reuveni H, Pliskin JS, Benenson I, Hatna E, Tal A (2006) Defining localities of inadequate treatment for childhood asthma: A GIS approach. Int J Health Geogr 5:3, available from http://www.ij-healthgeographics.com/content/5/1/3

Peterson MW, Strommer-Pace L, Dayton C (2001) Asthma patient education: Current utilization in pulmonary training programs. [Journal Article] J Asthma 38(3):261–267

Pew Internet and American Life (2006) More online, doing more. www.pewinternet.org/releases/release.asp?id = 15 (accessed 2006, Dec 19)

Porter SC, Cai Z, Gribbons W, Goldmann DA, Kohane IS (2004) The asthma kiosk: A patient-centered technology for collaborative decision support in the emergency department. J Am Med Inform Assoc 11(6):458–467

Porter SC, Kohane IS, Goldmann DA (2005) Parents as partners in obtaining the medication history. J Am Med Inform Assoc 12(3):299–305

Porter SC, Forbes P, Feldman HA, Goldmann DA (2006) Impact of patient-centered decision support on quality of asthma care in the emergency department. Pediatrics 117(1):e33–e42

Prochaska JO, Velicer WF (1997) The transtheoretical model of health behavior change. Am J Health Promot 12(1):38–48

Raat H, Mangunkusumo RT, Mohangoo AD, Juniper EF, Van Der Lei J (2007) Internet and written respiratory questionnaires yield equivalent results for adolescents. Pediatr Pulmonol 42(4):357–361

Rasmussen LM, Phanareth K, Nolte H, Backer V (2005) Internet-based monitoring of asthma: A long-term, randomized clinical study of 300 asthmatic subjects. J All Clin Immunol 115:1137–1142

Ray P, Vervloet D, Charpin D, Gautier V, Proudhon H, Redier H, Godard P (1995) Evaluation of atopy through an expert system: Description of the database. Clin Exp Allergy 25(11):1067–1073

Reddel HK, Ware SI, Salome CM et al (1998) Pitfalls in processing home electronic spirometric data in asthma. Eur Respir J 12:853–858

Redier H, Daures JP, Michel C et al (1995) Assessment of the severity of asthma by an expert system. Description and evaluation. Am J Respir Crit Care Med 151:345–352

Revere D, Dunbar PJ (2001) Review of computer-generated outpatient health behavior interventions. J Am Med Inform Assoc 8:62–79

Rhee H, Wyatt TH, Wenzel JA (2006) Adolescents with asthma: Learning needs and internet use assessment. Respir Care 51(12):1441–1449

Rhee H, Hollen PJ, Belyea MJ, Sutherland MA (2008) Decision-making program for rural adolescents with asthma: A pilot study. J Pediatr Nurs 23(6):439–450

Rhodes F, Fishbein M, Reis J (1997) Using behavioral theory in computer-based health promotion and appraisal. Health Educ Behav 24(1):20–34

Rietveld S, Oud M, Dooijes EH (1999) Classification of asthmatic breath sounds: Preliminary results of the classifying capacity of human examiners versus artificial neural networks. Comput Biomed Res 32(5):440–448

Rimal RN, Flora JA (1997) Interactive technology attributes in health promotion: Practical and theoretical issues. In: Lawrence Erlbaum Associates (ed) Health promotion and interactive technology: Theoretical applications and future directions. Mahwah, New Jersey, pp 19–38

Rob MA (2003) Applications of geographical information systems in understanding spatial distribution of asthma. Inform Sci J 6:89–99

Robinson TN, Patrick K, Eng TR, Gustafson D (1998) An evidence-based approach to interactive health communication: A challenge to medicine in the information age. J Am Med Assoc 280(14):1264–1269

Rodehorst TK, Wilhem SL, Jensen L (2005) Use of interdisciplinary simulation to understand perceptions of team members' roles. J Prof Nurs 21(3):159–166

Rogers EM (1995) Diffusion of innovations, vol 4. The Free Press, New York

Rosenstein AH (1999) Measuring the benefits of clinical decision support: Return on investment. Health Care Manage Rev 24(2):32–43

Rosser WW, Hutchison BG, McDowell I, Newell C (1992) Use of reminders to increase compliance with tetanus booster vaccination. CMAJ 146(6):911–917

Rubin DH, Leventhal JM, Sadock RT et al (1986) Educational intervention by computer in childhood asthma: A randomized clinical trial testing the use of a new teaching intervention in childhood asthma. Pediatrics 77:1–10

Rubin DH, Hecht AR, Marinangeli PC, Erenberg FG (1989) Asthma command. Am J Asthma Allergy Pediatricians 2(2):108–112

Ruchi SG, Weiss KB (2009) The 2007 National Asthma Educaiton and Prevention Program Asthma Guidelines: Accelerating their implementation and facilitating their impact on children with asthma. Pediatrics 123:S193–S198

Runge C, Lecheler J, Horns M, Tews J, Schaefer M (2006) Outcomes of a web-based patient education program for asthmatic children and adolescents. Chest 129(3):581–593

Sanders DL, Aronsky D (2006) Biomedical informatics applications for asthma care: A systematic review. J Am Med Inform Assoc 13:418–427

Schiller JS, Bernadel L (2004) Summary health statistics for the US population: National Health Interview Survey, 2002. Vital Health Stat 10(220):1–101

Schneider EC, Eisenberg JM (1998) Strategies and methods for aligning current and best medical practices. The role of information technologies. West J Med 168:311–318

Schunk DH (1983) Progress self-monitoring: Effects on children's self-efficacy and achievement. J Educ Psychol 51:89–93

Schunk DH (1986) Verbalization and children's self-regulated learning. Contemp Educ Psychol 11:347–369

Science Panel on Interactive Communication and Health (1999) Wired for health and well-being: The emergence of interactive health communication. In: Eng TR, Gustafson DH (ed) US Department of Health and Human Services, US Government Printing Office, Washington, DC

Serious Games Initiative (2006) Available at: http://www.seriousgames.org/index2.html. Accessed December 3

Shegog R, Sockrider MM, Bartholomew LK, Masse L, Parcel GS, Abramson SL (2001) Impact of a computer-assisted self-management education program on factors related to asthma self-management behavior. J Am Med Inform Assoc 8(1):49–61

Shegog R, Bartholomew LK, Czyzewski DI, Sockrider MM, Craver J, Pilney S, Mullen PD, Koeppl K, Gold RS, Fernandez M, Abramson SL (2004) Development of an expert system knowledge base: A novel approach to promote guideline congruent asthma care. J Asthma 41(4):385–402

Shegog R, Bartholomew LK, Sockrider MM, Czyzewski DI, Pilney S, Mullen P, Abramson SL (2006a) Computer-based decision-support for pediatric asthma management: Description and feasibility of the Stop Asthma Clinical System. Health Inform J 12(4):259–273

Shegog R, Bartholomew LK, Gold RS, Pierrel E, Parcel GS, Sockrider MM, Czyzewski DI, Fernandez ME, Berlin N, Abramson SL (2006b) Asthma management simulation for children: Translating theory, methods, and strategies to effect behavior change. Simul Healthcare Fall 1(3):151–159

Shiffman RN, Liaw Y, Brandt CA, Corb GJ (1999) Computer-based guideline implementation systems: A systematic review of functionality and effectiveness. J Am Med Inform Assoc 6:104–114

Shiffman RN, Freudigman KA, Brandt C, Liaw Y, Navedo DD (2000) A guideline implementation system using handheld computer for office management of asthma: Effects on adherence and patient outcomes. Pediatrics 105(4 Pt 1):767–773

Shiffman RN, Michel G, Essaihi A, Thornquist E (2004) Bridging the guideline implementation gap: A systematic, document-centered approach to guideline implementation. J Am Med Inform Assoc 11(5):418–426

Skinner CS, Kreuter M (1997) Using theories in planning interactive computer programs. In: Street R, Gold W, Manning T (eds) Health promotion and interactive technology: Theoretical applications and future directions. Lawrence Erlbaum Associates, Mahwah, NJ

Sly JL, Lombardi E, Kusel M, Sly PD (2006) Piloting a web-based continuing professional development program for asthma education. Int J Med Inform 75(10–11):708–713

Smith SE (1999a) Asthma care on the Internet. Inform Today 16(5):66

Smith SE (1999b) Asthma care on the Web, Part II. Inform Today 16(7):64

Smith SR, Jaffe DM, Fisher EB Jr, Trinkaus KM, Highstein G, Strunk RC (2004) Improving follow-up for children with asthma after an acute Emergency Department visit. J Pediatr 145(6):772–777

Sockrider MM, Abramson S, Brooks E, Caviness CA, Pilney S, Koerner C, Macias CG (2006) Delivering tailored asthma family education in a pediatric emergency department setting: A pilot study. Pediatrics 117(4):135–144

Spector SL, Nicklas RA (1995) Practice parameters for the diagnosis and treatment of asthma. J Allergy Clin Immunol 96:707–870

Staggers N, Thompson CB, Snyder-Halpern R (2001) History and trends in clinical information systems in the United States. J Nurs Scholarship 33(1):75–81

Starlight Foundation (2009) Quest For the Code®. Available at http://asthma.starlightprograms.org/, accessed February 2009

Stinson J, Wilson R, Gill N, Yamada J, Holt J (2008) A systematic review of Internet-based self-management interventions for youth with chronic conditions. J Pediatr Psychol 1–16, doi:10.1093/jpepsy/jsn115

Streel S, Lock S, Johnson N et al (2002) A feasibility study of remote monitoring of asthmatic patients. J Telemed Telecare 8(5):290–296

Street RL, Rimal RN (1997) Health promotion and interactive technology: A conceptual foundation. In: Street R, Gold W, Manning T (eds) Health promotion and interactive technology: Theoretical applications and future directions. Lawrence Erlbaum Associates, Mahwah, NJ

Sudre P, Jacquernet S, Uldry C, Perneger TV (1999) Objectives, methods, and content of patient education programmes for

adults with asthma: Systematic review of studies published between 1979 and 1988. Thorax 54:681–687
Sundberg R, Tunsater A, Palmqvist M, Ellbjar S, Lowhagen O, Toren K (2005) A randomized controlled study of a computerized limited education program among young adults with asthma. Respir Med 99:321–328
Takabayashi K, Tomita M, Tsumoto S, Suzuki T, Yamazaki S, Honda M, Satomura Y, Iwamoto I, Saito Y, Tomioka H (1999) Computer-assisted instructions for patients with bronchial asthma. Patient Educ Couns 38(3):241–248
Thomas KW, Dayton CS, Peterson MW (1999) Evaluation of Internet-based clinical decision support systems. J Med Internet Res 1(2):E6
Thoresen CE, Kirmil-Gray K (1983) Self-management psychology and the treatment of childhood asthma. J Allergy Clin Immunol 72(5):596–610
Tierney WM, Hui SL, McDonald CJ (1986) Delayed feedback of physician performance versus immediate reminders to perform preventive care. Effects on physician compliance. Med Care 24(8):659–666
Tierney WM, Miller ME, McDonald CJ (1990) The effect on test ordering of informing physicians of the charges for outpatient diagnostic tests. N Engl J Med 233(21):1499–1504
Tierney WM, Murray MD, Gaskins DL, Zhou X-H (1997) Using computer-based medical records to predict mortality risk for inner-city patients with reactive airways disease. JAMIA 4(4):313–321
Tierney WM, Overhage JM, Murray MD, Harris LE, Zhou XH, Eckert GJ, Smith FE, Nienaber N, McDonald CJ, Wolinsky FD (2005) Can computer-generated care suggestions enhance evidence-based management of asthma and chronic obstructive pulmonary disease? A randomized, controlled trial. Health Serv Res 40(2):477–497
Tinkelman DG, Lutz C, Conner B (1991) Methacholine challenges in the management of young children. Ann Allergy 66:225–230
Toelle BG, Ram FSF (2004) Written individualized management plans for asthma in children and adults. Cochrane Database Syst Rev CD002171
US DHHS (2003) Healthy people: National health promotion and disease prevention objectives. Available at http://www.healthypeople.gov
van der Ent CK, Brackel HJ, van der Laag J, Bogaard JM (1996) Tidal breathing analysis as a measure of airway obstruction in children three years of age and older. Am J Respir Crit Care Med 153(4):1253–1258
van der Meer V, van Stel HF, Detmar SB, Otten W, Sterk PJ, Sont JK (2007) Internet-based self-maangement offers an opportunity to achive better asthma control in adolescents. Chest 132:112–119
Velsor-Friedrich B, Srof B (2000a) Asthma self-management programs for children. Part 1: Description of the programs. J Child Fam Nurs 3(2):85–97
Velsor-Friedrich B, Srof B (2000b) Asthma self-management programs for children. Part 2: Empiric evaluation of programs and recommendations. J Child Fam Nurs 3(3):173–190
Vilozni D, Barker M, Jellouschek HG, Blau H (2001) An interactive computer-animated system (SpiroGame) facilitates spirometry in preschool children. Am J Respir Crit Care Med 164:2200–2205
Vollmer WM, O'Connor EA, Heumann M et al (2004) Searching multiple clinical information systems for longer time periods found more prevalent cases of asthma. J Clin Epidemiol 57(4):392–397
Wainright C, Wootton R (2003) A review of telemedicine and asthma. Dis Man Health Outcomes 11(9):557–563
Walton R, Dovey S, Harvey E, Freemantle N (1999) Computer support for determining drug dose: Systematic review and meta-analysis. BMJ 318:984–990
Wigal JK, Creer TL, Kotses H, Lewis P (1990) A critique of 19 self-management programs for childhood asthma: Part I. Development and evaluation of the programs. Pediatr Asthma Allergy Immunol 4(1):17–39
Williams RB, Boyles M, Johnson RE (1995) Patient use of a computer for prevention in primary care practice. Patient Educ Couns 25:283–292
Wjst M, Immervoll T (1998) An Internet linkage and mutation database for the complex phenotype asthma. Bioinformatics 14(9):827–828
Wolf FM, Guevara JP, Grum CM, Clark NM, Gates CJ. Educational interventions for asthma in children. *Cochrane Database Syst Rev* 2002; CD000326
Wolfenden LL, Diette GB, Krishnan JA, Skinner EA, Steinwachs DM, Wu AW (2003) Lower physician estimate of underlying asthma severity leads to undertreatment. Arch Intern Med 163(2):231–236
Woolcock A, Rubinfeld AR, Searle JP (1989) Thoracic Society of Australia and New Zealand asthma action plan. Med J Aust 151:650–653
Worstell M (2000) Asthma: Individual patient perspective and current unmet needs. Clin Exp Allergy 30(Suppl 1):11–15
Yawn BP, Algatt-Bergstrom PJ, Yawn RA, Wollan P, Greco M, Gleason M, Markson L (2000) An in-school CD-ROM asthma education program. J Sch Health 70(4):153–159
Yoo KH, Molis WE, Weaver AL, Jacobson RM, Juhn YJ (2007) The impact of electronic medical records on timeliness of diagnosis of asthma. Journal of Asthma. 44(9): 753–758
Zheng QT, Goryachev S, Weiss S, Sordo M, Murphy SN, Lazarus R (2006) Extracting principal diagnosis, co-morbidity and smoking status for asthma research: Evaluation of a natural language processing system. BMC Med Inform Decis Mak 6:30, available at http://www.biomedcentral.com/1472-6947/6/30
Zimmerman BJ (1986) Development of self-regulated learning: Which are the key subprocesses? Contemp Educ Psych 16:307–313
Zimmerman BJ (1989) Models of self-regulated learning and academic achievement. In: Zimmerman BJ, Schunk DH (eds) Self-regulated learning and academic achievement: Theory, research and practice. Springer, New York, pp 1–25
Zimmerman BJ, Ringle J (1981) Effects of model persistence and statements of confidence on children's efficacy and problem solving. J Educ Psychol 73:485–493

Part III
Asthma: A Social Ecological Perspective

Chapter 11
Asthma: A Lifespan Perspective

Tomas Tamulis and Monroe J. King

Introduction

Although many of the basic physiological processes are similar, there are sufficient differences between childhood and adult asthma to make the onset of disease, clinical symptoms, and psychosocial interactions unique to children and to adults with asthma. The impact of asthma on children and adults is also different, and these differences must be understood and considered in the development of various asthma control prevention strategies for lifespan disease management in children and adults. There are also differential concerns in terms of the burden of asthma in these populations. Moreover, the real impact of asthma in many cases is underestimated, and available estimates of the burden of asthma should be used with caution. In this chapter, we review the intermittent, variable, and reversible nature of asthma, and we adopt a lifespan approach in characterizing the burden of asthma in children, in adults, and to society. We also emphasize a lifespan perspective to the management of asthma. Asthma is a chronic disease that requires complex and multicomponent individualized case management interventions to improve physician practices, health outcomes, self-management of asthma, and overall quality of life in asthma patients.

T. Tamulis (✉)
College of Public Health, Kent State University, Kent, OH, USA
e-mail: tamulis@hawaii.edu

Definition of Asthma

The definition of disease is based on the current state of knowledge of the disease. Description of the symptoms, physical changes, and psychological status associated with asthma can be found in the ancient writings in China, dated as early as 2697 B.C., and in the writings of Hippocrates (460–370 B.C.) (Taitel et al. 1998). More recently, the National Asthma Education Expert Panel Report (NAEPP 1991) defined asthma as a disease with reversible airway obstruction; airway inflammation; and increased airway responsiveness to a variety of environmental triggers. As a chronic inflammatory disorder of the airways asthma involves many cells and cellular elements, in particular lymphocytes, macrophages, neutrophils, and epithelial cells (NAEPP 1997). The change in the definition of asthma over time – from a condition defined by physiological and functional parameters to one that emphasizes cellular and biochemical pathology – results from the substantial progress that has been made in our understanding of the disease and in the treatment of asthma. Unfortunately, the current definition of the disease is still far removed from a definition that captures meaningfully all asthma patients with respect to etiology, pathology, symptoms, or response to treatment.

Asthma is characterized by reversible constriction of the bronchial muscles, swelling of the bronchial tissues, mucus secretion, infiltration of inflammatory cells, or a combination of these factors, with prominent clinical symptoms of wheezing, coughing, chest tightness and shortness of breath (NAEPP 1997; American Lung Association 2004). Clinical symptoms may lead to fear, panic, aggressive behavior, anxiety, depression or fatigue. Asthma is a multifactorial disease explained by immunological, inflammatory and neurogenic

A. Harver and H. Kotses (eds.), *Asthma, Health and Society: A Public Health Perspective*, DOI 10.1007/978-0-387-78285-0_11, © Springer Science+Business Media, LLC 2010

mechanisms in combination with genetic, environmental, and psychosocial risk factors (Mannino et al. 1998). The underlying pathophysiology of asthma is airway inflammation of the large and small airways that may erupt from exposure to an allergen, cigarette smoke, or occupational aerosol; or by nonallergic stimuli such as exercise or cold air (Sandel and O'Connor 2002).

In one long-standing scheme, asthma is separated into "extrinsic" or "allergic" type (due to a specific allergen), and "intrinsic" or "nonallergic" type (when a specific antigen is unknown). "Extrinsic asthma" applies to the individual with hypersensitivity to a range of external environmental factors. Exposure to such allergens as the house dust mite, grass and tree pollen, household pets, and certain proteins in food may produce a variety of clinical symptoms from atopic dermatitis (eczema) and rhinitis to asthma or anaphylaxis. Skin-prick tests may confirm the allergen responsible for these reactions by the development of a wheal-and-flare reaction in the skin, and radioallergoimmunosorbant test (RAST) of the serum may be used to identify specific immunoglobulin-E (IgE) antigens.

There are a significant number of individuals with airflow obstruction with no known antigenic or chemical factor associated with airway inflammation. These individuals represent intrinsic or nonallergic asthma, and, as compared to extrinsic asthma, this condition usually is present later in the lifespan. Previous studies indicate that patients with intrinsic asthma may exhibit a poorer response to bronchodilators and may demonstrate a more rapid decrease in pulmonary function than those with extrinsic asthma (Ulrik et al. 1992). In the presence of a smoking history, these patients may be misdiagnosed with chronic obstructive pulmonary disease (COPD) and only additional medical tests may reveal a significant increase in blood and sputum eosinophils that is typical of asthma (Clark et al. 2000). Although there is difficulty in identifying environmental triggers of asthma in these patients, the underlying pathogenesis of intrinsic asthma is very similar to those of extrinsic asthma (Clark et al. 2000).

The latest research suggests that the terms "extrinsic" and "intrinsic" asthma may not be helpful in either the diagnosis or clinical confirmation of disease (Wray 1998). First, causal factors for intrinsic asthma remain unknown or could be defined only as any other factor not associated with extrinsic asthma. Second, the two categories are not helpful to determine specific treatment as the same person can experience both intrinsic and extrinsic asthma. There is also additional evidence available that an atopic tendency may decline with age, and negative skin-prick tests or low serum IgE levels in older patients may fail to demonstrate a previous allergic hypersensitivity to a well-known environmental allergen (Burrows 1995). In addition to "extrinsic" and "intrinsic" asthma, asthma associated with COPD can be separated as a third category. The term "chronic obstructive pulmonary disease," and the related terms of "chronic bronchitis," "emphysema," and "chronic obstructive airway disease" have caused much controversy and an unnecessary degree of redundancy in the terminology (Clark et al. 2000). The controversy has remained and continued largely because of insufficient knowledge about the differences between asthma and COPD.

Individuals with COPD demonstrate a progressive history of breathlessness over several years, have established smoking history, and generally are in their fifth decade or older. Pulmonary function testing shows an obstructive defect with little reversibility with inhaled β_2-agonists and may demonstrate abnormalities of reduced gas transfer with a large residual volume, suggesting air trapping. The typical patient is quite different from the typical asthma patient but challenges arise with the significant number of patients with breathlessness, wheezing, and airflow obstruction, and other clinical features compatible with both asthma and COPD. In addition, difficulties in differentiation and clinical diagnosis are exaggerated by the problem of defining the degree of reversibility that could be considered clinically relevant.

Intermittency, Variability and Reversibility of Asthma

The principal asthma characteristics of intermittence, variability, and reversibility define the content and goals of asthma self-management programs. The *intermittency* of asthma indicates that the frequency of asthma attacks for a single patient and from patient to patient over time, varies markedly. One patient may experience a series of attacks over a few days but remain episode free for several months or even years; another patient may experience episodes of asthma most days throughout the year. The intermittency of asthma is a function of physiological, health care, and individual variables (Creer and Bender 1993). Physiological variables include the number of different environmental factors that trigger asthma, and depend on the level of hyperreactivity of the airways. Health care variables relate to the access to asthma specialists and proper asthma treatment, and the degree of pharmacologic control over the disease. Knowledge of asthma, medication compliance and individual expectations make up the main categories of patient variables.

Variability of asthma refers to the severity and frequency of the disease. Asthmatic patients vary in the number of environmental stimuli to which they are sensitive, and to the level or degree of responsiveness to asthma "triggers." The response to stimuli can vary from mild symptoms such as difficulty in breathing to a severe response that requires the use of aggressive medical treatment or hospitalization. The range of sensitivity and degree of responsiveness will vary not only between individuals, but also within individuals. The severity of pre-existing airway obstruction also influences the subsequent response to a bronchodilator.

Several standard measures obtained through spirometry are used to assess airway obstruction, including the forced vital capacity (FVC), the forced expired volume in one second (FEV_1), and the FEV_1/FVC ratio. In patients with chronic obstructive pulmonary disorders the FEV_1/FVC value is less than 70% (Bush 2001). The FEV_1 may be a better marker of intermittent airway obstruction as compared to the FEV_1/FVC ratio and is commonly used to assess asthma severity. Because of spontaneous variability in airway function, however, there is no absolute threshold value to distinguish asthma. The expected 12% or 200 mL increase in FEV_1 levels following the administration of a bronchodilator, which is used in the diagnosis or exclusion of asthma, may be an unstable quantity (Clark et al. 2000). The National Asthma Education and Prevention Program (NAEPP) developed a general definition of severity based, in part, on the percent predicted value of FEV_1. In this scheme, asthma severity may be classified into four categories: mild intermittent, mild persistent, moderate persistent, or severe persistent (see Table 11.1) (NAEPP 2002). The 2007 NAEPP guidelines eliminated "mild intermittent" as patients with intermittent asthma may have severe exacerbations.

Asthma variability is also related to the perceived severity of the disease. Patient experiences are subjective by nature and are heavily influenced by the perceived severity of the disease (Kotses and Harver 1998). These experiences may influence future expectations of asthma control as a function of the perceived severity of asthma attacks. Failure to seek medical care for acute attacks that intensify in severity is an important factor contributing to the death from asthma (Kotses and Harver 1998).

The *reversibility* of asthma is an essential factor that distinguishes asthma from irreversible chronic respiratory disorders. Chronic obstruction of the airways can be differentiated from a reversible pulmonary disease on the basis of the FEV_1/FVC ratio (American Thoracic Society 1991). The high degree of reversibility in airflow obstruction to bronchodilators or anti-inflammatory medication is specific to asthma and is often used to differentiate asthma from COPD. The issue of irreversibility, however, may be relative and ambiguous. Although most patients with asthma show complete reversibility of airflow obstruction, many patients with asthma exhibit airway obstruction when they are asymptomatic. In addition, even intensive medical therapy may fail to completely reverse asthma in some patients.

Lifelong Impact of Asthma: Individual and Societal Perspectives

Asthma imposes a heavy financial burden on the individual patient and on society. In many cases, asthma is an easily treated inconvenient condition; but in some cases the disease may be debilitating or even fatal. Burden of illness can be characterized to include pain and suffering, changes in quality of life, lost productivity, direct and indirect financial costs resulting from primary and acute asthma care, and premature death. The overall impact of asthma reaches far beyond the individual patient to affect family, friends, colleagues, and the community.

The Impact of Asthma on the Individual

Unfortunately, a definition of asthma focused on the physiological and immunological changes occurring at a cellular level is too narrow to appraise the full impact of the disease on the individual. The day-to-day normal activities and social functioning of persons with asthma

Table 11.1 Asthma severity based on the frequency of symptoms and lung function before treatment

Asthma classification	Daytime and nighttime symptom frequency	Lung function
Intermittent asthma	2 days per week or less 2 nights per month or less	PEF or FEV_1: 80% or more of predicted values
Mild persistent asthma	More than 2 days per week but less than one time per day More than 2 nights per month	PEF or FEV_1: 80% or more of predicted values
Moderate persistent asthma	Daily More than 1 night per week	PEF or FEV_1: 60–80% of predicted values
Severe persistent asthma	Continual Frequent	PEF or FEV_1: 60% or less of predicted values

Adapted from: National Asthma Education and Prevention Program Second Expert Panel. Expert Panel Report 2: Guidelines for the diagnosis and management of asthma: expert panel 2. Bethesda, MD, NIH Publication No. 97-4051, 1997; and National Asthma Education and Prevention Program Expert Panel Report 3. Guidelines for the diagnosis and management of asthma. National Institutes of Health, NIH Publications No. 08-4051, 2007

is changed either by asthma symptoms or by the medical treatment required to control the disease. Limited normal daily activities can result in lower quality of life. The burden of asthma is not limited to physical symptoms; it not only disrupts regular daily activities but may also elicit anxiety, depression, and panic (Kotses and Harver 1998). Although very effective in controlling the disease, the common asthma medications may also be responsible for a number of adverse reactions. We briefly review the impact of asthma on the individual patient in terms of daily activities, psychological outcomes, and medical treatment side effects.

Regular Daily Activities

The most salient feature of asthma, interference with the conduct of regular daily activities, is the result of asthma symptoms including shortness of breath, chest tightness, wheezing, and coughing (Kotses and Harver 1998). Dyspnea, or difficulty breathing, is reported to be the most common reason for emergency room visits in asthma (Janson-Bjerklie et al. 1993; Janson-Bjerklie et al. 1992). Asthma is the leading cause of school absenteeism in children with asthma. The absenteeism associated with asthma may be due to frequent doctor visits, limited activity due to acute symptoms, or psychosocial problems brought on by the disease (Kotses and Harver 1998). Psychosocial problems may result from stress and a parent's belief that the child is too vulnerable to participate in some activities. Poor academic performance, restricted social development, and increased parent-child conflict emerge as physical limitations increase.

In adults, symptoms may lead to serious activity restrictions at work. Asthma is the third leading cause of work loss, behind only intervertebral disk and back disease (Blanc et al. 1993). Previous studies have disclosed that asthma has an equivalent effect on employment of young asthmatics of both genders (Sibbauld et al. 1992). Workers with current or past asthma were more likely to be unemployed, spend less time employed, hold more temporary jobs, and have spent less time in their most recent full-time positions compared to individuals without asthma. In addition, adults with asthma were found to represent a lower socioeconomic status group, and the reason for this may be that it is difficult to find and hold a position that would not be associated with asthma exacerbations. Employers may bias employment opportunities for individuals with asthma because of fear that they may miss workdays more often than other employees, or use more health benefits.

Psychological Outcomes

The most important psychological factors associated with asthma are panic, anxiety, denial, and depression (Kotses and Harver 1998). Panic symptoms such as chest pain, breathing difficulty, sweating, faintness, and shaking are also associated with acute asthma attacks. Panic symptoms may be the result of response to the clinical environment, including medical equipment, procedures, and personnel (Creer 1979) or lack of knowledge and confidence or self-control (Janson-Bjerklie et al. 1986; Gift 1991). Unfortunately, asthma knowledge is found to be very low among asthma patients and family members, which suggests that many panic attacks and symptoms may be controlled or reduced (Bucknall et al. 1988). Symptoms present during the panic attack are not only an important source of personal discomfort, but they also complicate and aggravate the asthma attack itself. The cumulative increase in panic symptoms and severity of acute asthma attack may result in hospitalization or even death (Kotses and Harver 1998).

Anxiety is the most common emotion associated with dyspnea during an asthma attack, and may develop before, together with, or following the attack (Creer 1979; Gift 1991). Anxiety may result from the unpredictability of an attack, or even fear of death (Creer 1979; Alt 1992). A lack of self-management skills and limited knowledge of asthma, and restricted access to medical care to reduce the severity of symptoms, may cause or increase anxiety levels during asthma episodes. In addition to panic and anxiety, hostility and aggressiveness may be exhibited as either verbal or physical abuse. Particularly among children, aggressive behaviors may originate from frustration and fear, and very often could be directed towards medical personnel.

Denial is another frequently reported psychological aspect of asthma (Creer 1979; Alt 1992). Denial in asthma can be described as more sporadic compliance or continuous refusal to comply with medical treatment and disease management by the patient with asthma. Denial may serve as a coping strategy for adapting to the disease, or for preserving self-esteem in the asthma patient.

Depression is not shown to be more prevalent among asthma patients than among individuals without asthma, however, the occurrence of depression symptoms may have a serious psychological effect on asthma patients (Janson-Bjerklie et al. 1993; Janson-Bjerklie et al. 1992; Janson et al. 1994). Depression in asthma may be associated with more frequent episodes of breathlessness after physical activity; disruption of normal sleep patterns and more frequent nocturnal waking with attacks of breathlessness; and inadequate perception of the danger or severity of the disease. Asthma negatively affects self-esteem, sense of control, and may lead to or aggravate depression. Increased perceived dependence on asthma medications may also be the result of depression in asthma patients. In the end, it should be noted that depressive symptoms in asthma may be resolved successfully or reduced with effective self-management and medical treatment strategies.

Continuous health problems associated with asthma may lead to frustration. The patience of even the most self-confident individual may be challenged by the constant vigilance required to control asthma; living with asthma may become a battle with constant frustration. The sources of frustration can include the discomfort or pain resulting from asthma symptoms, restrictions of daily physical activities, and decreases in overall quality of life (Quirk and Jones 1990).

Side Effects of Medical Treatment

The expected benefits must be weighted against potential side effects. The most serious clinical side effects may include weight gain, change in body fat distribution, change in adrenal function, cardiac arrhythmia, seizure, tremor, and change in sensory function. However, the use of inhaled, rather than oral, steroids reduces side effects greatly (Gross and Ponte 1998). The list of mild side effects includes nausea, anorexia, vomiting, nervousness, irritability, dizziness, confusion, sleep disturbance, sweating, headache, blood pressure elevation, and respiratory irritation (Gross and Ponte 1998). The cumulative effect of one or more of these conditions to the respiratory symptoms of acute asthma can contribute substantially to the burden of the disease for the individual patient.

Asthma in Children

Asthma is the most common chronic disease of childhood and the disruptions caused by asthma both in the individual child and in the family of the asthmatic child cannot be overemphasized (Bruce and Klinnert 1998). The dynamic interplay between social, family, and individual psychological factors can influence the onset, course, and severity of asthma. Although the onset of asthma may occur at any age, a great majority of children experience their first asthma symptoms before the age of 4–5 years (Behrman et al. 1987); more than half of the childhood patients develop their first symptoms before age 2 (Adams 1998). The most common root of asthma in children aged 6 months or younger is viral respiratory infection, such as viral bronchitis or pneumonia. It is extremely important that all members of the child's family be aware of the nature of the disease as well as of the existing options for disease management. For example, decreased school performance has been attributed to increased absences and to the effect of asthma medications, acute exacerbation, stress, and the perception of disease by teachers and parents. Children with asthma have high rates of school absences, but it is unclear whether these absences result in poor school performance or whether other neurocognitive or emotional problems associated with asthma account for existing differences in school performance for some children.

The overall impact of asthma on children includes physical and psychological effects. The physical impact of asthma includes limitations on physical activity and ability to cope with normal physical challenges without excessive fatigue. Previous studies document that children with asthma report the disease as the main reason for not being able to participate in sport programs (Donnelly et al. 1987; Coughlin 1988). Emphasis should be placed on maintaining as close as possible normal regular activities at home and school, including physical exercise.

Previous studies have demonstrated that behavioral and psychological factors play an important role in increasing or reducing the severity of symptoms, number of exacerbations, and in promoting more effective asthma self-management (Gustafsson et al. 1986; MacLean et al. 1992; Lask 1992). Unfortunately, asthma can negatively alter behaviors and attitudes, and levels of self-esteem. Asthma, like many other chronic conditions, is associated with a certain stigmata and loss of self-esteem that can influence how children perceive themselves and how they function in society (Mrazek 1992; Fritz et al. 1996). Asthmatic children may suffer embarrassment at school or play during flare-ups. Parents and physicians must reinforce a positive attitude in the child regarding asthma to avoid loss of self-esteem and development of poor self-image. Children with severe asthma who use emergency care services or who are frequently referred for hospital admissions may suffer increased anxiety and depression. There is no evidence that that these factors cause the disease; however, anxiety and depression aggravate the course of asthma.

Self-management of childhood asthma depends strongly on the parent-child interaction and on the direct involvement of parents or caretakers. Children are dependent on their parents for all or part of their asthma care, especially children with early asthma onset in the first few years of life. Parents typically select the physician, schedule and bring the child to medical appointments and the emergency department, administer prescribed medications, support and monitor home treatment, minimize exposure to known environmental triggers, and pay the costs of medical care. Parent-child interaction and parental functioning strongly influence the effectiveness of asthma management. Cognitive development advances rapidly, and at school age, children begin to assume responsibility for monitoring asthma symptoms, recognizing changes in respiratory status and selecting the most effective medical treatment. Asthmatic children of 6 years and older can use a handheld peak flow meter if provided with appropriate instructions and parental supervision.

As children progress toward adolescence, they become more responsible for self-management. The shift occurs over time in the context of innumerable parent-child interactions related to various tasks in asthma management. The impact of asthma on children's social functions and normal daily activities are important factors to estimate the overall burden of the disease. Asthmatic children very often experience various coexisting diseases and medical conditions, including allergic rhinitis and eczema, and emotional and behavioral problems, which will influence the overall burden of asthma symptoms. Effective asthma management involves not only taking medications on time but also developing a partnership with health-care providers, effective control of indoor and outdoor environmental asthma triggers, and recognition of asthma symptoms. The child and parent's knowledge of asthma and management strategies, and capacity to carry out disease management procedures, are important factors in successful childhood asthma management. Poverty, negative stressful life events, personality, comorbidities, and side effects of asthma medication may increase the risk for poorly controlled or severe asthma (Kotses and Harver 1998). Dysfunctional parent-child partnerships, spousal conflict, limited intellectual abilities, or financial limitations may interfere and endanger effective disease management processes.

Support groups for asthmatic children and parents are available in the form of "summer asthma camps" or year-round activities. "Multi-problem" families, with a variety of financial, social, and psychological needs and very often with children with severe and poorly controlled asthma, may require the active involvement of mental health or social service providers who can address these complicated interactions to improve overall disease management. Asthma-focused family therapy may be provided by a professional who is highly knowledgeable about asthma and who works in partnership with the physician of asthmatic child.

Individualized education may be important to address the problem of limited understanding of disease pathology, lifelong disease management strategies, and possible side effects of asthma medications. The study conducted by Liu et al. compared asthma patients with various methods of education (face-to-face, group and home-based video) and controls with no formal education to estimate the effect of individualized asthma education on clinical outcomes in children with asthma (Liu and Feekery 2001). The study concluded that all methods of education increased levels of parental asthma knowledge and immediately decreased child morbidity scores, but only face-to-face interactions reduced asthma severity in children. These finding could be considered in the design and format of future asthma education programs.

Asthma in Adults

Late-onset asthma differs substantially from early life asthma, and there is an unresolved controversy about the proportion of children who "outgrow" their asthma. Previous studies have revealed that approximately 25% of children diagnosed with asthma at 7 years of age will have persistent asthma at age 33 (Pellegrini 1990; Bender et al. 1995). Asthma can develop as a new diagnosis in an adult person with risk factors similar to childhood asthma. Adult asthma may be reactivated from the quiescent pediatric asthma as a result of persistent bronchial hyperresponsiveness (Barbee and Murphy 1998). However, it is less common to develop asthma as an adult, and the probability that the disease will disappear is also less common in adults than in children (Gershwin and Albertson 2001). Adult-onset asthma may be masked by other chronic respiratory illnesses, often associated with smoking history, and the symptoms of wheezing, shortness of breath, and chest tightness that are attributed to chronic bronchitis or emphysema.

Asthma in adults is very often under diagnosed because of its intrinsic nature and lack of common allergic characteristics that differentiate the disease in young patients with asthma. Adult asthma is less likely to be associated with atopy, as assessed by skin allergy testing and serum concentration of total or specific IgE (Braman et al. 1991). Although atopy may be important in the pathogenesis of elderly asthma, clinical sensitivity to allergens is less common in the elderly asthmatic group. Adult asthmatics are more likely to have a greater degree of airflow obstruction with limited reversibility that is often preceded by a diagnosis of chronic bronchitis or emphysema. Many older patients with COPD have both reversible and irreversible airflow obstruction. Older patients may attribute their symptoms to smoking, to previous occupational exposures, or to aging. Declines in lung function attributed to aging alone may lead physicians to ignore the importance of asthma symptoms in older patients. Therefore, the characterization of older asthma patients and differentiation of asthma by symptoms alone is inadequate and may result in misdiagnosis of the disease. Early diagnosis and delay of the onset of disability are crucial to sustaining quality of life in older patients. Aside from chronic bronchitis, emphysema, and congestive heart failure, symptoms of asthma in the elderly may also be mimicked by aspiration pneumonia, vocal cord dysfunction, endobronchial tumors, and drug-induced bronchial hyperactivity (Barbee and Bloom 1997).

Certain personal characteristics, along with social, economic, and environmental factors may influence disease management options and outcomes. As in childhood asthma, physical and psychological factors influence disease control and management in adults. Physical changes that might compete with asthma care are associated with both the aging process and with other chronic diseases that become more evident in older adults such as COPD, arthritis, diabetes, and hypertension (Bailey et al. 1992). Psychological changes that may compromise asthma management result from sleep disturbances, stroke, anemia, dementia, and thyroid dysfunction. Depression in elderly asthmatics can negatively affect both personal motivation and medication compliance. Severe asthma may not only lead to depression but depression by itself may contribute to poor disease management through reduced compliance and adherence with medical therapy. Depression may affect the perception of symptoms, ability to follow a treatment plan, and quality of life. Depression is more common in elderly persons with poorly controlled asthma, and may become more severe due to the treatment of asthma with increasing numbers of comorbid conditions such as Parkinsonism or hypertension. Memory lapses and neurological changes such as decreased visual acuity, color discrimination, and impaired hearing may affect communication in the elderly and the ability of the patient to consistently carry out a disease management program. Co-morbidities such as diabetes and cardiovascular disease may increase the number of daily medications the patient is required to track each day (Barbee and Bloom 1997). As in children, poor adherence with asthma therapy can result in disease exacerbations in adults (Milgrom et al. 1996).

Health-risk behaviors such as substance abuse and poor self-management of asthma may result in increased asthma morbidity and mortality. Abuse of alcohol and drugs has the potential to increase the risk of fatal episodes for the adult patient with asthma. The most common form of substance abuse is cigarette smoking that may trigger asthma attacks and may lead to worsening symptoms, decreased pulmonary function, and even respiratory infections (Weiss et al. 2000). On the other hand, positive asthma self-management strategies and interventions such as adherence with prescribed therapy, allergen avoidance, self-monitoring of symptoms, peak flow monitoring, and correct metered-dose inhaler (MDI) technique, which are based on both educational and behavioral modification models, may improve adult asthma management.

Effective asthma management usually requires external as well as internal resources. Social and economic factors that influence the management of adult asthma patients should be addressed by the family and social support networks. Such networks include but are not limited to spouse or families, neighbors, churches, and elderly care programs. Recommendations for both patient and family members to be an integral part of adult asthma self-management are of the same importance as for asthmatic children. However, older asthmatics usually do not live together and may not live close to other family members, and may experience less frequent family support. In addition, elderly asthmatics are more likely to have fixed or limited financial resources, which may affect health insurance options, and may result in restricted access to health care or lower adherence to medical therapy.

Asthma and the Workplace

Exposure in the workplace is a major environmental concern that may influence adult asthma. Occupational asthma arising from sensitization in the workplace represents a special subset of adult asthma. The person with asthma may have increased sensitivity to a variety of chemical and physical occupational stimuli, which makes him or her especially vulnerable to work-related exposures. Severe exacerbations and functional impairment may lead to decreased productivity, work loss, and disability. Imprecise differentiation and definition of impairment, disability, handicap, and quality of life have led to potential confusion in the interpretation of research on asthma-related work loss and have complicated the identification of main risk factors for work-related asthma. There are over 400 known causal risk factors associated with occupational asthma that can be divided into two broad groups: (1) biologically derived products, and (2) low molecular weight chemicals (Hall et al. 2000). Biological occupational exposure can be further divided into: fungal and bacterial antigens, such as *Cladosporium*, *Alternaria*, and *Didymella exitialis* fungi; arthropods, such as locust and grain mites; crustaceans, which workers get exposed to while handling or cooking fish or extracting meat from crabs, prawns, shrimps, and lobsters; animals, such as laboratory rats, mice, guinea pigs and rabbits; wood dust, especially hardwood and western red cedar; plants and plant products, such as flour, soya, and spices; cotton, which also increases the risk of occupational obstructive pulmonary disease in the same group of workers; inhaled enzymes, such as amylase and enzymes derived from Bacillus subtitles; and latex, which may cause anaphylactic reactions. Low molecular weight agents can be classified into: adhesives, such as acid anhydrides and isocyanates used as an epoxy resin and in polyurethane manufacture, respectively; drugs, such as antibiotics associated with developed extreme sensitivity; soldering fluxes, mainly colophony and aminoethylethanolamine present in noncorrosive electronic soldering fluxes and aluminum soldering; dyes, such as biological dyes and small molecular weight reactive dyes; metals, such as platinum salts, cobalt, chrome, aluminum, and zinc; reactive amines present in drugs, surface coating, and conventional photographic chemicals; and biocides and sterilizing agents, including formaldehyde, glutaraldehyde, chloramines, ethylene oxide, benzalkonium chloride, and chlorhexidine, which are usually present in many floor-cleaning household materials.

Specific causal relationships are usually defined when a worker with occupational asthma is exposed to a well-known or possible high risk environmental or occupational factor. Sometimes the individual with occupational asthma comes from a workplace without any known problems. In this case, identifying the specific IgE antibodies to a relevant occupational antigen by skin-prick or patch testing with characterized antigens may help to establish causal relationships. Older asthmatics are less likely to be exposed to occupational triggers of asthma compared to younger adult asthmatics. However, they may reside in older buildings or assisted living housing that results in greater exposure to such environmental irritants as indoor allergens, dust, humidity, mildew, institutional cleaning agents, and air pollutants (Barbee and Bloom 1997).

Pregnancy

Special considerations should be addressed in the self-management of asthma during pregnancy. Asthma may improve, worsen, or remain unchanged during pregnancy, and the mechanisms underlying these changes during pregnancy remain unknown (Hall et al. 2000). Asthma is also known to be one of the most common serious medical conditions to complicate pregnancy and accounts for up to 4% of all complicated pregnancies (NAEPP 1993). Hospitalizations for severe asthma may occur in almost half of asthmatic women, and acute asthma may be associated with maternal hypoxia, which may lead directly to fetal hypoxia (Cousines and Catanzarite 1998). Asthma in pregnancy may also be associated with dehydration, hypotension, hypertension, alkalosis, or hypocapnia (Hall et al. 2000). Uncontrolled asthma may reduce oxygen delivery to the fetus and lead to more serious complications. Optimal treatment and effective self-management strategies can reduce the likelihood of these adverse outcomes. Treatment of asthma during pregnancy is similar to the general treatment, and most of the regular asthma medications are safe and should be used during pregnancy. Unfortunately, the fear of serious side effects on the fetus has prompted many asthmatic women to discontinue their medical therapy, which could increase the risk of pregnancy-related complications. To reduce pregnancy complications that may adversely affect the mother and developing child, asthma should be well controlled before and during pregnancy. Daily asthma medication, such as cromolyn, inhaled corticosteroids, or theophylline, should be continued during pregnancy. In asthma patients who require regular corticosteroid treatment during pregnancy, corticosteroids for the stress of labor and delivery are recommended. Optimal treatment of severe asthma exacerbations should prevent maternal death and reduce the risk of fetal mortality. Finally, the risk of complications for pregnant asthmatics can be reduced dramatically through proper patient education and effective communication with the physician along with precautious use of asthma medications.

The Impact of Asthma on Society

Despite major advances in our knowledge and understanding of the pathogenesis and medical treatment of asthma, asthma is a common chronic disease with substantial morbidity and mortality rates. Data collected by the Centers for Disease Control and Prevention (CDC) reveal large and unexplained increases in asthma prevalence, hospitalization rates, and mortality over the last few decades in the United States (www.aafa.org). Asthma has been estimated to affect 17 million people or over 5% of the total population in the United States (www.cdc.gov/nchs/products/pubs/pubd/hestats/asthma/asthma.htm; Homa et al. 2002; Eggleston et al. 1999). The disease accounts for 10.4 million asthma-related office visits to medical care providers, 1.9 million emergency room visits, and 466,000 hospital admissions annually. The National Center for Health Statistics (NCHS) annually conducts the National Health Interview Survey (NHIS), which collects self-reported asthma prevalence, asthma office visits, asthma emergency room visits, asthma hospitalizations, and asthma deaths in subsets of the sample (www.aafa.org; Castro et al. 2001; Boss et al. 2001). The measurement of asthma prevalence was recently changed because of redesign of the NHIS in 1997. Because newer estimates cannot be easily compared with pre-redesign estimates, it will be necessary to follow asthma-related trends for several more years to determine whether asthma prevalence will decline, plateau, or continue to increase as they did through the 1980s and 1990s.

The burden and overall impact of asthma on society may be defined as a combination of both the individual patient and health-care perspectives. Principal components of the cost of asthma from the societal perspective can be divided into separate patient (indirect expenditures) and health-care (direct expenditures) categories (see Table 11.2). The indirect factors, important in the assessment of asthma burden from the patient point of view include: days lost from school or work; days of restricted activity at school, work or home; and the impact on family and society because of premature mortality (Hall et al. 2000). From the perspective of asthma patients, an acute event includes the immediate pain and suffering, and may include the period of disability as the patient begins to stabilize. The entire period of disability will include the time spent receiving emergency treatment as well as recovery time. Recovery time from an acute episode of asthma includes the time spent both at work and home when regular daily activities are restricted.

The economic burden of asthma is estimated to be $6 billion or $600 to $700 per single patient with asthma per year (Weiss et al. 1992; Smith et al. 1997). The current economic burden associated with asthma mortality most likely is over $1 billion per year in the United States (Hall et al. 2000). Annual number of workdays lost because of asthma has been estimated to range from 2.1 to 3 million days at an estimated annual cost between $222 and $346.3 million (Hall et al. 2000). School-loss estimates for children less than 18 years of age, have varied from 3.6 to 10 million days per year. The economic value of the caregiver time, when the child must miss school and stay at home, ranged from $195 to $900 million. Lost productivity by caregivers because of care provided to the most sensitive asthmatic children population group of 0–4 years of age, accounted for economic losses of $19 million annually (Smith et al. 1997). Restricted activity days, defined as a day when the patient due to asthma is unable to engage in usual daily activities for at least one-half day, have been estimated to account for 218 million days annually, at an economic value of $18.3 million (Smith et al. 1997).

Table 11.2 Main components of the burden of asthma from the societal perspective

Patient perspective (indirect expenditures)	Health system perspective (direct expenditures)
Work loss	Urgent physician office visits
School absence	Emergency department visits
Restricted activity	Hospital admissions
Mortality	Medications and medical supplies

The health system perspective is defined by utilization patterns and the cost of medical resources or services provided. These factors include: (1) utilization of emergency care (ED and hospital admissions); (2) ambulatory visits; (3) phone consultations; (4) medications and tests as a consequence of the acute event; and (5) cost of medical and nonmedical personnel involved in the period of treatment and post-treatment. The direct burden of asthma could be explained by the costs of emergency department (ED) visits and hospital admissions for asthma, which are responsible for approximately 60% of the overall annual direct expenditures for asthma (Hall et al. 2000). Although the number of ED visits for asthma decreased slightly from 1.8 million visits in 1985 to 1.6 million in 1994, the cost for emergency care increased from $200 million in 1985 to $483 million in 1994 (Weiss et al. 1992; Smith et al. 1997; Sullivan and Weiss 1998). The number of hospital admissions for asthma has been relatively constant at 450,000 hospitalizations per year during the period from 1985 to 1994. On the other hand, asthma hospitalization expenditures increased from $1 billion in 1985 to $1.7 billion in 1994. Together, these estimates suggest that direct medical expenditures for acute asthma have increased by 86% during this period despite little change in the number of ED visits or hospital admissions. The dramatic increases in medical expenditures may be the result of medical care inflation and the use of more costly new technologies or medical treatment.

Application of managed care principles in the ED may contribute to reduced hospitalization rates, length of stay and total cost (Roberts et al. 1997). Relatively stable hospitalization rates may also be the result of better management of disease with asthma medication. During 1985 and 1987, theophylline was the most frequently prescribed medication for asthma treatment, followed by β_2-agonists (Weiss et al. 1992; Smith et al. 1997). From 1988 to 1991, inhaled β_2-agonists were the most often prescribed medication, followed by oral corticosteroids; theophylline was the third most frequently prescribed medication (Roberts et al. 1997). The changes in treatment patterns was supported by recommendations from the U.S. National Treatment Guidelines for Diagnosis and Treatment of Asthma in

1991 (NAEPP 1991; National Heart, Lung and Blood Institute and World Health Organization 1995). Possibly, trends in hospitalization rates imply that patients are simply less likely to be admitted to the hospital over time because of changes in payer plans (Hall et al. 2000). This issue will be even more important in the future because more than 50% of all Americans are now enrolled in some kind of managed care plan (Health Care Financing Administration 1997).

Management of Asthma: A Lifespan Perspective

The accurate identification of a patient with asthma is the first step in successful disease management. A detailed medical history, physical examination, and lung function testing are used to identify and classify asthma patients. Based on the guidelines from the National Institutes of Health (NIH) Expert Panel on the Treatment and Diagnosis of Asthma (NAEPP 1993), these patients may be divided into intermittent or persistent asthma, and subsets of patients with mild, moderate, or severe persistent asthma. Once the diagnosis of chronic asthma has been established, the primary aim of periodic outpatient asthma management is to recognize whether the goals of therapy have been achieved. The principal goals of asthma therapy are summarized in Table 11.3.

The Expert Panel of the NIH Asthma Guidelines (NAEPP 1993) recommended that the following factors should be monitored and evaluated on a regular basis as an integral part of lifespan asthma management: (1) signs and symptoms of asthma; (2) asthma exacerbations; (3) pulmonary function through spirometry and peak flow values; (4) pharmacotherapy; (5) quality of life; and (6) patient-provider communication and patient satisfaction. Lifespan asthma management is based on effective daily control of known and probable risk factors, peak flow monitoring, pharmacotherapy, and patient education. Multiple previous studies have demonstrated that asthma knowledge and health outcomes can be improved by active participation in an asthma self-management program (Ruffin et al. 1991; Berg et al. 1997; Allen et al. 1995). Although all asthma self-management programs include patient and family education, numerous studies have indicated that education alone is not sufficient to modify complex behaviors (Kolbe et al. 1996). The possible explanatory mechanism for improved disease outcomes may be improved control of environmental triggers and increased adherence to medical treatment among patients (Hall et al. 2000). On the other hand, there are numerous potential obstacles to adequate disease management for asthma patients, including, but not limited to: severity of disease; patient and family belief systems; patient perceptions, fear and denial; poverty and education level; health-care access; and overall financial burden of the disease. Patients and their family members, and physicians and other lifelong asthma-care providers, must bear in mind that if these obstacles are not disclosed and resolved early on, then it is unlikely that asthma therapy will be effective and successful. Guidelines for lifelong asthma management are summarized in a number of reports, including the National Asthma Education Program (NAEPP 1997) and the Global Asthma Report (Global Initiative for Asthma 1995). The main emphasis of successful lifelong asthma management relies on four principal components: (1) objective measurement of lung function; (2) assessment and control of environmental triggers and irritants of asthma; (3) patient education; and (4) medical treatment.

Table 11.3 Principal goals of asthma therapy

Prevent chronic asthma symptoms (nocturnal dry cough, shortness of breath and constriction of airways)
Prevent recurrent exacerbations of asthma and minimize the need for emergency department visits and hospitalizations
Maintain stable normal or near-normal pulmonary function
Maintain normal daily activity levels (daily routine, work-related activities and exercise)
Provide optimal medical therapy with minimal or no adverse side effects
Assure satisfaction with asthma management and meet the expectations of patients and their family members

Adapted from: National Asthma Education Program Report of the Working Group on Asthma and Pregnancy: Management of asthma during pregnancy. National Institutes of Health, NIH Publication No. 93-3279A, September 1993

Measurement of Lung Function

The patient with asthma must take an active role in the self-management process in order for an asthma control strategy to succeed. Individuals who participate in their own care are generally more knowledgeable about their disease and interact better with the physician (Adams 1998). The peak flow meter is a relatively simple and inexpensive device that determines the maximum expiratory flow rate and can be used in and out of the home to monitor airflow obstruction. More sophisticated and expensive electronic peak flow meters, capable of storing several hundred peak flow measurements that can be downloaded to a personal computer or sent electronically to a health-care provider, are also available. Peak flow recordings can be used to evaluate the effectiveness of medical treatment or response to changes in pharmacotherapy, to identify environmental triggers or irritants at home and work, and to determine the need for urgent emergency management. Regular peak flow meter monitoring can direct a course of selected medical treatment. Changes in peak flow rates of 80% predicted, 60–80% predicted, and less than 60% predicted are typically used as benchmarks for assessing the severity of asthma and for adjusting treatment in a stepwise manner (Adams 1998).

Despite its attractiveness and acceptance, the value of peak flow monitoring in many cases is controversial, and may not always lead to improvements in asthma management (Kotses and Harver 1998). The ability to use a peak flow meter and individual factors such as age, severity of asthma, and physical and mental condition should be considered before the inclusion of regular peak flow monitoring as part of a personal self-management program. An alternative approach to personal peak flow monitoring is to increase sensitivity to acute changes in airflow obstruction in the patient with asthma (Kotses and Harver 1998). This approach could be used effectively in the early detection of asthma flare-ups. However, the clinical value of such an approach has not been fully evaluated and future studies are needed before considering this method as an integral component of asthma self-management programs.

Environmental Triggers and Irritants of Asthma

The factors that exacerbate asthma can be grouped into environmental asthma sensitizers and triggers. The sensitizers of asthma are those environmental agents that may induce airway inflammation and can increase disease risk. Viral infections are a notorious example of asthma provokers or sensitizers that may induce asthma exacerbations. Rhinovirus, respiratory syncytial virus, and influenza viruses are the main examples (Hall et al. 2000). Infants and children are more compromised by the inflammation caused by respiratory viruses than adults because the airways of infants and children are much smaller. Although many infants who wheeze during or after a viral infection will not develop chronic asthma, the reduction or complete elimination of environmental exposure to tobacco smoke, animal dander, and house dust mites should be considered as preventive measures for children with a family history of atopic disease (Hall et al. 2000). Increased severity of asthma due to respiratory viral infections in adults may be successfully prevented with an annual influenza vaccination (Centers for Disease Control and Prevention 1993).

Triggers of asthma exacerbations are different from inducers or sensitizers of asthma because they cause acute bronchoconstriction of the airways rather than latent inflammatory changes. In the presence of chronic inflammation, a trigger may cause a significant decrease in pulmonary function, and trigger avoidance should be considered an integral part of the prevention and management of asthma. Indoor and outdoor allergens – such as mold, cockroaches, house dust mites, and domestic pets – are important classes of environmental triggers that lead to asthma exacerbations (Hall et al. 2000). Many previous studies have found multiple allergens in homes, and multiple sensitivities to main allergens among residents with asthma (American Lung Association 2004). Case-control studies of adults in Wilmington, Delaware, and children in Atlanta, Georgia, revealed that subjects presenting with acute asthma exacerbations were substantially more likely than non-asthmatic controls to have multiple sensitivity to indoor allergens (cockroach, dust mite, or cat), and were more likely to have significant exposure to that allergen in their homes (Sandel and O'Connor 2002). In the latter study, asthmatic patients were exposed to high concentrations of home allergens: 79% of home dust samples contained excessive mite allergen, and 87% of samples contained excessive cockroach allergen levels. The National Co-operative Inner-City Asthma Study (NCICAS) involved eight major inner city areas and concluded that most inner-city children with asthma are exposed to multiple allergens, including cockroach. Asthma patients allergic to cockroach and exposed to high levels of cockroach allergens had significantly higher asthma hospitalization rates, more unscheduled annual medical visits for asthma, more missed school days, more days with wheezing, and more nights with disturbed sleep compared with other children (Custovic and Woodcock 2001; Crain et al. 2002). The physician examination followed by skin testing or testing for specific IgE in vitro are performed to determine the causal association and reduce or eliminate the exposure to specific triggers in the home or workplace. Confirmed positive or negative reactions to specific allergens are used to direct asthma management procedures toward disease control and also prevention of future exacerbations.

Environmental irritants such as tobacco smoke, changes in ambient temperature, fumes, smoke, and specific odors are common triggers of asthma. The detrimental effects of tobacco smoking on human health and lung tissue are particularly well known and zero exposure to direct or secondhand tobacco smoke is recommended by the NIH Expert Panel (NAEPP 1993). Unfortunately, this recommendation is not always followed by patients with asthma (Hall et al. 2000). Elimination of direct and secondhand tobacco smoke is one of the most critical factors in asthma management.

Exercise, cold air, and upper respiratory infections are well-known triggers of bronchoconstriction. Medical treatment with a bronchodilator prior to physical activity or even more aggressive control of chronic inflammation may be required to encourage exercise in patients (Hall et al. 2000). Both acute and chronic sinusitis and rhinitis may act as asthma triggers, and the treatment of these diseases should be an integral part of chronic asthma management. Nasal corticosteroids may reduce mucosal inflammation, and decrease lower airway bronchoconstriction and also control bronchial hyperresponsiveness (Hall et al. 2000). Antibacterial treatment of sinusitis or even surgical treatment of chronic sinusitis may also be required to reduce the inflammation of upper airways.

Patient Education

Patient education is a major part of any successful asthma management plan. The development and application of self-management programs may increase knowledge of asthma and improve overall disease management among patients. Medical treatment is useless unless patients are actively involved in the self-management process, and are aware when and how to use asthma medications. Asthma patients must understand the main characteristics and control of acute asthma exacerbations or disease remissions. Inhaled medications do not provide maximum therapeutic benefit unless they are administered properly, and used as intended. Patients should know the difference between long-term controller medications and short-term reliever medications. Special considerations should be given in the case of educational programs designed for parents or caregivers of very young children, for adolescents, and for elderly patients.

Identification of specific asthma triggers for individual patients is very important for successful asthma management. Tobacco smoke and pet allergen exposure tend to be the key elements that can be addressed in the environment to better control asthma. Patients who smoke or who are exposed to tobacco smoke should be educated about the direct effect of smoking on their disease and how smoking affects long-term management of disease. In addition, patients who are allergic to pets should be instructed on how to avoid contact with them, particularly if there is a pet in the house. There are many other interventions that may be discussed with patients, such as mattress and pillow covers, and carpet removal from the bedroom to reduce the exposure to such indoor allergens such as live house dust mites and mold.

Many patients with chronic asthma are poor judges of the degree of their airflow obstruction and could benefit from use of a peak flow meter. Patients should be carefully instructed where to record daily peak flow values, how to compare current values with previous estimates, and how to react if these values change significantly. By having this information, asthmatic patients should be able to self-monitor the progress of disease and initiate intervention therapy at the onset of increases in airflow obstruction. The panel of experts from the National Asthma Education Program (NAEP) formed by the National Heart, Lung, and Blood Institute (NHLBI) published comprehensive guidelines for the diagnosis and management of asthma, including the use of a "traffic light system" in combination with peak flow monitoring, in 1991 (NAEPP 1997). On the other hand, there is a general lack of research evidence to support the effectiveness and sensitivity of the zone system (Kotses and Harver 1998). For example, there are conflicting data about the interpretation of peak flow values, especially in the management of childhood asthma. Despite these concerns, the peak flow meter plays a significant role in the management of asthma and in the prevention of severe to fatal asthma.

Medical Management of Asthma

The medical treatment of asthma remains as one of the most important aspects of disease management. In 1979, the National Institute of Allergy and Infectious Diseases (NIAID) noted that treatment of asthma relied mainly on β_2-agonists, theophylline, cromolyn sodium, and corticosteroids (NIAID 1979). Major changes have occurred in the medical treatment and management of asthma since the report was published. In 2007, the NAEPP of the NHLBI at the NIH revised and updated previous standardized guidelines for the diagnosis and management of asthma in adults and children under 5 years of age (see Tables 11.4 and 11.5) (NAEPP 2002; NAEPP 1997; NAEPP 2007).

The main medical treatment goals for lifelong bronchial asthma are maintaining a normal lifestyle as well as regular daily activities. Effective medical treatment should sustain normal lung function, and should minimize symptoms such as shortness of breath, wheezing, and coughing. Treatment of asthma requires a step-by-step approach, which frequently begins with higher dosing levels to establish prompt control that are subsequently "stepped down" to minimize the risk of adverse effects of medications (Adams 1998). The "step-down" approach also ensures that medication will be given at the proper dosage and unnecessary medications will not be given to the patient. Asthma severity frequently guides the most appropriate medical treatment for asthma. It is important to stress that asthma severity varies from patient to patient and a crude definition of disease severity should not be employed rigidly. Asthma patients at any level may experience severe or life-threatening asthmatic attacks. In addition, severe asthma attacks may occur suddenly after long symptom-free periods with normal lung function.

Patients with mild persistent asthma may require anti-inflammatory agents such as inhaled corticosteroids, theophylline, cromolyn, nedocromil, or leukotriene modifiers. Patients with moderate persistent asthma require low-to-medium doses of inhaled corticosteroids and the addition of a long-acting inhaled β_2-adrenergic agonist, such as salmeterol or formoterol, administered on a regular basis. Patients continue to use short-acting β_2-agonists; however, the addition of a long-lasting β_2-agonist frequently may reduce the need of the short-acting agent. However, the overuse of short acting quick-relief medications and under use of long-acting anti-inflammatory medications still persists. Alternative agents for moderate persistent patients include theophylline, sustained-release β_2-agonist, and the anti-leukotrienes (Adams 1998). Patients who remain symptomatic with both reduced air flow rates and daily activity, despite the treatment with both a long-lasting β_2-agonist and inhaled corticosteroid, may require supplementary therapy with oral β_2-agonist, theophylline, or ipratropium bromide.

Patients with severe persistent asthma may require high doses of inhaled corticosteroids, long-acting β_2-agonist, theophylline, and frequent administrations of oral corticosteroids. Immunomodulators are also available and suggested as a new medication for long-term control of asthma (NAEPP 2007). Asthma self-management goals and potential side effects of oral corticosteroids should be addressed through the patient–physician interaction more frequently than in the case of mild or moderate asthma. Asthma patients with severe asthma, especially children, should consider the use of a home nebulizer to deliver not only β_2-adrenergic agonist preparations but also cromolyn sodium. A recent study conducted by Delaronde evaluated the effect of an intensive case management intervention and concluded that the case management intervention could be used successfully to identify persons who inappropriately used asthma medications, and to improve medication usage to achieve effective long-term control of asthma and improved quality of life (Delaronde 2002).

Available evidence from clinical trials suggests that there are no benefits from antibiotic therapy for acute severe exacerbations of asthma. The NAEPP Expert Panel did not recommend the use of antibiotics for the treatment of acute asthma exacerbations except as needed for such co-morbid conditions as pneumonia, purulent sputum with fever, or bacterial sinusitis (NAEPP 1997; NAEPP 2007).

Treatment of Children

The NAEPP Expert Panel opinion is that long-term therapy should be initiated in infants and young children with more than three annual episodes of wheezing that

Table 11.4 Stepwise approach for medical treatment of mild, moderate and severe asthma in adults and children older than 12 years of age

Severity of asthma	*Symptoms/day*Symptoms/night	Long-term medical treatment
Step 1: Intermittent asthma	*≤2 days/week*≤2 nights/month	Preferred treatment: No daily medication needed A course of systematic corticosteroids is recommended in cases of severe exacerbations, separated by long periods of normal lung function and no symptoms
Step 2: Mild persistent asthma	*2/week but ≤1/day*>2 nights/month	Preferred treatment: Low-dose inhaled corticosteroids Alternative treatment: Cromolyn, leukotriene modifier, nedocromolin, or theophylline to serum concentration of 5–15 mcg/mL
Step 3: Moderate Persistent Asthma	*Daily*>1 night/week	Preferred treatment: Low-dose inhaled corticosteroids and long-acting inhaled β_2-agonists. Alternative treatment: Increase inhaled corticosteroids within medium-dose range, OR Low-dose inhaled corticosteroids and either leukotriene receptor antagonist, zileuton, or theophylline
Step 4: Severe Persistent Asthma	*Continual*Frequent	Preferred treatment: Medium-dose inhaled corticosteroids, AND Long-lasting inhaled β_2-agonists, AND Oral corticosteroids (2 mg/kg/day but less than 60 mg per day, if needed) Alternative treatment: Medium-dose inhaled corticosteroids, AND EITHER leukotriene receptor antagonist, theophylline, OR zileuton
Step 5: Severe Persistent Asthma	*Continual*Frequent	Preferred treatment: High-dose inhaled corticosteroids, AND Long-lasting inhaled β_2-agonists, AND Omalizumab (preferred for patients who have allergies)
Step 6: Severe Persistent Asthma	*Continual*Frequent	Preferred treatment: High-dose inhaled corticosteroids, AND Long-lasting inhaled β_2-agonists, AND Oral corticosteroids, AND Omalizumab (preferred for patients who have allergies)

Adapted from: National Asthma Education and Prevention Program Third Expert Panel. Expert Panel Report 3: Guidelines for the diagnosis and management of asthma. Bethesda, MD, NIH Publication No. 08-4051, 2007

last more than 1 day and who have other risk factors for the development of asthma, such as parental history of asthma or physician-diagnosed atopic dermatitis, allergic rhinitis, wheezing except from colds, and peripheral blood eosinophilia (see Table 11.5) (NAEPP 2002; NAEPP 1997; NAEPP 2007). No daily medications are recommended for patients with mild intermittent asthma and a course of systematic corticosteroids should be administered only in a case of severe asthma exacerbations. Children under 5 years of age with mild

Table 11.5 Stepwise approach for medical treatment of mild, moderate and severe asthma in infants and young children of 5 years of age and younger with acute and chronic asthma

Severity of asthma	*Symptoms/day*Symptoms/night	Long-term medical treatment
Step 1: Intermittent asthma	*≤2 days/week*≤2 nights/ month	Preferred treatment: No daily medication needed, OR Inhaled short-acting inhaled β_2-agonists
Step 2: Mild persistent asthma	*2/week but ≤1/day*>2 nights/month	Preferred treatment: Low-dose inhaled corticosteroids (administered with nebulizer or MDI with holding chambers with or without mask or DPI) Alternative treatment: Cromolyn OR montelukast
Step 3: Moderate persistent asthma	*Daily*>1 night/week	Preferred treatment:Medium-dose inhaled corticosteroids
Step 4: Severe persistent asthma	*Continual*Frequent	Preferred treatment: Medium-dose inhaled corticosteroids, AND EITHER Long-lasting inhaled β_2-agonists, OR Montelukast
Step 5: Severe persistent asthma	*Continual*Frequent	Preferred treatment: High-dose inhaled corticosteroids, AND EITHER Long-lasting inhaled β_2-agonists, OR Montelukast
Step 6: Severe persistent asthma	*Continual*Frequent	Preferred treatment: High-dose inhaled corticosteroids, AND EITHER Long-lasting inhaled β_2-agonists, OR Montelukast Alternative treatment: Oral systemic corticosteroids

Adapted from: National Asthma Education and Prevention Program Third Expert Panel. Expert Panel Report 3: Guidelines for the diagnosis and management of asthma. NIH, Bethesda, MD, NIH Publication No. 08-4051, 2007

persistent asthma usually begin treatment with low-dose inhaled corticosteroids, administered via nebulizer or MDI with holding chamber, with or without a face mask. The NAEPP Expert Panel recommended that inhaled corticosteroids improve control of asthma for children with mild or moderate asthma as compared to prescribed as-needed β_2-agonists. The review of previous studies concluded that cromolyn, nedocromil, theophylline, or leukotriene receptor antagonists are not as effective as inhaled corticosteroids in improving asthma outcomes (NAEPP 2002; NAEPP 1997; NAEPP 2007).

Inhaled corticosteroids in dosages above 400 μg per day may affect adrenal function and bone growth in children but are considered safe up to this dose. The risk of side effects due to higher doses of inhaled corticosteroids in children should be considered against the negative effect and risk of uncontrolled asthma. Cromolyn is approved for children aged 5 and older. Children with moderate persistent asthma usually experience daily symptoms and have more than two asthma episodes per week. Thus, these pediatric patients require higher dosages of the inhaled corticosteroids and long-acting β_2-agonists. Theophylline may be administered in uncontrolled moderate asthma with precaution due to possible health side effects, such as nervousness, upset stomach, headache, and impaired learning abilities. Severe asthma in children requires the addition of higher doses of oral corticosteroids or long-acting inhaled β_2-agonists. The adverse effects are similar to those of adult asthmatics, but may be even more significant in younger patients. As in adult patients, children with mild asthma receiving nebulized or oral medication face a greater risk of such side effects as nervousness and tremor (Adams 1998). The overview of available scientific evidence disclosed that the use of inhaled corticosteroids at recommended doses do not have clinically significant effect on vertical growth, bone mineral density, ocular toxicity, or suppression of the hypothalamic-pituitary-adrenal (PAH) axis (NAEPP 2002; NAEPP 1997; NAEPP 2007). The NAEPP Expert Panel also concluded that the potential but small risk of delayed growth is overweighed by the effectiveness of inhaled corticosteroids in improving health outcomes for children with mild or moderate persistent asthma.

Treatment During Pregnancy

To reduce complications that may adversely affect the mother and developing child, asthma should be well controlled before and during pregnancy. Patients should also avoid exposure to allergens as much as possible. Daily peak flow measurements and regular medications should be maintained or adjusted accordingly. Uncontrolled asthma may significantly reduce the amount of oxygen delivered to the fetus and lead to serious complications. Treatment of asthma during pregnancy is similar to the general treatment plan and most of the asthma medications are safe to use during pregnancy. The inhaled β_2-agonists, such as albuterol, metaproterenol, pirbuterol, terbutaline, are the first-line bronchodilators during pregnancy. Theophylline may be also used with a close monitoring of blood levels that should not exceed 12 mg/L; newborns of women with high levels of theophylline may experience jitteriness, vomiting, and rapid heartbeat. Nonselective β_2-agonists are best avoided during pregnancy. Previous studies in animals and human observations raised many safety questions, and selective β_2-agonists should be preferred to nonselective medications during pregnancy. Cromolyn sodium and nedocromil sodium are nonsteroidal anti-inflammatory drugs with extremely low incidence of adverse side effects and may be the preferred anti-inflammatory therapy during pregnancy. On the other hand, inhaled and systemic corticosteroids may also serve as safe and effective anti-inflammatory agents to treat severe asthma exacerbations during pregnancy.

Final Thoughts

At this moment there are no easy methods for determining the true burden of asthma. Population-based longitudinal studies of the natural history of asthma would be useful to provide more accurate information on the true impact of asthma on the individual patient, family and society. However, these studies are not available and much of our understanding of the burden of asthma through a lifespan rests on proxy measures of emergency care visits, hospital admissions, and mortality. The estimated economic burden of asthma is significant, and the majority of the direct expenditures are a result of emergency room visits and hospitalizations for asthma. The majority of dollars spent for the treatment of asthma is used to control acute asthma rather than for early disease prevention. Well-treated asthma should be an illness with very little acute health-care needs. The available information on the burden of asthma suggests a failure to efficiently allocate the necessary health-care resources toward preventing asthma exacerbations that would reduce the social, psychological, and economic burden of asthma.

There is no single solution to improve lifelong asthma management. Despite the progress made in the medical treatment of the disease, the management of asthma still poses a challenge and expenditures for asthma have continued to rise in recent years. Contemporary medical treatment guidelines emphasize an aggressive step-down approach with the use of anti-inflammatory medication to achieve long-term control of asthma. Development of more safe and effective asthma medications that are affordable, easily monitored by both physicians and patients, and associated with minimal adverse side effects will facilitate adherence to individual asthma therapy and disease self-management.

Effective lifelong asthma management requires a commitment from both patient and physician. The partnership between physician and patient will continue to play a significant role in future self-management programs and overall management of asthma. Patient education can empower persons with asthma to begin guided self-management of their disease. Such shared responsibility may help to ensure a favorable clinical outcome and an improved quality of life. Widespread use of asthma self-management techniques may be the best solution to reverse the current trends. Effective asthma self-management techniques reduce asthma symptoms and ultimately reduce the overall financial burden of the disease.

Future lifelong asthma management strategies must be focused on the personalization of asthma self-management. Increased motivation, self-esteem and behavioral changes in patients with asthma through education will remain as a significant component of disease management. Although much remains to be discovered about the role of social and economic factors in controlling asthma, variability in asthma outcomes are strongly influenced by socio-economic status. There are significant differences in exposure to exacerbating factors, especially indoor allergens

(Weiss et al. 2000). The regulation of indoor and outdoor environmental triggers and control of environmental allergen exposure is an important step in successful asthma management. The management of asthma is influenced by important socio-economic disparities and inequities in the access to and quality of health care received.

Finally, asthma is a chronic disease that requires complex and multicomponent individualized, case management interventions to improve physician practices, health outcomes, self-management of asthma, and overall quality of life of asthma patients. The combination of three main components – long-term control medication, patient education, and guided self-management – can decrease disease severity and improve lifelong management of asthma.

References

Adams FV (1998) The asthma sourcebook: everything you need to know, 2nd edn. Lowell House, Los Angeles

Allen RM, Jones MP, Oldenburg B (1995) Randomised trial of an asthma self-management program for adults. Thorax 50:731–738

Alt H (1992) Psychiatric aspects of asthma. Chest 101:415–416

American Lung Association (2004) Trends in asthma morbidity and mortality. American Lung Association, Epidemiology and Statistics Unit, Research and Scientific Affairs. April 2004, www.lungusa.org

American Thoracic Society (1991) Lung function testing: selection of reference values and interpretive strategies. Am Rev Respir Dis 144:1202–1218

Bailey WC, Richards JM Jr, Brooks CM et al (1992) Features of asthma in older adults. J Asthma 29:21–28

Barbee RA, Bloom JW (1997) Asthma in the Elderly. Marcel Dekker, New York, p 94

Barbee RA, Murphy S (1998) The natural history of asthma. J Allergy Clin Immunol 102:s65–s72

Behrman RE, Vaughan VC, Nelson WE (eds) (1987) Nelson textbook of pediatrics. WB Saunders, Philadelphia, PA, p 495

Bender B, Milgrom H, Bowry P et al (1995) Asthmatic children's adherence with aerosolized medications. Am J Respir Crit Care Med 151:352

Berg J, Dunbar-Jacob J, Sereika SM (1997) An evaluation of a self-management program for adult with asthma. Clin Nurs Res 6:225–238

Blanc PD, Jones M, Besson C, Katz P, Yelin E (1993) Work disability among adults with asthma. Chest 104:1371–1377

Boss LP, Kreutzer RA, Luttinger D et al (2001) The public health surveillance of asthma. J Asthma 38(1):83

Braman SS, Kaemmerlen JT, Davis SM (1991) Asthma in the elderly: a comparison between patients with recently acquired and long standing disease. Am Rev Respir Dis 143:336–340

Bruce GB, Klinnert MD (1998) Psychological correlates of asthma severity and treatment outcome in children. In: Kotses H, Harver A (eds) Self-management of asthma. Lung biology in health and disease, vol 113. Marcel Dekker, New York, p 63

Bucknall CE, Robertson C, Moran F, Stevenson RD (1988) Management of asthma in the hospital: a prospective audit. BMJ 296:1637–1639

Burrows B (1995) Allergy and the development of asthma and bronchial hyperresponsiveness. Clin Exp Allergy 25:15–16

Bush RK (2001) Environmental asthma. Marcel Dekker, New York, p 186

Castro M, Schechtman KB, Halstead J, Bloomberg G (2001) Risk factors for asthma morbidity and mortality in a large metropolitan city. J Asthma 38(8):625–635

Centers for Disease Control and Prevention (1993) Prevention and control of influenza. Recommendations of the Advisory Committee on Immunization Practices (ACIP). MMWR Recomm Rep 42(6):1–14

Clark TJH, Godfrey S, Lee TH, Thomson NC (2000) Asthma, 4th edn. Oxford University Press, New York, pp 4–5

Coughlin SP (1988) Sports and the asthmatic child: a study of exercise-induced asthma and the resultant handicap. J R Coll Gen Pract 38:253–255

Cousines L, Catanzarite VA (1998) Fetal oxygenation, acidbase balance and assessment of well-being in the pregnancy complicated by asthma or anaphylaxis. In: Schatz M, Zeiger RS, Claman HN (eds) Asthma and immunologic diseases in pregnancy and early infancy. Marcel Dekker, New York, p 27

Crain EF, Walter M, O'Connor GT et al (2002) Home and allergic characteristics of children with asthma in seven US urban communities and design of an environmental intervention: the Inner-City Asthma Study. Environ Health Perspect 110:939–945

Creer TL (1979) Asthma therapy: a behavioral health care system for respiratory disorders. Springer, New York

Creer TL, Bender BG (1993) Asthma. In: Gatchel RJ, Blanchard EB (eds) Psychophysiological disorders: research and clinical applications. American Psychological Association, Washington, DC, pp 151–208

Custovic A, Woodcock A (2001) On allergens and asthma (again): does exposure to allergens in homes exacerbate asthma? (editorial). Clin Exp Allergy 31:670–673

Delaronde S (2002) Using case management to increase anti-inflammatory medication use among a managed care population with asthma. J Asthma 39(1):55–63

Donnelly JE, Donnelly WJ, Thong YH (1987) Parental perceptions and attitudes toward asthma and its treatment: a controlled study. Soc Sci Med 24:431–437

Eggleston PA, Buckley TJ, Breysse PN et al (1999) The environment and asthma in US inner cities. Environ Health Perspect 107(3):439–450

Fritz GK, Wamboldt MZ (1998) Pediatric asthma: psychosomatic interactions and symptom perception. In: Kotses H, Harver A (eds) Self-management of asthma. Lung biology in health and disease, vol 113. Marcel Dekker, New York, p 195

Fritz GK, Yeung A, Wambodt MZ, Spirito A, McQuaid EL, Klein R, Seifer R (1996) Conceptual and methodologic issues in quantifying perceptual accuracy in childhood asthma. J Pediatr Psychol 21:153–173

Gershwin ME, Albertson TE (2001) Bronchial asthma. Principles of diagnosis and treatment. Humana Press, Totowa, NJ

Gift A (1991) Psychologic and physiologic aspects of acute dyspnea in asthmatics. Nurs Res 40:196–199

Global Initiative for Asthma (1995) Global strategy for asthma management and prevention. National Institutes of Health, Bethesda, MD, NIH Publication No. 95-3659

Gross KM, Ponte CD (1998) New strategies in the medical management of asthma. Am Fam Physician 58(1):1–17

Gustafsson PA, Kjellman NIM, Cederblad M (1986) Family therapy in the treatment of severe childhood asthma. J Psychosom Res 30:369–374

Hall JB, Corbridge TC, Rodrigo C, Rodrigo GJ (2000) Acute asthma. McGraw-Hill, New York, p 242, p 281, p 297.

Health Care Financing Administration (1997) Office of the Actuary: Data from the Office of National Health Statistics. Health Care Financing Administration, Washington, DC

Homa DM, Mannino DM, Redd SC (2002) Regional differences in hospitalizations for asthma in the United States, 1988–1996. J Asthma 39(5):449–455

Janson C, Bjornsson E, Hetta J, Boman G (1994) Anxiety and depression in relation to respiratory symptoms and asthma. Am J Respir Crit Care Med 149:930–940

Janson-Bjerklie S, Carrieri VK, Hudes M (1986) The sensation of pulmonary dyspnea. Nurs Res 35:154–159

Janson-Bjerklie S, Ferketich S, Benner P, Becker G (1992) Clinical markers of asthma severity and risk: importance of subjective as well as objective factors. Heart Lung 21:265–272

Janson-Bjerklie S, Ferketich S, Benner P (1993) Predicting the outcomes of living with asthma. Res Nurs Health 16:241–250

Kolbe J, Vamos M, Fergusson W, Elkind G, Garrett J (1996) Differential influences on asthma self-management knowledge and self-management behavior in acute severe asthma. Chest 110:1463–1468

Kotses H, Harver A (1998) Self-management of asthma. Marcel Dekker, New York

Lask B (1992) Psychological treatments for childhood asthma. Arch Dis Child 67:891

Liu C, Feekery C (2001) Can asthma education improve clinical outcomes? An evaluation of a pediatric asthma education program. J Asthma 38(3):269–278

MacLean WE, Perrin JM, Gortmaker S, Pierre CB (1992) Psychological adjustment of children with asthma: effects of illness severity and recent stressful life events. J Pediatr Psychol 17(2):159–171

Mannino MD, Homa DM, Petrowsky CA, Ashizawa A, Nixon LL, Jahnson CA, Ball LB, Jack E, Kang DS (1998) Surveillance for asthma – Unites States, 1960–1995. MMWR CDC Surveill Summ 47:1–28

Milgrom H, Bender B, Ackerson L, Bowry P, Smith B, Rand C (1996) Noncompliance and treatment failure in children with asthma. J Allergy Clin Immunol 98:1051–1057

Mrazek DA (1992) Psychiatric complications of pediatric asthma. Ann Allergy 69:285–294

NAEPP (1991) National Asthma Education and Prevention Program Expert Panel Report. Guidelines for the diagnosis and management of asthma. National Institutes of Health, Bethesda, MD, National Institutes of Health Publication No. 91-3042

NAEPP (1993) National Asthma Education Program Report of the Working Group on Asthma and Pregnancy: management of asthma during pregnancy. National Institutes of Health, Bethesda, MD, NIH Publication No. 93-3279A

NAEPP (1997) National Asthma Education and Prevention Program Expert Panel Report 2. Guidelines for the diagnosis and management of asthma. National Institutes of Health National Heart, Lung, and Blood Institute. Bethesda, MD, National Institutes of Health Publication No. 97-4051

NAEPP (2002) National Asthma Educational Program Expert Panel Report 2. Guidelines for the diagnosis and management of asthma – update on selected topics 2002. National Institutes of Health National Heart, Lung, and Blood Institute. National Institutes of Health, Bethesda, MD, National Institutes of Health Publication No. 02-4052

NAEPP (2007) National Asthma Education and Prevention Program Expert Panel Report 3. Guidelines for the diagnosis and management of asthma. National Institutes of Health, Bethesda, MD, NIH Publications No. 08-4051

National Heart, Lung and Blood Institute, World Health Organization (1995) Global strategy for asthma management and prevention; workshop report. National Institute of Health, Bethesda, MD

NIAID (1979) Asthma and other allergic diseases. NIAID Task Force Report. National Institutes of Health, Bethesda, MD, NIH Publication No. 79-387

Pellegrini DS (1990) Psychosocial risk and protective factors in childhood. J Dev Behav Pediatr 11:201–209

Quirk FH, Jones PW (1990) Patients' perception of distress due to symptoms and effects of asthma on daily living and an investigation of possible influential factors. Clin Sci (Lond) 79:17–21

Roberts RR, Zalenski RJ et al (1997) Costs of an emergency department accelerated diagnostic protocol vs. hospitalization in patients with chest pain: a randomized controlled trial. JAMA 278(20):1670–1676

Ruffin RE, Latimer KM, Schembri DA (1991) Longitudinal study of near fatal asthma. Chest 99(1):77–83

Sandel M, O'Connor G (2002) Inner-city asthma. Immunol Allergy Clin North Am 22:737–752

Sibbauld B, Anderson HR, McGuigan S (1992) Asthma employment in young adults. Thorax 47:19–24

Smith DH, Malone DC et al (1997) A national estimate of the economic costs of asthma. Am J Respir Crit Care Med 156:787–793

Sullivan SD, Weiss KB (1998) Estimates from the National Ambulatory Medical Care Survey (unpublished data)

Taitel MS, Allen L, Creer TL (1998) The impact of asthma on the patient, family, and society. In: Kotses H, Harver A (eds) Self-management of asthma. Marcel Dekker Inc, New York, pp 3–16

Ulrik CS, Backer V, Dirksen A (1992) A 10 year follow-up of 180 adults with bronchial asthma: factors important for the decline in lung function. Thorax 47:14–18

Weiss KB, Gergen PJ et al (1992) An economic evaluation of asthma in the united states. N Engl J Med 326:862–866

Weiss KB, Buist AS, Sullivan SD (2000) Asthma's impact on society. Marcel Dekker, New York

Wray BB (1998) Taking charge of asthma: a lifetime strategy. Wiley, New York, p 7

A close look at asthma. Asthma and Allergy Foundation of America/ National Pharmaceutical Council, www.aafa.org

CDC National Center for Health Statistics. New asthma estimates: tracking prevalence, health care, and mortality. www.cdc.gov/nchs/products/pubs/pubd/hestats/asthma/asthma.htm

Chapter 12
Adolescents and Asthma

David R. Naimi and Andrea J. Apter

Introduction

Adolescence is a time of rapid development where children undergo marked physical, intellectual, and psychosocial growth. This transitional period between childhood and adulthood usually encompasses the second decade of life, although its onset and duration can vary. In children with chronic illness including asthma, adolescence is an important period for establishing proper self-management and coping skills. In fact, asthma is the most common chronic illness of adolescence (Mannino et al. 1998; 2002). The capacity to manage one's disease is an essential component of asthma care and is influenced by adolescents' increasing maturity; growing need for independence and engagement in health risk behaviors. Consequently, effective communication between the adolescent patient, their family, school and health care provider is essential to achieve optimal control. This chapter will review these influences on asthma self-management and discuss their implications for effective patient-provider communication.

Epidemiology of Adolescent Asthma

Over the last two decades, the prevalence of asthma among children of all ages has been on the rise, although new data suggests that it may have reached a plateau in recent years (Akinbami and Schoendorf 2002). Determining asthma prevalence in adolescents requires some estimation, since data is reported using different age ranges. For example, according to the 2005 Youth Risk Behavior Surveillance System (YRBSS), 17% of students had ever been told by a doctor or nurse that they had asthma. The survey found the prevalence of lifetime asthma higher in 11th grade males compared with females (18.2% vs. 14.6%), although in 9th graders the prevalence in females was higher (18.7% vs. 14.6%) (Eaton et al. 2006). Thus, approximately 15% of adolescents have been told at some point in their lives that they have asthma.

According to the latest CDC survey (2002b) of 10–17 year olds, asthma prevalence differs by demographic group and socioeconomic status. American Indians/Alaska Natives have the highest prevalence of lifetime asthma diagnoses (21%), followed by non-Hispanic blacks (18%), non-Hispanic whites (15%), Hispanics (13%), and Asians (7%) (CDC/NCHS 2002a). However, it should be noted that among all ethnicities, Puerto Ricans have the highest prevalence of lifetime asthma (27%) (CDC/NCHS 2002a). The relatively lower total percentage of affected Hispanics is attributed to the Mexican population who demonstrated a lifetime asthma diagnoses of 11% (CDC/NCHS 2002a). Morbidity and mortality rates associated with asthma are significantly higher among racial and ethnic minority groups than nonminority groups (Schwartz et al. 1990). In 2002, the mortality rate for non-Hispanic black children was more than twice than the non-Hispanic whites (CDC/NCHS 2002b). Puerto Ricans have greater asthma mortality rates than non-Hispanic whites, but there is less data for the adolescent age group, for other Latino groups, and other minority groups. Children from low-income families (14%) are more likely to have ever been diagnosed

D.R. Naimi (✉)
Clinical Assistant Professor of Pediatrics, University of Washington, Northwest Asthma & Allergy Center, Suite 200, Springbrook Professional Center, 4540 Sand Point Way NE, Seattle, WA, 98105-3941, USA
e-mail: dnaimi@nwasthma.com

A. Harver and H. Kotses (eds.), *Asthma, Health and Society: A Public Health Perspective*,
DOI 10.1007/978-0-387-78285-0_12,

with asthma and to have more severe asthma than children from more affluent families (12%) (Bloom and Dey 2006; Chen et al. 2003b).

Adolescence is the time of cognitive growth and psychosocial development, which includes formation of identity. This age is also characterized by risky behaviors that threaten health including unprotected sexual activity, cigarette smoking, substance abuse, and poor nutrition all of which can affect adherence and potentially complicate the management of asthma (Bender 2006; Hovell et al. 2003). According to the 2005 YRBSS, 37% of sexually active high school students did not use condoms, 23% had smoked cigarettes in the 30 days before the survey, 43% had drunk alcohol, and 2% had injected an illegal drug (Eaton et al. 2006). Additionally, 80% had not eaten the recommended fruits and vegetables during the 7 days preceding the survey. Along with their nonasthmatic peers, adolescents with asthma have been shown to participate in risk behaviors such as smoking and substance abuse (Bender 2006; Forero et al. 1996; Zbikowski et al. 2002).

Of potential comorbidities in asthmatic adolescents, obesity and depression may be the most significant. Depression affects up to 17% of adolescents (Hankin 2006), and 8.4% of adolescents have attempted suicide (Eaton et al. 2006). In adolescents with asthma, depression may increase the likelihood of risk behaviors such as smoking, which may in turn contribute to poor asthma control (Bender 2006). Additionally, more than 30% of children between 6 and 19 years are overweight or above the 85th percentile for weight (Hedley et al. 2004).

Low-income and minority adolescents are at increased risk for asthma, obesity, and symptoms of depression (Miech et al. 2006; Rushton et al. 2002). Thus, adolescents from low income minority groups are at risk for several comorbidities that can threaten their health.

Asthma as a Chronic Disease

Adolescents with a chronic disease appear to have more difficulty with psychological adjustment, more behavioral disorders, and lower self-esteem (Suris et al. 2004). In general, the impact of a chronic disease on psychosocial development, feelings of well-being, and perception by others is related to the severity of the disease and the intrusiveness of the required treatment (Suris et al. 2004). One survey of elementary school teachers found that asthma is perceived by asthmatic adolescents, their peers, and teachers to have less impact on their lives than other chronic diseases like cystic fibrosis or epilepsy (Olson et al. 2004), although the physical impact of significant asthma was perceived equivalently with diabetes in another study (Wirrell et al. 2006). In that study, teens without asthma regarded asthma as primarily affecting exercise ability of asthmatic peers. Exercise ability may be particularly important to the adolescent age group, but only 4% of surveyed "normal" teens reported any reluctance to befriend a peer with asthma (Wirrell et al. 2006). This suggests that mild asthma is likely to have little psychosocial impact. Nevertheless, feelings of loneliness, unhappiness, depression, and somatic complaints were more frequent in asthmatic adolescents than healthy controls in some but not in all studies (Forero et al. 1996). As in other chronic diseases, the impact of asthma may be more significant with severe disease.

Effect of Asthma on Growth and Puberty

Delayed growth and puberty is common in severe chronic illnesses, particularly in those characterized by chronic inflammation and malnutrition such as cystic fibrosis and inflammatory bowel disease. While permanent growth loss may occur (Kelly et al. 2003), chronic illnesses that are less severe may cause a transient growth delay, ultimately resulting in normal adult height after catch-up growth.

With regards to asthma, the Childhood Asthma Management Program (CAMP) examined whether mild to moderate persistent asthma sufficient to produce a decrease in baseline lung function, is associated with an adverse effect on growth and bone mineral density (BMD) in children. This secondary analysis (the primary analysis was a randomized controlled trial comparing chronic nedocromil with inhaled budesonide) was a cross-sectional study of 1,041 children (32% ethnic/racial minorities and 40% female). The investigators found that in children aged 5–12 years with mild-moderate asthma of as long as 4–7 years' duration did not demonstrate an adverse effect on linear growth or BMD (Kelly et al. 2003). However, a small, transient reduction in growth velocity was observed (The CAMP Research Group 2000). The past use of corticosteroids did not adversely affect either growth or BMD. Other analyses of CAMP data demonstrated no effects of chronic inhaled steroid (budesonide) treatment on the hypothalamic-pituitary-adrenal axis function over a 3-year period (Bacharier et al. 2004). Certainly, in moderate to severe asthma that may require higher doses of inhaled corticosteroids as well as frequent courses of oral steroids, the impact on growth and development may be significant.

Adolescents with delayed puberty, as may occur in severe asthma, may be treated differently by adults and peers, resulting in difficulties in school and work due to their apparent immaturity (Power and Manor 1995). The potential impact of delayed puberty caused by chronic illnesses can affect a child's psychosocial development, altering self-image, and causing emotional immaturity and a subsequent difficulty in separating from parents (Suris et al. 2004).

Barriers to Asthma Control

There are many barriers to asthma control, but some are unique to the adolescent age group and will be reviewed in the following sections. These include cognitive, identity, risk taking, body image, mood, peer and family relationships, socioeconomic, racial/ethnic, and community factors. While exposures to infectious agents and seasonal and perennial allergens are important causes of asthma exacerbations, they are not unique to this age group and are covered thoroughly in other texts (Adkinson et al. 2003). Since self-management skills tend to be deficient in teens (Bruzzese et al. 2004), this manuscript will focus on psychosocial influences of particular importance for asthma self-management that are unique to adolescents (Bruzzese et al. 2004). These barriers can be considered arising from a variety of levels: individual, family and peer interactions, and neighborhood and larger community influences.

Individual Influences

Chronic illnesses including moderate or severe asthma require constant medical management but are also typically characterized by a variable course marked by periods of acute crisis (LeBlanc et al. 2003). There are also asymptomatic periods, occurring more frequently in milder asthma, when medications must be continued. Thus, asthma may require an individual of any age to adjust to frequent medical visits, physical changes, daily medical regimens, and to prepare for recurring acute medical emergencies (Eiser 1990). For adolescents, these accommodations must be achieved in a context of growing independence, increasing ability to understand concepts related to health, and the new assumption of responsibility for self-management. Accommodations for asthma self-management also must occur in the setting of some important health-beliefs unique to this age group surrounding invincibility and pre-occupation with body image (Radzik et al. 2002). Co-morbidities are relatively infrequent in this age group. Nevertheless, in adolescents with asthma, mood fluctuations, behavioral disorders, depression, and obesity are among the most common that are likely to influence asthma outcome.

Adolescent Thinking

Unlike younger children, adolescents can integrate and consider several concepts at once, think abstractly and logically, and solve problems (Radzik et al. 2002). They can understand different perspectives and have an increased capacity to acquire new knowledge (Bruzzese et al. 2004). Adolescents are also able to describe and evaluate their own thinking (Bruzzese et al. 2004). These evolving cognitive skills provide the potential for successful management.

Adolescent Identity

Development of an identity is a key task of adolescence (Radzik et al. 2002). Identity comprises an individual's perceived defining features, values, beliefs, strengths, and weaknesses; is influenced by parents and increasingly by peers; involves formation of self-image and ego and includes significant attention to body image as part of one's identity. Adolescent identity also tends to include beliefs surrounding invulnerability. These perceptions of invulnerability and body image are particularly relevant to the overall health of the adolescent with asthma.

Invulnerability and Risk-Taking Behavior

Perceptions of invulnerability, orientation to the present (Sawyer and Aroni 2005), and lack of impulse control (Radzik et al. 2002) may underlie adolescents' tendency to engage in risky behavior more commonly than adults. Risky behaviors, a leading cause of morbidity and mortality among youth and adults, include unprotected sexual activity, cigarette smoking, abuse of alcohol and other substances, unsafe driving practices, and even poor diet (Eaton et al. 2006; Neinstein et al. 2002). Although preventable, these patterns of risk-behaviors are often established during childhood and peak in mid-adolescence, but may extend into adulthood (Eaton et al. 2006). Reckless behavior has been understood to be a function of the egocentrism of adolescence (Harris et al. 2002), peer-pressure, and other aspects of social environment. Harris et al. (2002) have suggested that a "nothing to lose" attitude is associated with risky behavior. In particular, adolescents with low expectations about their future may have little regard to the consequences of such behavior. It is hypothesized that individuals who do not experience academic success may be at increased risk of engaging in such thinking, while those who go on to college have better expectations of the future and are perhaps, less likely to engage in risky behavior (Harris et al. 2002).

Along with their healthy peers, adolescents with asthma have been shown to participate in risk-taking behaviors such as smoking and substance abuse (Bender 2006; Zbikowski et al. 2002). In fact, smoking rates in adolescents with asthma have been shown to be higher than their healthy peers (Forero et al. 1996; Tyc and Throckmorton-Belzer 2006; Zbikowski et al. 2002). In one community-based study of 4,550 11–17 year olds from Australia, tobacco use and alcohol consumption were higher in asthmatic adolescents (Forero et al. 1996). In another study of asthmatics aged 18–29 years presenting to an emergency department with acute asthma, approximately 33% smoked daily (Silverman et al. 2003). This information is undoubtedly concerning since asthma is particularly recalcitrant to treatment in current smokers (Tomlinson et al. 2005; Tyc and Throckmorton-Belzer 2006).

Risk-taking behaviors may be associated with poor treatment adherence and depression (Bender 2006; Hovell et al. 2003; Kilpatrick et al. 2003). This latter association is important since depression, like risk-taking behavior, is also associated with poor adherence and together may further increase the risk of poor asthma outcome (Bender 2006; DiMatteo et al. 2000). In fact, deaths from asthma are often associated with nonadherence to medications, psychological dysfunction (Jorgensen et al. 2003; Sturdy et al. 2002), denial of symptoms, and poor asthma management (Kravis 1987; Strunk 1987).

Body Image

Body dissatisfaction and distortion of body image peak during adolescence, particularly in females (Bruzzese et al. 2004; Littleton and Ollendick 2003; Radzik et al. 2002). Adolescents with chronic illness report higher dissatisfaction with body image (Suris and Parera 2005). Also, dissatisfaction with body image is common in obese adolescents (Wardle and Cook 2005). This dissatisfaction may result in unhealthy eating behaviors to preserve thinness (Radzik et al. 2002; Suris and Parera 2005). In fact, 12.5% of high school students in the United States had a recent history of going without eating for more than 24 h to lose weight or to keep from gaining weight (Eaton et al. 2006). Body image problems have been observed to lead to an increase in sexual behavior and unsafe practices, which may be increased in adolescents with chronic disease (Suris et al. 2004).

For adolescents with asthma, concern about body image may influence self-care and asthma control. Fear of changes in appearance related to systemic steroids and the perception of change due to inhaled steroids may influence adherence to asthma medications. Concern about appearance may be related to emphasis on athletic achievement (McCreary and Sasses 2000), which may be impaired by significant asthma. Finally, body dissatisfaction has been found to be associated with low self-esteem and negative emotions (Littleton and Ollendick 2003) including depression (Poli et al. 2003; Kelsay et al. 2005), which can also influence asthma outcomes as discussed below.

Behavioral and Mood Disturbances

Behavioral disturbances and depression are common in adolescents. As many as between 20% and 50% of teens report some level of depressive symptoms (Hankin 2006; Sarles and Neinstein 2002). In fact, these conditions are reported to be more common in those with chronic illnesses (LeBlanc et al. 2003). Disease severity and the complexity of its treatment may increase the likelihood of behavioral disturbance (Engström 1999).

Nevertheless, it is well to remember that this finding is not universal (Kean et al. 2006). Studies examining psychological difficulties in children and adolescents with chronic disease including asthma have produced contrasting results, with some finding such a link (Creer et al. 1983; Forero et al. 1996; Forrest et al. 1997; Hambley et al. 1989) and others finding no increase in psychological problems (Bender et al. 2000a, b; Suris et al. 1996; Wamboldt et al. 1998). For example, Wamboldt et al. (1998), in a study of 337 children aged 7–19 years, demonstrated that children and adolescents with severe asthma did not rate themselves as having higher levels of anxiety than those with mild or moderate asthma or healthy controls. However, in a cross-sectional survey conducted on a school sample of more than 3,000 U.S. teenagers, Forrest et al. (1997) found that those with asthma and recent wheezing had more physical and emotional symptoms, poorer functional status, lower perceived well-being, more negative behaviors that threatened to disrupt social development, and a greater number of co-morbidities.

The conflicting findings in these studies may in part be explained by the differences in the subject populations. The studies that found relatively little psychological difficulty among adolescents and children with asthma largely consisted of subjects from outpatient clinical sites (Bender et al. 2000a, b) who likely have milder asthma than those requiring prolonged hospitalizations for asthma (Creer et al. 1983; Hambley et al. 1989). The data from all of these studies suggests that in asthma, as in other chronic illnesses, severity of disease is associated with a greater adverse impact on psychological functioning.

Several studies suggest that adolescents with asthma can be more vulnerable to panic symptoms (Perna et al. 1997; Rietveld et al. 2005; Goodwin et al. 2004; Gillaspy et al. 2002). Also, both adolescents with asthma and parents of adolescents who have experienced a life-threatening asthma exacerbation may have high levels of posttraumatic stress symptoms, which can accompany functional impairment due to asthma (Kean et al. 2006). Thus, asthma symptoms can be frightening to patients and their caretakers, resulting in symptoms that can mimic asthma accompanied by symptoms that are manifestations of poor asthma control.

Depression often begins in adolescence (Hankin 2006) and may occur with other disorders, particularly anxiety and disruptive behavioral disorders (Hankin 2006). Depression and anxiety, common in patients with asthma, can be associated with an increase in risky behaviors such as smoking and substance abuse and negatively correlated with treatment adherence (Bender 2006; DiMatteo et al. 2000; Kilpatrick et al. 2003). According to a 21-year longitudinal study in adolescents and young adults, asthma was associated with an increased likelihood of major depression, panic attacks, and any anxiety disorders when compared with individuals without asthma (Goodwin et al. 2004).

The mechanistic link behind the statistical association of asthma with depressive and anxiety disorders is complex and unclear. These associations could reflect the fact that asthma may provoke depression or anxiety disorders, or that depression and anxiety disorders may provoke asthma (Goodwin et al. 2004). In addition, other confounding factors such as genetic vulnerability (Wright et al. 2005) or distressed caretaker–child relationships and other negative events may account for some of the comorbidity of asthma and depressive/anxiety disorders, rather than a direct causal link (Goodwin et al. 2004).

Obesity

Besides depression, the comorbidity most likely to impact adolescent asthma is obesity (Hedley et al. 2004). As the overall prevalence of asthma in children and adolescents has increased over the last two decades (Mannino et al. 2002), so has the prevalence of obesity in this age group (Hedley et al. 2004). Among adolescents (12–19 years) and younger children (6–11 years) 16% are overweight according to the 1999–2002 data from the National Center for Health Statistics (Hedley et al. 2004). These numbers are triple the rate of obesity for adolescents in 1980 (Hedley et al. 2004). An additional 15% was considered at risk of becoming overweight defined as between the 85th and 95th percentile of sex-specific Body Mass Index (BMI) (Hedley et al. 2004). Overweight adolescents are at increased risk of developing diabetes as an adolescent. They are also at risk for becoming overweight as an adult, and acquiring the obesity-related health problems of adults including diabetes and cardiovascular disease (Hedley et al. 2004). Additionally, in adolescents, obesity is a risk factor for depression and depression is a risk factor for obesity (McElroy et al. 2004); and as a result, the combination adds to a risk of poor asthma control.

The increased prevalence of obesity among children in the United States is highest among Mexican–American (23%) and non-Hispanic black adolescents (21%) when compared to non-Hispanic white adolescents (14%) (Hedley et al. 2004). Thus, the groups at increased risk for asthma and obesity overlap. The recent dramatic increase in both high BMI and asthma has led to the hypothesis that increased weight causes asthma (Flaherman and Rutherford 2006).

Although a number of studies have shown a statistical association between asthma and obesity in children, adolescents, and adults, the finding is not universal (Beuther et al. 2006; Chinn 2003; Ford et al. 2004). Some studies have been limited by self-report data of BMI or asthma (Gilliland et al. 2003; Gold et al. 2003; Flaherman and Rutherford 2006; Guerra et al. 2004). Some of these studies had cross-sectional designs (Figueroa-Muñoz et al. 2001) that do not allow conclusions about whether asthma predicts obesity, and obesity is associated with future asthma, or if a causal relationship is lacking. A randomized trial would provide excellent support for a causal relationship but such studies are rarely feasible or practical.

Several longitudinal studies have examined the relationship between asthma and obesity in children and adolescents. Gold et al. (2003) in a large study of 6–14 year olds followed for 5 years, found an increased risk of asthma (parent report of doctor-diagnosed asthma with persistent wheeze) in obese children. Gilliland et al. (2003) in a large study of 7–18 year olds followed for 4 years also found the risk of developing asthma was higher in those who were obese. In a population-based cohort study, Guerra et al. (2004) found that being overweight at age 11 was associated with a threefold increased risk for persistence of infrequent wheezing after the onset of puberty and with a twofold increased risk for persistent asthma. Finally, in a recent meta-analysis of the effect of high weight on asthma, high body weight among school-aged children increased the risk of future asthma by approximately 50% (Flaherman and Rutherford 2006). Although these studies were longitudinal, they were also observational and used self-report of a doctor's diagnosis of asthma without more stringent diagnostic criteria such as spirometry.

The biological basis for a causal relationship between asthma and obesity is not clear but several possibilities have been suggested. Some have postulated that dietary components associated with hypercholesterolemia (Al-Shawwa et al. 2006) or increased intake of polyunsaturated fats might provide links between obesity and asthma (Flaherman and Rutherford 2006). A more detailed theory is that leptin, increased in obese humans, is a promoter of inflammation in which its structure is similar to interleukin-6 (IL-6), a promoter of T-cell proliferation and activation (Beuther et al. 2006). Other possible links of asthma and obesity may be the presence of gastroesophageal reflux (which is prevalent in both conditions), hormonal influences, atopy, chronic systemic inflammation, and the mechanical effects of obesity (Beuther et al. 2006; Flaherman and Rutherford 2006; Shore and Fredberg 2005). Finally, excess weight may cause shortness of breath and exercise intolerance that may be mistaken for asthma.

To support the hypothesis that weight plays a role in the persistence of asthma symptoms, studies are needed to demonstrate that weight reduction among individuals with well-characterized asthma results in improvements in lung function and decreased symptoms (Guerra et al. 2004). However, to date, there are relatively few published reports of such research. One trial of 14 adults, randomized subjects to a very restrictive diet for a short duration of time (Hakala et al. 2000; Stenius-Aarniala et al. 2000). Other studies have examined the effects of bariatric surgery in adults. While improvement in respiratory comorbidities have been described (Spivak et al. 2005), many of the studies of bariatric surgery patients have been observational without strict criteria for asthma (Ahroni et al. 2005; Spivak et al. 2005). In summary, an explanation of how obesity could cause asthma has not been established. Moreover, most of the limited research is in adults, and the application of these findings to adolescents who do not undergo surgery is unclear.

Family and Peer Interactions

Adolescence is characterized by increasing separation from caregivers and increasing dependency on peers. Family well-being influences asthma in adolescents while severe asthma can reciprocally impact family functioning. The growing influence of peers on the adolescent can also influence asthma outcomes.

Separation from Caregivers

Emerging autonomy allows adolescents the potential for responsible self-management. However, the demands of managing a significant chronic illness can instead increase dependence on the family and caregivers at a time when an adolescent should be gaining more independence (Eiser and Berrenberg 1995). The desire for autonomy and independence may lead adolescents to consider caregiver input nagging, which may cause adolescents to avoid taking their medicine (Penza-Clyve et al. 2004). Medical personnel may hold parents accountable for adherence behaviors of their teenagers, while also encouraging adolescents to assume responsibility for their illness (Sawyer and Aroni 2005). Parents may feel accused of being overprotective when, from their perspective, they are fulfilling their parental obligations (Sawyer and Aroni 2005).

Impact of Asthma on Family

Chronic illness is not only a problem for the child or adolescent to endure, but also for the family. The presence of an adolescent with a chronic condition imposes an increased burden on the caregivers (Cadman et al. 1991). Given that the severity of chronic illnesses varies and that measures of family function are not standardized, it is not surprising that researchers' findings of the impact of such illnesses on family dynamics is not uniform (Suris et al. 2004). Some families adequately cope with this situation while others are overwhelmed by the problems brought on by the condition (Suris et al. 2004).

Since asthma is a chronic disease, it places increased demands on parental time and energy (Kurnat and Moore 1999). Lack of knowledge about the disease, fear of their child dying, and anxiety about their child's health contribute to increased levels of stress and anxiety among parents of asthmatics (Jerrett and Costello 1996). Parental loss of workdays owing to their children's asthma is substantial. During one 12-month study, nearly 30% of caregivers of asthmatic children lost workdays during the study because of their child's illness, and more than 13% of caregivers lost more than 5 days (Sherman and Milgrom 2005). Caregiver absenteeism significantly correlated with all components of asthma control (use of relievers, nocturnal symptoms, impairment of activities, and asthma crises) (Sherman and Milgrom 2005). A significant eightfold risk of losing more than 5 workdays by caregivers was observed when the child's asthma was poorly controlled (Sherman and Milgrom 2005). As indicated in the next section, how well the family copes with the child's asthma ultimately influences the asthma outcome.

Impact of the Family on Asthma

There is a tendency for families of severely asthmatic adolescents to have psychological disturbances (Chesson et al. 2004; Kaugars et al. 2004; Klinnert et al. 1994; Klinnert et al. 2001; Mrazek et al. 1999; Wamboldt et al. 1996). Klinnert et al. (2001) found that parenting difficulties early in a child's infancy predict asthma onset and persistence. The mental health status of a child's caretaker has also been shown to be a significant factor when predicting hospitalizations due to asthma in a study of 4–9 year olds (Weil et al. 1999). In a study of 115 children, aged 4–18, Chen et al. (2003a) found that repeat hospitalizations for asthma were associated with characteristics of a child's caretaker: a lower sense of mastery and being less emotionally bothered by their child's asthma. These investigators also found that a history of hospitalizations for asthma was associated with greater family strain, conflict, and financial difficulties.

Kaugars et al. (2004) hypothesized two pathways that may explain the relationship between family characteristics and asthma outcomes: (1) that family conflict and stressors can affect the asthma management behaviors of a family, and (2) that there may be an association between family characteristics, physiologic (hypothalamic pituitary axis and autonomic nervous system) functioning, and asthma outcomes. The relationship between family dynamics and stressors, physiologic factors, and asthma control needs further study in order to fully understand the complexities involved in pediatric asthma.

Influence of Peers

As adolescents separate from their families and form their individual identity, their reliance on peers increases (Bruzzese et al. 2004). These peer relationships and friendships play a critical role in the development of the adolescent's identity (Ladd 1999;

Radzik et al. 2002). Adolescents exchange ideas and feelings, and develop values, attitudes and behaviors with peers (Suris et al. 2004). Self-image also evolves under the influence of peers.

In children with chronic illness, the development of peer relationships and self-image issues may be in conflict with the demands of chronic illness treatment regimens or the disability itself (Suris et al. 2004). Furthermore, young people with chronic conditions may become excluded from their peer group, especially in those with taxing medical conditions or those that mark them out as very different (Manworren 1996). Difficulty with peers can lead to anxiety or emotional disturbance and may impact the teens' ability to manage their asthma.

Peer groups can either hinder or facilitate adolescents' asthma management (Bruzzese et al. 2004). As social relationships develop, adolescents may choose not to take medications in certain circumstances due to social barriers (McQuaid et al. 2003; Penza-Clyve et al. 2004). Whereas a younger child may feel less embarrassed in making a quick visit to the school nurse for medication, a teenager might not want to leave the lunchroom for fear of "standing out" (McQuaid et al. 2003). Adolescents may need to take their asthma medications in public places, which may be embarrassing (Slack and Brooks 1995). Thus, some teens with chronic lung disease may struggle with peer relationships because of having the fear of peer rejection and isolation occurring as a result of social, emotional and physical consequences of their underlying lung disease and its treatment (Fitzgerald 2001).

If adolescents with asthma are able to be part of peer groups that have positive attitudes regarding asthma, the outcome may be positive for the adolescent (Bruzzese et al. 2004). For example, when friends accept the potential need for visible treatment for asthma, adolescents are more likely to adhere to the treatment plans (Bruzzese et al. 2004). A small study assessing peer relationships in children with asthma demonstrated that asthmatic children (ages 8–13) had peer relationships that were equivalent to those of their classmates, although they were seen as being sicker and missing more school (Graetz and Shute 1995). Those children who experienced more hospitalizations were less preferred as playmates, perceived as more sensitive, isolated, and lonely (Graetz and Shute 1995).

The Influence of the Larger Community: Socioeconomic Status (SES) and Racial and Ethnic Disparities in Asthma Care in Adolescents

The social environment, that is, the community in which an adolescent lives, can have a profound effect on a teen's health (Leventhal et al. 2005). Race and socioeconomic resources significantly influence asthma outcome and the impact of each is usually difficult to separate from the other. Discrimination against racial and ethnic minorities influences access to socioeconomic resources, including health care. A recent Institute of Medicine report, Unequal Treatment (Smedley et al. 2003), found differences in health care provided to patients on the basis of their race-ethnicity even when access related factors such as patients' insurance status and income were controlled. That is, the poorer health outcomes seen in minority groups could be attributed, in part, to differences in the health care provided and to access to that care.

Access to healthcare in poor communities is more difficult to obtain than in more affluent communities. Availability of medical facilities, practices with specific expertise in caring for asthma, and pharmacies may be limited. Features of area medical practices such as the lack of evening hours may limit access. In a study of characteristics of primary care practices serving Medicaid patients, Lowe et al. (2005) found that emergency department use was lower in practices with evening hours and a lower ratio of number of active patients per clinician-hour of practice time. In some communities, there may be no accommodations made for language and cultural differences, which can impair communication. Lieu et al. (2004), in a prospective cohort study of Medicaid-insured children with asthma, found practice sites that promote cultural competence (e.g., recruits ethnically diverse and bilingual staff, offers training to minimize cultural barriers and promotes communication), use reports to clinicians (e.g., lists of asthma patients, registries that prompt clinicians about medications, feedback reports to clinicians, reminders to clinicians of guideline recommendations), and promote access and continuity (encourages appointments for preventive chronic asthma management, provides telephone advice including evenings and weekends, ensures primary care follow-up after an urgent visit) gave higher quality of care.

Within the health care facilities, there is evidence that poor and minority patients including adolescents are less likely to get the same quality of care as white patients (Elster et al. 2003; Smedley et al. 2003; Wallace et al. 2004). Specifically with respect to asthma, several studies of Medicaid-insured children with asthma found that Black and Latino children had worse asthma status than white children but were less-likely to receive and use inhaled anti-inflammatory medication (Ferris et al. 2006; Lieu et al. 2002).

At the larger neighborhood level, there are other factors that may influence asthma outcomes. African-American and Latino children are approximately three times more likely than non-Hispanic white children to come from poor families (Leventhal et al. 2005). Families that are poor and minority, particularly those in urban areas, are more likely to live in poor neighborhoods (Leventhal et al. 2005). Such communities have fewer resources such as hospitals, high quality schools, public transportation, and grocery stores (Evans 2004; Atkins et al. 2006). Schools in poorer communities are likely to have less health education, and less availability of on-site nurses (Hillemeier et al. 2006). Children from these communities are more likely to be exposed to violence, which can impact their academic performance, and result in high rates of depression and disruptive behavior (Schwartz and Gorman 2003). Poorer neighborhoods may be targeted for more advertising of tobacco and alcohol; smoking may be more prevalent in these neighborhoods (Dell et al. 2005); thus, these teens are more likely to be exposed to smoking behavior.

Low SES has been associated in children with more frequent exposure to violence and other stressful events. Poor housing and living conditions can be stressful. One study found that children of Latino and African-American families in urban public housing communities are two to four times more likely to suffer from chronic physical and mental conditions than the general population (Bazargan et al. 2005). Exposure to violence predicted in a graded fashion more symptom days in children with asthma and more nights of lost sleep by their caretakers, even when controlling for SES, housing deterioration and negative life events (e.g., death of a family member) (Wright et al. 2004). Chen et al. (2006) demonstrated that, in children with asthma, lower SES was associated with higher levels of stress and threat perception. These findings were associated with increased production of interleukin-5 (IL-5), interleukin-13 (IL-13), and higher eosinophil counts.

Many studies on the relationship between SES and asthma focus on children over a large age span. There is a relative paucity of data aimed at clarifying this relationship specifically in adolescents. The contribution of community factors to health compared with individual and family factors requires further research not only in children, but also more specifically in adolescents. Provided the adolescent has access to medications like inhaled steroids and necessary health services, the impact of these individual, family and peer, and neighborhood/community barriers to asthma control are frequently mediated by adherence.

Adherence

The World Health Organization recently defined adherence to long-term therapy, as "the extent to which a person's behavior – taking medication, following a diet, and/or executing lifestyle changes, corresponds with agreed recommendations from a health care provider," Rand 1993). This definition emphasizes agreement and communication between patient and provider and stresses a broader range of activities in addition to medication taking. Adherence therefore involves self-management, but extends beyond a discussion of taking medication to include other behaviors like keeping appointments, refilling medications, and abstinence from smoking. Nevertheless, much of the available research on adherence in asthma including adolescents is centered on taking medication.

Although older children have been shown to know more about asthma and assume more responsibility for disease management than their younger counterparts (McQuaid et al. 2003), adherence in adolescents is poorer than for younger children (Bender et al. 2000a, b; McQuaid et al. 2003). In one study, electronic monitors were placed on daily asthma inhalers for 1 month and subjects were told that medication use was recorded (McQuaid et al. 2003). In the 14–16 year old subjects, the mean adherence calculated as the number of recorded daily doses divided by number of prescribed doses averaged over a month, was 42% ± 29%.

In considering the individual barriers presented earlier, the orientation of adolescents to the present and their tendency to feel invulnerable are likely to limit the incentive for taking chronic medications like inhaled steroids. Concern about body image and fear of weight gain may motivate some adolescents to avoid taking oral or inhaled corticosteroids.

At the family level, taking medications may become part of the battle for independence with parents (Logan et al. 2003). Family habits, pressures, lack of cohesiveness, and upheaval are associated with low adherence (Bender 2006; DiMatteo 2004a, b). Mood disorders, high risk behaviors, and nonadherence tend to accompany one another and together make asthma control problematic (Bender 2006). In fact, deaths from pediatric asthma have been shown to be associated with denial of symptoms, poor asthma management and adherence, intense family conflict, and psychological dysfunction (Strunk et al. 1985).

Activities with peers may interfere with medication taking. If adolescents are engaged in an activity with peers that they do not want to interrupt, some may forget to take their medications (Penza-Clyve et al. 2004). More important, adolescents may not take medications because of concerns that they would be viewed unfavorably by peers if it was known that they have asthma or take medicine.

Minority and poor adolescents with asthma have been reported to be less likely to adhere to medication regimens. Cooper and Hickson (2001) found black youth less likely than white youth to fill a prescription for corticosteroids after an emergency department visit for asthma. Black and Hispanic children were shown to be significantly less likely than white children to use daily inhaled anti-inflammatory medication (Lieu et al. 2002). Emergency department use for asthma has been reported to be greater among black children than compared to white children, while black children were also less likely than were white children to have an office visit for asthma (Lozano et al. 1995). However, further research is necessary to completely understand the relative impact of the myriad of barriers to adherence that adolescents with asthma face at all levels (e.g., neighborhood stresses, family stresses, difficulty scheduling appointments and accessing health care).

Many health-related behavioral patterns formed in adolescence continue into adulthood (van Es et al. 2001). Therefore, intervening in adolescence has the potential to instill in youth a preventive style of asthma management that is likely to continue into adulthood (Bruzzese et al. 2004).

Unique Influences of Asthma on the Life of Adolescents

While previous sections have demonstrated the importance of the social environment on asthma control, reciprocally, there are unique features of adolescent life affected by asthma control: school, sleep, and exercise.

Influences of Asthma on School and Sports

Success in school is important for an individual's subsequent vocational and academic success and eventual financial independence (Suris et al. 2004). School experiences influence self-image (Harris et al. 2002); it is where peer pressure is applied, popularity or lack of it is experienced, romantic and platonic relationships emerge, and where classes and sports activities lead to success or failure. It may also be a place where teens may be exposed to violence, tobacco, and drugs, which if pursued can influence adherence and asthma control.

Across illness types, children and teenagers with chronic conditions are more likely than their healthy peers to miss school due to their condition or its treatment (Fowler et al. 1985; Suris et al. 2004). They are also more likely to skip school (Charlton et al. 1991; Suris et al. 2004). According to the National Health Interview Survey in 2002, children and adolescents of 5–17 years of age missed 14.7 million school days due to asthma and had more absences than nonasthmatic children (CDC/NCHS 2002b).

There is conflicting evidence about the impact of asthma on school performance (Fowler et al. 1992). Some studies show that children with asthma are at higher risk for problems with academic achievement (Fowler et al. 1992). US data from the National Health Interview Survey in 1988 suggest that after adjusting for age, sex, race/ethnicity, maternal education, and income, asthmatic children have similar risks of grade failure and suspension/expulsion, but increased risk of having a learning disability (Fowler et al. 1992). Also, children with asthma from low-income families had twice the odds of grade failure when compared with well-equipped children (Fowler et al. 1992).

Sleep disturbance is more common in adolescent asthmatics (Yeatts and Shy 2001). Diette et al. (2000)

determined that the presence of nocturnal asthma symptoms in children and adolescents was associated with decreased school attendance and performance, as well as with missed work in their parents. Thus, it has been hypothesized that asthma, by impairing a child and adolescent's sleep patterns, can result in school absence which threatens academic and career success.

Studies reporting low school performance or learning disabilities in children and adolescents with asthma have often relied on subjective measures, such as parental surveys about their child's school performance (Diette et al. 2000; Fowler et al. 1992). Many parents believe that asthma or asthma medications can cause learning problems in their child, when in fact these children's objective scores on achievement tests were as high as those of their peers (Roder et al. 2003). However, when objective measures have been used to evaluate school performance via standardized tests, the results generally do not support the conclusion that asthma or its treatment places children at risk for a learning disability or low school performance (MacLean et al. 1992; Roder et al. 2003; Silverstein et al. 2001). In fact, children and adolescents with asthma tend to have higher standardized scores than national norms (Silverstein et al. 2001). Nevertheless, physicians should ensure that families are aware of the potential impact of asthma on academics, and school absenteeism and encourage appropriate planning and coordination between family and school (LeBlanc et al. 2003).

Exercise-Induced Bronchospasm (EIB) in the Adolescent

Uncontrolled asthma interferes with participation in sports or other physical activities, thus compromising relations with peers (Bruzzese et al. 2004). Sports and physical activity play an important role in the life of an adolescent, yet adolescents with asthma are 20 times more likely to have limitations on physical activity than asymptomatic adolescents (Yeatts and Shy 2001). Approximately 50–90% of all individuals with asthma have airways that are hyper-reactive to exercise and up to 38% of athletes have been reported to have EIB (Rundell and Jenkinson 2002). Thus, individuals with asthma may limit their participation in aerobic activities (Garfinkel et al. 1992), which may impair their quality of life (Hallstrand et al. 2003).

It has been reported that asthmatics as a group have a decreased level of physical fitness because of their relative inactivity (Mannix et al. 2004). Interestingly, this limited fitness level in asthmatic subjects seems not to be related to their degree of obstruction, but rather to their decreased levels of habitual activity (Lucas and Platts-Mills 2005). Therefore, exercise conditioning in asthmatics is said to be an important part of the management and treatment for all cases of asthma (Lucas and Platts-Mills 2005). The benefits of conditioning on asthma are both subjective (increased participation in activities, improved emotional status, and decreased intensity of wheezing attacks) and objective (improved running performance and increased aerobic fitness) (Lucas and Platts-Mills 2005).

EIB may go unrecognized if an adolescent is reluctant to report symptoms to their parents or coaches or to seek a physician's advice (Rupp et al. 1993). Sometimes symptoms of EIB such as coughing, wheezing, and chest tightness are perceived as normal responses to exercise (Mannix et al. 2004). In addition, because athletes are generally fit and healthy, the presence of a significant medical problem may not be considered (Parsons and Mastronarde 2005). It is important to note that occasionally, a death occurring in close association with a sporting event or physical activity is attributed to asthma (Becker et al. 2004). On the other hand, adolescents such as those who are obese or otherwise out-of-shape may experience shortness of breath with exercise that is then incorrectly attributed to asthma.

Caring for the Adolescent with Asthma

Adolescents must have a voice in their own health care (Ginsburg et al. 2002). That is, adolescents, particularly those with chronic disease, want their physicians to be honest with them, allow them the opportunity to participate in their own care, and have their viewpoints and concerns taken seriously (Britto et al. 2004; Ginsburg et al. 1995). The characteristics of the provider are a major determinant as to whether an adolescent will seek preventive care (Ginsburg et al. 2002). Adolescents want a strong interpersonal relationship with their health care provider, a sense of emotional and physical safety, and a trustworthy provider who can offer counseling, privacy (Ginsburg et al. 2002) and clear communication (DiMatteo et al. 2004). Indeed, effective communication has been shown to promote adherence (DiMatteo et al. 2004b).

Once trust and communication are established, providers should explore the psychosocial environment of the adolescent with asthma as summarized in Table 12.1. The environment should be assessed at the level of individual factors, family and peer dynamics, as well as community and neighborhood characteristics. For example, on an individual level, the adolescent should be asked about risk-taking behavior, mood or behavioral disorders (Smith and Shuchman 2005), sleep quality, body image, risk factors for obesity, activity limitation, and adherence. It is important to assess the psychological functioning of the adolescent particularly when asthma is severe. Family interactions, caretaker mental health (DiMatteo et al. 2004; Kaugars et al. 2004; LeBlanc et al. 2003; Weil et al. 1999), and peer dynamics also must be explored. On the community level, the teen's progress in school, school attendance, and other resources within the larger community in which the teen lives should be analyzed.

Table 12.1 Factors to consider in the psychosocial assessment of adolescents with asthma

Individual factors
Trends in physical growth, development, and onset of puberty
Defining characteristics of the adolescent's identity
Cognitive skills, ability to problem-solve
Perception of invulnerability
Impulse control
Risk-taking behavior such as
Smoking and the use of other substances
Unprotected sexual activity
Unsafe driving
Perception of body image
Presence of obesity and eating disorders
Activity limitation
Mood disorders and depression
Psychological stressors
Sleep quality
Adherence
Family and peer relations
Functioning within the family
Gaining independence from the family
Availability of family resources: financial, social, environmental
Caretaker mental health
Quality of peer relationships
Community and neighborhood resources
School performance and attendance
Availability of resources for health, learning, recreation, transportation
Membership in religious and other community groups
Exposure to violence

Adolescents comprise a unique patient group in that they are undergoing a transition from childhood to adulthood, while experiencing rapid changes in cognitive and physical development. As in all chronic diseases, risk taking behaviors, peer group pressures, family relationships, psychological stressors, socioeconomic status, and race/ethnicity can all potentially play a role in complicating disease management. During a single clinic visit, it can be a daunting task to address all of the needs of an adolescent patient. Realistically, establishing a relationship with effective communication between the adolescent and provider can take a number of visits. This is particularly important for the adolescent severely affected by asthma. Such a physician–teen relationship will benefit the adolescent for years to come and facilitate a smooth transition from pediatric to adult centered health care. At the same time, this relationship will be intensely rewarding for the clinician.

Acknowledgements We gratefully acknowledge Bruce G. Bender, PhD, Head, Pediatric Behavioral Health, National Jewish Medical and Research Center for his invaluable review and suggestions.

References

Adkinson FN, Yunginger JW, Busse WW, Bochner BS, Holgate ST, Simons EF (2003) Middleton's allergy principles and practice. Mosby, Philadelphia

Ahroni JH, Montgomery KF, Watkins BM (2005) Laparoscopic adjustable gastric banding: weight loss, co-morbidities, medication usage and quality of life at one year. Obes Surg 15(5):641–647

Akinbami LJ, Schoendorf KC (2002) Trends in childhood asthma: prevalence, health care utilization, and mortality. Pediatrics 110(2 Pt 1):315–322

Al-Shawwa B, Al-Huniti N, Titus G, Abu-Hasan M (2006) Hypercholesterolemia is a potential risk factor for asthma. J Asthma 43(3):231–233

Atkins MS, Frazier SL, Birman D, Adil JA, Jackson M, Graczyk PA, Talbott E, Farmer AD, Bell CC, McKay MM (2006) School-based mental health services for children living in high poverty urban communities. Adm Policy Ment Health 33(2):146–159

Bacharier LB, Raissy HH, Wilson L, McWilliams B, Strunk RC, Kelly HW (2004) Long-term effect of budesonide on hypothalamic-pituitary-adrenal axis function in children with mild to moderate asthma. Pediatrics 113(6):1693–1699

Bazargan M, Calderon JL, Heslin KC, Mentes C, Shaheen MA, Ahdout J, Baker RS (2005) A profile of chronic mental and physical conditions among African-American and Latino children in urban public housing. Ethn Dis 15(4 Suppl 5):S5-3-9.

Becker JM, Rogers J, Rossini G, Mirchandani H, D'Alonzo GE Jr (2004) Asthma deaths during sports: report of a 7-year experience. J Allergy Clin Immunol 113(2):264–267

Bender BG (2006) Risk taking, depression, adherence, and symptom control in adolescents and young adults with asthma. Am J Respir Crit Care Med 173(9):953–957

Bender BG, Annett RD, Ikle D, DuHamel TR, Rand C, Strunk RC (2000a) Relationship between disease and psychological adaptation in children in the Childhood Asthma Management Program and their families. CAMP Research Group. Arch Pediatr Adolesc Med 154(7):706–713

Bender B, Wamboldt FS, O'Connor SL, Rand C, Szefler S, Milgrom H, Wamboldt MZ (2000b) Measurement of children's asthma medication adherence by self report, mother report, canister weight, and Doser CT. Ann Allergy Asthma Immunol 85(5):416–421

Beuther DA, Weiss ST, Sutherland ER (2006) Obesity and asthma. Am J Respir Crit Care Med 174(2):112–119

Bloom B, Dey AN (2006) Summary health statistics for U.S. children: National health interview survey, 2004. National Center for Health Statistics, Vital Health Stat 10(227):1–85

Britto MT, DeVellis RF, Hornung RW, DeFriese GH, Atherton HD, Slap GB (2004) Health care preferences and priorities of adolescents with chronic illnesses. Pediatrics 114(5):1272–1280

Bruzzese JM, Bonner S, Vincent EJ, Sheares BJ, Mellins RB, Levison MJ, Wiesemann S, Du Y, Zimmerman BJ, Evans D (2004) Asthma education: the adolescent experience. Patient Educ Couns 55(3):396–406

Cadman D, Rosenbaum P, Boyle M, Offord DR (1991) Children with chronic illness: family and parent demographic characteristics and psychosocial adjustment. Pediatrics 87(6):884–889

Centers for Disease Control and Prevention, National Center for Health Statistics, Hyattsville, MD. (2002) Asthma prevalence, health care use, and mortality. http://www.cdc.gov/nchs/fastats/asthma.htm 7 Apr 2006

Centers for Disease Control and Prevention, National Center for Health Statistics, Hyattsville, MD. (2002–2004) Health Data for All Ages (HDAA). http://www.cdc.gov/nchs/fastats/asthma.htm. 18 Aug 2006

Charlton A, Larcombe IJ, Meller ST, Morris Jones PH, Mott MG, Potton MW, Tranmer MD, Walker JJ (1991) Absence from school related to cancer and other chronic conditions. Arch Dis Child 66(10):1217–1222

Chen E, Bloomberg GR, Fisher EB Jr, Strunk RC (2003a) Predictors of repeat hospitalizations in children with asthma: the role of psychosocial and socioenvironmental factors. Health Psychol 22(1):12–18

Chen E, Fisher EB, Bacharier LB, Strunk RC (2003b) Socioeconomic status, stress, and immune markers in adolescents with asthma. Psychosom Med 65(6):984–992

Chen E, Hanson MD, Paterson LQ, Griffin MJ, Walker HA, Miller GE (2006) Socioeconomic status and inflammatory processes in childhood asthma: the role of psychological stress. J Allergy Clin Immunol 117(5):1014–1020

Chesson RA, Chisholm D, Zaw W (2004) Counseling children with chronic physical illness. Patient Educ Couns 55(3):331–338

Chinn S (2003) Obesity and asthma: evidence for and against a causal relation. J Asthma 40(1):1–16

Cooper WO, Hickson GB (2001) Corticosteroid prescription filling for children covered by Medicaid following an emergency department visit or a hospitalization for asthma. Arch Pediatr Adolesc Med 155(10):1111–1115

Creer TL, Ipacs J, Creer PP (1983) Changing behavioral and social variables at a residential treatment facility for childhood asthma. J Asthma 20(1):11–15

Dell JL, Whitman S, Shah AM, Silva A, Ansell D (2005) Smoking in 6 diverse Chicago communities – a population study. Am J Public Health 95(6):1036–1042

Diette GB, Markson L, Skinner EA, Nguyen TT, Algatt-Bergstrom P, Wu AW (2000) Nocturnal asthma in children affects school attendance, school performance, and parents' work attendance. Arch Pediatr Adolesc Med 154(9):923–928

DiMatteo MR (2004a) Social support and patient adherence to medical treatment: a meta-analysis. Health Psychol 23(2):207–218

DiMatteo MR (2004b) The role of effective communication with children and their families in fostering adherence to pediatric regimens. Patient Educ Couns 55(3):339–344

DiMatteo MR, Lepper HS, Croghan TW (2000) Depression is a risk factor for noncompliance with medical treatment: meta-analysis of the effects of anxiety and depression on patient adherence. Arch Intern Med 160(14):2101–2107

Eaton DK, Kann L, Kinchen S, Ross J, Hawkins J, Harris WA, Lowry R, McManus T, Chyen D, Shanklin S, Lim C, Grunbaum JA, Wechsler H (2006) Youth risk behavior surveillance – United States, 2005. J Sch Health 76(7):353–372

Eiser C (1990) Psychological effects of chronic disease. J Child Psychol Psychiatry 31(1):85–98

Eiser C, Berrenberg JL (1995) Assessing the impact of chronic disease on the relationship between parents and their adolescents. J Psychosom Res 39(2):109–114

Elster A, Jarosik J, VanGeest J, Fleming M (2003) Racial and ethnic disparities in health care for adolescents: a systematic review of the literature. Arch Pediatr Adolesc Med 157(9):867–874

Engström I (1999) Inflammatory bowel disease in children and adolescents: mental health and family functioning. J Pediatr Gastroenterol Nutr 28(4):S28–S33

Evans GW (2004) The Environment of childhood poverty. Am Psychol 59(2):77–92

Ferris TG, Kuhlthau K, Ausiello J, Perrin J, Kahn R (2006) Are minority children the last to benefit from a new technology? Technology diffusion and inhaled corticosteriods for asthma. Med Care 44(1):81–86

Figueroa-Muñoz JI, Chinn S, Rona RJ (2001) Association between obesity and asthma in 4–11 year old children in the UK. Thorax 56(2):133–137

Fitzgerald D (2001) Non-compliance in adolescents with chronic lung disease: causative factors and practical approach. Paediatr Respir Rev 2(3):260–267

Flaherman V, Rutherford GW (2006) A meta-analysis of the effect of high weight on asthma. Arch Dis Child 91(4):334–339

Ford ES, Mannino DM, Redd SC, Mokdad AH, Mott JA (2004) Body mass index and asthma incidence among USA adults. Eur Respir J 24(5):740–744

Forero R, Bauman A, Young L, Booth M, Nutbeam D (1996) Asthma, health behaviors, social adjustment, and psychosomatic symptoms in adolescence. J Asthma 33(3):157–164

Forrest CB, Starfield B, Riley AW, Kang M (1997) The impact of asthma on the health status of adolescents. Pediatrics 99(2):E1

Fowler MG, Johnson MP, Atkinson SS (1985) School achievement and absence in children with chronic health conditions. J Pediatr 106(4):683–687

Fowler MG, Davenport MG, Garg R (1992) School functioning of US children with asthma. Pediatrics 90(6):939–944

Garfinkel SK, Kesten S, Chapman KR, Rebuck AS (1992) Physiologic and nonphysiologic determinants of aerobic fitness in mild to moderate asthma. Am Rev Respir Dis 145(4 Pt 1):741–745

Gillaspy SR, Hoff AL, Mullins LL, Van Pelt JC, Chaney JM (2002) Psychological distress in high-risk youth with asthma. J Pediatr Psychol 27(4):363–371

Gilliland FD, Berhane K, Islam T, McConnell R, Gauderman WJ, Gilliland SS, Avol E, Peters JM (2003) Obesity and the risk of newly diagnosed asthma in school-age children. Am J Epidemiol 158(5):406–415

Ginsburg KR, Slap GB, Cnaan A, Forke CM, Balsley CM, Rouselle DM (1995) Adolescents' perceptions of factors affecting their decisions to seek health care. JAMA 273(24):1913–1918

Ginsburg KR, Forke CM, Cnaan A, Slap GB (2002) Important health provider characteristics: the perspective of urban ninth graders. J Dev Behav Pediatr 23(4):237–243

Gold DR, Damokosh AI, Dockery DW, Berkey CS (2003) Body-mass index as a predictor of incident asthma in a prospective cohort of children. Pediatr Pulmonol 36(6):514–521

Goodwin RD, Fergusson DM, Horwood LJ (2004) Asthma and depressive and anxiety disorders among young persons in the community. Psychol Med 34(8):1465–1474

Graetz B, Shute R (1995) Assessment of peer relationships in children with asthma. J Pediatr Psychol 20(2):205–216

Guerra S, Wright AL, Morgan WJ, Sherrill DL, Holberg CJ, Martinez FD (2004) Persistence of asthma symptoms during adolescence: role of obesity and age at the onset of puberty. Am J Respir Crit Care Med 170(1):78–85

Hakala K, Stenius-Aarniala B, Sovijarvi A (2000) Effects of weight loss on peak flow variability, airways obstruction, and lung volumes in obese patients with asthma. Chest 118(5):1315–1321

Hallstrand TS, Curtis JR, Aitken ML, Sullivan SD (2003) Quality of life in adolescents with mild asthma. Pediatr Pulmonol 36(6):536–543

Hambley J, Brazil K, Furrow D, Chua YY (1989) Demographic and psychosocial characteristics of asthmatic children in a Canadian rehabilitation setting. J Asthma 26(3):167–175

Hankin BL (2006) Adolescent depression: description, causes, and interventions. Epilepsy Behav 8(1):102–114

Harris KM, Duncan GJ, Boisjoly J (2002) Evaluating the Role of "Nothing to Lose" Attitiudes on Risky Behavior in Adolescents. Soc Forces 80(3):1005–1039

Hedley AA, Ogden CL, Johnson CL, Carroll MD, Curtin LR, Flegal KM (2004) Prevalence of overweight and obesity among US children, adolescents, and adults, 1999–2002. JAMA 291(23):2847–2850

Hillemeier MM, Gusic ME, Bai Y (2006) Rural and urban children with asthma: are school health services meeting their needs? Pediatrics 118(3):1097–1103

Hovell MF, Sipan CL, Blumberg EJ, Hofstetter CR, Slymen D, Friedman L, Moser K, Kelley NJ, Vera AY (2003) Increasing Latino adolescents' adherence to treatment for latent tuberculosis infection: a controlled trial. Am J Public Health 93(11):1871–1877

Jerrett MD, Costello EA (1996) Gaining control: parents' experiences of accommodating children's asthma. Clin Nurs Res 5(3):294–308

Jorgensen IM, Jensen VB, Bulow S, Dahm TL, Prahl P, Juel K (2003) Asthma mortality in the Danish child population: risk factors and causes of asthma death. Pediatr Pulmonol 36(2):142–147

Kaugars AS, Klinnert MD, Bender BG (2004) Family influences on pediatric asthma. J Pediatr Psychol 29(7):475–491

Kean EM, Kelsay K, Wamboldt F, Wamboldt MZ (2006) Posttraumatic stress in adolescents with asthma and their parents. J Am Acad Child Adolesc Psychiatry 45(1):78–86

Kelly HW, Strunk RC, Donithan M, Bloomberg GR, McWilliams BC, Szefler S (2003) Growth and bone density in children with mild-moderate asthma: a cross-sectional study in children entering the Childhood Asthma Management Program (CAMP). J Pediatr 142(3):286–291

Kelsay K, Hazel NA, Wamboldt MZ (2005) Predictors of body dissatisfaction in boys and girls with asthma. J Pediatr Psychol 30(6):522–531

Kilpatrick DG, Ruggiero KJ, Acierno R, Saunders BE, Resnick HS, Best CL. J Consult Clin Psychol. 2003 Aug;71(4): 692–700. Violence and risk of PTSD, major depression, substance abuse/dependence, and comorbidity: results from the National Survey of Adolescents.

Klinnert MD, Mrazek PJ, Mrazek DA (1994) Early asthma onset: the interaction between family stressors and adaptive parenting. Psychiatry 57(1):51–61

Klinnert MD, Nelson HS, Price MR, Adinoff AD, Leung DY, Mrazek DA (2001) Onset and persistence of childhood asthma: predictors from infancy. Pediatrics 108(4):E69

Kravis LP (1987) An analysis of fifteen childhood asthma fatalities. J Allergy Clin Immunol 80(3 Pt 2):467–472

Kurnat EL, Moore CM (1999) The impact of a chronic condition on the families of children with asthma. Pediatr Nurs 25(3):288–292

Ladd GW (1999) Peer relationships and social competence during early and middle childhood. Annu Rev Psychol 50:333–359

LeBlanc LA, Goldsmith T, Patel DR (2003) Behavioral aspects of chronic illness in children and adolescents. Pediatr Clin North Am 50(4):859–878

Leventhal T, Fauth RC, Brooks-Gunn J (2005) Neighborhood poverty and public policy: a 5-year follow-up of children's educational outcomes in the New York City moving to opportunity demonstration. Dev Psychol 41(6):933–952

Lieu TA, Lozano P, Finkelstein JA, Chi FW, Jensvold NG, Capra AM, Quesenberry CP, Selby JV, Farber HJ (2002) Racial/ethnic variation in asthma status and management practices among children in managed Medicaid. Pediatrics 109(5):857–865

Lieu TA, Finkelstein JA, Lozano P, Capra AM, Chi FW, Jensvold N, Quesenberry CP, Farber HJ (2004) Cultural competence policies and other predictors of asthma care quality for Medicaid-insured children. Pediatrics 114(1):e102–e110

Littleton HL, Ollendick T (2003) Negative body image and disordered eating behavior in children and adolescents: what places youth at risk and how can these problems be prevented? Clin Child Fam Psychol Rev 6(1):51–66

Logan D, Zelikovsky N, Labay L, Spergel J (2003) The Illness Management Survey: identifying adolescents' perceptions of barriers to adherence. J Pediatr Psychol 28(6):383–392

Lowe RA, Localio AR, Schwarz DF, Williams S, Tuton LW, Maroney S, Nicklin D, Goldfarb N, Vojta DD, Feldman HI

(2005) Association between primary care practice characteristics and emergency department use in a medicaid managed care organization. Med Care 43(8):792–800

Lozano P, Connell FA, Koepsell TD (1995) Use of health services by African-American children with asthma on Medicaid. JAMA 274(6):469–473

Lucas SR, Platts-Mills TA (2005) Physical activity and exercise in asthma: relevance to etiology and treatment. J Allergy Clin Immunol 115(5):928–934

MacLean WE Jr, Perrin JM, Gortmaker S, Pierre CB (1992) Psychological adjustment of children with asthma: effects of illness severity and recent stressful life events. J Pediatr Psychol 17(2):159–171

Mannino DM, Homa DM, Pertowski CA, Ashizawa A, Nixon LL, Johnson CA, Ball LB, Jack E, Kang DS (1998) Surveillance for asthma – United States, 1960–1995. MMWR CDC Surveill Summ 47(1):1–27

Mannino DM, Homa DM, Akinbami LJ, Moorman JE, Gwynn C, Redd SC (2002) Surveillance for asthma – United States, 1980–1999. MMWR CDC Surveill Summ 51(1):1–13

Mannix ET, Roberts MA, Dukes HJ, Magnes CJ, Farber MO (2004) Airways hyperresponsiveness in high school athletes. J Asthma 41(5):567–574

Manworren RC (1996) Developmental effects on the adolescent of a temporary ileostomy. J Wound Ostomy Continence Nurs 23(4):210–217

McCreary DR, Sasses DK (2000) An exploration of the drive for muscularity in adolescent boys and girls. J Am Coll Health 48(6):297–304

McElroy SL, Kotwal R, Malhotra S, Nelson EB, Keck PE, Nemeroff CB (2004) Are mood disorders and obesity related? A review for the mental health professional. J Clin Psychiatry 65(5):634–651

McQuaid EL, Kopel SJ, Klein RB, Fritz GK (2003) Medication adherence in pediatric asthma: reasoning, responsibility, and behavior. J Pediatr Psychol 28(5):323–333

Miech RA, Kumanyika SK, Stettler N, Link BG, Phelan JC, Chang VW (2006) Trends in the association of poverty with overweight among US adolescents, 1971–2004. JAMA 295(20):2385–2393

Mrazek DA, Klinnert M, Mrazek PJ, Brower A, McCormick D, Rubin B, Ikle D, Kastner W, Larsen G, Harbeck R, Jones J (1999) Prediction of early-onset asthma in genetically at-risk children. Pediatr Pulmonol 27(2):85–94

Neinstein LS, MacKenzei RG, Morris RE (2002) High risk and out-of-control behavior. In: Neinstein LS (ed) Adolescent health care, a practical guide. Lippincott Williams & Wilkins, Philadelphia, pp 1402–1406

No Author. Long-term effects of budesonide or nedocromil in children with asthma. The Childhood Asthma Management Program Research Group. (2000). N Engl J Med, 343(15), 1054–1063.

Olson AL, Seidler AB, Goodman D, Gaelic S, Nordgren R (2004) School professionals' perceptions about the impact of chronic illness in the classroom. Arch Pediatr Adolesc Med 158(1):53–58

Parsons JP, Mastronarde JG (2005) Exercise-induced bronchoconstriction in athletes. Chest 128(6):3966–3974

Penza-Clyve SM, Mansell C, McQuaid EL (2004) Why don't children take their asthma medications? A qualitative analysis of children's perspectives on adherence. J Asthma 41(2):189–197

Perna G, Bertani A, Politi E, Colombo G, Bellodi L (1997) Asthma and panic attacks. Biol Psychiatry 42(7):625–630

Poli P, Sbrana B, Marcheschi M, Masi G (2003) Self-reported depressive symptoms in a school sample of Italian children and adolescents. Child Psychiatry Hum Dev 33(3):209–226

Power C, Manor O (1995) Asthma, enuresis, and chronic illness: long term impact on height. Arch Dis Child 73(4):298–304

Radzik M, Sherer S, Neinstein LS (2002) Psychosocial development in normal adolescents. In: Neinstein LS (ed) Adolescent health care, a practical guide. Lippincott Williams & Wilkins, Philadelphia, pp 52–58

Rand CS (1993) Measuring adherence with therapy for chronic diseases: implications for the treatment of heterozygous familial hypercholesterolemia. Am J Cardiol 72(10):68D–74D

Rietveld S, van Beest I, Prins PJ (2005) The relationship between specific anxiety syndromes and somatic symptoms in adolescents with asthma and other chronic diseases. J Asthma 42(9):725–730

Roder I, Kroonenberg PM, Boekaerts M (2003) Psychosocial functioning and stress-processing of children with asthma in the school context: differences and similarities with children without asthma. J Asthma 40(7):777–787

Rundell KW, Jenkinson DM (2002) Exercise-induced bronchospasm in the elite athlete. Sports Med 32(9):583–600

Rupp NT, Brudno DS, Guill MF (1993) The value of screening for risk of exercise-induced asthma in high school athletes. Ann Allergy 70(4):339–342

Rushton JL, Forcier M, Schectman RM (2002) Epidemiology of depressive symptoms in the National Longitudinal Study of Adolescent Health. J Am Acad Child Adolesc Psychiatry 41(2):199–205

Sarles RM, Neinstein LS (2002) Adolescent depression. In: Neinstein LS (ed) Adolescent health care, a practical guide. Lippincott Williams & Wilkins, Philadelphia, pp 1432–1441

Sawyer SM, Aroni RA (2005) Self-management in adolescents with chronic illness. What does it mean and how can it be achieved? Med J Aust 183(8):405–409

Schwartz D, Gorman AH (2003) Community violence exposure and children's academic functioning. J Educ Psychol 95(1):163–173

Schwartz J, Gold D, Dockery DW, Weiss ST, Speizer FE (1990) Predictors of asthma and persistent wheeze in a national sample of children in the United States. Association with social class, perinatal events, and race. Am Rev Respir Dis 142(3):555–562

Sherman R, Milgrom H (2005) Asthma and activities of daily living. Clin Rev Allergy Immunol 29(2):159–164

Shore SA, Fredberg JJ (2005) Obesity, smooth muscle, and airway hyperresponsiveness. J Allergy Clin Immunol 115(5):925–927

Silverman RA, Boudreaux ED, Woodruff PG, Clark S, Camargo CA Jr (2003) Cigarette smoking among asthmatic adults presenting to 64 emergency departments. Chest 123(5): 1472–1479

Silverstein MD, Mair JE, Katusic SK, Wollan PC, O'Connell EJ, Yunginger JW (2001) School attendance and school performance: a population-based study of children with asthma. J Pediatr 139(2):278–283

Slack MK, Brooks AJ (1995) Medication management issues for adolescents with asthma. Am J Health Syst Pharm 52(13):1417–1421

Smedley BD, Stith AY, Nelson AR (2003) Summary. In Unequal treatment, confronting racial and ethnic disparities in health care. The National Academies, Washington, D.C

Smith BA, Shuchman M (2005) Problem of nonadherence in chronically ill adolescents: strategies for assessment and intervention. Curr Opin Pediatr 17(5):613–618

Spivak H, Hewitt MF, Onn A, Half EE (2005) Weight loss and improvement of obesity-related illness in 500 U.S. patients following laparoscopic adjustable gastric banding procedure. Am J Surg 189(1):27–32

Stenius-Aarniala B, Poussa T, Kvarnstrom J, Gronlund EL, Ylikahri M, Mustajoki P (2000) Immediate and long term effects of weight reduction in obese people with asthma: randomised controlled study. BMJ 320(7238):827–832

Strunk RC (1987) Asthma deaths in childhood: identification of patients at risk and intervention. J Allergy Clin Immunol 80(3 Pt 2):472–477

Strunk RC, Mrazek DA, Fuhrmann GS, LaBrecque JF (1985) Physiologic and psychological characteristics associated with deaths due to asthma in childhood. A case-controlled study. JAMA 254(9):1193–1198

Sturdy PM, Victor CR, Anderson HR, Bland JM, Butland BK, Harrison BD, Peckitt C, Taylor JC (2002) Psychological, social and health behavior risk factors for deaths certified as asthma: a national case-control study. Thorax 57(12):1034–1039

Suris JC, Parera N (2005) Sex, drugs and chronic illness: health behaviours among chronically ill youth. Eur J Public Health 15(5):484–488

Suris JC, Parera N, Puig C (1996) Chronic illness and emotional distress in adolescence. J Adolesc Health 19(2):153–156

Suris JC, Michaud PA, Viner R (2004) The adolescent with a chronic condition. Part I: developmental issues. Arch Dis Child 89(10):938–942

Tomlinson JE, McMahon AD, Chaudhuri R, Thompson JM, Wood SF, Thomson NC (2005) Efficacy of low and high dose inhaled corticosteroid in smokers versus non-smokers with mild asthma. Thorax 60(4):282–287

Tyc VL, Throckmorton-Belzer L (2006) Smoking rates and the state of smoking interventions for children and adolescents with chronic illness. Pediatrics 118(2):e471–e487

van Es SM, Nagelkerke AF, Colland VT, Scholten RJ, Bouter LM (2001) An intervention programme using the ASE-model aimed at enhancing adherence in adolescents with asthma. Patient Educ Couns 44(3):193–203

Wallace JC, Denk CE, Kruse LK (2004) Pediatric hospitalizations for asthma: use of a linked file to separate person-level risk and readmission. Prev Chronic Dis 1(2):A07

Wamboldt MZ, Weintraub P, Krafchick D, Wamboldt FS (1996) Psychiatric family history in adolescents with severe asthma. J Am Acad Child Adolesc Psychiatry 35(8):1042–1049

Wamboldt MZ, Fritz G, Mansell A, McQuaid EL, Klein RB (1998) Relationship of asthma severity and psychological problems in children. J Am Acad Child Adolesc Psychiatry 37(9):943–950

Wardle J, Cook L (2005) The impact of obesity on psychological well-being. Best Pract Res Clin Endocrinol Metab 19(3):421–440

Weil CM, Wade SL, Bauman LJ, Lynn H, Mitchell H, Lavigne J (1999) The relationship between psychosocial factors and asthma morbidity in inner-city children with asthma. Pediatrics 104(6):1274–1280

Wirrell E, Cheung C, Spier S (2006) How do teens view the physical and social impact of asthma compared to other chronic diseases? J Asthma 43(2):155–160

Wright RJ, Mitchell H, Visness CM, Cohen S, Stout J, Evans R, Gold DR (2004) Community violence and asthma morbidity: the Inner-City Asthma Study. Am J Public Health 94(4): 625–632

Wright RJ, Cohen RT, Cohen S (2005) The impact of stress on the development and expression of atopy. Curr Opin Allergy Clin Immunol 5(1):23–29

Yeatts KB, Shy CM (2001) Prevalence and consequences of asthma and wheezing in African-American and white adolescents. J Adolesc Health 29(5):314–319

Zbikowski SM, Klesges RC, Robinson LA, Alfano CM (2002) Risk factors for smoking among adolescents with asthma. J Adolesc Health 30:279–287

Chapter 13
Asthma and the Family

Elizabeth L. McQuaid and Deborah Friedman

Introduction

Regardless of whether patients are young children, adolescents, or adults, the management and course of asthma most often takes place within the context of a family. Parents of young children with asthma monitor and treat asthma symptoms, parents and older children negotiate management of asthma with one another, and spouses and/or caretakers of older adults with asthma can support or hinder efforts toward appropriate symptom management and trigger control. Family systems theory emphasizes how, for chronic illnesses, family members' attitudes and behaviors regarding the illness do not exist in a static system, but mutually influence one another within and across contexts (Kazak 1989). For example, family dysfunction, including family conflict and parental mental health problems, is a risk factor for mental and physical health problems in children (Fiese et al. 2000). On the other side of the continuum, family strengths, such as family cohesion and competent parenting, may serve a protective function, enabling a child with asthma to demonstrate resilience (Koinis Mitchell et al. 2004).

Early conceptualizations of asthma emphasized the role of the mother–child relationship in symptom development (French and Alexander 1941). This view declined in popularity as understanding of the underlying allergic and inflammatory processes of the disease increased. Nevertheless, the role of the family, particularly in pediatric asthma management, continued to receive attention. For example, one early case control study comparing children who had died due to asthma to a matched sample of children who had not died identified the existence of family conflict as one factor distinguishing the two groups (Strunk et al. 1985). More recent conceptualizations emphasize the complex interactions between behavioral and biological factors (Miller and Wood 2003) and reciprocal influences between parent and child in disease management and outcomes (Kaugars et al. 2004).

There exists a burgeoning literature regarding family factors and asthma, including investigations of how family variables relate to the onset and course of asthma (Klinnert et al. 1994), new methods for assessing how families manage asthma (Fiese and Wamboldt 2003; McQuaid et al. 2005), and research regarding how asthma influences quality of life indicators for families (Asmussen et al. 1999). This chapter will provide an overview of research in the areas of asthma and the family. We review the role of parents in childhood asthma, the assessment of family variables in asthma management and care, and the effectiveness of family interventions in asthma education and management. As the large majority of research in this area investigates pediatric asthma, much of this review addresses research with children. Relevant family research on adults with asthma, specifically, spousal support in chronic illness and asthma management, is also covered. New directions for research and clinical interventions will be highlighted throughout.

Asthma Onset: The Role of the Family

A growing body of research indicates that heredity plays a central role in the development and expression of asthma (Wills-Karp and Ewart 2004). Psychosocial

E.L. McQuaid (✉)
Child Psychiatry, Bradley Hasbro Research Center, Brow Medical School
1 Hoppin Street, Providence, RI, 02903, USA
e-mail: elizabeth_mcquaid@brown.edu

A. Harver and H. Kotses (eds.), *Asthma, Health and Society: A Public Health Perspective*, DOI 10.1007/978-0-387-78285-0_13, © Springer Science+Business Media, LLC 2010

factors and family context, however, have also been demonstrated to play a role in the age of onset of asthma symptoms. For example, maternal smoking during pregnancy is associated with increased risk of asthma (Environmental Protection Agency 1992), and, conversely, some research indicates that breastfeeding may serve a protective function in asthma development (Oddy 2004). Work by Klinnert, Mrazek, and colleagues (Klinnert et al. 1994; Klinnert et al. 2001) examining factors that prospectively predict the onset and persistence of asthma provide evidence of the importance of caregiver psychological functioning for child asthma onset and early course. For children with a family history of asthma, mothers' reports of parenting difficulties (e.g., post partum depression), when their children were 3 weeks of age, and had not yet experienced the onset of respiratory or wheezing illnesses, predicted early asthma onset prior to age 3 years, as well as asthma diagnosis at ages 6–8 (Klinnert and Mrazek 1994; Klinnert et al. 2001). Another recent study of early onset asthma and wheezing in a group of 2–3 year old children documented early risk factors of exposure to violence and maternal anxiety, as well as the potential protective impact of social support (Berz et al. 2007). In short, findings suggests that family characteristics, particularly caretaker functioning, are an important factor in predicting asthma onset, and that the infant care-giving environment is critical to asthma outcomes for children who are at-risk for developing asthma (Klinnert et al. 2001).

Caregiver Mental Health and Asthma Course

As described above, caregiver functioning is a factor that is predictive of the development of a child's asthma. The actual mechanism by which caregiver psychological functioning and parenting difficulties during infancy translates into an increased risk for development of asthma is not completely clear. Several different pathways, both psychosocial and physiological, could be involved. For example, in accordance with Kaugars' model (Kaugars et al. 2004), maternal depression may affect asthma outcomes via physiological processes by increasing the stress of the overall family climate in a way that negatively affects the developing child's immune system. Once asthma has been diagnosed, maternal depressive symptoms may influence the course of asthma disease by interfering with the parent's ability to engage in effective asthma management practices. More research that accounts for alternate psychosocial and environmental risk factors (e.g., poverty), which may account for both symptoms of depression as well as increased risk for asthma, is needed to elucidate these pathways further. In addition, interpretations of research findings in this area must be tempered by the fact that most studies have utilized mothers' reports of both their own psychological functioning and asthma outcomes for their child, such that significant associations between the two may be accounted for by reporting biases (Kaugars et al. 2004).

There is considerable evidence that once asthma has been diagnosed, maternal mental health has a bearing on disease course. The association between maternal mental health problems and poor asthma outcomes has been demonstrated across different populations, including low income, inner city families (Bartlett et al. 2001; Shalowitz et al. 2001), as well as Island Puerto Rican families (Ortega et al. 2004). The presence of maternal depressive symptoms, in particular, has been identified as a risk factor for poor health outcomes in children with asthma. For example, in one sample of children in subspecialty care, maternal depressive symptoms, along with life stressors reported by the mother, were found to have strong associations with asthma morbidity (Shalowitz et al. 2001). In a sample of urban, at-risk families, maternal depression was also found to be linked with increased asthma disease activity (as measured both objectively and by parent-report). This association operated indirectly through the impact of maternal depression on child psychological dysfunction (Lim et al. 2008).

Maternal depression has also been linked to higher levels of health care utilization for pediatric asthma patients. One group of researchers found that children whose parents had high levels of mental health problems had twice the rate of hospitalizations for asthma (Weil et al. 1999). Another study of African-American inner-city children with asthma found that mothers with a high level of self-reported depressive symptoms were 30% more likely to report having taken their child to the emergency department for asthma, even after controlling for such factors as asthma symptoms and age of the mother. Depressive symptoms were high in this particular sample, with nearly half of mothers reporting significant levels of depression (Bartlett et al. 2001).

Maternal depression has also been associated with beliefs and attitudes that may have an influence on effective asthma management practices and adherence to asthma medications. For example, African-American mothers living in the inner-city who reported a high level of depressive symptoms also reported significantly more problems with proper inhaler use, forgetting doses, and less confidence in asthma medications. They also reported increased emotional distress, and interference due to asthma with daily activities, and less self-efficacy in coping with acute episodes. Moreover, they were much more likely to report poor communication with health care providers. Specifically, mothers with depressive symptoms were eight times more likely to report that their child's doctor had not adequately explained the rationale for, or proper use of, asthma medicines (Bartlett et al. 2004). Of note, little research has investigated middle-to upper income families, or non-Latino whites, and measures of depression appear to be limited to screening instruments that indicate symptom levels, and not clinical diagnoses.

Features of the Parent–Child Relationship

Several studies have examined how specific characteristics of the parent–child relationship may influence asthma outcomes. *Parent–child attachment status* and *parental expressed emotion* have received the most attention. Attachment status has been shown to influence symptom-reporting, health care utilization, and the restriction of activities in children who have a chronic illness (Feeney 2000). Those studies examining the parent–child relationship specifically in children with asthma have found links between measures of attachment and asthma status as well. One study found that preschoolers with severe asthma were more likely to be insecurely attached than preschoolers without asthma (Mrazek et al. 1987). In one promising theoretical model, attachment is proposed as a central factor linking family processes with both emotional regulation and disease activity in children with asthma (Wood et al. 2000). Results from a small study testing this model indicated that an insecure father–child attachment relationship, as reported by the child, was linked both to child-reported feelings of hopelessness as well as increased vagal activation, one mechanism of airway compromise in asthma (Wood et al. 2000).

Parental expressed emotion, and parental criticism in particular, have also been linked to asthma outcomes in childhood. Parental expressed emotion is typically measured in clinical research through rating the emotional content of a brief interview in which the parent is asked to express his or her thoughts and feelings about the ill child (Wamboldt and Wamboldt 2000). A high degree of parental criticism, as measured through the expressed emotion paradigm, has been found to be highly predictive of relapse in several psychiatric populations (Wamboldt et al. 1996). A few studies have found that parental criticism may impact outcomes for children with asthma as well. Specifically, both mothers and fathers of children with asthma were found to have a more critical attitude toward their child when compared with families of children without asthma (Schobinger et al. 1992), and maternal critical attitude was related to decreased child compliance with the medical regimen (Schobinger et al. 1993). Fathers' attitudes appear to play a role as well. An additional study found that paternal criticism was associated with increased school absences for children with asthma (Gartland and Day 1999).

Parental Beliefs

The belief system of parents regarding asthma and the usefulness of medication also likely influences the manner in which the child's asthma is managed at home. For example, findings from one study indicated that many families who were frequent users of the emergency department for their child's asthma held beliefs about the ineffectiveness of medications (Wasilewski et al. 1996). Similarly, another study reported that one of the most frequent barriers to asthma care in urban children was parental beliefs about the ineffectiveness or potential harmfulness of medication use. Many parents reported that they modified the asthma management plan prescribed by their health care provider due to their concerns, leading to suboptimal treatment of the child's asthma (Mansour et al. 2000). Parental self-efficacy, or the parent's belief in their own ability to manage their child's asthma, has also been related to asthma outcomes in a sample of families who were primarily from lower income and minority backgrounds. Parents with increased feelings of helplessness tended to have children with greater asthma-related morbidity, and parents with decreased self-efficacy to manage asthma tended to have children who missed more school due to asthma episodes (Grus et al. 2001). Similarly, a parent's perception of the child's vulnerability to illness was associated with increased health service utilization and more frequent school absences, even when controlling for the frequency and intensity of the child's asthma symptoms (Spurrier et al. 2003.). These studies suggest that open communication between regarding parents' beliefs and concerns may enhance the treatment of childhood asthma.

Overall Family Functioning: Conflict, Organization, and Support

In addition to examining specific parenting factors, such as caregiver psychological functioning and parent–child relationship quality, researchers have also found associations among global family functioning variables and child asthma outcomes. Global family functioning variables are those that capture interaction patterns among the family as a whole. For example, in one study, multiple dimensions of family functioning, including the quality of affective relationships among family members, were associated with the child's self report of the extent to which he or she is burdened by asthma, even after controlling for the frequency of asthma symptoms (Sawyer et al. 2001). Negative family emotional climate, as rated by parents, was also found to be associated with child-reported depressive symptoms, which in turn were associated with asthma disease severity (Wood et al. 2007).

Family conflict has been identified as a risk factor for mental and physical health problems for children in general, and several studies have demonstrated the negative influence of high levels of family conflict on the course of childhood asthma (Kaugars et al. 2004; Repetti et al. 2002). In one early case-controlled study, Strunk et al. (Strunk et al. 1985) found that high levels of family conflict were a key risk variable associated with asthma mortality in a pediatric population. In a more recent study of children hospitalized for asthma, family conflict was found to be associated with a lifetime history of multiple hospitalizations (Chen et al. 2003).

Research has also consistently demonstrated the importance of factors related to family organization, structure, and support in effective family asthma management. For example, the frequency and richness of family rituals and routines appear to serve a protective function for children with asthma in two-parent families, particularly during times of high stress (Markson and Fiese 2000). Interestingly, gender differences have been found in the ways in which family rituals exert a positive influence on child adjustment, such that mothers' endorsement of the meaning of family rituals and fathers' endorsement of the regularity and assignment of roles within family rituals were both associated with lower levels of anxiety for the child with asthma (Markson and Fiese 2000). Family rituals may be protective for several reasons. They may provide stability for families disrupted by illness and other chronic stressors, and they may also provide a greater structure in which the routines and responsibilities of asthma management could be more easily integrated (Markson and Fiese 2000).

The ways in which families allocate responsibility for asthma care tasks is an area of potential coordination or disruption in the family's management of asthma. Typically, children take on increasing self-management responsibility as they age (McQuaid, et al. 2001). Ideally, parents involve children in asthma management in a developmentally appropriate manner with a dynamic progression of increasing autonomy based on factors such as age and indications of social, emotional, and cognitive maturity. Preadolescent children may be able to assume responsibility for symptom management, but parents may still have primary responsibility for preventive care. Adolescents may be able to take on the larger share of responsibility for their own care, but likely will continue to require active support and guidance from parents.

Research in this area shows that older children do in fact demonstrate greater knowledge about asthma and take on more responsibility for asthma care than younger children. Older children, however, also demonstrate lower levels of medication adherence (McQuaid et al. 2003). When parents and children have both been asked to report on the allocation of asthma care tasks, the two reports tend to be only moderately correlated (McQuaid et al. 2001; Walders et al. 2000; Wade et al. 1999). In two separate studies, children tended to report having a greater degree of responsibility for asthma care tasks than parents perceived them to have (McQuaid et al. 2001; Wade et al. 1999). This discrepancy may reflect parents' lack of awareness of children's asthma care skills outside the home, such as with friends or at school. Large discrepancies between parental and child perceptions of the allocation of asthma care tasks, however, may be an indicator of increased risk for ineffective management. In one study of African-American adolescents and their caregivers, parental overestimation of the level of adolescent responsibility for asthma self-care predicted increased nonadherence and greater functional morbidity (Walders et al. 2000). Little is known about how parents and children negotiate the balance of responsibility of asthma management as the child develops, and what factors may facilitate a successful transition. More research is needed on the development of self-management skills given that the transition to adolescence appears to be a period of increased risk (Bender et al. 1998). In addition, results of existing research in this area suggest that discrepancies between parent and child perceptions of responsibility for asthma tasks may be a fruitful area of clinical intervention (McQuaid et al. 2001; Wade et al. 1999).

While research on asthma and families has typically focused almost exclusively on the role of mothers, significant effects have been found regarding fathers when they have been included in research designs (Gartland and Day 1999; Markson and Fiese 2000). Clinical impressions indicate that mothers tend to have responsibility for the majority of asthma management tasks as compared to fathers. There are some data, however, to suggest that fathers represent an important source of support in families, and that their involvement in asthma care may be instrumental. A few studies have examined the role of fathers in disease management in a sample of children with chronic illnesses, including a subset of children with asthma (Wysocki and Gavin 2004; Gavin and Wysocki 2006; Wysocki and Gavin 2006). One of these studies showed that fathers' participation in disease management tasks occurred on 25–50% of available opportunities. Mothers' reports of the helpfulness of fathers' involvement was higher than fathers' reports of their own perceptions of their helpfulness suggesting that fathers may underestimate what their involvement may mean within families (Wysocki and Gavin 2004). Amount of father involvement was also shown to have a positive association with family functioning and marital satisfaction, and mothers' ratings of the helpfulness of fathers' involvement was associated with fewer self-reported maternal psychiatric symptoms and less perceived impact of the chronic illness on family functioning (Gavin and Wysocki 2006). Higher levels of paternal involvement were also associated with more favorable self-reported adherence to medical regimens and quality of life among chronically ill adolescents (Wysocki and Gavin 2006).

Asthma's Impact on the Family

As reviewed in the previous section, parenting and family factors may greatly influence asthma outcomes. It is also important, however, to consider the other side of this equation – the impact that asthma has on family processes. The entire family is likely to be affected by a child's asthma diagnosis. Along with the emotional stress that may accompany having a child who is chronically ill, parents are often relied upon to negotiate various illness-related issues throughout the child's development, from providing direct asthma management to balancing the requirements of the child's health issues with other family needs.

Considering these ways in which a child's illness can place additional stress on the family, it is not surprising that families of children with chronic illness are at an increased risk for psychosocial difficulties (Kazak et al. 1995). Research shows that parents of a child with chronic medical conditions report greater psychological distress than parents of healthy children (Kazak 1989; Kazak et al. 1995). Factors related to the illness condition as well as psychosocial factors may moderate the impact of child chronic illness on parent functioning (Silver et al. 1998). For example, one study found that the severity of a child's asthma symptoms was related to the parental report of quality of life (Halterman et al. 2004).

Asthma symptoms have been shown to predict family relational patterns as well (Gustafsson et al. 1994). In a sample of infants who were at risk for allergic disease due to a strong family history, dysfunctional family interaction patterns did not predict onset of illness during the first 18 months of life. Dysfunctional family interaction patterns, however, were predicted by the development of wheezing in the child, with the majority of families classified as exhibiting dysfunctional patterns displaying a disengaged style with chaotic interactions and little closeness among family members (Gustafsson et al. 1994).

Whereas, it is clear that families may experience stress or disruption as a result of a child's asthma, it is important to note that chronic illness appears to have selective effects on family processes. As reviewed by Wamboldt and Wamboldt (2000) and Kazak et al. (1995), the risk for parental mental health problems may increase but generally not into the clinical range, and areas of disruption may coexist with areas of increased resilience.

Adults with Asthma and the Impact of Familial Support

Although adults with asthma are typically responsible for their own symptom management, self-management behaviors generally continue to occur within the context of a family system. For example, adults with asthma may need to implement trigger control strategies in a household that is shared by a spouse or other family members, who may or may not have asthma themselves. While there is little research on the impact of family factors on asthma outcomes in adults, there is a wide body of literature that highlights the positive and protective influences of social support on physical and mental health outcomes for adults more generally. There is some evidence to suggest that social support may influence asthma outcomes through its effect on physiological processes or its effect on self-management behaviors. For example, marital status (i.e., in this case being married) was found to be associated with better adherence for adults with asthma (Clark et al. 1999).

One comprehensive meta-analysis of 81 research studies found that social support was reliably related to several different physiological processes, including immune function, across healthy adults (Uchino et al. 1996). Many different sources of social support were examined, but there was some evidence that familial support may be particularly important. In addition, while pulmonary processes were not specifically examined in this review, one may speculate that social support could potentially affect asthma outcomes via its influence on immune system functioning.

A second review paper provided evidence for the positive effects of social support on self-management behaviors for adults with chronic illness in general (Gallant 2003). This report included studies of social support and self-management of a variety of illnesses, with diabetes being the most frequently represented. Across studies, the sources and types of social support were often not specifically delineated. It seems likely, however, that spouses and/or family members caring for older adults may be particularly influential with regard to supporting or hindering positive self-management behaviors. Spouses and caretakers may provide support for effective self-management of asthma by sharing the responsibility or burden of specific asthma-related tasks, or by providing emotional support and encouragement around self-management of the illness. They may help to create a living environment that is conducive to effective management, for example, by facilitating trigger control strategies (e.g., implementing a household smoking ban, or choosing not to have pets). Spouses and caretakers of adults may also provide effective self-management support indirectly by increasing general motivation or improving quality of life. Across a variety of studies, small to moderate effect sizes were found for the association between social support and illness self-management (Gallant 2003). As noted in this review, however, more research is needed to further understand this relationship.

A number of limitations in this research area make it difficult to draw definitive conclusions regarding the role of spousal or caretaker support in adult asthma management. Most of the research has addressed individual factors that influence behavior, such as self-efficacy, and relatively few studies have examined social factors that may play a role in adult self-management capability. In addition, the research that exists tends to focus on the positive influences of social support, and little is known about how the unsupportive behaviors of spouses or significant others (e.g., continued smoking) may negatively influence self-management efficacy and subsequent health outcomes. Furthermore, Gallant's (Gallant 2003) review was unable to make any conclusions about the type of support that may be important (i.e., illness-specific support behaviors vs. general support), or the relevance of the match of support to actual need or desire for support. Hence, the mechanisms that may explain how social support influences self-management remain largely unknown (Gallant 2003).

One recent, prospective study following a small sample involved in an intervention to promote self-management of asthma and diabetes looked at the influence of different types of spousal support on health and self-efficacy. Spousal support involving active engagement or overprotection did not appear to have an effect, but protective buffering, described as "hiding concerns" and "denying worries" had a significant negative impact on mental and physical health as reported by patients (De Ridder et al. 2005). Further research employing prospective designs, and addressing an array of potentially supportive and/or unsupportive behaviors is needed.

Future Directions: Reciprocal Influences

Although the majority of the literature addresses how family factors influence asthma outcomes, or conversely, how aspects of asthma influence family functioning, most researchers acknowledge that there are multiple, bidirectional levels of influence between family factors and disease processes (Kaugars et al. 2004; Wamboldt and Wamboldt 2000). Recently, some researchers have implemented longitudinal designs to begin to assess relationships between family level and disease level variables over time. In one study using latent growth modeling, reciprocal relationships were found in the interplay between family adaptation to medical illness and use of medications over time. Families where infants initially presented with more severe symptoms showed greater positive change over time with regard to adapting to the demands of illness management. A second model showed that families who initially demonstrated better illness management practices, and where infants had more severe initial symptoms, were more likely to use medications consistent with more intense treatment over time (Kaugars et al. 2008). More such longitudinal research is needed to assess how individual, family, and disease factors influence one another dynamically over time.

Assessment of Family Variables in Asthma

A vast array of general measures of family functioning and adjustment exist. A smaller, yet still substantial number of measures exist to assess child- or parent-specific measures of asthma, such as child knowledge (Cummings et al. 2004), parent and child self-efficacy to manage asthma (Bursch et al. 1999), and asthma related quality of life from child (Juniper et al. 2004) and parent (Juniper et al. 1996) perspectives. Far fewer instruments, however, have been developed to assess family-specific aspects of asthma, such as asthma management within the family context, or the effects of asthma on general family functioning. Current existing measures provide methods for measuring the division of responsibility for asthma management tasks within the family (McQuaid et al. 2001; Wade et al. 1999), family asthma management skills (McQuaid et al. 2005) and routines (Fiese and Wamboldt 2003), and effects of asthma on family activities (Asmussen et al. 1999).

Identifying who is responsible for asthma management tasks within the family may be a critical prerequisite to pinpoint management difficulties and structuring interventions. Wade et al. (1999) developed the Asthma Responsibility Interview (ARI), a structured interview, that has versions for children and caretakers, which assesses the division of responsibilities for asthma tasks within the family. The interview identifies all potential individuals responsible for asthma care (including the parent, child, or others), and then probes the extent to which each makes decisions or implements treatments in various areas of asthma management. The ARI has been used with children ages 6–9 (Wade et al. 1999), and with African-American adolescents (Walders et al. 2000). The ARI includes a visual analog scale that can be used with young children (Wade et al. 1999). A ten-item questionnaire to assess the division of responsibility for asthma management tasks among parents and children, the Asthma Responsibilities Questionnaire (ARQ), has also been developed and validated (McQuaid et al. 2001). The ARQ demonstrated convergent validity through associations with measures of general independence and asthma self-efficacy (McQuaid et al. 2001).

There are two interviews available to assess overall approaches to family management of pediatric asthma. Fiese and Wamboldt (Fiese and Wamboldt 2003) developed the Asthma Impact Interview (AII), a 20-min parent interview regarding how asthma has affected the family, and how the family managed challenging situations in asthma care. Transcripts are coded and family management approaches are classified as either reactive (i.e., anxiety leads to action), coordinated care (i.e., the family follows health care providers' directions), or family partnerships (i.e., plans for asthma management are based on multiple sources of information). These three management styles were associated with objective measures of medication adherence at the time of interview and at the 1-year follow-up. The authors suggest that the interview may have useful clinical applications in identifying families who might be at risk for poor adherence or who might need extra support in following complex directions for asthma care (Fiese and Wamboldt 2003).

The family asthma management system scale (FAMSS) is a semi-structured interview comprised of a series of open-ended questions that are designed to assess several areas of asthma management, such as disease knowledge, medication adherence, and trigger control (Klinnert et al. 1997; McQuaid, et al. 2005). The interview can be administered to parents alone, if the child is younger than eight years. Children of the age group of eight and older, however, can participate together with their parents, because school aged children may provide unique perspectives regarding asthma management outside the home such as in school.

FAMSS interviews are coded using a standard manual, which provides rating instructions and a series of rating guidelines for each scale. Scales are given a nine-point rating, from 1 (ineffective or harmful management) to 9 (highly adaptive management). A summary score (mean of all scale scores) can also be derived. A recent study indicated the FAMSS has convergent validity with measures of asthma knowledge, asthma self-efficacy, and objective indices of medication adherence (McQuaid et al. 2005). Additionally, the FAMSS summary score was related to functional morbidity at baseline and prospectively, and explained additional variance in concurrent asthma morbidity beyond self-reports or objective adherence monitoring. One drawback is that the interview takes between 25 min and an hour to administer, depending on the version implemented, which limits its practical use in fast-paced clinical settings. An in-depth interview such as the FAMSS also requires training to assure reliable administration and rating of the scales. Therefore, The FAMSS may be more appropriate for use as a baseline interview to identify particular treatment targets prior to clinical intervention.

Multiple quality of life (QOL) measures have been used to assess the impact of asthma on adult functioning (Juniper et al. 2004), as well as the effects of pediatric asthma on child (Asmussen et al. 1999) and parental (Juniper et al. 1996) functioning. One more recent QOL measure, specifically developed for pediatric populations, includes an assessment of whether asthma has affected family functioning. This measure, the Children's Health Survey for Asthma (Asmussen et al. 1999) yields five domain scores, including impact of asthma on family activities and effects of asthma on family emotional health. It has demonstrated good internal consistency and test-retest reliability. A subsequent study indicated that CHSA scores were significantly associated with changes in asthma symptoms and health care utilization over the course of one year (Sharek et al. 2002).

Family-Based Interventions

A wealth of programs exist to provide education to children with asthma, and enhance self-management strategies (see Wolf et al. 2003, for a review). These programs tend to be targeted directly to the individual with asthma. There are also numerous interventions that provide education to parents of children with asthma, particularly those with young children (e.g., Brown et al. 2002). Some approaches incorporate education for *both* the parent and child with asthma (e.g., Georgiou et al. 2003). Programs have also been developed to provide education, support, and management strategies for adults with asthma (see Gibson et al. 2002, and Powell and Gibson 2003 for reviews). Of the interventions discussed above for both children and adults, very few have been designed specifically using a family-centered approach, and most do not incorporate all members of the patient's family. Here, we provide a brief review of the existing family-based interventions for asthma, highlighting some innovative features of such programs that could be adapted and applied for clinical use.

Given the historical emphasis on the effect of family dynamics on the development and course of asthma, some early programs utilized family therapy in the treatment of pediatric asthma, specifically for more severe groups. In one early study, Lask and Matthew (Lask and Matthew 1979) compared the effects of a relatively brief course of family therapy (6 h over four months) and medical treatment to the effects of standard medical treatment alone. Results were mixed, with no differences on many of the disease variables, except for some modest effects on day-wheeze score and thoracic lung volume. In a later study, Gustafsson and colleagues also evaluated the effects of longer-term family therapy in comparison to standard medical care for severe asthma (Gustafsson et al. 1986). Children who received conventional treatment demonstrated no change in symptoms and pulmonary function scores, whereas children in the family therapy condition improved in the general pediatric assessment of overall health, a key measure of overall functioning. There was some heterogeneity in response to treatment in the experimental group, however, with a proportion of children (12 of 18) improving on numerous measures (e.g. peak expiratory flow, days with functional impairment, doses of quick-relief medication), and others evidencing little change with treatment. Results of these early studies suggest that outpatient family therapy may serve an important adjunctive role to medical treatment for some children with asthma, specifically those with severe illness. The cost and time required to implement family treatment, however, needs to be considered.

Some interventions for pediatric asthma have integrated family treatment as part of an inpatient hospitalization or medical residential program. Weinstein et al. (1992) implemented a family-centered, short-term residential program incorporating medical and behavioral components. They found a significant reduction in subsequent health care utilization (emergency visits and hospitalizations), as well as improvements in lung function and symptom presentation. One limitation to this approach, however, is the difficulty in implementing a randomized, controlled format in evaluating a multi-component inpatient program. Hence, it is not clear, which components of treatment were most effective (medical vs. behavioral), and there is no control group against which to evaluate outcomes.

One more recent study evaluated the effects of an intensive, 3-month family based intervention for asthma management in urban families in contrast to a usual care control (Bonner et al. 2002). This approach combined family workshops and individualized sessions by a family coordinator to facilitate family-physician communication and promote family awareness of asthma as a chronic health condition through behavioral strategies (e.g., symptom monitoring and review). The experimental group demonstrated significant improvements on many measures of knowledge, health beliefs, self-efficacy, and self-reported adherence. Decreases in symptom persistence and activity restriction were also evident. Given the high morbidity and higher risk of mortality typically evidenced in urban, minority groups (Mannino et al. 1998), an intensive, family-based approach such as this one may be more effective than standard group-based asthma education.

In sum, there are very few family-based interventions for pediatric asthma. In a recent review of the literature, we were unable to locate any family-oriented interventions for adults with asthma. Our brief review of the existing literature suggests that family-based approaches may be quite useful, however given the intensity of time and resources needed to implement such interventions, targeting specific patient populations (e.g., patients with more severe asthma and/or with a high degree of medical utilization) may be the most fruitful approach.

Conclusion

There is a wealth of research indicating that families shape the onset and progression of asthma disease course, and are, in turn, shaped by a family member having asthma. Although the majority of assessment instruments specific to asthma are geared toward individual beliefs, attitudes, and behaviors, some selected questionnaires and interviews are available to assess aspects of family functioning specific to asthma management and the effects of asthma on the family. Family-based interventions may be costly, yet have the potential to be uniquely helpful in cases of more severe disease or complex psychosocial situations. Research should continue to attempt to capture the complex picture of the role of asthma in the family by utilizing prospective, longitudinal designs that map the influence of individual, family, and disease variables over time.

References

Asmussen L, Olson L, Grant E, Fagan J, Weiss K (1999) Reliability and validity of the Children's Health Survey for Asthma. Pediatrics 104:71

Bartlett SJ, Kolodner K, Butz AM, Eggleston P, Malveaux F, Rand C (2001) Maternal depressive symptoms and emergency department use among inner-city children with asthma. Arch Pediatr Adolesc Med 155:347–353

Bartlett SJ, Krishnan JA, Riekert KA, Butz AM, Malveaux FJ, Rand CS (2004) Maternal depressive symptoms and adherence to therapy in inner-city children with asthma. Pediatrics 113(2):229–237

Bender B, Milgrom H, Rand C, Ackerson L (1998) Psychological factors associated with medication nonadherence in asthmatic children. J Asthma 35:347–353
Berz JB, Carter AS, Wagmiller RL, Horwitz SM, Murdock KK, Briggs-Gowan M (2007) Prevalence and correlates of early onset asthma and wheezing in a healthy birth cohort of 2- to 3-year olds. J Pediatr Psychol 32(2):154–166
Bonner S, Zimmerman BJ, Evans D, Clark NM, Feldman CH, Irigoyen M, Resnick D, Mellins RB (2002) An individualized intervention to improve asthma management among urban Latino and African-American families. J Asthma 39(2): 167–179
Brown JV, Bakeman R, Celano MP, Demi AS, Kobrynski L, Wilson SR (2002) Home-based asthma education of young low-income children and their families. J Pediatr Psychol 27(8):677–688
Bursch B, Schwankovsky L, Gilbert J, Zeiger R (1999) Construction and validation of four childhood asthma self-management scales: parent barriers, child and parent self-efficacy and parent belief in treatment efficacy. J Asthma 36(1):115–128
Chen E, Bloomberg GR, Fisher EGJ, Strunk RC (2003) Predictors of repeat hospitalizations in children with asthma: the role of psychosocial and socioenvironmental factors. Health Psychol 22:12–18
Clark N, Jones P, Keller S, Vermeire P (1999) Patient factors and compliance with asthma therapy. Respir Med 93(12):856–862
Cummings L, Mobley CN, McQuaid EL, Celano M, Penza-Clyve S, Kopel S (2004) Developement and validation of the child asthma knowledge questionnaire across two sites. Paper presented at the National Conference on Child Health Psychology, Charleston, SC
De Ridder DTD, Schreurs KMG, Kuijer RG (2005) Is spousal support always helpful to patients with asthma or diabetes? A prospective study. Psychol Health 20(4):497–508
Environmental Protection Agency (1992) Respiratory Health Effects of Passive Smoking: Lung cancer and other disorders (EPA Publication EPA/600/6-90-006F). Environmental Protection Agency, Washington, DC
Feeney JA (2000) Implications of attachment style for patterns of health and illness. Child Care Health Dev 26(4):277–288
Fiese BH, Wamboldt FS (2003) Tales of pediatric asthma management: family-based strategies related to medical adherence and health care utilization. J Pediatr 143(4):457–462
Fiese BH, Wilder J, Bickham NL (2000) Family context in developmental psychopathology. In: Sameroff AJ, Lewis M, Miller SM (eds) Handbook of developmental psychopathology, 2nd edn. Kluwer Academics Publishers, Dordrecht, Netherlands, pp xxxi, pp 813
French TM, Alexander F (1941) Psychogenic factors in bronchial asthma. Psychosom Med 4:2
Gallant MP (2003) The influence of social support on chronic illness self-management: a review and directions for research. Health Educ Behav 30(2):170–195
Gartland HJ, Day HD (1999) Family predictors of the incidence of children's asthma symptoms: Expressed emotion, medication, parent contact, and life events. J Clin Psychol 55:573–584
Gavin L, Wysocki T (2006) Associations of paternal involvement in disease management with maternal and family outcomes in families of children with chronic illness. J Pediatr Psychol 31:481–489
Georgiou A, Buchner DA, Ershoff DH, Blasko KM, Goodman LV, Feigin J (2003) The impact of a large-scale population-based asthma management program on pediatric asthma patients and their caregivers. Ann Allergy Asthma Immunol 90(3):308–315
Gibson PG, Powell H, Coughlan J, Wilson AJ, Hensley MJ, Abramson M, Bauman A, Walters EH (2002) Limited (information only) patient education programs for adults with asthma. Cochrane Database Syst Rev 2. CD001005
Grus CL, Lopez-Hernandez C, Delameter A, Appelgate B, Brito A, Wurm G, Wanner A (2001) Parental self-efficacy and morbidity in pediatric asthma. J Asthma 38:99–106
Gustafsson PA, Kjellman NI, Cederblad M (1986) Family therapy in the treatment of severe childhood asthma. J Psychosom Res 30:369–374
Gustafsson PA, Bjorksten B, Kjellman NI (1994) Family dysfunction in asthma: a prospective study of illness development. J Pediatr 125(3):493–498
Halterman JS, Yoos HL, Conn KM, Callahan PM, Montes G, Neely TL, Szilagyi PG (2004) The impact of childhood asthma on parental quality of life. J Asthma 41(6):645–653
Juniper EF, Guyatt GH, Feeny DH, Ferrie PJ, Griffith LE, Townsend M (1996) Measuring quality of life in the parents of children with asthma. Qual Life Res 5(1):27–34
Juniper EF, Svensson K, Mork AC, Stahl E (2004) Measuring health-related quality of life in adults during an acute asthma exacerbation. Chest 125(1):93–97
Kaugars AS, Klinnert MD, Bender BG (2004) Family influences on pediatric asthma. J Pediatr Psychol 29:475–491
Kaugars A, Klinnert MD, Robinson J, Ho M (2008) Reciprocal influences in children's and families' adaptation to early childhood wheezing. Health Psychol 27(2):258–267
Kazak AE (1989) Families of chronically ill children: A systems and social-ecological model of adaptation and challenge. J Consult Clin Psychol 57:25–30
Kazak AE, Segal-Andrews AM, Johnson K (1995) Pediatric psychology research and practice: A family/systems approach. In: Roberts MC (ed) Handbook of pediatric psychology. Guilford, New York
Klinnert M, Mrazek D (1994) Early asthma onset: The interaction between family stressors and adaptive parenting. Psychiatry 57:51–61
Klinnert M, Mrazek P, Mrazek D (1994) Early asthma onset: The interaction between family stressors and adaptive parenting. Psychiatry 57(1):51–61
Klinnert MD, McQuaid EL, Gavin L (1997) Assessing the family management system. J Asthma 34:77–88
Klinnert M, Nelson H, Price M, Adinoff A, Leung D, Mrazek D (2001) Onset and persistence of childhood asthma: Predictors from infancy. Pediatrics 108(4):e69–e77
Koinis Mitchell D, Murdock KM, McQuaid EM (2004) Risk and resilience in urban children with asthma. Children's Health Care 33(4):275–298
Lask B, Matthew D (1979) Childhood asthma. A controlled trial of family psychotherapy. Arch Dis Child 54(2):116–119
Lim J, Wood BL, Miller BD (2008) Maternal depression and parenting in relation to child internalizing symptoms and asthma disease activity. J Fam Psychol 22(2):264–273
Mannino DM, Homa DM, Pertowski CA, Ashizawa A, Nixon LL, Johnson CA, Ball LB, Jack E, Kang DS (1998)

Surveillance for asthma: United States, 1960–1995. Morb Mortal Wkly Rev 47:1–27

Mansour M, Lanphear B, DeWitt T (2000) Barriers to asthma in urban children: parent perspectives. Pediatrics 106:512–519

Markson S, Fiese BH (2000) Family rituals as a protective factor for children with asthma. J Pediatr Psychol 25(7):471–480

McQuaid EL, Penza-Clyve S, Nassau JH, Fritz GK, Klein R, O'Conner S, Wamboldt FS, Gavin L (2001) Sharing family responsibility for asthma management tasks. Children's Health Care 30(3):183–199

McQuaid E, Kopel SJ, Klein RB, Fritz GK (2003) Medication adherence in pediatric asthma: reasoning, responsibility, and behavior. J Pediatr Psychol 28:323–333

McQuaid E, Walders N, Kopel S, Fritz G, Klinnert M (2005) Pediatric asthma management in the family context: The family asthma management system scale. J Pediatr Psychol 30:492–502

Miller BD, Wood BL (2003) Emotions and family factors in childhood asthma: psychobiologic mechanisms and pathways of effect. Adv Psychosom Med 24:131–160

Mrazek DA, Casey B, Anderson I (1987) Insecure attachment in severely asthmatic preschool children: Is it a risk factor? J Am Acad Child Adolesc Psychiatry 26(4):516–520

Oddy WH (2004) A review of the effects of breastfeeding in respiratory infection, atopy and childhood asthma. J Asthma 41:605–621

Ortega A, McQuaid EL, Canino G, Goodwin RD, Fritz GK (2004) Comorbidity of asthma and anxiety and depression in Puerto Rican children. Psychosomatics 45(2):93–99

Powell H, Gibson PG (2003) Options for self-management education for adults with asthma. Cochrane Database Syst Rev 1. CD004107

Repetti RL, Taylor SE, Seeman TE (2002) Risky families: family social environments and the mental and physical health of offspring. Psychol Bull 128(2):330–366

Sawyer MG, Spurrier N, Kennedy D, Martin J (2001) The relationship between the quality of life of children with asthma and family functioning. J Asthma 38(3):279–284

Schobinger R, Florin I, Zimmer C, Lindemann H, Winter H (1992) Childhood asthma: paternal critical attitude and father-child interaction. J Psychosom Res 36(8):743–750

Schobinger R, Florin I, Reichbauer M, Lindemann H, Zimmer C (1993) Childhood asthma: mother's affective attitude, mother-child interaction and children's compliance with medical requirements. J Psychosom Res 37(7):697–707

Shalowitz MU, Berry CA, Quinn KA, Wolf RL (2001) The relationship of life stressors and maternal depression to pediatric asthma morbidity in subspecialty practice. Ambulatory Pediatrics 1(4):185–193

Sharek P, Mayer M, Loewy L, Robinson T, Shames R, Umetsu D, Bergman D (2002) Agreement among measures of asthma status: a prospective study of low-income children with moderate to severe asthma. Pediatrics 110(4):797–804

Silver EJ, Westbrook LE, Stein REK (1998) Relationship of parental psychological distress to consenquences of chronic health conditions in children. J Pediatr Psychol 23(1):5–15

Spurrier NJ, Staugas R, Sawyer MG, Wakefield MA, Ruffin RE, Jureidini J, Arney F, Baghurst P (2003) Health-service use by children with asthma over a 6-month period. J Paediatr Child Health 39(1):15–21

Strunk R, Mrazek DA, Wofson Fuhrmann GS, LaBreque JF (1985) Physiological and psychological characteristics associated with deaths due to asthma in childhood: A case-controlled study. J Am Med Assoc 254:1193–1198

Uchino BN, Cacioppo JT, Kiecolt-Glaser JK (1996) The relationship between social support and physiological processes: a review with emphasis on underlying mechanisms and implications for health. Psychol Bull 119(3):488–531

Wade SL, Islam S, Holden G, Kruszon-Moran D, Mitchell H (1999) Division of responsibility for asthma management tasks between caregivers and children in the inner city. J Dev Behav Pediatr 20:93–98

Walders N, Drotar D, Kercsmar C (2000) The allocation of family responsibility for asthma management tasks in African-American adolescents. J Asthma 37:89–99

Wamboldt MZ, Wamboldt FS (2000) Role of the family in the onset and outcome of childhood disorders: selected research findings. J Am Acad Child Adolesc Psychiatry 39(10):1212–1219

Wamboldt MZ, Weintraub P, Krafchick D, Wamboldt FS (1996) Psychiatric family history in adolescents with severe asthma. J Am Acad Child Adolesc Psychiatry 35(8):1042–1049

Wasilewski Y, Clark N, Evans D, Levison M, Levin B, Mellins R (1996) Factors associated with emergency department visits by children with asthma: implications for health education. Am J Public Health 86:1410–1415

Weil C, Wade SL, Bauman LJ, Lynn H, Mitchell H, Lavigne J (1999) The relationship between psychosocial factors and asthma morbidity in inner-city children with asthma. Pediatrics 104:1274–1280

Weinstein AG, Faust DS, McKee L, Padman R (1992) Outcome of short-term hospitalization for children with severe asthma. J Allergy Clin Immunol 90:66–75

Wills-Karp M, Ewart SL (2004) Time to draw breath: asthma-susceptibility genes are identified. Nat Rev Genet 5(5):376–387

Wolf FM, Guevara JP, Grum CM, Clark NM, Cates CJ (2003) Educational interventions for asthma in children. Cochrane Database Syst Rev 6(4):106–107

Wood BL, Klebba KB, Miller BD (2000) Evolving the biobehavioral family model: the fit of attachment. Fam Process 39(3):319–344

Wood BL, Lim J, Miller BD, Cheah PA, Simmens S, Stern T, Waxmonsky J, Ballow M (2007) Family emotional climate, depression, emotional triggering of asthma, and disease severity in pediatric asthma: Examination of pathways of effect. J Pediatr Psychol 32(5):542–551

Wysocki T, Gavin LA (2004) Psychometric properties of a new measure of father's involvement in the management of pediatic chronic diseases. J Pediatr Psychol 29:231–240

Wysocki T, Gavin L (2006) Paternal involvement in the management of pediatric chronic diseases: Associations with adherence, quality of life, and health status. J Pediatr Psychol 31: 501–511

Chapter 14
Asthma in the Schools

Joan M. Mangan, Sarah Merkle, and Lynn B. Gerald

Introduction

As other chapters in this text have illustrated, asthma is affected by a myriad of social and economic factors. It is also greatly influenced by factors in the physical environment of a person with asthma. As children spend a significant amount of time at school, the conditions at school are important for their asthma control. For example, they may experience asthma symptoms or exacerbations while at school and need to take medication. Moreover, they may need to use preventive medication before engaging in physical education activities or take steps to avoid other asthma triggers throughout the day. These precautions often require support from school administrators and assistance from school staff.

Over ten million children under age 18 (14%) have ever been told by a health care professional that they have asthma (Bloom and Cohen 2009). Within this group, almost 7 million (10%) report a current asthma diagnosis. Therefore, on average, one of every ten students in the United States has asthma. In 2006, these children made nearly four million outpatient health care visits and 593,000 emergency department visits, and asthma accounted for 155,000 pediatric hospitalizations (Akinbami et al. 2009). Thus, asthma is the leading cause of hospitalizations among children. Fortunately, deaths from asthma are rare; in 2005 the total reported number of deaths due to asthma among children in the United States was 131 (Akinbami et al. 2009). Asthma morbidity is disproportionately higher among low-income, minority, and inner-city children. Lack of access to consistent, high-quality health care and greater exposure to allergens, environmental triggers, stress, and other factors may contribute to the reported disparities.

A variety of studies have demonstrated that asthma can significantly affect school attendance and students' academic performance. The National Health Interview Survey, conducted in 2003, determined that children with at least one asthma attack (4 million) in the previous year missed 12.8 million school days due to asthma (Akinbami 2006). A more recent industry-funded survey indicated that 54% of children aged 4–18 with asthma had missed school in the past year as a result of their asthma, and 9% had missed more than 2 weeks because of asthma (Schulman, Ronca, and Bucuvalas, Inc. [SRBI] 2004). Parents reported that their children with asthma missed 3.7 days of school on average each year. (SRBI 2004). If this number is applied to almost 7 million children with asthma in this age group, then an estimated total of almost 26 million school days are missed per year.

Asthma may also affect students' academic performance in less obvious ways (Clark et al. 2004; Diette et al. 2000). Studies have found that many children experience regular disruptions during their sleep because of their asthma. A study by Diette et al. (2000) indicated that more than 40% of children with asthma had nocturnal awakenings from asthma in the 4-week period immediately before the survey, and disrupted sleep was associated with missed school days. Furthermore, missed sleep is associated with poor recall memory and increased attention difficulties (Dahl 1996; Raidy and Scharff 2005; Stores et al. 1998), lack of concentration, mood swings (Dahl 1996), and behavioral problems (Sadeh et al. 2002). Even less severe asthma symptoms that might not

L.B. Gerald (✉)
Mel and Enid Zuckerman College of Public Health, University of Arizona, 1295 N. Martin Ave, PO Box 245163, Tucson, AZ, 85724, USA
e-mail: lgerald@email.arizona.edu

A. Harver and H. Kotses (eds.), *Asthma, Health and Society: A Public Health Perspective*, DOI 10.1007/978-0-387-78285-0_14, © Springer Science+Business Media, LLC 2010

prompt a parent to seek care for a child can also interfere with a child's ability to get a good night's sleep, play, or fully participate in school activities. For these reasons, asthma has emerged as an important health problem that schools must address.

Strategies for Managing Asthma

Over the past decade, the school setting has increasingly received attention from federal, state, and local groups that seek to improve the diagnosis, treatment, and self-management of childhood asthma and provide asthma education to children, their caregivers, and school personnel. During the "Asthma Prevention, Management, and Treatment: Community-based Approaches for the New Millennium" conference sponsored by the American Lung Association and Kaiser Permanente in 2000, an expert panel was convened to develop the key elements required for school-based asthma education and intervention. Later, the Centers for Disease Control and Prevention (CDC) used these key elements to outline six strategies for schools to use to create a healthy, safe environment conducive to learning for students with asthma. Specifically, these strategies propose that schools accomplish the following (CDC 2005):

Strategy 1: Establish management and support systems for asthma-friendly schools.
Strategy 2: Provide appropriate school health and mental health services for students with asthma.
Strategy 3: Provide asthma education and awareness programs for students and school staff.
Strategy 4: Provide a safe and healthy school environment to reduce asthma triggers.
Strategy 5: Provide safe, enjoyable physical education and activity opportunities for students with asthma.
Strategy 6: Coordinate school, family, and community efforts to better manage asthma symptoms and reduce school absences among students with asthma.

A detailed list of recommended tactics for each of these strategies and complementary resources that stakeholders may employ to implement these approaches are available through the CDC, the American Lung Association, and the National Asthma Education and Prevention Program (CDC 2005).

Although these strategies and recommended tactics provide a comprehensive and admirable approach, implementation of all six strategies would be a very ambitious undertaking for most schools or school districts. Furthermore, not every strategy may be appropriate or feasible for a particular school. Yet, even small changes can have a significant impact on the health of children with asthma. Therefore, when considering how to improve asthma care, program planners need to examine the resources or services that are currently available and identify barriers or problems with current approaches to the provision of appropriate care. This process, often called a "formal needs assessment," can help program planners to determine the met and unmet needs for asthma services. (A *met need* is a service within a school or district that is currently being addressed through existing resources. An *unmet need* is a service that is not currently being addressed through existing services and activities, either because no services are currently available or available services may be inappropriate or inaccessible.) Identifying unmet needs enables planners to pinpoint "gaps" or discrepancies between the ideal situation and current conditions. Planners can then establish and prioritize the objectives for a program and select the CDC strategies and corresponding tactics to employ. CDC's *School Health Index* (CDC 2005) is one tool that could be used to conduct a needs assessment.

Implementing Recommended Asthma Strategies

This chapter is organized around the six comprehensive strategies for asthma management in schools. The following sections highlight some of the tactics for implementing these strategies within an individual school or across an entire district, a few pragmatic suggestions for groups seeking to initiate an asthma program, and several factors that program planners may need to consider as they strive to put these strategies into practice.

Management and Support Systems

The CDC strategies acknowledge that asthma, like other chronic health problems, requires the systems to be in place to support a child with asthma and facilitate asthma self-management practices. This entails an initial assessment of existing asthma needs, resources, and potential barriers as described in the previous section. This needs assessment should be followed by the development and implementation of written policies and procedures for asthma education and management (CDC 2005). Optimally, one person, such as the health coordinator of the school or district, is designated to coordinate these activities.

Once these policies and procedures are in place, school records can be used or adapted to identify students who have a physician diagnosis of asthma. Priority should be given to identifying and intervening with those students who have poorly managed asthma. (Bonilla et al. 2005; Bruzzese et al. 2006; Moonie et al. 2006; Taras and Potts-Datema 2005; Vargas et al. 2006; Yawn 2006; Yawn et al. 2003).These students may be identified by (1) monitoring children who have frequent absences to determine whether the absences are health related; (2) monitoring students' health care seeking behaviors while at school; (3) monitoring the number of times students are sent home because of asthma; and (4) having discussions with teaching staff and (5) having students with asthma periodically complete a validated assessment of their asthma control (NAEPP 2007). Schools may also consider monitoring school-initiated calls for emergency services and parental reports of emergency room visits and hospitalizations.

It is important to note that the CDC and partner organizations do not advocate that schools engage in mass screening or mass case detection programs with screening tools, questionnaires, or pulmonary function testing to identify children with asthma. These approaches are time and resource intensive and have not been shown to improve health outcomes (Boss et al. 2003; CDC 2005; Wheeler et al. 2004; Wheeler and Boyle 2006; Yawn 2006; Yawn et al. 2003). Currently, the CDC and organizations such as the American Thoracic Society recommend that schools consider using a case identification system to identify students who have asthma (Gerald et al. 2007). This approach entails using information or documents that many schools require as part of enrollment, such as health history cards, physical examination reports from health care providers, or emergency contact cards, to create a list of students with various health concerns (Wheeler et al. 2004). Recent research has indicated that the addition of two simple questions – (1) Has a doctor ever said your child has asthma? and (2) In the past 12 months has your child taken asthma medicine (pills, inhalers, or puffers) prescribed by a doctor? – to a school health form can be used to identify children who have asthma with 96% specificity and 66% sensitivity (Gerald et al. 2004). Finally, the actions that schools take to accommodate a student's health needs or activity limitations may be outlined in Individualized Education Plans (IEP) or 504 Plans.

Before these activities begin, any group or organization seeking to initiate a program must actively garner the support of school administrators. This includes the leadership at the district level such as the superintendent of schools and assistant superintendents; the directors of facilities, student health, and student enrollment and attendance; and the leaders within individual schools including the principal, vice principals, school nurse, and custodial staff supervisors. The support of these leaders can facilitate the (1) recruitment of school personnel willing to support the program, (2) time commitment to asthma-specific activities, (3) coverage for school-based team members to attend meetings, and (4) school-wide staff participation in a program (Forbis et al. 2006; Langenfeld et al. 2006). These leaders can also help program planners accomplish the following: (1) gain program approval from the school board, (2) identify proper forms or paperwork that must be completed relative to planned activities in accordance with the policies and procedures of state or local boards of education (e.g., forms authorizing students to self-carry asthma medication), and (3) collect outcome data.

Without the support of school leaders, a program may fail to launch at the onset or the objectives of the program may not be completely realized. Programs that have successfully gained the support of these leaders have done so by discussing measures for which schools and their leaders are held accountable, including student factors such as attendance, academic achievement, participation in physical activity, and attainment of physical fitness, as well as facilities management for environmental safety, staff development, and parental involvement (Langenfeld et al. 2006). To further illustrate the need to address asthma in schools, successful programs have provided school administrators with baseline data such as the number of students with asthma in the school or district, the average absenteeism for students with and without asthma, the numbers of children with and without emergency asthma action plans, and the number of children with quick-relief medications available within the school. With permission from the students' parent, asthma program staff may also consider providing school administrators information related to students' physician or clinic office visits, 911 calls, and telephone calls the school has made to parents regarding their children's asthma, if such data are available (Langenfeld et al. 2006). If this information is not readily available, data from previous studies or data collected through national surveys may be substituted and used as a benchmark to evaluate program efforts. One data set that may be particularly helpful is the CDC's School Health Policies and Programs Study, which is a survey conducted periodically to assess school health policies and programs at the state, district, school, and classroom level (CDC 2001).

School administrators are only one group of stakeholders from whom program planners should have input and commitment to ensure the successful implementation of these strategies. Stakeholders are all persons with a direct interest or investment in addressing asthma in the school environment. Other stakeholders include, but are not limited to, teachers, coaches, school environmental services staff, school nurses, students, parents, local medical personnel, asthma coalitions, and agencies or organizations vested in decreasing asthma symptoms. Each stakeholder group will have a slightly different perspective on the strategies listed above and may set priorities differently from their colleagues. These differing perspectives and roles will influence the selection and implementation of priorities for a coordinated asthma management program as well as the manner in which a program is evaluated. For these reasons, potential stakeholders should be identified and recruited early in the planning process.

Another factor frequently cited as a key to success in implementing these strategies is the identification of an "asthma champion," or a person who enthusiastically supports the aims of an asthma program (Byrne et al. 2006; Guglielmo and Little 2006). Often, these are people who have close ties with the schools and personal experiences with asthma. Many "asthma champions" either have a diagnosis of asthma themselves or have a close family member or child who has been diagnosed with the disease. As a result, they are able to put their own experiences into the context of the school setting. Potential "asthma champions" will usually present themselves to program leaders when plans to initiate a program are announced. They may be a school administrator, a faculty member, part of the school's support personnel, or a volunteer who works closely with the school staff, such as the president of the parent–teacher association. Primarily, "asthma champions" help motivate their colleagues or school staff to initiate and sustain program activities. Consequently, they too should be considered important stakeholders for program leaders to engage in the planning process.

Health and Mental Health Services

Reductions in asthma morbidity and subsequent improvements in school attendance and performance are seldom feasible without access to appropriate medical care and pharmacotherapy. The collective experience of past and current programs has demonstrated that those programs that provide care directly or establish a relationship between the school and the students' healthcare providers have more success in reducing asthma morbidity than those programs that have not provided links to medical care (Anderson et al. 2004; Barbot et al. 2006; Bartholomew et al. 2006; Byrne et al. 2006; Forbis et al. 2006; Frankowski et al. 2006; Guglielmo and Little 2006; Halterman et al. 2004; Jones et al. 2005; Levy et al. 2006; Liao and Galant 2004; Liao et al. 2006; Lwebuga-Mukasa and Dunn-Georgiou 2002; Millard et al. 2003; Murphy et al. 2006; Richmond et al. 2006; Taras et al. 2004; Tinkelman and Schwartz 2004; Webber et al. 2003; Wheeler et al. 2006).

In addition to providing appropriate health services, schools and programs must strive to make mental health services readily accessible to children with asthma. As with other chronic diseases, asthma is associated with psychological factors such as depression, anxiety, panic, and embarrassment. In fact, youth with asthma have an almost twofold higher prevalence of anxiety and depressive disorders compared with control youth (Katon 2007).

Asthma symptoms and exacerbations, as well as perceptions of a dependence on asthma medications, can cause asthma patients to feel different from their peers or experience depressive states, anxiety, panic, or embarrassment (Anderson et al. 2005; SRBI 2004; Taitel et al. 1998). In a survey of 801 children with asthma, in which the parent or caregiver was interviewed if the child was 4–15 years of age and children 16–18 years of age were interviewed directly, 30% of respondents reported that they often or sometimes felt fearful as a result of their asthma, 30% often or sometimes felt angry, and 20% often or sometimes felt depressed (SRBI 2004). In a subset of adolescent respondents ($n=226$) who reported not always admitting that asthma was the reason they did not participate in an activity, 32% reported not wanting others to worry and 23% reported that embarrassment prevented them from admitting that asthma was the underlying reason (SRBI 2004). Emotional responses to asthma may cause a child with asthma to have more trouble than a child without asthma adjusting to the school environment and establishing relationships with peers and teachers (McQuaid et al. 2001; Weil et al. 1999). School health teams and asthma program staff can support the social and emotional health of students by teaching all students to support classmates and others with asthma. Asthma education programs and after-school asthma clubs can provide peer support for students with asthma and may help students feel more comfortable talking about their frustrations and fears related to having the chronic disease.

The primary tactic a school can adopt to decrease the physical impact of asthma is to obtain a copy of a written asthma action plan developed by the student's healthcare provider from the parents of all students who have been diagnosed with asthma. Optimally, action plans include a list of the student's asthma triggers, instructions for peak flow monitoring, instructions for medications, and an individualized emergency plan with emergency contact information (NAEPP 2007). If a student does not have a personal asthma action plan, standardized emergency procedures for children who experience respiratory distress may be developed using recommendations from local health officers or national organizations (CDC 2005). Additionally, schools must ensure that students have immediate access to their prescribed medications at all times. To achieve this, administrators may contemplate allowing students to self-carry and self-administer inhaled asthma medications. It is recommended, however, that the decision to allow a student to carry and administer his or her own medicine be determined on a case-by-case basis and that the school personnel, the child's health care provider, and parents have a role in the decision (CDC 2005; Jones and Wheeler 2004; National Asthma Education and Prevention Program 2005).

A review of the literature indicates that a proactive approach is needed to realize these strategies. Significant school resources, such as school nursing time, will be needed to get appropriate forms and quick-relief medications to the school and to encourage coordination among the school, the family, and the health care provider (Wheeler et al. 2006). Reports indicate that, on average, schools receive written asthma action plans for less than 50% of students who have been diagnosed with asthma, and among children who seek care at school for an asthma episode, action plans are on file or available approximately 25% of the time (McLaughlin et al. 2006; SRBI 2004; Whalen et al. 2004). Common challenges to obtaining these items include an inability to contact parents, parents' poor understanding of good asthma control, and parents' lack of compliance with school policies (Anderson et al. 2005; Dozier et al. 2006; Forbis et al. 2006; Wheeler et al. 2006). Moreover, parents may not report their child's asthma to the school, so that schools are often unaware of students who have a physician diagnosis of asthma or who carry asthma medications on their person (Bartholomew et al. 2006). To rectify these problems, some programs have included asthma information in new-student packets, school newsletters, and school websites (Langenfeld et al. 2006). Other strategies have included parent workshops of asthma, presentations during parent–teacher association meetings or parent–teacher conferences, or displays with asthma information. The availability of a nebulizer and stock quick-relief medications with spacers in first aid kits at school can also serve as an incentive for parents and school nurses to get a signed order for treatment at school, especially if the school's policy is to send students home if they have an asthma episode and if a medication order is not available (Byrne et al. 2006; Wheeler et al. 2006).

As mentioned earlier in this section, some asthma programs have worked to connect children with health care providers to confirm an asthma diagnosis, provide medical therapy, create personalized asthma action plans, and teach parents and their children asthma self-management. It is important to note that these labor-intensive approaches have yielded mixed results (Bartholomew et al. 2006;

Gerald et al. 2006). Regrettably, some programs that have offered good access to medical care and pharmacotherapy report that even when care is available, it is often not used. Barriers to establishing links to appropriate care include a lack of family involvement, poor understanding that asthma can seriously affect their child's school activities and that asthma can be better controlled (Ayala et al. 2006; Dozier et al. 2006; Yawn et al. 2003), transportation issues, and problems with cost and availability of medications or health care providers (Wheeler et al. 2006). Strategies that have helped to overcome these barriers include the establishment of working relationships between school nurses and community asthma care clinicians (Barbot et al. 2006; Bergman et al. 2008; Frankowski et al. 2006; Guglielmo and Little 2006; Levy et al. 2006; Richmond et al. 2006; Tinkelman and Schwartz 2004; Wheeler et al. 2006; Wilson et al. 2009) or area hospitals (Bartholomew et al. 2006; Byrne et al. 2006; Halterman et al. 2004; Lwebuga-Mukasa and Dunn-Georgiou 2002), a school-based asthma specialist (Bartholomew et al. 2006; Millard et al. 2003), a school-based health center (Webber et al. 2003), or a mobile asthma care clinic (Halterman et al. 2004; Jones et al. 2005; Liao et al. 2006).

The provision of school nurse case management for those children with significant asthma morbidity has been successful in improving medical care of children with asthma (Byrne et al. 2006; Richmond et al. 2006; Taras et al. 2004). This form of case management may entail meeting with or calling parents and clinicians, providing individual health counseling to students, and ensuring that all proper medications and forms are available at the school (Barbot et al. 2006; Frankowski et al. 2006; Guglielmo and Little 2006; Levy et al. 2006; Splett et al. 2006; Taras et al. 2004; Wheeler and Boyle 2006; Wheeler et al. 2006). Although case management programs are ideal, they require frequent communication between asthma care clinicians, parents, and school staff. Unfortunately, school nurses are not present in every school. Instead, one nurse may be responsible for many students in a number of schools. This staffing design often leads to an overwhelming student-to-nurse ratio, restricts the time and attention a nurse may provide to a school, and limits his or her ability to deliver comprehensive services or provide timely communication to asthma care clinicians and parents.

A simple strategy to decrease asthma exacerbations that has proven effective in schools without full time nurses is the daily supervision of inhaled corticosteroids in children with persistent asthma (Gerald et al. 2009). Among children, rates of adherence to daily controller medications range from 18 to 65% (Boychuk et al. 2006; Milgrom et al. 1996) with most reports indicating less than 50% adherence. Directly observed therapy can ensure adherence (Osterberg and Blaschke 2005) and also help establish the habit of taking daily medication even when symptoms are not present. In a study involving 290 children with persistent asthma in 36 schools, the likelihood of experiencing an episode of poor asthma control among students whose inhaled steroids were not supervised at school was 57% higher than for students whose inhaled steroids were supervised at school. Daily supervision of medication was accomplished using only seven part-time staff. Although many schools do not have full-time nurses, approximately 5% of children receive daily medication at school (McCarthy et al. 2000). Medication supervision is often accomplished through trained medication teams, which may consist of office personnel or other trained school personnel. Once-daily dosing of inhaled steroids has been found to be as effective as the more commonly prescribed twice daily dosing (Mallol and Aguirre 2007; Moller et al. 1999; Campbell et al. 1998; Herjavecz et al. 1999) and greatly facilitates the supervision of this medication at school. Therefore, it is feasible that this type of intervention could be effectively established in schools without full-time nurses.

Regardless of the availability of school nurses, it is judicious for all asthma programs to develop a system to facilitate communication between schools, clinicians, and parents regarding asthma episodes that occur at school. Schools can provide important information that can assist clinicians in providing more appropriate care and can increase parental awareness of any difficulties that their child may be experiencing (Wheeler et al. 2006).

Asthma Education

An asthma education and awareness campaign can make a significant contribution to a school asthma program. For students and their parents, these campaigns can help to provide a better understanding of an asthma diagnosis, recommended medication regimens, and the skills needed to better manage the disease (Bernard-Bonnin et al. 1995; Lorig et al. 1999; Parcel et al. 1986). Additionally, educational campaigns have the capacity to modify peoples' attitudes and beliefs regarding asthma and its treatment, as well as the practices necessary to avoid and control asthma episodes. This is important because misperceptions related to asthma are not uncommon. For example, many parents and children report significant levels of asthma symptoms but consider the asthma to be well controlled (Dozier et al. 2006). Parents and students also frequently underestimate the severity of asthma or the impact it may have on a child's participation at school (Dozier et al. 2006; Yawn et al. 2006). These views may be a major yet unrecognized barrier to asthma control.

It is important to note that education that focuses primarily on providing information about asthma is not sufficient to improve asthma management or morbidity (Hilton et al. 1986). Although a baseline level of knowledge is necessary to enable some actions such as proper inhaler technique to occur, after this threshold has been met, additional factual information does not automatically cause additional changes in people's behaviors (Green and Marshall 1991). To be most effective, educational interventions must expand beyond factual knowledge about the disease and focus on applied knowledge, such as how to avoid triggers or how to respond appropriately to an asthma episode. Furthermore, without links to appropriate medical care, educational interventions are unlikely to be successful in reducing asthma exacerbations.

As part of their efforts to provide effective asthma education for their students, some schools and their asthma programs have incorporated lessons specific to asthma into health and physical education curricula, tobacco programs, or environmental health programs for the general student body (Langenfeld et al. 2006). Other schools have initiated school-based asthma clubs that meet regularly during the academic year for students with asthma, have started peer-led educational programs, or have offered one of a number of evidence-based educational programs developed specifically for students and school staff (Brasler and Lewis 2006; CDC, *Potentially Effective Interventions for Asthma;* Cicutto et al. 2005; Patterson et al. 2005; Shah et al. 2001). Because many of these programs have been broadly disseminated and assessed, developing new materials is usually unnecessary. Evaluations of these programs have revealed improvements in students' knowledge, self-efficacy to manage their asthma, asthma symptoms, school absenteeism, skills using inhaler medications and peak flow meters, activity limitations, and emotional function (Asthma Health Outcomes Project Final Report 2007).

Despite the benefits of educational interventions, school administrators, teachers, and parents have pointed to several drawbacks regarding programs provided specifically for students with asthma. Often these tailored programs require participants to miss regularly scheduled classes or stay after school, necessitate the use of limited space within the school, and require parental consent. These factors add to the work load of initiating such a program. Additionally, some stakeholders may be concerned that the students who participate in specific or "special" programs may be seen as being "different" or having a "problem," which can cause them to be ostracized by their peers (Lurie et al. 1998). These issues highlight the need for flexibility in program scheduling (Langenfeld et al. 2006; Wheeler et al. 2006), especially if a school is under pressure to improve student performance on standardized tests of core academic skills. Asthma program planners also need to accept constructive criticism from school staff and may need to adapt planned program activities in response to the input provided.

For school personnel, asthma educational activities and awareness campaigns may help to facilitate appropriate and timely responses of the staff in the event of a child experiencing an asthma exacerbation and can help to diminish or eliminate triggers within the school environment. School administrators, classroom teachers, physical education teachers and coaches, front office staff, facility and maintenance staff, and bus drivers often report an interest in, and a need for, education related to asthma and its management (Anderson et al. 2005). These staff members frequently report being unsure of what policies exist in relation to asthma, how to respond appropriately to a child exhibiting signs of respiratory distress, when and how to use asthma medications, and when to call emergency medical services for students in distress (Anderson et al. 2005). For these reasons, authorities agree that training for school staff should focus on providing information about the following: (1) the disease itself, (2) preventive medication use, (3) medication use for asthma symptoms, (4) environmental control measures, (5) knowledge of and access to health care services, and (6) how to respond in the event of an emergency (CDC 2005; Lurie et al. 1998). Programs that have offered training in these topics reported that the staff members who participated often felt better prepared and more competent to handle students' asthma exacerbations (Szczepanski et al. 2001). To further increase staff interest in asthma and the likelihood of program support, planners might want to assess staff perceptions and concerns about asthma at school before the training session and incorporate these issues into the curriculum. Additionally, program planners might consider working with school administrators or state education officials to have training sessions approved for inclusion in professional development plans or as a source of continuing-education credit (CDC 2005; Keysser et al. 2006; Langenfeld et al. 2006). As a tactic to boost attendance, training sessions may be delivered during regularly scheduled professional development days before or during the academic year. Finally, the information provided at these training sessions can be streamlined and posted as bulletins in the school or on school district websites to further increase the visibility of asthma messages and to prompt staff recall of policies or plans of action to initiate when students experience respiratory distress.

Safe and Healthy School Environment

Seasonal worsening of asthma has been well documented in the literature. While the fewest asthma exacerbations are reported during the middle of the summer, an increased incidence of exacerbations among school-age children has been reported in the late summer and early fall in numerous industrialized nations (Fleming et al. 2000; Johnston et al. 2006; Silverman et al. 2005; Silverman et al. 2003; Weiss, 1990). Research suggests that this seasonality in children is primarily related to viral respiratory tract infections (Freymuth et al. 1999; Johnston et al. 1995; Johnston et al. 2005; Monto 2002; Rakes et al. 1999; Thumerelle et al. 2003). Furthermore, recent research suggests an interaction between viral infections and allergens such that viral infection can increase the airway response to allergens (Calhoun et al. 1994; Green et al. 2002; Murray et al. 2006; Schwarze et al. 1997). The primary means of spreading respiratory viruses is through hand-to-hand contact or from handling objects that have been touched by someone with a cold (Gwaltney and Hendley 1978, 1982). Regular hand washing has been widely recognized as the most effective means to combat the spread of infectious illnesses, including the viral infections that can trigger asthma symptoms (Boyce et al. 2002). Thus, schools must ensure that soap dispensers are functional and filled and that hand dryers are operable for hand washing throughout the school day and school year.

The apparent relationship between worsening asthma and the opening of school has led researchers to also study indoor allergens within school environments. Eight indoor allergens have been "causally related" or "associated" with asthma exacerbations among school-age children (Institute of Medicine 2000). These allergens include rhinovirus, cockroach, dust mite, cat, dog, fungi, environmental tobacco, and nitrogen oxides. On average, studies of these allergens indicate that their concentrations in schools are usually under the risk levels for symptoms or sensitization, although many schools contain at least one location, such as the cafeteria, library, or classrooms, where concentrations exceed these risk levels (Tranter 2005). Studies also suggest that compared with children's homes, schools often have lower levels of allergens (Tortolero et al. 2002). Yet even allergen concentrations below accepted risk levels can increase the risk for some children with asthma (Tranter 2005). Therefore, from a public health perspective, it is vital to ensure that school environments are safe and healthy so that students can learn and engage in physical and social activities. For these reasons, the school environment is acknowledged in the strategies outlined by the CDC and is often a high priority for many school-based asthma programs.

A review of indoor allergens from samples obtained in school settings indicates that dust mite, cockroach, and dog and cat allergens can be found on all types of room furnishings, such as chairs, tables, shelving units, curtains, and flooring. A range of factors can influence the levels of allergens present in school facilities, including the type of furnishings used, the age of these items, the age of the facility, the frequency of cleaning, the use of wet (mopping) or dry (sweeping) cleaning techniques, and the types of cleaners used. For example, carpets contain significantly higher levels of allergens than does smooth flooring (Dybendal et al. 1989;

Tranter 2005; Zock and Brunekreef 1995), and upholstered furniture may contain higher levels of allergens than do carpeted floors (Custovic et al. 1994; Tranter 2005). In addition, allergen levels vary by grade level of the child (Abramson et al. 2006). Rooms used by students in lower grade levels typically contain higher allergen concentrations because of the way in which these classrooms are often equipped. For example, pillows, upholstered pads, or blankets used during story or nap times are frequently found in kindergarten rooms.

The sources of allergens in schools may be the students and school staff, who bring pet allergens into the school attached to their clothing (i.e., pet hairs) or shed virus particles; humidity in the environment (dust mites thrive in humid, damp conditions or seasons); the geographic location of the school (mite and cockroach species vary by geography); and poor ventilation within the school (Abramson et al. 2006; Almqvist et al. 2001; Tortolero et al. 2002; Tranter 2005).

The CDC encourages schools to improve indoor air quality by taking steps to reduce or eliminate allergens and irritants that can trigger asthma symptoms. Air quality may be improved by the following tactics: increasing the frequency, efficiency, and thoroughness of cleaning; maintaining indoor temperatures and humidity at appropriate levels; performing regular maintenance of HVAC (heating, ventilation, and air conditioning) systems; immediately cleaning up leaks and mold; using integrated pest management techniques; and banning smoking at all times on all school property, during school-sponsored events, and in vehicles used for the transportation of students (CDC 2005; Tortolero et al. 2002; Tranter 2005). To systematically identify problems or areas that require special attention within a school, program planners should consider using a variety of checklists to initially or routinely assess school and individual classroom environments. These checklists are available from the National Heart, Lung, and Blood Institute, the Environmental Protection Agency, and the American Lung Association (Dautel et al. 1999; Environmental Protection Agency 2005).

Physical Education and Activity

Asthma should not preclude children from participating in physical activities when they are well, and students with asthma should be encouraged to join their classmates. However, poor asthma control does force many children to avoid or limit their participation in activities that are important to them. In a survey by Schulman, Ronca, and Bucuvalas, Inc. (SRBI 2004), nearly two-thirds of the children with asthma reported that they were limited "a lot" or "some" in playing organized sports, engaging in outdoor activities, playing with friends, participating in school activities, or doing things with their families.

Schools can optimize the number of days students are well and capable of engaging in the same activities as their peers by ensuring access to preventive medications before the start of these activities and immediate access to the medications in the event asthma symptoms arise during an activity. Schools may need to modify outdoor activities according to air quality readings and temperature to accommodate not only children with asthma, but also children and staff with other respiratory problems. Another tactic is to provide students with modified activities as outlined in a 504 Plan or IEP as appropriate. Across the United States, between 55% and 91% of schools (median 85%) have provided modified physical education and physical activities as indicated by students' asthma action plans (Grunbaum et al. 2005).

Coordinated School, Family, and Community Efforts

One of the most important strategies is to coordinate school, family, and community efforts to improve asthma outcomes for school-age children. Coordination involves the organization of multiple elements, such as the school health program, medical services, and the school environment, into an integrated operation. Coordination is the "glue" that connects initiatives and creates a system that supports students and their families. A coordinated system of care prevents duplication of effort and ensures that various activities are delivering similar educational messages. In addition, a coordinated effort is necessary to achieve the lofty goal of improving asthma care. However, such a system is dependent on partnerships between service providers, families, teachers, community programs, and others who may provide care for the child with asthma. This coordinated care team can then work together to ensure that each child has an individualized plan.

Multicomponent asthma interventions that address health services, patient education, and staff professional development on asthma basics and emergency response procedures are likely to be more successful than programs that address only one of these areas (CDC 2005; Keysser et al. 2006; Wheeler et al. 2006), and these types of programs are best accomplished through coordinated school, family, and community efforts. Several multicomponent programs have reported promising results (Anderson et al. 2005; Clark et al. 2004), whereas others reported minimal or no effects on asthma outcomes or school performance (Bartholomew et al. 2006; Gerald et al. 2006). One of the features of school asthma programs that can limit their effectiveness is a poor link between the school and health care provider. Communication among the child's family, school, and health care provider is one of the most important collaborative efforts, but is often difficult to achieve. Some methods for achieving communication among such partners have been described earlier in this chapter, such as establishing and sharing asthma action plans for each child. Other tactics include having parents give permission for the school and the child's health care provider to share health information directly (CDC 2005) or using Internet data systems to share information on asthma events that occur at school (Mangan and Gerald 2006). Programs that provide asthma care directly at school or provide case management have used community collaborations to eliminate the frequently cited gap between schools and medical management of children with asthma (Barbot et al. 2006; Bartholomew et al. 2006; Frankowski et al. 2006; Gerald et al 2009; Guglielmo and Little 2006; Halterman et al. 2004; Jones et al. 2005; Levy et al. 2006; Liao and Galant 2004; Liao et al. 2006; Millard et al. 2003; Richmond et al. 2006; Splett et al. 2006; Taras et al. 2004; Webber et al. 2003). Another way to coordinate asthma activities and programs at the school with community initiatives is to appoint a professional at the school or district level who is responsible for accomplishing these objectives.

Coordinating asthma resources and programs that have traditionally been disjointed can allow consolidation and reallocation of resources rather than lead to new costs. As discussed earlier, community partners are key stakeholders in any school asthma program. When community partners and organizations are committed stakeholders in a school program, they may become motivated to provide staffing and funding, which would enable schools to continue such initiatives with limited resources. Collaborations with hospitals, universities, community organizations, local asthma coalitions, parents, physicians, respiratory therapists, and others are particularly important for schools with limited resources (Wheeler et al. 2006). Community partners can also support schools in providing asthma education (Brasler and Lewis 2006) and appropriate health resources, such as stock albuterol and nebulizers (Byrne et al. 2006).

In addition to coordinating the activities of schools, families, and community organizations, program planners should think about coordinating asthma programs with other school health programs and activities. Linking programs to existing school schedules creates time for planning and program delivery. Programs should remain flexible and work within the activities that schools have already planned, such as open houses, student registration, parent–teacher conferences, professional development activities, grade-level team meetings, classroom curricula, websites, and newsletters (Langenfeld et al. 2006). Furthermore, the CDC and other organizations recommend a coordinated school health approach. Such an approach embraces the idea that health is not just the absence of disease, but is complete physical, mental, and social well-being. Each health or disease component should make a unique contribution to student health while also complementing the others, ultimately creating a whole that is more than just the sum of its parts (Marx et al. 2000; Marx et al. 1998). In such an approach, asthma would be a single component of a more comprehensive school health program.

Evaluation of School-based Asthma Programs

Regardless of the kind of strategies chosen to address asthma, school-based asthma programs must be evaluated to demonstrate their benefits, to document strengths and weaknesses, and to help strategize program improvements. Evaluation results may also be used to justify continued support of a program or the expansion of services and resources dedicated to a program. If financial support has been obtained to initiate a program, funders are more likely to continue their support if the impact of a program has been verified (Wheeler et al. 2006).

The outcomes examined often reflect the results most important to individuals or groups involved in supporting or implementing a program and assess the immediate and continuing changes that a program may create. Immediate changes may include the development, approval, and implementation of asthma-friendly policies, as well as changes in students' or staff members' asthma knowledge and ability to respond appropriately to an asthma exacerbation. Continuing changes may be physical or social–behavioral in nature. An example of a physical change is an improvement in daily peak flow rate among students after removal of carpeting from classroom areas. Other examples include decreases in health-room visits for asthma symptoms, fewer students sent home early due to asthma, fewer 911 calls, fewer case management encounters, and decreases in students' use of school health resources (Wheeler et al. 2006). An example of a social–behavioral change would be students' adherence to a daily controller medication.

Optimally, planning for program evaluation begins at the same time as planning for the program itself. A meaningful evaluation requires active participation by appropriate staff, students, and families, and the use of adequate and appropriate outcome measures. However, participation in evaluation activities is often difficult to obtain. Some researchers have increased parental participation on asthma symptom questionnaires to 98% by providing small incentives for students (pencils and stickers), as well as incentives for the teacher who obtained the questionnaires (Gerald et al. 2006). Likewise, choosing appropriate outcome measures can be challenging. Access to school records related to absences, grades, and health care utilization is often difficult to obtain, and these records may be incomplete for evaluation purposes. School records often do not state the reason for absences, making it difficult to assess the impact of a program on absences due to asthma. Furthermore, when school records are not computerized, their retrieval is costly and time-consuming (Wheeler et al. 2006). When student turnover is high, the percentage of attendance is needed (not simply days absent) because students are not always enrolled in a specific school for an entire school year (Wheeler et al. 2006). To limit these confounding variables, planners may consider comparing the total percentages of attendance (or percentages of absenteeism) for students with and without asthma (Splett et al. 2006; Wheeler et al. 2006). This method can also be applied to the number of health room visits, 911 calls, or early dismissals (Wheeler et al. 2006). If planners intend to assess students' academic performance, they must contemplate several factors, such as the quality of teachers, class size, and specific education programs, as these factors also have the potential to influence students' grades. Finally, capturing health care utilization and medical data is time-consuming and expensive (Gerald et al. 2006). The two most common methods used to collect these data are parental report and medical record review. Parental reporting requires staff to contact parents regularly for interviews. Medical record review is a complex task, particularly in areas with multiple health care facilities that children may access for care. Furthermore, obtaining consent is often complicated (Ayala et al. 2006; Gerald et al. 2006; Wheeler et al. 2006). Because of these logistical difficulties, planners may choose to focus their evaluation on a smaller, more targeted group of students, such as those with poorly controlled asthma, or evaluate the feasibility and success of one or two program changes (Wheeler et al. 2006). Nonetheless, for an evaluation to be useful, program planners must be methodical in their approach. The first step is to identify the goals of the evaluation and how to use the information gained. The next steps include determining decisions concern which outcomes will be evaluated, what design will be used, when and what data will be collected, and how these data will be gathered and reported to program stakeholders.

Conclusions

Although asthma is one of the most common chronic diseases among children, many schools receive minimal support or resources to address asthma-related issues (McGhan et al. 2002). Instead, competing priorities supersede the development or maintenance of "asthma-friendly" schools. However, there is growing recognition that health, social conditions, and environmental factors are inextricably tied to academic performance. The strategies used to address asthma in schools reinforce the overall mission of our schools and can have a positive impact on the academic and health indicators by which schools are judged. Therefore, asthma-friendly schools benefit not only children with asthma, but the entire student body as well (McGhan et al. 2002; Wheeler et al. 2006).

To help schools overcome the challenges associated with establishing and sustaining an initiative to address asthma in schools, a variety of guidance documents have been created over the last decade. Additionally, several programs have been launched through the National Heart, Lung, and Blood Institute, the CDC, the Environmental Protection Agency, and the National Asthma Education and Prevention Program to foster and sustain asthma-friendly schools (CDC 2005; National Asthma Education and Prevention Program 2006; U.S. Environmental Protection Agency 2005). These documents and programs have led to the development, implementation, and evaluation of an array of tools for school administrators, teachers, and students. Products include self-management education programs and comprehensive asthma health programs designed to be delivered in the school setting, materials to help schools identify and remediate environmental factors that exacerbate asthma and targeted materials and education programs for widespread dissemination through partnerships with schools, professional organizations, asthma coalitions, and asthma organizations (CDC 2005). National organizations such as the American Lung Association and the Asthma and Allergy Foundation of America have also aided the development and dissemination of these products. At the local level, school health nurses and educators, community-based asthma coalitions, healthcare professionals, and parents have worked diligently together to make their schools asthma-friendly.

This work has generated several lessons that future efforts must heed if further advances in coordinated school health programs and asthma control are to be realized. These lessons are provided below (Wheeler et al. 2006):

- Self-assessment tools, such as the CDC's School Health Index, help schools to identify the strengths and weaknesses of their health and safety policies and programs, inform key administrators, and create tailored plans of action (CDC, *School Health Index: A Self-Assessment and Planning Guide*).
- State and district school health programs should establish asthma-friendly policies and procedures. These policies can increase the sustainability of an asthma management program, even in the event of staff turnover. The support of school leaders and staff training are required to facilitate implementation of these policies, and regular monitoring is needed to ensure that schools are enforcing established policies.
- To identify children with poorly controlled asthma and help programs evaluate the impact of their efforts, data related to school-associated morbidity should be collected for students with asthma. Morbidity measures include, among others, percentage absenteeism, health room visits, 911 calls, and number of times sent home sick from school.
- School-based asthma programs need to ensure that students are connected with high-quality medical care. Programs must work around staffing deficiencies to help students with asthma receive good medical care through case management, active communication, and collaboration among students, parents, school nurses and other health service staff, and asthma care clinicians.
- To conserve limited resources, school asthma programs should use evidence-based materials rather than recreate existing materials.
- It is critical that schools, asthma programs, community members, and local groups collaborate with one another to procure the resources necessary to address the needs of students with asthma, such as working toward every school having a full-time nurse.
- Promising ideas for programs must be evaluated and the results published, whether or not a strong research design is possible. Collaborations among schools, community groups, and researchers can help to support these evaluation efforts.

References

Abramson SL, Turner-Henson A, Anderson L, Hemstreet MP, Bartholomew LK, Joseph CL, Tang S, Tyrrell S, Clark NM, Ownby D (2006) Allergens in school settings: results of environmental assessments in 3 city school systems. J Sch Health 76(6):246–249

Akinbami LJ. The state of childhood asthma, United States, 1980–2005. Advance data from vital and health statistics; no 381, Hyattsville, MD: National Center for Health Statistics. 2006

Akinbami LJ, Moorman JE, Garbe PL, Sondik EJ (2009) Status of childhood asthma in the United States, 1980–2007. Pediatrics 123:S131–S145

Almqvist C, Wickman M, Perfetti L, Berglind N, Renstrom A, Hedren M, Larsson K, Hedlin G, Malmberg P (2001) Worsening of asthma in children allergic to cats, after indirect exposure to cat at school. Am J Respir Crit Care Med 163:694–698

Anderson EW, Valerio M, Liu M, Benet DJ, Joseph C, Brown R, Clark NM (2005) Schools' capacity to help low-income minority children to manage asthma. J Sch Nurs 21(4):236–242

Anderson ME, Freas MR, Wallace AS, Kempe A, Gelfand EW, Liu AH (2004) Successful school-based intervention for inner-city children with persistent asthma. J Asthma 41(4):445–453

Asthma Health Outcomes Project Final Report (December 2007) Center for Managing Chronic Disease, University of Michigan. Available at: http://cmcd.sph.umich.edu/assets/files/final_AHOP_report.pdf. Accessed 22 Feb 2009.

Ayala GX, Miller D, Zagami E, Riddle C, Willis S, King D (2006) Asthma in middle schools: what students have to say about their asthma. J Sch Health 76(6):208–214

Barbot O, Platt R, Marchese C (2006) Using pre-printed rescue medication order forms and health information technology to monitor and improve the quality of care for students with asthma in New York City public schools. J Sch Health 76(6):329–332

Bartholomew LK, Sockrider MM, Abramson SL, Swank PR, Czyzewski DL, Tortolero SR, Markham CM, Fernandez ME, Shegog R, Tyrrell S (2006) Partners in school asthma management: evaluation of a self-management program for children with asthma. J Sch Health 76(6):283–289

Bergman DA, Sharek PJ, Ekegren K, Thyne S, Mayer M, Saunders M (2008) The use of telemedicine access to schools to facilitate expert assessment of children with asthma. Int J Telemed Appl

Bernard-Bonnin AC, Stachenko S, Bonin D, Charette C, Rousseau E (1995) Self-management teaching programs and morbidity of pediatric asthma: a meta-analysis. J Allergy Clin Immunol 95(1 Pt 1):34–41

Bloom, B., Cohen, R.A. (2009). Summary health statistics for US children: National health interview survey, 2008. National Center for Health Statistics. Vital Health Stat. 10(244).

Bonilla S, Kehl S, Kwong KYC, Morphew T, Kachru R, Jones CA (2005) School absenteeism in children with asthma in a Los Angeles inner city school. J Pediatr 147(6):802–806

Boss LP, Wheeler LS, Williams PV, Bartholomew LK, Taggart VS, Redd SC (2003) Population-based screening or case detection for asthma: are we ready? J Asthma 40(4):335–342

Boyce JM, Pittet D, Healthcare Infection Control Practices Advisory Committee, HICPAC/SHEA/APIC/IDSA Hand Hygiene Task Force (2002) Guideline for hand hygiene in health-care settings. Recommendations of the Healthcare Infection Control Practices Advisory Committee and the HICPAC/SHEA/APIC/IDSA Hand Hygiene Task Force. Society for Healthcare Epidemiology of America/Association for Professionals in Infection Control/Infectious Diseases Society of America. MMWR Recomm Rep 51(RR-16):1–45

Boychuk RB, Demesa CJ, Kiyabu KM et al (2006) Change in approach and delivery of medical care in children with asthma: results from a multicenter emergency department educational asthma management program. Pediatrics 117(4):S145–S151

Brasler M, Lewis M (2006) Teens: taking control of asthma. J Sch Health 76(6):269–271

Bruzzese JM, Evans D, Wiesemann S, Pinkett-Heller M, Levison MJ, Du Y, Fitzpatrick C, Krigsman C, Ramos-Bonoan C, Turner L, Mellins RB (2006) Using school staff to establish a prevention network of care to improve elementary school students' control of asthma. J Sch Health 76(6):307–312

Byrne J, Schreiber ME, Nguyen TQ (2006) Community hospital-school partnership to treat asthma episodes at school and improve management. J Sch Health 76(6):336–339

Calhoun WJ, Dick EC, Schwartz LB, Busse WW (1994) A common cold virus, rhinovirus 16, potentiates airway inflammation and segmental allergen bronchoprovocation in allergic subjects. J Clin Invest 94:2200–2208

Campbell LM, Bodalia B, Gogbashian CA, Gunn SD, Humphreys PJ, Powell JP (1998) Once daily budesonide: 400 micrograms once daily is as effective as 200 micrograms twice daily in controlling childhood asthma. Int J Clin Pract 52(4):213–219

Centers for Disease Control and Prevention. Potentially effective interventions for asthma. Available at: http://www.cdc.gov/asthma/interventions/default.htm. Accessed 28 Apr 2006

Centers for Disease Control and Prevention. School health index: a self-assessment and planning guide (2005). Available at: http://www.cdc.gov/HealthyYouth/SHI. Accessed 28 Apr 2006

Centers for Disease Control and Prevention (2001) School Health Policies and Programs Study (SHPPS) 2000: a summary report. J Sch Health 71(7):249–350

Centers for Disease Control and Prevention (2005) Strategies for addressing asthma within a coordinated school health program, with updated resources. Centers for Disease Control and Prevention, National Center for Chronic Disease Prevention and Health Promotion, Atlanta, GA. Available at: http://www.cdc.gov/HealthyYouth/asthma/pdf/strategies.pdf. Accessed 28 Apr 2006.

Cicutto L, Murphy S, Coutts D, O'Rourke J, Lang G, Chapman C, Coates P (2005) Breaking the access barrier: evaluating an asthma center's efforts to provide education to children with asthma in schools. Chest 128(4):1928–1935

Clark NM, Brown R, Joseph CLM, Anderson EW, Liu M, Valerio MA (2004) Effects of a comprehensive school-based asthma program on symptoms, parent management, grades, and absenteeism. Chest 125(5):1674–1679

Custovic A, Taggart SC, Woodcock A (1994) House dust mite and cat allergen in different indoor environments. Clin Exp Allergy 24:1164–1168

Dahl RE (1996) The impact of inadequate sleep on children's daytime cognitive function. Semin Pediatr Neurol 3(1):44–50

Dautel PJ, Whitehead L, Tortolero S, Abramson S, Sockrider MM (1999) Asthma triggers in the elementary school environment: a pilot study. J Asthma 36(8):691–702

Dey AN, Schiller JS, Tai DA (2004) Summary health statistics for U.S. children: National Health Interview Survey, 2002. Vital Health Stat 10(221):1–78

Diette GB, Markson L, Skinner EA, Nguyen TT, Algatt-Bergstrom P, Wu AW (2000) Nocturnal asthma in children affects school attendance, school performance, and parents' work attendance. Arch Pediatr Adolesc Med 154(9):923–928

Dozier A, Aligne CA, Schlabach MB (2006) Parents' perception of children's asthma control. J Sch Health 76(6):215–218

Dybendal T, Vik H, Elsayed S (1989) Dust from carpeted and smooth floors. II. Antigenic an allergenic content of dust vacuumed from carpeted and smooth floors in schools under routine cleaning schedules. Allergy 44:401–411

Fleming DM, Cross KW, Sunderland R, Ross AM (2000) Comparison of the seasonal patterns of asthma identified in general practitioner episodes, hospital admissions, and deaths. Thorax 55:662–665

Forbis S, Rammell J, Huffman B, Taylor R (2006) Barriers to care of inner-city children with asthma: school nurse perspective. J Sch Health 76(6):205–207

Frankowski BL, Keating K, Rexroad A, Delaney T, McEwing SM, Wasko N, Lynn S, Shaw J (2006) Community collaboration: concurrent physician and school nurse education and cooperation increases the use of asthma action plans. J Sch Health 76(6):303–306

Freymuth F, Vabret A, Brouard J, Toutain F, Verdon R, Petitjean J, Gouarin S, Duhamel JF, Guillois B (1999) Detection of viral, Chlamydia pneumoniae and Mycoplasma pneumoniae infections in exacerbations of asthma in children. J Clin Virol 13:131–139

Gerald LB, McClure LA, Mangan JM, Harrington K, Gibson L, Erwin S, Atchison J, Grad R (2009) Effectiveness of a school based supervised asthma therapy program. Pediatrics 123:466–474

Gerald LB, Sockrider MM, Grad R, Bender BG, Boss LP, Galant SP, Gerritsen J, Joseph CLM, Kaplan RM, Madden JA, Mangan JM, Redding GJ, Schmidt DK, Schwindt CD, Taggart VS, Wheeler LS, Van Hook KN, Williams PV, Yawn BP, Yuksel B, on behalf of the ATS Ad Hoc Committee on Issues in Screening for Asthma in Children (2007) An Official ATS Workshop Report: Issues in screening for asthma in children. Proc Am Thorac Soc 4:133–141

Gerald LB, Redden D, Wittich AR, Hains C, Turner-Henson A, Hemstreet MP, Feinstein R, Erwin S, Bailey WC (2006) Outcomes for a comprehensive school-based asthma management program. J Sch Health 76(6):291–296

Gerald LB, Turner-Henson A, Hains C, Tang S, Feinstein R, Wille K, Erwin S, Grad R (2004) Validation of a multi-stage asthma case detection procedure for elementary school children. Pediatrics 114(4):e459–e468

Green LW, Marshall K (1991) Health promotion planning, an educational and environmental approach. Mayfield Publishing Company, Mountain View, CA

Green RM, Custovic A, Sanderson G, Hunter J, Johnston SL, Woodcock A (2002) Synergism between allergens and viruses and risk of hospital admission with asthma: a case-control study. Br Med J 324:763–768

Grunbaum JA, Di Pietra J, McManus T, Hawkins J, Kann L (2005) School health profiles: characteristics of health programs among secondary schools (profiles 2004). Centers for Disease Control and Prevention, Atlanta, GA. Available at: http://www.cdc.gov/HealthyYouth/profiles/2004/report.pdf. Accessed 29 Sept 2006

Guglielmo C, Little A (2006) Tragedy in a beachfront community: a proactive school district responds to asthma. J Sch Health 76(6):297–299

Gwaltney JM, Hendley JO (1978) Rhinovirus transmission. One if by air, two if by hand. Am J Epidemiol 107(5):357–361

Gwaltney JM, Hendley JO (1982) Transmission of experimental rhinovirus infection by contaminated surfaces. Am J Epidemiol 116:828–833

Halterman JS, Szilagyi PG, Yoos HL, Conn KM, Kaczorowski JM, Holzhauer RJ, Lauver SC, Neely TL, Callahan PM, McConnochie KM (2004) Benefits of a school-based asthma treatment program in the absence of secondhand smoke exposure: results of a randomized clinical trial. Arch Pediatr Adolesc Med 158(5):460–467

Herjavecz I, Blomqvist P, Serrano A (1999) Efficacy of once- and twice-daily administration of budesonide via Turbuhaler as initial therapy in patients with mild persistent asthma. Respir Med 93(4):230–235

Hilton S, Sibbald B, Anderson HR, Freeling P (1986) Controlled evaluation of the effects of patient education on asthma morbidity in general practice. Lancet 1(8471):26–29

Institute of Medicine, National Academy of Sciences (2000) Clearing the air: asthma and indoor air exposures. National Academy Press, Washington, DC

Johnston NW, Johnston SL, Ducan JM, Greene JM, Kebadze T Keith PK, Roy M, Waserman S, Sears MR (2005) The September epidemic of asthma exacerbations in children: a search for etiology. J Allergy Clin Immunol 115: 132–138

Johnston NW, Johnston SL, Norman GR, Dai J, Sears MR (2006) The September epidemic of asthma hospitalization: school children as disease vectors. J Allergy Clin Immunol 117(3):557–562

Johnston SL, Pattemore PK, Sanderson G, Smith S, Lampe F, Josephs L, Symington P, O'Toole S, Myint SH, Tyrrell DA, Holgate ST (1995) Community study of role of viral infections in exacerbations of asthma in 9–11 year old children. Br Med J 310:1225–1229

Jones CA, Clement LT, Hanley-Lopez J, Morphew T, Kwong KY, Lifson F, Opas L, Guterman JJ (2005) The Breathmobile™ program: structure, implementation, and evolution of a large-scale, urban, pediatric asthma disease management program. Dis Manag 8(4):205–222

Jones SE, Wheeler L (2004) Asthma inhalers in schools: rights of students with asthma to a free, appropriate education. Am J Public Health 94(7):1102–1108

Katon W, Lozano P, Russo J, McCauley E, Richardson L, Bush T. (2007) The prevalence of DSM-IV anxiety and depressive disorders in youth with asthma compared with controls. J Adolesc Health 41:455–463

Keysser J, Splett PL, Ross S, Fishman E (2006) Statewide asthma training for Minnesota school personnel. J Sch Health 76(6):264–268

Langenfeld NA, Bonaiuto MM, Edmonds EO (2006) Garnering administrative support for school-based asthma education programs. J Sch Health 76(6):250–254

Levy M, Heffner B, Stewart T, Beeman G (2006) The efficacy of asthma case management in reducing school absences, symptomatology, and hospitalizations in an urban school district. J Sch Health 76(6):320–324

Liao O, Galant S (2004) Demographics and outcomes of a school-based breathmobile program in Orange, Co. CA. J Allergy Clin Immunol 113(suppl 2):S285

Liao O, Morphew T, Amaro S, Galant SP (2006) The Breathmobile™: a novel comprehensive school-based mobile asthma care clinic for urban underprivileged children. J Sch Health 76(6):313–319

Lorig KR, Sobel DS, Stewart AL, Brown BW Jr, Bandura A, Ritter P, Gonzalez VM, Laurent DD, Holman HR (1999) Evidence suggesting that a chronic disease self-management program can improve health status while reducing hospitalization: a randomized trial. Med Care 37(1):5–14

Lurie N, Straub MJ, Goodman N, Bauer EJ (1998) Incorporating asthma education into a traditional school curriculum. Am J Public Health 88(5):882–883

Lwebuga-Mukasa J, Dunn-Georgiou E (2002) A school-based asthma intervention program in the Buffalo, NY schools. J Sch Health 72(1):27–32

Mallol J, Aguirre V (2007) Once versus twice daily budesonide metered-dose inhaler in children with mild to moderate asthma: effect on symptoms and bronchial responsiveness. Allergol Immunopathol (Madr) 35(1):25–31

Mangan J, Gerald LB (2006) Asthma agents: monitoring asthma in school. J Sch Health 76(6):255–258

Marx E, Northrop D, Pierce JD (2000) Talking about health is academic. Teachers College Press, New York

Marx E, Wooley SF, Northrop D (eds) (1998) Health is academic: a guide to coordinated school health programs. Teachers College Press, New York

McCarthy AM, Kelly MW, Reed D (2000) Medication administration practices of school nurses. J Sch Health 70(9):371–376

McGhan SL, Reutter LI, Hessel PA, Melvin D, Wilson DR (2002) Developing a school asthma policy. Public Health Nurs 19(2):112–123

McLaughlin T, Maljanian R, Kornblum R, Clark P, Simpson J, McCormack K (2006) Evaluating the availability and use of asthma action plans for school-based asthma care: a case study in Hartford Connecticut. J Sch Health 76(6): 325–328

McQuaid EL, Kopel SJ, Nassau JH (2001) Behavioral adjustment in children with asthma: a meta analysis. J Dev Behav Pediatr 22(6):430–440

Milgrom H, Bender B, Ackerson L, Bowry P, Smith B, Rand C (1996) Noncompliance and treatment failure in children with asthma. J Allergy Clin Immunol 98(6):1051–1057

Millard MW, Johnson PT, McEwen M, Neatherlin J, Lawrence G, Kennerly DK, Bokovoy JL (2003) A randomized controlled trial using the school for anti-inflammatory therapy in asthma. J Asthma 40(7):769–776

Moller C, Stromberg L, Oldaeus G, Arwestrom E, Kjellman M (1999) Efficacy of once-daily versus twice daily administration of budesonide by Turbuhaler in children with stable asthma. Pediatr Pulmonol 28(5):337–343

Monto AS (2002) The seasonality of rhinovirus infections and its implications for clinical recognition. Clin Ther 24(12):1987–1997

Moonie SA, Sterling DA, Figgs L, Castro M (2006) Asthma status and severity affects missed school days. J Sch Health 76(1):18–24

Murphy KR, Hopp RJ, Kittelson EB, Hansen G, Windle ML, Walburn JN (2006) Life threatening asthma and anaphylaxis in schools: a treatment model for school-based programs. Ann Allergy Asthma Immunol 96(3):398–405

Murray CS, Poletti G, Kebadze T, Morris J, Woodcock A, Johnston SL, Custovic A (2006) A study of modifiable risk factors for asthma exacerbations: virus infection and allergen exposure increase the risk of asthma hospitalizations in children. Thorax 61(5):376–382

National Asthma Education and Prevention Program (2007) Expert Panel Report 3: Guidelines for the Diagnosis and Management of Asthma. U.S. Department of Health and Human Services, National Heart, Lung, and Blood Institute. Bethesda, MD.

National Asthma Education and Prevention Program (2005) When should students with asthma or allergies carry and self-administer emergency medications at school? Guidance for health care providers who prescribe emergency medications. National Asthma Education and Prevention Program, National Heart, Lung and Blood Institute, Bethesda, MD. Available at: http://www.nhlbi.nih.gov/health/prof/lung/asthma/emer_medi.htm. Accessed 28 Apr 2006

National Asthma Education and Prevention Program, National Heart, Lung, and Blood Institute (2008) How asthma-friendly is your school? Available at: http://www.nhlbi.nih.gov/health/public/lung/asthma/friendhi.htm. Accessed 25 August 2009

Osterberg L, Blaschke T (2005) Adherence to medication. N Engl J Med 353(5):487–497

Parcel GS, Bartlett EE, Bruhn JG (1986) The role of health education in self-management. In: Holroyd KA, Creer TL (eds) Self-management of chronic disease: handbook of clinical interventions and research. Academic, London, pp 3–27

Patterson EE, Brennan MP, Linskey KM, Webb DC, Shields MD, Patterson CC (2005) A cluster randomized intervention trial of asthma clubs to improve quality of life in primary school children: the School Care and Asthma Management Project (SCAMP). Arch Dis Child 90:786–791

Raidy DJ, Scharff LF (2005) Effects of sleep deprivation on auditory and visual memory tasks. Percept Mot Skills 101(2):451–467

Rakes GP, Arruda E, Ingram JM, Hoover GE, Zambrano JC, Hayden FG, Platts-Mills TA, Heymann PW (1999) Rhinovirus and respiratory syncytial virus in wheezing children requiring emergency care. Am J Respir Crit Care Med 159:785–790

Richmond CA, Sterling DA, Huang XH, Wilson K, Pike E (2006) Asthma 411 – addition of a consulting physician to enhance school health. J Sch Health 76(6):333–335

Sadeh A, Gruber R, Raviv A (2002) Sleep, neurobehavioral functioning, and behavior problems in school-age children. Child Dev 73(2):405–417

Schulman, Ronca, and Bucuvalas, Inc. (SRBI) on behalf of GlaxoSmithKline (February–May 2004) Children and asthma in America. Available at: http://www.asthmainamerica.com/children_index.html. Accessed 10 Jul 2006

Schwarze J, Hamelmann E, Bradley KL (1997) Respiratory syncytial virus results in airway hyperresponsiveness and enhanced airway sensitization to allergen. J Clin Invest 100:226–233

Shah S, Peat JK, Mazurski EJ, Wang H, Sindhusake D, Bruce C, Henry RL, Gibson PG (2001) Effect of peer led programme for asthma education in adolescents: cluster randomized controlled trial. Br Med J 322:583–587

Silverman RA, Ito K, Stevenson L, Hastings HM (2005) The relationship of fall school opening and emergency department asthma visits in a large metropolitan area. Arch Pediatr Adolesc Med 159:818–823

Silverman RA, Stevenson L, Hastings H (2003) Age-related seasonal patterns of emergency department visits for acute asthma in an urban environment. Ann Emerg Med 42:577–586

Splett PL, Erickson CD, Belseth SB, Jensen C (2006) Evaluation and sustainability of the healthy learners asthma initiative. J Sch Health 76(6):276–282

Stores G, Ellis AJ, Wiggs L, Crawford C, Thomson A (1998) Sleep and psychological disturbance in nocturnal asthma. Arch Dis Child 78(5):413–419

Szczepanski R, Brockmann G, Friede G (2001) Dealing with asthma for teachers: needs and possibilities. Pneumologie 55(11):512–519

Taitel MS, Allen L, Creer TL (1998) The impact of asthma on the patient, family, and society. In: Kotses H, Harver A (eds) Self management of asthma. Marcel Dekker, Inc., New York, pp 3–19

Taras H, Potts-Datema W (2005) Childhood asthma and student performance at school. J Sch Health 75(8):296–312

Taras H, Wright S, Brennan J, Campana J, Lofgren R (2004) Impact of school nurse case management on students with asthma. J Sch Health 74(6):213–219

Thumerelle C, Deschildre A, Bouquillon C, Santos C, Sardet A, Scalbert M, Delbecque L, Debray P, Dewilde A, Turck D, Leclerc F (2003) Role of viruses and atypical bacteria in exacerbations of asthma in hospitalized children: a prospective study in the Nord-Pas de Calais region (France). Pediatr Pulmonol 35:75–82

Tinkelman D, Schwartz A (2004) School-based asthma disease management. J Asthma 41(4):455–462

Tortolero SR, Bartholomew LK, Tyrrell S, Abramson SL, Sockrider MM, Markham CM, Whitehead LW, Parcel GS (2002) Environmental allergens and irritants in schools: a focus on asthma. J Sch Health 72(1):33–38

Tranter DC (2005) Indoor allergens in settled school dust: a review of findings and significant factors. Clin Exp Allergy 35:126–136

U.S. Environmental Protection Agency (2005) Indoor air quality tools for schools kit, 3rd edn. U.S. Environmental Protection Agency, Washington, DC, EPA 402-K-95-001. Available at: http://www.epa.gov/iaq/schools/toolkit.html. Accessed 30 Sept 2006.

Vargas PA, Magee JS, Bushmiaer M, Jones CA, Field CR, Jones SM (2006) School-based asthma case finding: the Arkansas experience. J Sch Health 76(6):223–226

Webber MP, Carpiniello KE, Oruwariye T, Lo Y, Burton WB, Appel DK (2003) Burden of asthma in inner-city elementary schoolchildren. Do school-based health centers make a difference? Arch Pediatr Adolesc Med 157(2):125–129

Weil CM, Wade SL, Bauman LJ, Lynn H, Mitchell H, Lavigne J (1999) The relationship between psychosocial factors and asthma morbidity in inner-city children with asthma. Pediatrics 104(6):1274–1280

Weiss KB (1990) Seasonal trends in US asthma hospitalizations and mortality. J Am Med Assoc 263:2323–2328

Whalen LG, Grunbaum JA, Kann L, Hawking J, McManus T, Davis KS (2004) School heath profiles: surveillance for characteristics of health programs among secondary schools (profiles 2002). Centers for Disease Control and Prevention, Atlanta, GA

Wheeler LS, Boss LP, Williams PV (2004) School-based approaches to identifying students with asthma. J Sch Health 74(9):378–380

Wheeler LS, Boyle S (2006) Attempting to use a district-wide asthma case identification system for asthma prevalence. J Sch Health 76(6):219–222

Wheeler LS, Merkle SL, Gerald LB, Taggart VS (2006) Managing asthma in schools: lessons learned and recommendations. J Sch Health 76(6):340–344

Wilson KD, Moonie S, Sterling DA, Gillespie KN, Kurz RS (2009) Examining the consulting physician model to enhance the school nurse role for children with asthma. J Sch Health 79:1–7

Yawn BP (2006) Asthma screening, case identification and treatment in school-based programs. Curr Opin Pulm Med 12(1):23–27

Yawn BP, Wollan P, Kurland M, Bertram S (2006) Comparison of parent and student responses to asthma surveys: two different experiences with similar results. Students grades 3–12 and their parents, from a suburban private school setting. J Sch Health 76(6):241–245

Yawn BP, Wollan P, Scanlon PD, Kurland M (2003) Outcome results of a school-based screening program for undertreated asthma. Ann Allergy Asthma Immunol 90(5):508–515

Zock JP, Brunekreef B (1995) House dust mite allergen levels in dust from schools with smooth and carpeted floors. Clin Exp Allergy 25:549–553

Chapter 15
Women and Asthma

Jan Warren-Findlow, Larissa R. Brunner Huber, Melanie J. Rouse, and Andrew Harver

Introduction

This chapter focuses on women who have asthma, the factors that influence the onset and exacerbation of asthma in women, and the resulting health consequences of the disease and its treatments. Research on women's health is frequently deficient because we fail to separate out the effects of sex, defined as female biology, and gender, the socially constructed roles and behaviors that women perform (Krieger 2003); thus many studies use the terms "sex" and "gender" interchangeably (Krieger 2003; Phillips 2005). Few researchers have successfully wrestled with how to measure the social construct of gender and how it affects women's health and their coping responses to disease states (Phillips 2005). This is particularly important because of the vast political, economic, and social power differentials between women and men that affect women's access to health care and contribute to the feminization of poverty (Phillips 2005; World Health Organization 1998). Both sex and gender have a significant influence on women's exposure to disease risk factors, disease outcomes, health seeking behaviors, and the ability to follow treatment regimens (Krieger 2003). These issues make sex and gender particularly relevant with respect to asthma in women (Clark et al. 2008; McCallister and Mastronarde 2008; Melgert et al. 2007; Postma 2007).

We attempt to distinguish, whenever possible, whether a body of literature is referring to either sex effects or to gender effects. The chapter is organized along the following lines: the epidemiology of women and asthma; asthma over the life course as it relates to changes in sex-steroids (puberty and menopause); asthma and the menstrual cycle; asthma during pregnancy; and women's utilization of health care resources for asthma. We conclude with a discussion of methodological issues and directions for future research.

Asthma Prevalence, Morbidity, and Mortality Among Women

In the United States, 24 million people are affected by asthma (Pleis and Lethbridge-Cejku 2007). Though the prevalence of asthma has increased for both men and women, women have experienced the greatest increase. Among the United States women, the prevalence of asthma increased 82% from a prevalence rate of 2.9% in 1982 to 5.4% in 1992 (Weiss et al. 1992). During the same time frame, prevalence rates for men increased 29% (4.0–5.4%). More recent national data from 2006 indicate that among the women who are the age group of 18 and above, 12.5% reported ever having physician-diagnosed asthma and 8.9% reported that they are still suffering from asthma (Pleis and Lethbridge-Cejku 2007). In comparison, 9.5% of men reported ever being diagnosed with asthma and only 5.6% reported that they still have asthma.

An increase in asthma morbidity and mortality has accompanied the increased prevalence of asthma. Annually there are approximately 11 million medical visits for asthma (Cherry et al. 2008), including over 200,000 emergency department visits related to asthma (Pitts et al. 2008). Women with asthma have hospitalization rates 2.5–3.0 times that of men (Skobeloff et al.

J. Warren-Findlow (✉)
Department of Public Health Sciences, University of North Carolina at Charlotte, 9201 University City Blvd., Charlotte, 28223, NC, USA
e-mail: jwarren1@uncc.edu

A. Harver and H. Kotses (eds.), *Asthma, Health and Society: A Public Health Perspective*, DOI 10.1007/978-0-387-78285-0_15, © Springer Science+Business Media, LLC 2010

1992) and report a lower quality of life than men (Bousquet et al. 1994). In addition, women have higher asthma-related mortality rates than men. Approximately 16 deaths per million population are attributed to asthma for women versus 10 deaths per million population for men (Minino et al. 2007). In 2004, nearly 64% of asthma deaths occurred in women (Minino et al. 2007).

Epidemiologic Studies of Asthma

Defining asthma in the context of an epidemiologic study can be challenging. Consequently, many studies rely on self-reported information including self-reports of physician diagnosed asthma, the presence of asthma symptom(s), and the severity of asthma (Eder et al. 2006). The use of different definitions for asthma makes it difficult to compare studies and to generalize results to other populations. Though clinical objective measures for pulmonary function, such as spirometry, can be used, they are costly, and unavailable for large-scale or community-based studies.

In addition to problems with defining asthma, many studies also consider sex to be a confounder of exposure-asthma associations. While sex may be a confounder of some associations, it is also likely that sex is an effect modifier of many of the observed exposure-asthma associations. When associations are not separated out by sex, many important relationships can be obscured. To date, epidemiologic investigations on risk factors for asthma among women are sparse.

Studies that have been conducted among cohorts of women have found that obesity is associated with an increased risk of asthma (Camargo et al. 1999; Coogan et al. 2009; Romieu et al. 2003). Specifically, overweight and obese women have nearly twice the risk of asthma as compared to women with a normal body mass index (BMI). In addition, an increase in body silhouette after menarche has also been found to be related to an increased risk of asthma in adulthood (RR = 1.6; 95% CI: 1.18–2.32).

Studies conducted with populations of men and women indicate that socioeconomic, lifestyle, and environmental factors are associated with an increased risk of asthma. Specifically, low income, lower education level, and non-Hispanic black race/ethnicity have been found to be associated with an increased risk of asthma (Arif et al. 2003; Bandiera et al. 2008; Drake et al. 2008; Grant et al. 2000; Litonjua et al. 1999). Though it has been suggested that associations that have been seen between race/ethnicity and asthma may be largely explained by factors like income, area of residence, and education level, researchers have found race/ethnicity to be an independent risk factor for asthma (Litonjua et al. 1999). However, data from the 2006 National Health Interview Survey did not indicate that the prevalence of ever having physician-diagnosed asthma differed considerably between non-Hispanic black women and non-Hispanic white women (Pleis and Lethbridge-Cejku 2007). Specifically, 12.8% of non-Hispanic white women reported ever having asthma as compared to 13.9% of non-Hispanic black women. Hispanic women had the lowest asthma prevalence (10.8%).

A family history of asthma (Lugogo and Kraft 2006; Sunyer et al. 1997) and diet have also been implicated as risk factors for asthma in populations of men and women. In particular, low dietary intakes of Vitamin E and n-3 polyunsaturated fatty acids (found in oily fish and leafy, green vegetables) and high dietary intakes of n-6 polyunsaturated fatty acids (found in vegetable oils) are associated with an increased risk of asthma (Black and Sharpe 1997; Hodge et al. 1996; Raper et al. 1992; Seaton et al. 1994). Environmental factors such as secondhand tobacco smoke and exposure to chemicals, and materials used in home improvement activities or industries, including beauty salons, also affect asthma risk (Arif et al. 2009; Becklake and Kauffmann 1999; Chan-Yeung and Malo 1995; Delclos et al. 2007; Gold et al. 1996; Masi et al. 1988; Xu and Wang 1994; Xu et al. 1994).

Concluding Remarks

Women are more likely to report adult onset of asthma than men (Becklake and Kauffmann 1999; Caracta 2003; De Marco et al. 2000; Flattery et al. 2001; Janson et al. 2001; Nicolai et al. 2003; PausJenssen and Cockcroft 2003), and demonstrate higher asthma-related hospitalization and mortality rates than men (Kochanek et al. 2002; McCaig and Burt 2005; Minino et al. 2007; Pitts et al. 2008; Skobeloff et al. 1992). One explanation for these observations relates to the hormonal changes that affect asthma risk in women. In particular, women's airways are subject to cyclical variations in sex hormones which occur in relation to circadian rhythms, menstrual cycles, hormonal contraceptive use, pregnancy, and menopause (Alberts 1997; Chandler et al. 1997; Edwards et al. 1996; Eliasson et al. 1986; Lieberman et al. 1995; Murphy and Gibson 2008; Schatz et al. 1988; Shanies et al. 1997; Skobeloff et al. 1992; Stenisu-Aarniala 1996; Tan et al. 1997; Troisi et al. 1995). Despite the indication that asthma risk is quite different for men and women, many studies of adulthood asthma treat sex as a confounder of any observed associations. Future studies need to investigate possible risk factors for asthma separately for men and women.

Asthma and Changes in Female Sex-Steroid Hormones Over the Life Course

Asthma in women has been hypothesized to be related to natural changes in sex-steroid hormone levels during a woman's life course; thus, the onset of puberty, the beginning of perimenopause, and the completion of menopause are biological transition points when asthma may begin or change. Whether these transition points trigger the onset of asthma, exacerbate existing asthma symptoms and severity, or relieve asthma is still being researched. It is clear that for many women with asthma, fluctuations in endogenous hormone levels are correlated with changes in their asthmatic condition.

Puberty

The onset of puberty potentially plays a critical role in the development of asthma and its symptoms in females. Observational evidence supporting this are the differences in prevalence rates of asthma between boys and girls prior to puberty, with boys having a significantly higher prevalence of asthma than girls (9.6% vs. 7.4%). This trend then reverses post-puberty with women having a significantly higher prevalence than men in the age group of 18 and above (8.4% vs. 4.9%) (Centers for Disease Control and Prevention 2003). Researchers suspect that hormonal factors are the dominant determinant of the asthma prevalence seen in adult women (Becklake and Kauffmann 1999). Young girls have lower rates of asthma as compared to boys, and around the time of puberty asthma rates are essentially equal in boys and girls. However, after puberty, women have increased rates of developing asthma as compared to men. When considered in 5-year intervals, this reversal is first seen in the 15–20 year age group when women have 1.38 times the rate of asthma as compared to men (95% CI: 1.02–1.88), and becomes more dramatic as age increases (De Marco et al. 2000). Among adults 40–45 years of age, women have nearly six times the rate of developing asthma when compared to men (95% CI: 2.31–15.26). Testosterone appears to have an anti-inflammatory effect, whereas estrogen has a pro-inflammatory effect (Osman 2003). However, researchers are not in agreement on whether puberty is associated with increased risk of asthma, with some supporting an association (Haggerty et al. 2003) and others refuting it (Zannolli and Morgese 1997). There is some suggestion that social and cultural factors may play a role, resulting in girls being under-diagnosed with asthma (Haggerty et al. 2003) and boys being more likely to be diagnosed because they have increased severity of asthma at younger ages resulting in hospitalizations (Balzano et al. 2001; Haggerty et al. 2003).

The actual biological mechanism by which puberty in girls would influence asthma onset and severity has not been explored, although we can infer from studies of asthma and the menstrual cycle that increasing levels of estradiol, follicle stimulating hormone (FSH) and luteinizing hormone (LH) related to menarche and other bodily changes would have some effect. Women who experienced menarche before age 12, had twice the risk of experiencing asthma post-puberty (Salam et al. 2006). Increasing rates of obesity in children may also be a factor that needs to be examined in the future since BMI and asthma are associated in women (Camargo et al. 1999; Romieu et al. 2003).

Menopause

Onset of Asthma

At the other end of the reproductive life cycle, if increasing levels of estradiol precipitate the onset of asthma during puberty, then logically we should see a reversal in asthma severity as women go through menopause (Balzano et al. 2001; Barr and Camargo 2004); but this has not proved to be the case (Gómez Real et al. 2006).

Prevalence of asthma in women continues to increase with age as 9.2% of women in the age group of 45–64 report having asthma and these rates do not decline until women are over 65 (6.8%) (Centers for Disease Control and Prevention 2003). Postmenopausal women have significantly lower levels of sex-steroid hormones than pre-menopausal women, but asthmatic postmenopausal women have even lower levels of estradiol and estrone than non-asthmatic women in menopause (Haggerty et al. 2003). Research on post-menopausal women and asthma has not examined the natural transition into menopause with concomitant tracking of clinical measures of reproductive hormones and clinical measures of pulmonary function in asthmatic and non-asthmatic women who are not taking hormone replacement therapy (Haggerty et al. 2003). Rather, the tendency has been to examine how hormone replacement therapy (HRT) affects asthma symptoms and severity; thus HRT and asthma have become entwined without first examining the main effects of changes in endogenous sex steroids and its association with pulmonary functioning. A recent study examining this issue, has included only the women who are not HRT users (Gómez Real et al. 2008). This cross-sectional study revealed that menopausal women had decreased lung function (as measured by FEV_1 and forced vital capacity) and increased respiratory symptoms (OR = 1.82; CI: 1.27–2.61) as compared to women who were still menstruating. These results were especially pronounced among lean women with BMI <23 kg/m^2. This analysis underscores the need for a prospective epidemiology study to address this tremendous gap in the science on asthma and menopause.

While there have been no prospective studies examining the natural transition to menopause and pulmonary function, studies that have considered the relationship between asthma and HRT use in relation to menopause are revealing. Four studies have been made and they have concluded that users of HRT have a higher risk of asthma than never users of HRT (Barr et al. 2004; Gómez Real et al. 2006; Lange et al. 2001; Troisi et al. 1995). In a preliminary analysis from the Nurses Health Study, postmenopausal women who had never taken HRT had a statistically significantly lower, age-adjusted risk of asthma than pre-menopausal women. When duration of HRT use was considered, women who had ever used HRT for 10 or more years had twice the risk of asthma as compared to never users of HRT (Troisi et al. 1995). A subsequent analysis controlled for differences in current versus past hormone use in postmenopausal women and found that current estrogen use and current estrogen and progestin use are each associated with increased rates of asthma in comparison to women who have never used hormones (Barr et al. 2004).

In a similar analysis of postmenopausal women in the Copenhagen City Heart Study (Lange et al. 2001), there was a significantly higher prevalence of asthma ($p = 0.004$) and the need to use asthma medication ($p = 0.018$), in never smokers who used HRT than in current smokers. Overall, the association between HRT use and self-reports of asthma (OR = 1.42; 95% CI: 0.95–2.12), asthma symptoms (wheezing [OR = 1.29; 95% CI: 1.02–1.64] and coughing upon exertion [OR = 1.34; 95% CI: 1.01–1.77]), and medication use (OR = 1.45; 95% CI: 0.97–2.18) were categorized as "consistent but weak" and the authors concluded that no change in HRT protocol was necessary. In a recent study that examined the interaction of HRT and BMI with asthma in perimenopausal women, Gómez Real et al. (2006) found that in women aged 46–54 who were not taking exogenous hormones, increasing BMI was associated with a greater risk of asthma, supporting the findings of Camargo and colleagues (1999). In women taking HRT, there was a significant increased risk of asthma (Barr et al. 2004). Thus, both HRT and BMI have significant and independent associations with increased risk of asthma. However, when the HRT users are stratified by BMI, the increased risk of asthma is only significant for lean women (Jarvis and Leynaert 2008); thus BMI may act as an effect modifier of the HRT-asthma association. Gómez Real et al. (2006) hypothesize that the pro-inflammatory effects of insulin resistance, which is associated with BMI, may be an important factor in explaining the HRT and BMI interaction.

These findings suggest that physiologically natural low levels of estrogen may be protective against asthma. Thus, lean women, who often tend to be White, wealthier and more educated, should theoretically have reduced rates of asthma. However, these are the same women who are likely taking HRT (Troisi et al. 1995), either because of concerns about reduced bone density (prevalent in lean women), or because they suffer from menopausal symptoms because of their reduced fatty tissue and reduced estrogen levels. These data suggest that research should examine hypotheses relating to whether women with low body fat percentages such as athletes and dancers, women who are excessively thin, or women with amenorrhea, have lower rates of asthma. Similarly, girls with low body fat and delayed onset of puberty might experience delayed onset of asthma.

Hormone Replacement Therapy and Pulmonary Function

Given the recent controversial findings about HRT and its effects in women in relation to heart disease, breast cancer and stroke (Cauley et al. 2003; Chlebowski et al. 2003; Rossouw et al. 2002), a renewed interest in examining HRT and its effects on asthma in women should be a key priority. Early studies examining the association between estrogen replacement therapy and respiratory function revealed a statistically significant reduction in peak expiratory flow (PEF) in postmenopausal asthmatic women and a self-reported increase in bronchodilator inhaler use (Lieberman et al. 1995), but no corresponding decrease in women's subjective measures of well-being. Thus, the authors concluded that there were sub-clinical effects, but that these effects were not sufficient to influence women's well-being. These findings do not take into account the cumulative long term effects of these sub-clinical markers. In addition, this study did not control for confounders such as tobacco exposure, allergy status, pollution, and respiratory infection among others (Haggerty et al. 2003). In a later study, designed to duplicate the research of Lieberman et al. (1995), Hepburn and colleagues (2001) found no significant changes in forced expiratory volume at 1 s (FEV_1) or use of β-agonist bronchodilators in postmenopausal asthmatic women who ceased HRT and then re-initiated it after 28 days.

In contrast, more recent studies have shown that asthmatic postmenopausal women have significantly lower levels of estradiol and estrone concentration than non-asthmatic women (Kos-Kudla et al. 2000); adjusting these levels through the introduction of exogenous hormones may alleviate asthma symptoms. Kos-Kudla et al. (2000) found that a 6-month intervention with HRT increased estrogen and estrone levels in lean, postmenopausal, non-smoking women. Participants reported decreased psychosomatic symptoms of menopause, reductions in the use of inhaled glucocorticoids, and improved spirometry during the HRT intervention (Kos-Kudla et al. 2001).

These positive effects of an HRT intervention on asthmatic women are supported by other observational studies. In a German study examining HRT use with bronchial hyper-responsiveness (BHR) in postmenopausal women (Mueller et al. 2003), HRT users are significantly less likely to demonstrate BHR in comparison to non-HRT users, suggesting that HRT may relax bronchial smooth muscle. This confirms a large scale cross-sectional analysis of 2,353 postmenopausal HRT users and non-users, who are 65 years and older, which has found that current HRT users have higher FEV_1 than former or never users, and less pulmonary obstruction (Carlson et al. 2001). This study has been able to control for several confounding variables including: smoking status, BMI, other respiratory problems, race, age, years of education, and dose and formulation of HRT; however, the study was limited by the small number of asthmatic women in the project. Additionally, the duration of current or former HRT use, which may be a confounding factor, was not considered. While this study had a sample that was 17% non-White, it is important to remember that Black women with asthma are more likely to die before ever reaching age 65; thus, in this cross-sectional study a survival bias may have occurred.

Despite these studies, no definitive, consistently replicable results have been found (see Haggerty et al. 2003 for a brief review) and BMI may be an effect modifier on the association between HRT and asthma (Gómez Real et al. 2006). Similarly, estrogen dosage in HRT is much less than that found in oral contraceptives and may not be sufficient to demonstrate a dose–response relationship with pulmonary function. The other elements complicating these findings are the various formulations of estrogen therapy and asthma severity. Early studies were conducted using only estrogen therapy while later studies used formulations including progesterone. Early HRT interventions were also of short duration (14–28 days) versus later studies that evaluated HRT duration of 6 months (Kos-Kudla et al. 2000).

Greater efforts to enroll asthmatic, postmenopausal women of all races and of younger ages should be a top priority in future studies of HRT use. Studies also need to be prospective and of sufficient length to examine long term effects and trends of respiratory function and duration of HRT use. As we have seen from the Women's Health Initiative study (Chlebowski et al. 2003; Cushman et al. 2004; Rossouw et al. 2002), duration of HRT use is particularly important in evaluating disease risk.

Consequences of Asthma in Postmenopausal Women

One-third of the published research on menopause and asthma has examined the effects of corticosteroid use on bone mineral density (BMD) and fractures in perimenopausal and postmenopausal women. The prevalence of this condition has resulted in the term "corticosteroid-induced osteoporosis" (Saag et al. 2006; Tsugeno et al. 2002; Walsh et al. 2002). Typically, this condition is associated with the use of oral glucocorticoid steroids such as prednisone or its equivalents. As inhaled corticosteroids (ICS) have more recently become the "gold standard" treatment for asthma (Dahl 2006) and other lung diseases, and as asthma is a chronic condition, the long term, cumulative effects of ICS usage are a significant health issue. Similarly the use of oral corticosteroids, while no longer the primary/daily form of treatment for asthma, has also been examined for its long term effects, including its well-established negative effects on BMD and fractures (Angeli et al. 2006; National Institutes of Health Osteoporosis and Related Bone Diseases ~ National Resources Center 2005; Walsh et al. 2002).

Both oral and inhaled corticosteroids are absorbed systemically into the circulation system with the former occurring through the gastrointestinal tract and the latter being absorbed through the lung. However, some percentage of ICS are swallowed and the level of absorption of inhaled medications are dependent upon the particular agent, the inhaler device, and inhaler technique (Tattersfield et al. 2004). Drug absorption is particularly salient for women, as they metabolize drugs differently than men (Gandhi et al. 2004; Jochman et al. 2005; Martin 2006; Morris et al. 2003).

Multiple empirical studies of varying designs and sample sizes have found a statistically significant, inverse association between ICS use and BMD (Israel et al. 2001; Langhammer et al. 2004; Toogood et al. 1995; Wong et al. 2000) and this finding is further supported in review articles (Dahl 2006; Tattersfield et al. 2004). However, the specific biological mechanism, dosage, particular drug used, duration of use, cumulative dosage, age of participants, and other factors are not consistent across these studies and no clear dose–response relationship has been established or replicated.

Earlier studies found no significant reduction in BMD with inhaled corticosteroid use (Laatikainen et al. 1999; Luengo et al. 1997) and other reviews have also concluded that ICS use is generally safe with respect to bone density (Jones et al. 2002; Peters 2006). Two recent, separate meta-analyses examining use of inhaled corticosteroids and BMD (Halpern et al. 2004; Sharma et al. 2003) also concluded that use of ICS for asthma was not associated with significant decreases in BMD. The two studies had no overlap between the articles included in their respective meta-analyses and had small sample sizes ($n<10$). The Cochrane Review article (Jones et al. 2002), while not finding any statistically significant negative effects, did indicate that their conclusions were very narrowly defined to conventional doses of ICS and over the short or medium term (2–3 years) in younger adults (i.e., premenopausal women). More prospective, randomized clinical trials are needed with attention to specific factors related to bone density such as diet and time of assay collection. Studies with postmenopausal women will be complicated by HRT use, which appears to counteract the potential negative effects of ICS on BMD (Toogood et al. 1995). HRT use has been shown to increase BMD in osteoporotic women, although it is not recommended for treatment of existing disease because of the other health risks associated with it (Cauley et al. 2003).

To summarize, no definitive conclusions can be reached about the long term effects of inhaled corticosteroids on BMD and risk of fracture. While there does appear to be a decrease in BMD with possible increase in risk of fracture, findings do not consistently achieve clinical or statistical significance. The role of HRT appears to modify the risk of ICS, but HRT is no longer recommended as a disease preventative and should only be used in cases of severe menopausal symptoms and for the shortest possible duration.

Summary

Evidence exists that changes in sex steroid levels in women are associated with changes in asthma; however, the direction and magnitude of change is inconsistent. Interaction effects between asthma and weight, and asthma and use of exogenous hormones, complicate comparisons between studies. While changes in endogenous hormone levels are related to biology and life course transitions, the use of exogenous hormones is often related to gender, thus sex and gender need to be examined separately. The need for prospective cohort studies to examine the natural transition points of puberty and menopause are crucial to understand the sex-related issues with asthma in women.

Asthma and the Menstrual Cycle

The exacerbation of asthma in women associated with the menstrual cycle has been explored by researchers beginning as early as 1931 (Tan 2001). Several of these studies have been able to demonstrate that asthma exacerbation related to the menstrual cycle, particularly the perimenstrual phase of the cycle, can be a severe and life threatening event (Martinez-Moragon et al. 2004; Nakasato et al. 1999; Oguzulgen et al. 2002). Because of the potential severity of the phenomenon, it is important that asthma etiology and pathology are understood in order to effectively treat the condition. Most of the studies had small sample sizes and explored this association using retrospective study designs in which asthma severity was self-reported through questionnaires. Objective measures of pulmonary function and airway inflammation have been used in these studies only with in the last 30 years. Although asthma associated with the menstrual cycle has been known to affect women for over 70 years, the prevalence, etiology, and pathology of the association remain unclear (Vrieze et al. 2003).

Prevalence

Estimated prevalence rates of menstrual cycle linked asthma have varied across studies, as the timing of the menstrual cycle phase has been more related to the asthma exacerbation. Zimmerman et al. (2000) were able to demonstrate that only 13% of women reported reproductive factors as triggers of their asthma. A number of studies have demonstrated no significant differences in asthma exacerbation rates across the various intervals of the menstrual cycle, while others were able to demonstrate that the perimenstrual phase of the menstrual cycle can be associated with up to 46% of the cases of asthma exacerbation (Agarwal and Shah 1997; Brenner et al. 2005; Martinez-Moragon et al. 2004; Skobeloff et al. 1996; Zimmerman et al. 2000). Gómez Real et al. (2007) found that irregular menstrual cycles are associated with asthma exacerbation based on self-reports. Despite the variance that can be found in the prevalence and timing of menstrual cycle linked asthma, the most consistent finding is that asthma exacerbations most often occur during the perimenstrual phase of the menstrual cycle, followed by the periovulatory phase (Vrieze et al. 2003).

Etiology and Pathophysiology

There are several hypotheses relating to the etiology and pathophysiology of menstrual cycle related asthma exacerbations. The most common of these hypotheses relates asthma exacerbations to the cyclical changes in sex hormone levels in women, including significant decreases in estrogen, progesterone and estradiol levels during the follicular and luteal phases of the menstrual cycle. Findings from human and animal models suggest that progesterone and estrogen may improve lung function in women, by reducing contractility of bronchial smooth muscle and by strengthening airway muscles (Matsubara et al. 2008; Popovic and White 1998; Skobeloff 1995). It has also been demonstrated that estrogen withdrawal causes an increase in bronchial smooth muscle contractility, thereby decreasing lung function (Haggerty et al. 2003). Sex hormone levels in women have also been thought to be associated with lung inflammation, which increases the risk of asthma exacerbation. Morishita and colleagues (1999) found that estradiol and progesterone inhibit human peripheral monocyte production of interlukin-1. Interlukin-1 has been found to be a mediator of inflammation. Other studies have also been able to demonstrate that estradiol exhibits anti-inflammatory properties (Litonjua et al. 1999).

Other hypotheses relating to the pathophysiology of menstrual cycle related asthma exacerbations center around mediators and manifestations of airway inflammation in asthma. Previous research has demonstrated that prostaglandins are mediators of airway inflammation (Smith et al. 1992). Metabolites of prostaglandins have been found to increase in women during ovulation and pre-menstrually. The peaking of the metabolites of prostaglandins is important to the pathology of asthma exacerbations related to the menstrual cycle because they have been shown to be effective bronchoconstrictors that may trigger or at the very least increase the risk of asthma exacerbations (Koullapis and Collins 1980).

Bronchial hyperresponsiveness (BHR) is a manifestation of the airway inflammation process and triggers much of the symptomatology of asthma exacerbation (Tan 2001). Studies examining the presence of BHR among women with menstrual cycle related asthma have found varying results. Tan et al. (1997) found that BHR increased during the luteal phase of the menstrual cycle. Other studies have found that there are no cyclical changes in BHR (Juniper et al. 1987; Weinmann et al. 1987).

Additional hypotheses refer to the effects that endogenous female sex steroids have on the vasorelaxant and bronchorelaxant effects of catecholamines (Tan 2001). Many of the studies exploring these hypotheses have focused on β_2-adrenoceptor function and regulation. It has been demonstrated that women have more β_2-adrenoceptor responses to β_2-agonists than men, suggesting that female sex hormones may facilitate β_2-adrenoceptor function and regulation (Rahman et al. 1992). It has also been demonstrated that there are cyclical changes in β_2-adrenoceptor function. A study by Wheeldon et al. (1994) found that there is greater β_2-adrenoceptor density during the luteal phase of the menstrual cycle when the sex hormone levels are high.

Psychological factors may also influence physiological reactivity in women with menstrual cycle related asthma. The results of studies exploring potential psychological factors have varied (Dorhofer and Sigmon 2002; Mirdal et al. 1998). Dorhofer and Simon (2002) explored the relationship between anxiety and other psychological symptoms and the menstrual cycle in women with and without a diagnosis of asthma. While the investigators did not find any significant differences in psychological measures with menstrual cycle phase as a factor, they did find that women with asthma and a history of panic attacks typically experienced more psychological distress than did the other women in the study. Experiencing more psychological distress has been suggested to be a factor in the exacerbation of asthma during the perimenstrual phase. Mirdal and colleagues (1998) were able to demonstrate a relationship between lower resistance to stress and infections and increases in bronchial hyperresponsiveness during the perimenstrual phase. These findings suggest that in addition to the physiological changes that occur during the menstrual cycle, psychological factors can also play a role in increasing risks of asthma exacerbation related to the menstrual cycle.

Oral Contraceptives

Because it has been demonstrated that some female asthmatics experience menstrual cycle related asthma exacerbation as a result of cyclical changes in female sex hormone levels, the way in which exogenous female sex hormones influence asthma and asthma-like symptoms is important, particularly in the case of oral contraceptive use. In non-asthmatic women, using oral contraceptives increased risk of current wheeze (OR = 1.75; 95% CI: 1.15–2.65) (Salam et al. 2006), but in contrast, a study of Tasmanian women found that each year of oral contraceptive use decreased the risk of current asthma by 7% (95% CI: 0–13%) (Jenkins et al. 2006). Oral contraceptives reduce the amount of fluctuations in female sex hormone levels throughout the menstrual cycle (Forbes 1999). Consequently, it is easy to hypothesize that the use of oral contraceptives would reduce the presence of menstrual cycle related asthma exacerbations (Forbes 1999). Studies investigating the relationship between the use of oral contraceptives and asthma exacerbations, however, have found varying results.

Of the studies that have explored the relationship between the use of oral contraceptives and asthma, only some were able to demonstrate significant differences in asthma symptoms, and severity between women taking oral contraceptives and those who did not take them. However, even among the studies that found significant differences between groups, there is some variance in the specific findings (Forbes 1999). One such study was able to demonstrate that there is an increase in airway reactivity and in peak expiratory flow rates during the luteal phase of the menstrual cycle among women not receiving oral contraceptives (Tan et al. 1997). The participants that received the oral contraceptives did not have significant increases in airway reactivity or in peak expiratory flow rates during the luteal phase, suggesting a decrease in asthma symptoms as a result of oral contraceptive use (Tan et al. 1997). Other studies demonstrating improvements in asthma symptoms as a result of oral contraceptive use in women with more severe menstrual cycle related asthma exacerbations have also been reported (Matsuo et al. 1999; Salam et al. 2006).

In contrast to the studies mentioned above, Forbes et al. (1999) were able to demonstrate that the use of oral contraceptives can have either a negative or positive influence on asthma symptoms. The results of their study demonstrated that only 6% of women taking oral contraceptives reported that their use of contraceptives influenced asthma severity. Surprisingly, of those women stating that their use of oral contraceptives influenced asthma severity, nearly two-thirds stated that their symptoms worsened as a result of the contraceptives. The remaining women reported improvements in their asthma symptoms.

Other studies have been able to show that there are no significant differences between women receiving oral contraceptives and those not receiving them and their resulting asthma severity. These studies, however, explored a limited subset of asthma symptoms and they did not investigate differences between women receiving monophasic and triphasic oral contraceptives (Lange et al. 2001; Murphy and Gibson 2008; Tan et al. 1998). Tan et al. (1998) investigated β_2-adrenoceptor regulation and function without examining other asthma symptoms. In a similar manner, Lange and colleagues (2001) questioned their participants on the presence of wheeze, cough on exertion, and use of asthma medication without exploration of the underlying causes of these asthma symptoms. These limitations in the methods may have influenced the researchers' ability to demonstrate any differences in asthma symptoms and severity among the study groups.

Summary

While there have been several studies examining the association between asthma exacerbation and the menstrual cycle throughout the last 70 years, the details regarding the phenomenon remain unclear (Chhabra 2005). Despite the inconsistent findings of studies investigating asthma and the menstrual cycle, the results of studies that demonstrate an association between the menstrual cycle and asthma exacerbations suggest that the menstrual cycle can be a factor in asthma exacerbation in some women, although the exact prevalence, etiology, and pathophysiology is still uncertain (Tan 2001). The inconsistencies in the results of these studies also suggest that menstrual related asthma exacerbations may be dependent upon other non-menstrual related factors in the individual female, particularly with regards to the use of oral contraceptives, which have been shown to have varying effects on asthma exacerbations (Forbes et al. 1999).

It is possible that much of the confusion about asthma and the menstrual cycle results from the limitations of the studies exploring the disease. These studies often had small sample sizes that may not have allowed for enough power to identify any significant differences. In addition, many of the studies used participant self-report to measure asthma symptoms and severity which may not have allowed for full exploration of the disease. Also, the limitations in the measures used may have allowed for some important underlying causes of asthma exacerbations to be ignored.

Asthma and Pregnancy

Because this chapter is focused on women *with* asthma, the relationship between asthma and pregnancy is considered from the perspective of the effect of asthma on pregnant women and subsequent maternal outcomes (preeclampsia, gestational hypertension, oligohydramnios, etc…), but not fetal outcomes. There are several excellent recent articles on the subject of maternal asthma and fetal outcomes (Dombrowski 2006; Hanania and Belfort 2005; Rudra et al. 2006; Sheiner et al. 2005), but these will not be discussed here.

The prevalence of asthma among pregnant women in the U.S. is estimated to be between 3.7% and 8.4% based on self-reports in national datasets (Kwon et al. 2003). African Americans have a 38% higher prevalence of asthma than do Whites (American Lung Association 2005), and thus we should expect a higher prevalence among pregnant women as well. Parity may play a role in the onset of asthma. Risk of current asthma has been found to increase with each birth (OR = 1.50; 95% CI: 1.01–2.23) (Jenkins et al. 2006). However, in the same study, women with a solo birth had a lower risk of current asthma than nulliparous women (OR = 0.46; 95% CI: 0.2–1.06).

Based on empirical studies, there is a direct relationship between a woman's asthma severity classification and her experience of severe asthma exacerbations during pregnancy (Murphy et al. 2005, 2006; Schatz et al. 2003). In a recent meta-analysis, 20% of pregnant women experienced an asthma exacerbation requiring medical intervention (Murphy et al. 2006). In both the Asthma During Pregnancy Study (ADPS) (Schatz et al. 2003) and an Australian study (Murphy et al. 2005), modeled on the ADPS, the percentage of asthmatic women experiencing severe asthma exacerbations (as defined by hospital admission, emergency department visit, unscheduled physician visit or treatment with oral steroids for asthma) increased with increasing asthma severity classification. In women with mild asthma, 8% and 12.6% experienced exacerbations (ADPS study and Australia study respectively). Severe exacerbations during the course of pregnancy were experienced by 25.7% (ADPS) to 47% (Australia) of women with moderate asthma and by 51.9% (ADPS) to 65% (Australia) of women with severe asthma. There were some slight differences between the study protocols and the proportions of women in the various asthma severity categories. Overall, 36% of women in the Australia study experienced severe exacerbations versus only 20% in the ADPS. Notably, the ADPS had a large percentage of African American participants (55%), who typically experience a higher prevalence of asthma and more severe asthma. Differences in the health care systems of Australia and the U.S. may also explain variation in the findings. Australia has a government financed, universal health care system; in the U.S., women may underutilize health care depending upon their health insurance status.

The Yale Asthma Study enrolled 873 pregnant asthmatic women and 1,333 women with no asthma history (Bracken et al. 2003). In women with diagnosed asthma, 49% were classified as mild severity, 24.6% had mild persistent asthma severity, 15.2% had moderate persistent severity, and 11.2% had severe persistent asthma severity. In addition, 34% of non-asthmatic women experienced asthma symptoms or used asthma medication during pregnancy. Severe asthma during pregnancy was associated with younger age, unmarried, Hispanic and black ethnicity, lower education, higher prepregnancy weight, smoking during pregnancy, and consuming 150 mg or more of caffeine during pregnancy.

A recent and comprehensive retrospective chart review of pregnant white and black women enrolled in Medicaid in Tennessee (Carroll et al. 2005), found that in comparison to white women, black women had a significantly higher risk of asthma exacerbations including: emergency room visits for asthma (adjusted RR = 1.89; 95% CI: 1.57–2.27), hospital admission (adjusted RR = 1.73; 95% CI: 1.34–2.24), or filling a rescue corticosteroid prescription (adjusted RR = 1.35; 95% CI: 1.14–1.61). In this study, Blacks were more likely to be single, urban, non-smoking and to receive substandard pre-natal care.

Asthma Improvement During Pregnancy

In the ADPS, some women experienced improvements in their asthma during pregnancy (23%), whereas 30% demonstrated increasing asthma severity (Schatz et al. 2003). In a subset analysis of the ADPS using data from the San Diego site, 33.6% of pregnant women experienced improvements in their asthma during the course of pregnancy based on self-assessments and 36.4% experienced worsening of their asthma (Kircher et al. 2002). Changes in asthma were directly related to self-reported changes in rhinitis. A recent study prospectively measured peak flow values in 43 racially and ethnically diverse, asthmatic pregnant women (Beckmann 2008) and found a statistically significant increase in peak flow between the first and third ($p < 0.005$) and second and third trimesters ($p < 0.01$).

Studies examining the underlying causes of asthma exacerbation during pregnancy have investigated the following factors: sex of the infant (Bakhireva et al. 2008; Firoozi et al. 2009), maternal weight gain, maternal pre-pregnancy BMI, maternal smoking during pregnancy, panic-fear hypotheses, infant birth weight, use of corticosteroids, and seasonality. There are conflicting results for all of these variables. For example, Kircher and colleagues (2002) analyzed a subset of ADPS data ($n = 568$) and found no association between pre-pregnancy weight and asthma exacerbations during pregnancy, whereas Hendler et al. (2006), analyzing the full ADPS data set ($n = 1{,}699$) found that obesity was significantly related to asthma exacerbations during pregnancy (OR = 1.3; 95% CI: 1.1–1.7).

It has been hypothesized that many asthma exacerbations during pregnancy are the result of women not adhering to their asthma drug therapy for fear of harming the fetus. Non-adherence is a distinctly gendered response by women based on the medicalization of pregnancy and social norms about motherhood. Enriquez et al. (2006) in a retrospective review of Medicaid claims data of over 8,000 pregnant women with asthma, found that women decreased asthma medication use in the first trimester (23% decrease in ICS, 13% decrease in β-agonists and 54% decline in rescue therapies). These findings are similar to patients of a managed care organization (Chambers 2003). If true, health care providers require training to educate women about the course and progression of asthma during pregnancy and the safety of ICS.

Adverse Maternal Outcomes in Pregnant Women with Asthma

Obesity is associated with pregnancy complications (gestational hypertension, gestational diabetes and caesarean section), regardless of the presence of asthma (Hendler et al. 2006). But in a recent analysis of the ADPS and an additional dataset for an asthma medication randomized control trial, lower FEV_1 in asthmatic women during pregnancy was significantly associated with increased gestational hypertension, gestational diabetes and premature birth (Schatz et al. 2006b). Similarly, pregnant women with moderate-to-severe asthma have an increased risk of caesarean delivery as compared to nonasthmatic controls (adjusted OR = 1.4; 95% CI: 1.1–1.8) (Dombrowski et al. 2004).

Treatment of Asthma During Pregnancy

There are two consistently definitive findings in studies on asthma and pregnancy: first, inhaled corticosteroids are safe to use during pregnancy and there are no significant adverse maternal, fetal or infant outcomes as a result of ICS use; second, use of oral steroids increases adverse perinatal outcomes. In the Yale Asthma Study (Bracken et al. 2003), pregnant women with and without asthma and pregnant women without a diagnosis of asthma but with asthma symptoms were prospectively monitored from weeks 20 through postpartum. There was no increased risk of pre-term delivery or intrauterine growth restriction (IUGR) with ICS use. Preterm delivery was 50% more likely in asthmatic women, however, there was no increased risk of preterm delivery associated with increasing levels of asthma severity as determined by the Global Initiative for Asthma criteria. A recent review of ICS use during pregnancy concluded that ICSs were safe to use, but the authors noted the low statistical power of the current published studies (Breton et al. 2008).

Summary

Based on the few available studies, pregnancy does change the severity of asthma in many women, but the direction of the change is not predictable. Those women experiencing an asthma exacerbation during pregnancy may be at increased risk for adverse maternal outcomes. Increased exacerbations of asthma may be due to reduced use of asthma medications, even though evidence-based research supports the safety of inhaled corticoid steroids during pregnancy with no significant adverse maternal or fetal outcomes.

Women and Health Care Utilization

Although gender differences in the incidence and prevalence of asthma among children have been recognized throughout the last 20 years, gender differences among adults have not been explored as thoroughly. Most studies that have explored gender differences among adults with asthma have focused on the use of health care due to asthma exacerbations. These studies have demonstrated that women are more likely than men to present to the emergency department with complaints of asthma exacerbation and to be admitted to the hospital, despite similar prevalence rates of asthma among both groups (Cydulka et al. 2001; DiMarco 1989; Prescott et al. 1997; Rowe et al. 2009). These findings agree with the results of previous research exploring gender differences in health care utilization. Bertakis and colleagues (2000) were able to demonstrate that women tend to utilize health care services more than men, particularly emergency room, primary care, and diagnostic services. The gender differences that have been shown in health care use related to asthma are thought to be caused by differences in severity of the disease and symptom experience (Prescott et al. 1997; Schatz et al. 2006a).

Upon presentation to the emergency room, women have been found to report more severe symptoms in terms of symptom frequency, intensity, and resulting activity limitations than do men (Cydulka et al. 2001). While self-reports of symptoms indicate that women experience more severe asthma than men, analysis of objective measures of asthma severity such as forced expiratory volume in 1 s and peak expiratory flow rates demonstrate that men more often present to the emergency room with more clinically severe asthma exacerbations (Awadh et al. 1996; Cydulka et al. 2001; Schatz et al. 2006a; Singh et al. 1999). In particular, women with clinically moderate asthma exacerbations were found to be much more likely than men to report severe activity limitations. In males and females reporting to the emergency department for acute asthma, women were more likely than men to report an ongoing asthma exacerbation or relapse (Rowe et al. 2008; Singh et al. 1999).

The differences found in self-report of symptoms and objective clinical measures indicate that differences in symptom experience between men and women may explain the differences in health care use (Cydulka et al. 2001). Gender differences in symptom experiences that result in differences in health care utilization for asthma exacerbations may be due to several factors including clinical factors (e.g., the natural history of asthma), and psychosocial issues (Cydulka et al. 2001), and education related to sex and gender and asthma (Clark et al. 2008).

Studies exploring clinical factors that may influence gender differences in symptom experience have varied in their results. Burden and colleagues (1982) were able to demonstrate that asthmatic patients with a longer history of airflow obstruction were more likely to have a lower awareness of airway obstruction. These findings were found to occur independently of gender, suggesting that the propensity for women to develop asthma at a later age then men may cause them to have a higher perception of airway obstruction during an exacerbation (Burdon et al. 1982). Other studies have shown that female sex, along with younger age and more severe airway responsiveness, is associated with an increased perception of airway obstruction (Brand et al. 1992). In contrast, Boulet and colleagues (1994) found that high or low perception of obstruction and breathlessness were similar across age, gender, and baseline level of airway obstruction and responsiveness.

Psychosocial issues as related to gender differences in symptom experience and health care utilization have not been explored in detail. Studies that have explored these issues in adults with asthma have demonstrated that women, compared to men, more often exhibit elevated levels of psychological distress and anxiety (Belloch et al. 2003; Tovt-Korshynska et al. 2001). These elevated levels of distress occur across all levels of clinical severity and duration of asthma and are often reflected in somatic and psychological complaints, such as dyspnea, insomnia, and lack of energy (Belloch et al. 2003). These findings suggest that women react to the presence of the disease and the somatic symptoms of their psychological distress and not necessarily the severity of the disease. In contrast, levels of distress in men have been shown to increase as the clinical severity and duration of the disease increases, demonstrating that they react to the physiological exacerbation of the disease (Tovt-Korshynska et al. 2001).

Other hypotheses regarding the source of the gender differences in symptom experience and health care utilization have been proposed. One hypothesis is that women are more aware of, and attentive to, bodily changes than men (Redline and Gold 1994) and thus may be more likely to seek clinical help for less severe asthma symptoms. It has also been suggested that gender differences in health care utilization may result from men being more reluctant to seek health care and/or acknowledge symptoms until the severity of the exacerbation has reached a point that it is unable to be ignored (Cydulka et al. 2001). Further investigation of these hypotheses will be important in developing a greater understanding of gender differences in symptom experience and subsequent health care utilization. Clark et al. (2007) have demonstrated that an asthma disease-management program targeted to women with asthma can improve women's quality of life ($p=0.0005$), self-regulation ($p=0.03$), and asthma self-efficacy ($p=0.001$).

Discussion

The majority of asthma research with women, similar to other health research with women, has focused on the biological mechanisms that influence the onset and course of asthma, primarily changes in sex-steroid levels. These studies have had conflicting findings, but it is clear that fluctuations in sex-steroid levels, whether because of exogenous or endogenous hormones, are associated with changes in asthma severity in many women. However, *the direction* of the change is inconsistent, and thus there may be additional biological factors underlying these relationships that have yet to be determined. The existing research base is limited by the lack of prospective studies examining women at different stages of the menstrual cycle; at all phases of pregnancy, both pre- and postpartum; and at menopause and its transitions.

Given that asthma exacerbations reported during pregnancy may be due to women's decreased medication usage, more research is needed to examine women's gendered responses to motherhood and pregnancy. The increasing focus on in utero influences on fetal development and health can be embodied by women as a "blame the mother" mentality. Medical and societal strictures on women in relation to alcohol use, smoking, food intake, and drug and medication use during pregnancy, and now even pre-pregnancy, are increasing and can carry social stigma and even criminal penalties. These social strictures have resulted in some women being tested for drug use without their knowledge or consent and then being arrested for child abuse (Dailard and Nash 2000). In Oklahoma, the state took custody of a woman's fetus because she was found in an environment where drugs were manufactured. Despite the fact that the woman tested drug free, she was incarcerated where ironically she was denied milk and prenatal vitamins for 2 weeks (Cooper 2003). While these are admittedly extreme cases and focus on women who are poor and often African American, at the other end of the spectrum are upper middle-class White women who continue to drink alcohol during pregnancy (albeit at reduced rates) with the endorsement of their physicians (Moskin 2006). Given these double standards, societal norms about motherhood, and persistence advice from physicians, websites, and pregnancy books to avoid medications that are contraindicated during pregnancy, (Andrade et al. 2004) it is understandable that women may respond in a manner that they perceive to be protective or conservative, with the result that women choose to avoid all medications, even those that may be deemed safe such as inhaled corticosteroids. In that context, the decreased use of asthma medications during pregnancy is a logical gendered response.

Similarly, women's use of HRT has gendered connotations. Many women approach menopause with concerns about their appearance and sexuality deteriorating when they are surrounded by a culture that values youth and beauty. For years, HRT was marketed as the wonder drug to forestall aging and sexual decline. With new research that now highlights the negative effects of HRT on women's health and risk profiles, we have seen large numbers of women stop taking HRT with a corresponding drop in the incidence of breast cancer (Clarke et al. 2006). This decline in HRT use increases the need to understand the relationship between the perimenopause and menopause transition, and asthma, now that these conditions will be uncomplicated by HRT use.

Gender influences how and when women access the health care system. In contrast to other research that demonstrates that women tend to delay seeking health care treatment, such as with myocardial infarction (Rosenfeld et al. 2005; Schoenberg et al. 2003) and stroke (Mandelzweig et al. 2006), where delay is associated with more severe cases of disease and thus the need for hospitalization and emergency care, the research on asthma suggests that women are more likely to seek health care with only mild or moderate asthma flare-ups. However, women are still more likely to be hospitalized than men who have more severe asthma. This finding has gender implications, both on the part of the patients and their symptom interpretation, but also the physicians who admit them. The role of the physician and potential gender bias with respect to asthma has not been studied.

Possibly the most troubling gap in the research on women and asthma is the lack of research on African American women who have asthma mortality rates that are reportedly 2.5 times higher than white women (National Institute on Allergy and Infectious Diseases 2001). The most recent statistics available on asthma mortality rates for black females indicate that black women over age 65 had the highest crude asthma mortality rates (Moorman and Mannino 2001), but these numbers are now over a decade old. Given the number of co-morbidities that African American women have, the low socioeconomic status of many of these women, and lack of health care access, all of which are significantly associated with asthma, this population subgroup deserves special attention in order to reduce the health disparities associated with asthma morbidity and mortality.

Future asthma research needs to address multiple methodological issues such as the reliance on self-reports as opposed to clinical measures of respiratory function; the lack of prospective studies examining natural sex-steroid transition points; and the need to test various formulations of HRT and oral contraceptives including monophasic and triphasic pill formulations (Haggerty et al. 2003); and the myriad hormone delivery mechanisms (pill, patch, and cream) now available to women. In sum, research on women and asthma is still in its infancy with many avenues yet to be explored. These issues are unfortunately becoming more, not less, complicated as we untangle sex differences from gender differences in women's health research.

References

Agarwal AK, Shah A (1997) Menstrual-linked asthma. J Asthma 34(6):539–545

Alberts WM (1997) Circa menstrual rhythmicity and asthma. Chest 111(4):840–842

American Lung Association. (2005). Lung disease data in culturally diverse communities: 2005 http://www.lungusa2.org/embargo/lddcdc/LDD.pdf.

Andrade SE, Gurwitz JH, Davis RL, Chan KA, Finkelstein JA, Fortman K et al (2004) Prescription drug use in pregnancy. Am J Obst Gynecol 191(2):398–407

Angeli A, Guglielmi G, Dovio A, Capelli G, de Feo D, Giannini S et al (2006) High prevalence of asymptomatic vertebral fractures in post-menopausal women receiving chronic glucocorticoid therapy: a cross-section outpatient study. Bone 39(2):253–259

Arif AA, Delclos GL, Lee ES, Tortolero SR, Whitehead LW (2003) Prevalence and risk factors of asthma and wheezing among US adults: An analysis of the NHANES III data. Eur Respir J 21(5):827–833

Arif AA, Delclos GL, Serra C (2009) Occupational exposures and asthma among nursing professionals. Occup Environ Med 66(4):274–278

Awadh N, Shu S, Grunfeld A, Simpson K, Fitzgerald JM (1996) Comparison of males and females presenting with acute asthma to the emergency department. Respir Med 90(8):485–489

Bakhireva LN, Schatz M, Jones KL, Tucker CM, Slymen DJ, Klonoff-Cohen HS, Gresham L, Johnson D, Chambers CD, the OTIS Collaborative Research Group (2008) Fetal sex and maternal asthma control in pregnancy. J Asthma 45(5): 403–407

Balzano G, Fuschillo S, Melillo G, Bonini S (2001) Asthma and sex hormones. Allergy 56(1):13–20

Bandiera FC, Periera DB, Arif AA, Dodge B, Asal N (2008) Race/ethnicity, income, chronic asthma, and mental health: a cross-sectional study using the behavior risk factor surveillance system. Psychosom Med 70(1):77–84

Barr RG, Camargo CA Jr (2004) Hormone replacement therapy and obstructive airway diseases. Treat Respir Med 3(1):1–7

Barr RG, Wentowski CC, Grodstein F, Somers SC, Stampfer MJ, Schwartz J et al (2004) Prospective study of postmenopausal hormone use and newly diagnosed asthma and chronic obstructive pulmonary disease. Arch Int Med 164(4):379–386

Becklake MR, Kauffmann F (1999) Gender differences in airway behavior over the human life span. Thorax 54(12): 1119–1138

Beckmann CA (2008) Peak flow values by gestation in women with asthma. Clin Nurs Res 17(3):174–181

Belloch A, Perpina M, Martinez-Moragon E, de Diego A, Martinez-Frances M (2003) Gender differences in health-related quality of life among patients with asthma. J Asthma 40(8):945–953

Bertakis KD, Azari R, Helms LJ, Callahan EJ, Robbins JA (2000) Gender differences in the utilization of health care services. J Fam Pract 49(2):147–152

Black PN, Sharpe S (1997) Dietary fat and asthma: is there a connection? Eur Respir J 10(1):6–12

Boulet LP, Leblanc P, Turcotte H (1994) Perception scoring of induced bronchoconstriction as an index of awareness of asthma symptoms. Chest 105(5):1430–1433

Bousquet JJ, Knani J, Dhivert H, Richard A, Chicoye A, Ware JE et al (1994) Quality of life asthma. I. Internal consistency and validity of the SF-36 questionnaire. Am J Respir Crit Care Med 149(2):371–375

Bracken MB, Triche EW, Belanger K, Saftlas A, Beckett WS, Leaderer BP (2003) Asthma symptoms, severity, and drug therapy: a prospective study of effects on 2205 pregnancies. Obstet Gynecol 102:739–752

Brand PL, Rijcken B, Schouten JP, Koëter GH, Weiss ST, Postma DS (1992) Perception of airway obstruction in a random population sample. Relationship to airway hyperresponsiveness in the absence of respiratory symptoms. Am Rev Respir Dis 146(2):396–401

Brenner BE, Holmes TM, Mazal B, Camargo CA (2005) Relation between phase of the menstrual cycle and asthma presentations in the emergency department. Thorax 60(10):806–809

Breton M, Martel M, Vilain A, Blais L (2008) Inhaled corticosteroids during pregnancy: a review of methodologic issues. Respir Med 102(6):862–875

Burdon JGW, Juniper EF, Killian KJ, Hargreave FE, Campell EJM (1982) The perception of breathlessness in asthma. Am Rev Respir Dis 126:825–828

Camargo CA Jr, Weiss ST, Zhang S, Willett WC, Speizer FE (1999) Prospective study of body mass index, weight change, and risk of adult-onset asthma in women. Arch Int Med 159(21):2582–2588

Caracta CF (2003) Gender differences in pulmonary disease. Mt Sinai J Med 70(4):215–224

Carlson CL, Cushman M, Enright PL, Cauley JA, Newman AB (2001) Hormone replacement therapy is associated with higher FEV1 in elderly women. Am J Respir Crit Care Med 163(2):423–428

Carroll KN, Griffin MR, Gebretsadik T, Shintani A, Mitchel E, Hartert TV (2005) Racial differences in asthma morbidity during pregnancy. Obstet Gynecol 106(1):66–72

Cauley JA, Robbins J, Chen Z, Cummings SR, Jackson RD, LaCroix AZ et al (2003) Effects of estrogen plus progestin on risk of fracture and bone mineral density: The Women's

Health Initiative Randomized Trial. J Am Med Assoc 290(13):1729–1738

Centers for Disease Control and Prevention (2003) Health data for all ages. http://www.cdc.gov/nchs/health_data_for_all_ages.htm. Accessed 5 Jul 2006

Chambers K (2003) Asthma education and outcomes for women of childbearing age. Case Manager 14(6):58–61

Chandler MHH, Schuldheisz S, Phillips BA, Muse KN (1997) Premenstrual asthma: the effect of estrogen on symptoms, pulmonary function, and Beta-2 receptors. Pharmacotherapy 17(2):224–234

Chan-Yeung M, Malo JL (1995) Occupational asthma. N Engl J Med 333(2):107–112

Cherry DK, Hing E, Woodwell DA, Rechtsteiner EA (2008) National Ambulatory Medical Care Survey: 2006 Summary. Natl Health Stat Report 6(3):1–39

Chhabra SK (2005) Premenstrual asthma. Indian J Chest Dis Allied Sci 47(2):109–116

Chlebowski RT, Hendrix SL, Langer RD, Stefanick ML, Gass M, Lane D et al (2003) Influence of estrogen plus progestin on breast cancer and mammography in healthy postmenopausal women: The Women's Health Initiative Randomized Trial. J Am Med Assoc 289(24):3243–3253

Clark NM, Gong ZM, Wang SJ, Lin X, Bria WF, Johnson TR (2007) A randomized trial of a self-regulation intervention for women with asthma. Chest 132:88–97

Clark NM, Valerio MA, Gong ZM (2008) Self-regulation and women with asthma. Curr Opin Allergy Clin Immunol 8(3):222–227

Clarke CA, Glaser SL, Uratsu CS, Selby JV, Kushi LH, Herrinton LJ (2006) Recent declines in hormone therapy utilization and breast cancer incidence: clinical and population-based evidence. J Clin Oncol 24(33):e49–e50

Coogan PF, Palmer JR, O'Connor JT, Rosenberg L (2009) Body mass index and asthma incidence in the Black Women's Health Study. J Allergy Clin Immunol 123:89–95

Cooper CL (2003) Pregnant and punished. Ford Foundation Report (Winter), 34(1):28–31

Cushman M, Kuller LH, Prentice R, Rodabough RJ, Psaty BM, Stafford RS et al (2004) Estrogen plus progestin and risk of venous thrombosis. J Am Med Assoc 292(13):1573–1580

Cydulka RK, Emerman CL, Rowe BH, Clark S, Woodruff PG, Singh AK et al (2001) Differences between men and women in reporting of symptoms during an asthma exacerbation. Ann Emerg Med 38(2):123–128

Dahl R (2006) Systemic side effects of inhaled corticosteroids in patients with asthma. Respir Med 100:1307–1317

Dailard C, Nash E (2000) State responses to substance abuse among pregnant women. Guttmacher Rep Public Policy 3(6):3–6

De Marco R, Locatelli F, Sunyer J, Burney P (2000) Differences in incidence of reported asthma related to age in men and women: a retrospective analysis of the data of the European Respiratory Health Survey. Am J Respir Crit Care Med 162(1):68–74

Delclos GL, Gimeno D, Arif AA, Burau KD, Carson A, Lusk C et al (2007) Occupational risk factors and asthma among health care professionals. Am J Respir Crit Care Med 175(7):667–675

DiMarco AF (1989) Asthma in the pregnant patient: a review. Ann Allergy 62(6):527–533

Dombrowski MP (2006) Outcomes of pregnancy in asthmatic women. Immunol Allergy Clin North Am 26(1):81–92

Dombrowski MP, Schatz M, Wise R, Momirova V, Landon M, Mabie W et al (2004) Asthma during pregnancy. Obstet Gynecol 103(1):5–12

Dorhofer DM, Sigmon ST (2002) Physiological and psychological reactivity in women with asthma: the effects of anxiety and menstrual cycle phase. Behav Res Ther 40(1):3–17

Drake KA, Galanter JM, Burchard EG (2008) Race, ethnicity and social class and the complex etiologies of asthma. Pharmacogenomics 9(4):453–462

Eder W, Ege MJ, von Mutius E (2006) The asthma epidemic. N Engl J Med 355(21):2226–2235

Edwards AL, Rose MS, Donovan LE, Ford GT (1996) Premenstrual exacerbation of life-threatening asthma: effect of gonadotropin releasing hormone analogue therapy. Can Respir J 3(3):203–206

Eliasson O, Scherzer HH, DeGradd ACJ (1986) Morbidity in asthma in relation to the menstrual cycle. J Allergy Clin Immunol 77(1):87–94

Enriquez R, Wu P, Griffin MR, Gebretsadik T, Shintani A, Mitchel E et al (2006) Cessation of asthma medication in early pregnancy. Am J Obstet Gynecol 195(1):149–153

Firoozi F, Ducharme FM, Lemière C, Beauchesne M, Perreault S, Forget A, Blais L (2009) Effect of fetal gender on maternal asthma exacerbations in pregnant asthmatic women. Respir Med 103(1):144–151

Flattery J, Davis L, Rosenman KD, Harrison R, Lyon-Callo S, Filios M (2001) The proportion of self-reported asthma associated with work in three states: California, Massachusetts, and Michigan. J Asthma 43(3):213–218

Forbes L (1999) Do exogenous oestrogens and progesterone influence asthma? Thorax 54(3):265–267

Forbes L, Jarvis D, Burney P (1999) Do hormonal contraceptives influence asthma severity? Eur Respir J 14(5):1028–1033

Gandhi M, Aweeka F, Greenblatt RM, Blaschke TF (2004) Sex differences in pharmacokinetics and pharmacodynamics. Annu Rev Pharmacol Toxicol 44:499–523

Gold DR, Wang X, Wypij D, Speizer FE, Ware JH, Dockery DW (1996) Effects of cigarette smoking on lung function in adolescent boys and girls. N Engl J Med 335(13):931–937

Gómez Real F, Svanes C, Bjornsson EH, Franklin KA, Gislason D, Gislason T et al (2006) Hormone replacement therapy, body mass index and asthma in perimenopausal women: a cross sectional survey. Thorax 61(1):34–40

Gómez Real FG, Svanes C, Omenaas ER, Antò JM, Plana E, Jarvis D et al (2007) Menstrual irregularity and asthma and lung function. J Allergy Clin Immunol 120(3):557–564

Gómez Real FG, Svanes C, Omenaas ER, Antò JM, Plana E, Jarvis D et al (2008) Lung function, respiratory symptoms, and the menopausal transition. J Allergy Clin Immunol 121(1):72–80

Grant EN, Syltte CS, Weiss KB (2000) The relation of socioeconomic factors and racial/ethnic differences in US asthma mortality. Am J Public Health 90(12):1923–1925

Haggerty CL, Ness RB, Kelsey S, Waterer GW (2003) The impact of estrogen and progesterone on asthma. Ann Allergy Asthma Immunol 90(3):284–291

Halpern MT, Schmier JK, Van Kerkhove MD, Watkins M, Kalberg CJ (2004) Impact of long-term inhaled corticosteroid therapy on bone mineral density: results of a meta-analysis. Ann Allergy Asthma Immunol 92:201–207

Hanania NA, Belfort MA (2005) Acute asthma in pregnancy. Crit Care Med 33(10 Suppl):S319–S324

Hendler I, Schatz M, Momirova V, Wise R, Landon M, Mabie W et al (2006) Association of obesity with pulmonary and nonpulmonary complications of pregnancy in asthmatic women. Obstet Gynecol 108(1):77–82

Hepburn MJ, Dooley DP, Morris MJ (2001) The effects of estrogen replacement therapy on airway function in postmenopausal, asthmatic women. Arch Int Med 161(22):2717–2720

Hodge L, Salome CM, Peat JK, Haby MM, Xuan W, Woolcock AJ (1996) Consumption of oily fish and childhood asthma risk. Med J Aust 164(3):137–140

Israel E, Banerjee TR, Fitzmaurice GM, Kotlov TV, LaHive K, LeBoff MS (2001) Effects of inhaled glucocorticoids on bone density in premenopausal women. N Engl J Med 345(13):941–947

Janson C, Antò J, Burney P, Chinn S, de Marco R, Heinrich J et al (2001) The European Community Respiratory Health Survey: what are the main results so far? Eur Respir J 18(3):598–611

Jarvis D, Leynaert B (2008) The association of asthma, atopy and lung fuction with hormone replacement therapy and surgical cessation of menstruation in a population-based sample of English women. Allergy 63:95–102

Jenkins MA, Dharmage SC, Flander LB, Douglass JA, Ugoni AM, Carlin JB et al (2006) Parity and decreased use of oral contraceptives as predictors of asthma in young women. Clin Exp Allergy 36:609–613

Jochman N, Stangl K, Garbe E, Baumann G, Stangl V (2005) Female-specific aspects in the pharmacotherapy of chronic cardiovascular diseases. Eur Heart J 26(16):1585–1595

Jones A, Fay JK, Burr M, Stone M, Hood K, Roberts G (2002) Inhaled corticosteroid effects on bone metabolism in asthma and mild chronic obstructive pulmonary disease. Cochrane Database Syst Rev (1): CD003537

Juniper EF, Kline PA, Roberts RS, Hargreave FE, Daniel EE (1987) Airway responsiveness to methacholine during the natural menstrual cycle and the effect of oral contraceptives. Am Rev Respir Dis 135(5):1039–1042

Kircher S, Schatz M, Long L (2002) Variables affecting asthma course during pregnancy. Ann Allergy Asthma Immunol 89:463–466

Kochanek KD, Murphy SL, Anderson RN, Scott C (2002) Deaths: final data for 2002, National Vital Statistics Report, vol. 53. National Center for Health Statistics, Hyattsville, MD.

Kos-Kudla B, Ostrowska Z, Marek B, Ciesielska-Kopacz N, Sieminska L, Kajdaniuk D et al (2000) Hormone replacement therapy in postmenopausal asthmatic women. J Clin Pharm Ther 25(6):461–466

Kos-Kudla B, Ostrowska Z, Marek B, Ciesielska-Kopacz N, Kajdaniuk D, Kudla M (2001) Effects of hormone replacement therapy on endocrine and spirometric parameters in asthmatic postmenopausal women. Gynecol Endocrinol 15(4):304–311

Koullapis E, Collins L (1980) The concentration of 13-14-di-OH-15-OXO prostaglandin F2-alpha in peripheral venous plasma throughout the normal ovarian and menstrual cycle. Acta Endocrinol 93(1):123–128

Krieger N (2003) Genders, sexes, and health: What are the connections – why does it matter? Int J Epidemiol 32:652–657

Kwon HL, Belanger K, Bracken MB (2003) Asthma prevalence among pregnant and childbearing-aged women in the United States: estimates from national health surveys. Ann Epidemiol 13(5):317–324

Laatikainen AK, Kröger HPJ, Tukiainen HO, Honkanen RJ, Saarikoski SV (1999) Bone mineral density in perimenopausal women with asthma: a population-based cross-sectional study. Am J Respir Crit Care Med 159:1179–1185

Lange P, Parner J, Prescott E, Ulrik CS, Vestbo J (2001) Exogenous female sex steroid hormones and risk of asthma and asthma-like symptoms: a cross sectional study of the general population. Thorax 56(8):613–616

Langhammer A, Norjavaara E, de Verdier MG, Johnsen R, Bjermer L (2004) Use of inhaled corticosteroids and bone mineral density in a population based study: the Nord-Trondelag Health Study (the HUNT Study). Pharmacoepidemiol Drug Saf 13(8):569–579

Lieberman D, Kopernik G, Porath A, Lazer S, Heimer D (1995) Sub-clinical worsening of bronchial asthma during estrogen replacement therapy in asthmatic post-menopausal women. Maturitas 21:153–157

Litonjua AA, Carey VJ, Weiss ST, Gold DR (1999) Race, socioeconomic factors, and area of residence are associated with asthma prevalence. Pediatr Pulmonol 28(6):394–401

Luengo M, del Río L, Pons F, Picardo C (1997) Bone mineral density in asthmatic patients treated with inhaled corticosteroids: a case-control study. Eur Respir J 10:2110–2113

Lugogo NL, Kraft M (2006) Epidemiology of asthma. Clin Chest Med 27(1):1–15

Mandelzweig L, Goldbourt U, Boyko V, Tanne D (2006) Perceptual, social, and behavioral factors associated with delays in seeking medical care in patients with symptoms of acute stroke. Stroke 37:1248–1253

Martin CM (2006) Gender-specific pharmacology: implications for therapy. Consult Pharm 21(8):620–622 631–624

Martinez-Moragon E, Plaza V, Serrano J, Picado C, Galdiz JB, Lopez-Vina A et al (2004) Near-fatal asthma related to menstruation. J Allergy Clin Immunol 113(2):242–244

Masi MA, Hanley JA, Ernst P, Becklake MR (1988) Environmental exposure to tobacco smoke and lung function in young adults. Am Rev Respir Dis 138(2):296–299

Matsubara S, Swasey CH, Loader LE, Dakhama A, Joetham A, Ohnishi H et al (2008) Estrogen determines sex differences in airway responsiveness after allergen exposure. Am J Respir Cell Mol Biol 38(5):501–508

Matsuo N, Shimoda T, Matsuse H, Kohno S (1999) A case of menstruation-associated asthma: treatment with oral contraceptives. Chest 116(1):252–253

McCaig LF, Burt CW (2005) National Hospital Ambulatory Medical Care Survey: 2003 emergency department summary. National Center for Health Statistics, Hyattsville, Maryland

McCallister JW, Mastronarde JG (2008) Sex differences in asthma. J Asthma 45:853–861

Melgert BN, Ray A, Hylkema MN, Timens W, Postma DS (2007) Are there reasons why adult asthma is more common in females? Curr Allergy Asthma Rep 7:143–150

Minino AM, Heron MP, Murphy SL, Kochanek KD (2007) Deaths: Final data for 2004. Natl Vital Stat Report 55(19):1–119

Mirdal GM, Peterssen B, Weeke B, Vibits A (1998) Asthma and menstruation: the relationship between psychological and bronchial hyperreactivity. Br J Med Psychol 71(1):47–55

Moorman JE, Mannino DM (2001) Increasing U.S. asthma mortality rates: who is really dying? J Asthma 38(1):65–71

Morris ME, Lee HJ, Predko LM (2003) Gender differences in the membrane transport of endogenous and exogenous compounds. Pharmacol Rev 55(2):229–240

Morshita M, Miyagi M, Iwamoto Y (1999) Effects of sex hormones on production of interleukin-1 by human peripheral monocytes. J Periodontol 70(7):757–760

Moskin J (2006) The weighty responsibility of drinking for two. The New York Times, November 29

Mueller JE, Frye C, Brasche S, Heinrich J (2003) Association of hormone replacement therapy with bronchial hyper-responsiveness. Respir Med 97:990–992

Murphy VE, Gibson P (2008) Premenstrual asthma: prevalence, cycle-to-cycle variability and relationship to oral contraceptive use and menstrual symptoms. J Asthma 45(8):696–704

Murphy VE, Gibson P, Talbot PI, Clifton VL (2005) Severe asthma exacerbations during pregnancy. Obstet Gynecol 106(5 Pt 1):1046–1054

Murphy VE, Clifton VL, Gibson PG (2006) Asthma exacerbations during pregnancy: incidence and association with adverse pregnancy outcomes. Thorax 61:169–176

Nakasato H, Ohrui T, Sekizawa K, Matsui T, Yamaya M, Tamura G et al (1999) Prevention of severe premenstrual asthma attacks by leukotriene receptor antagonist. J Allergy Clin Immunol 104(3 Pt 1):585–588

National Institute on Allergy and Infectious Diseases (2001) Asthma: A concern for minority populations. National Institutes of Health.

National Institutes of Health Osteoporosis and Related Bone Diseases ~ National Resources Center (2005) What people with asthma need to know about osteoporosis. http://www.niams.nih.gov/bone/hi/osteoporosis_asthma.htm. Accessed 19 Jul 2006

Nicolai T, Pereszlenyiova-Bliznakova L, Illi S, Reinhardt D, von Mutius E (2003) Longitudinal follow-up of the changing gender ratio in asthma from childhood to adulthood: role of delayed manifestation in girls. Pediatr Allergy Immunol 14(4):280–283

Oguzulgen IK, Turktas H, Erbas D (2002) Airway inflammation in premenstrual asthma. J Asthma 39(6):517–522

Osman M (2003) Therapeutic implications of sex differences in asthma and atopy. Arch Dis Child 88:587–590

PausJenssen ES, Cockcroft DW (2003) Sex differences in asthma, atopy, and airway hyperresponsiveness in a university population. Ann Allergy Asthma Immunol 91(1):34–37

Peters SP (2006) Safety of inhaled corticosteroids in the treatment of persistent asthma. J Natl Med Assoc 98(6):851–861

Phillips SP (2005) Defining and measuring gender: a social determinant of health whose time has come. Int J Equity Health 4(11):1–4

Pitts SR, Niska RW, Xu J, Burt CW (2008) National Hospital Ambulatory Medical Care Survey: 2006 emergency department summary. Natl Health Stat Report 6(7):1–38

Pleis JR, Lethbridge-Cejku M (2007) Summary health statistics for US adults: National Health Interview Survey, 2006. Vital Health Stat 10(235):1–153

Popovic RM, White DP (1998) Upper airway muscle activity in normal women: influence of hormonal status. J Appl Physiol 84(3):1055–1062

Postma DS (2007) Gender differences in asthma development and progression. Gend Med 4(Suppl B):S133–S146

Prescott E, Lange P, Vestbo J (1997) Effect of gender on hospital admissions for asthma and prevalence of self-reported asthma: a prospective study based on a sample of the general population. Copenhagen City Heart Study Group. Thorax 52(3):287–289

Rahman A, McDevitt D, Struthers A, Lipworth BJ (1992) Sex differences in hypokalaemic and electrocardiographic effects of inhaled terbutaline. Thorax 47(12):1056–1059

Raper NR, Cronin FJ, Exler J (1992) Omega-3 fatty acid content of the US food supply. J Am Coll Nutr 11(3):304–308

Redline S, Gold D (1994) Challenges in interpreting gender differences in asthma. Am J Respir Crit Care Med 150(5):1219–1221

Romieu I, Avenel V, Leynaert B, Kauffmann F, Clavel-Chapelon F (2003) Body mass index, change in body silhouette, and risk of asthma in the E3N Cohort Study. Am J Epidemiol 158(2):165–174

Rosenfeld AG, Lindauer A, Darney BG (2005) Understanding treatment-seeking delay in women with acute myocardial infarction: descriptions of decision-making patterns. Am J Crit Care 14(4):285–293

Rossouw JE, Anderson GL, Prentice RL, LaCroix AZ, Kooperberg C, Stefanick ML et al (2002) Risks and benefits of estrogen plus progestin in healthy postmenopausal women: principal results from the Women's Health Initiative randomized controlled trial. J Am Med Assoc 288(3): 321–333

Rowe BH, Villa-Roel C, Sivilotti ML, Lang E, Borgundvaag B, Worster A et al (2008) Relapse after emergency department discharge for acute asthma. Acad Emerg Med 15(8):709–717

Rowe BH, Voaklander DC, Wang D, Senthilselvan A, Klassen TP, Marrie TJ et al (2009) Asthma presentations by adults to emergency departments in Alberta, Canada: a large population-based study. Chest 135(1):57–65

Rudra CB, Williams MA, Frederick IO, Luthy DA (2006) Maternal asthma and risk of preeclampsia: a case-control study. J Reprod Med 51(2):94–100

Saag KG, Gehlbach SH, Curtis JR, Youket TE, Worley K, Lange JL (2006) Trends in prevention of glucocorticoid-induced osteoporosis. J Rheumatol 33(8):1651–1657

Salam MT, Wenten M, Gilliland FD (2006) Endogenous and exogenous sex steroid hormones and asthma and wheeze in young women. J Allergy Clin Immunol 117:1001–1007

Schatz M, Harden K, Forsythe A, Chilingar L, Hoffman C, Sperling W et al (1988) The course of asthma during pregnancy, post partum, and with successive pregnancies: a prospective analysis. J Allergy Clin Immunol 81(3):509–517

Schatz M, Dombrowski MP, Wise R, Thom EA, Landon M, Mabie W et al (2003) Asthma morbidity during pregnancy can be predicted by severity classification. J Allergy Clin Immunol 112(2):283–288

Schatz M, Clark S, Camargo CA (2006a) Sex differences in the presentation and course of asthma hospitalizations. Chest 129:50–55

Schatz M, Dombrowski MP, Wise R, Momirova V, Landon M, Mabie W et al (2006b) Spirometry is related to perinatal outcomes in pregnant women with asthma. Am J Obstet Gynecol 194(1):120–126

Schoenberg NE, Peters JC, Drew EM (2003) Unraveling the mysteries of timing: women's perceptions about time to treatment for cardiac symptoms. Soc Sci Med 56:271–284

Seaton A, Godden DJ, Brown K (1994) Increase in asthma: a more toxic environment or a more susceptible population? Thorax 49(2):171–174

Shanies JM, Vnkataraman MT, Peter T (1997) Reversal of intractable acute severe asthma by first-trimester termination of pregnancy. J Asthma 34(2):169–172

Sharma PK, Malhotra S, Pandhi P, Kumar N (2003) Effect of inhaled steroids on bone mineral density: a meta-analysis. J Clin Pharmacol 43:193–197

Sheiner E, Mazor M, Levy A, Wiznitzer A, Bashiri A (2005) Pregnancy outcome of asthmatic patients: a population-based study. J Matern Fetal Neonatal Med 18(4):237–240

Singh AK, Cydulka RK, Stahmer SA, Woodruff PG, Camargo CA (1999) Sex differences among adults presenting to the emergency department with acute asthma. Arch Int Med 159(11):1237–1243

Skobeloff EM (1995) Estrogen withdrawal alters bronchial muscle response in a rabbit asthmatic model. Ann Emerg Med 25(1):128–129

Skobeloff EM, Spivey WH, St. Clair SS, Schoffstall JM (1992) The influence of age and sex on asthma admissions. J Am Med Assoc 268(24):3437–3440

Skobeloff EM, Spivey WH, Silverman R, Eskin BA, Harchelroad F, Alessi TV (1996) The effect of the menstrual cycle on asthma presentations in the emergency department. Arch Int Med 156(16):1837–1840

Smith HR, Larsen GL, Cherniak RM, Wenzel SE, Voelkel NF, Westcott JY et al (1992) Inflammatory cells and eicosanoid mediators in subjects with late asthmatic responses and increased airway responsiveness. J Allergy Clin Immunol 89(6):1076

Stenius-Aarniala BSM, Hedman J, Teramo KA (1996) Acute asthma during pregnancy. Thorax 51(4):411–414

Sunyer J, Anto JM, Kogevinas M, Barcelo MA, Soriano JB, Tobias A et al (1997) Risk factors for asthma in young adults. Eur Respir J 10(11):2490–2494

Tan KS (2001) Premenstrual asthma: epidemiology, pathogenesis and treatment. Drugs 61(14):2079–2086

Tan KS, McFarlane LC, Lipworth BJ (1997) Modulation of airway reactivity and peak flow variability in asthmatics receiving the oral contraceptive pill. Am J Respir Crit Care Med 155(4):1273–1277

Tan KS, McFarlane LC, Lipworth BJ (1998) Beta2-adrenoceptor regulation and function in female asthmatic patients receiving the oral combined contraceptive pill. Chest 113(2):278–282

Tattersfield AE, Harrison TW, Hubbard RB, Mortimer K (2004) Safety of inhaled corticosteroids. Proc Am Thorac Soc 1:171–175

Toogood JH, Baskerville JC, Markov AE, Hodsman AB, Fraher LJ, Jennings B et al (1995) Bone mineral density and the risk of fracture in patients receiving long-term inhaled steroid therapy for asthma. J Allergy Clin Immunol 96:157–166

Tovt-Korshynska MI, Dew MA, Chopey IV, Spivak MY, Lemko IS (2001) Gender diffferences in psychological distress in adults with asthma. J Psychosom Res 51(5):629–637

Troisi RJ, Speizer FE, Willett WC, Trichopoulos D, Rosner B (1995) Menopause, postmenopausal estrogen preparations, and the risk of adult-onset asthma. A prospective cohort study. Am J Respir Crit Care Med 152(4 Pt 1):1183–1188

Tsugeno H, Tsugeno H, Fujita T, Goto B, Sugishita T, Hosaki Y et al (2002) Vertebral fracture and cortical bone changes in corticosteroid-induced osteoporosis. Osteoporos Int 13(8):650–656

Vrieze A, Postma DS, Kerstjens HA (2003) Perimenstrual asthma: a syndrome without known cause or cure. J Allergy Clin Immunol 112(2):271–282

Walsh LJ, Lewis SA, Wong CA, Cooper S, Oborne J, Cawte SA et al (2002) The impact of oral corticosteroid use on bone mineral density and vertebral fracture. Am J Respir Crit Care Med 166(5):691–695

Weinmann GG, Zacur H, Fish JE (1987) Absence of changes in airway responsiveness during the natural menstrual cycle and the effect of oral contraceptives. J Allergy Clin Immunol 79(4):634–638

Weiss KB, Gergen PJ, Hodgson TA (1992) An economic evaluation of asthma in the United States. N Engl J Med 326(13):862–866

Wheeldon N, Newnham D, Coutie W, Peters JA, McDevitt DG, Lipworth BJ (1994) Influence of sex-steroid hormones on the regulation of lymphocyte Beta2 adrenoceptors during the menstrual cycle. Br J Clin Pharmacol 37(6):583–588

Wong CA, Walsh LJ, Smith CJP, Wisniewski AF, Lewis SA, Hubbard R et al (2000) Inhaled corticosteroid use and bone-mineral density in patients with asthma. Lancet 355:1399–1403

World Health Organization (1998) Gender and health: Technical Paper (No. WHO/FRH/WHD/98.16). World Health Organization, Geneva, Switzerland

Xu X, Wang L (1994) Gender differences in smoking effects on adult pulmonary function. Eur Respir J 7(3):477–483

Xu X, Weiss ST, Rijcken B, Schouten JP (1994) Smoking, changes in smoking habits, and rate of decline in FEV: new insight into gender differences. Eur Respir J 7(6):1056–1061

Zannolli R, Morgese G (1997) Does puberty interfere with asthma? Med Hypotheses 48:27–32

Zimmerman JL, Woodruff PG, Clark S, Camargo CA (2000) Relation between phase of menstrual cycle and emergency department visits for acute asthma. Am J Respir Crit Care Med 162(2):512–515

Chapter 16
Asthma in Minority Populations

Alexander N. Ortega, Daphne Koinis-Mitchell, and Peter J. Gergen

Introduction

This chapter presents information on asthma in the minority population in the United States. The asthma literature is vast with over 4,000 new studies being added each year. Despite this impressive number of publications, the asthma literature on ethnic and racial minorities is sufficient enough only to discuss the black and Latino experiences. Furthermore, most asthma studies include children, since asthma is the most common childhood chronic disease. Thus, we focus most of our review on asthma in children. The observations for minority children and adults are similar. In brief, Latino and black children and adults have higher prevalence rates of asthma, have a higher likelihood of being hospitalized for asthma, have asthma symptoms that are poorly controlled and managed, and have higher asthma-related mortality rates than their white counterparts (Canino et al. 2006; Hunninghake et al. 2006; Mannnino et al. 1998; Ortega and Calderon 2000; Rhodes et al. 2003; Shapiro and Stout 2002).

While the asthma literature on minority populations is quite voluminous, and thus difficult to capture fully in one chapter, this chapter will focus on a handful of key risk factors for minority populations including environmental factors, psychosocial factors, psychiatric disorders, obesity, genetics, and cultural factors. We then discuss issues in asthma management and control for minority populations, and we review the importance of considering cultural factors and the application of broad-based intervention approaches.

Epidemiology of Asthma in Minority Populations

Minority children and adults suffer a disproportionate burden of asthma morbidity and mortality. For example, Lara et al. (2006) recently analyzed the National Health Interview Survey (NHIS) and reported that 13% of youth ages 2–17 years had a parent-reported lifetime asthma diagnosis. Approximately 12.7% of white youth, 15.8% of black youth, and 12.4% of Latino youth had a lifetime diagnosis of asthma (Lara et al. 2006). When the Latino group was disaggregated, 25.8% of Puerto Rican youth, 10.1% of Mexican youth, 14.9% of Cuban youth, and 14.9% of Dominican youth had a lifetime diagnosis. It should be noted that while Mexican-American children have a lower proportion of parent-reported asthma diagnosis in the population, the public health impact is very significant. Mexican-Americans represent the highest *frequency* of Latino children with asthma, given that they are the largest ethnic subgroup in the population.

For minority populations, asthma is associated with high levels of impairment, many missed days from school and work, hospitalizations, and increased odds for mortality when compared with whites (Akinbami et al. 2005; Cohen et al. 2006; Mannino et al. 2002). Minorities are also less likely to be on appropriate asthma management plans, and, thus, they are more

A.N. Ortega (✉)
School of Public Health and Institute for Social Research, University of California Los Angeles, 2134 Rolfe Hall, Los Angeles, CA, 90095-1484, USA
e-mail: aortega@ucla.edu

A. Harver and H. Kotses (eds.), *Asthma, Health and Society: A Public Health Perspective*,
DOI 10.1007/978-0-387-78285-0_16, © Springer Science+Business Media, LLC 2010

likely to have their asthma poorly controlled (Lieu et al. 2002; Ortega et al. 2002a). For Latinos, high rates of asthma and its consequences appear specific to Puerto Ricans both on the U.S. mainland and on the island. Puerto Ricans have been shown, in multiple probability studies, to have the highest prevalence of self- or parent-reported asthma than any other racial or ethnic group (Carter-Pokras and Gergen 1993; Rhodes et al. 2003; Lara et al. 2006; Ortega et al. 2002b; Perez-Perdomo et al. 2003; Rose et al. 2006), and Puerto Ricans have demonstrated to have more morbidity, as measured by missed days of school, clinic visits and emotional impact (Cohen et al. 2006; Lieu et al. 2002).

Understanding the Asthma Differences

Given the differences reported in morbidity and mortality of asthma among the various racial/ethnic groups, it is logical to ask if these differences simply reflect the economic disparities which exist in the U.S., or are they just the indication of underlying biologic differences in asthma among different groups. For instance, Smith et al. (2005) used the National Health Interview Survey to examine the prevalence of childhood asthma by race and ethnicity and income, and they reported that income modified the association between race and asthma, where black children were at higher odds of asthma than white children but only among the very poor. Race, ethnicity, and poverty are important determinants of asthma morbidity and mortality. In the US, the various racial, ethnic, and poverty groups tend to be geographically segregated. Large concentrations of poverty and minority populations are disproportionately present in inner-cities. It is difficult to explore the role of race and ethnicity in the pathogenesis of asthma, since there are many confounding factors (i.e., income levels, educational status, insurance status, zone of residence). We can, however, indirectly approach the study of the phenomenon by examining what is known about asthma clinical course, risk factors, genetics, and treatment response in order to understand if there are consistent differences found.

Atopy

Atopy is a consistent risk factor for the development and severity of asthma. Allergen skin tests and total and/or specific IgE are commonly used measurements of atopy. Population surveys of allergen skin test reactivity report higher rates of skin test reactivity among minorities (Arbes et al. 2005). Looking specifically at allergens associated with asthma (cockroach, dust mite, Alternaria), black and Mexican-American children are found to have higher levels of reactivity to these specific allergens than whites (Stevenson et al. 2001). Higher levels of total IgE have also been found in black and Latina women (Lester et al. 2001; Litonjua et al. 2005). The development of atopy is a complex interaction of genetic predisposition and environmental exposures. Environmental exposures can vary greatly on a number of different factors such as urban versus rural and socioeconomic gradient. Different environmental exposure could explain these differences or they could reflect yet unknown genetic differences.

Pulmonary Function

Asthma is a lung disease. Certain lung characteristics such as lung size or airway size may predispose a group to more readily develop asthma. Racial and ethnic differences do exist for pulmonary function and bronchoreactivity. Spirometric reference standards created from healthy population samples find that even after adjusting for height, an important determinant of pulmonary function, blacks have lower FEV_1, a measure of air flow in the lung, than Latinos or whites (Hankinson et al. 1999). Further, bronchoreactivity, a measure of how easily airways will constrict and impede airflow, is increased in blacks as compared with whites (Joseph et al. 2000; Sherman et al. 1993). The reason for this increase in bronchoreactivity is unclear. Adjusting for known risk factors of bronchoreactivity, such as IgE, has explained this increase in some (Sherman et al. 1993) but not all studies (Joseph et al. 2000). The lower flow rates and increased bronchoreactivity could clinically manifest in certain groups reacting to lower levels of asthmogenic agents such as allergens or pollution. This lowered sensitivity would manifest as more asthma activity and severity.

Asthma Attacks

Lara et al. (2006) reported on 12-month parent-reported asthma attacks in the NHIS, and they found that approximately 6% of all youth had an asthma attack in the past year. About 5.7% of white youth, 7.5% of black youth, and 5.1% of Latino youth had a 12-month asthma attack. For the Latino youth, 11.8% of Puerto Ricans, 4% of Mexicans, 5.9% of Cubans, and 5.3% of Dominicans had a 12-month asthma attack. With reported morbidity and mortality consistently elevated in minorities, particularly for blacks and Puerto Ricans, it raises the question: Are asthma attacks more severe in these populations? A number of studies looking at children and adults with asthma attacks presenting to emergency rooms provide information on this question. In a large study of children presenting to the emergency room with an acute asthma attack, asthma severity at presentation, emergency room management, and post-discharge outcomes were similar for black, Latino, and white children (Boudreaux et al. 2003a). Similar findings for adults were reported by this same group (Boudreaux et al. 2003b). Another study of adults presenting with acute asthma to an emergency room found that blacks presented with lower pulmonary flow rates than whites during an acute attack (El-Ekiaby et al. 2006). For the most part, an asthma attack appears to have the same range of intensity among the various racial/ethnic groups.

Response to Therapy

Another aspect of an acute attack which could contribute to racial/ethnic group differences is the response to therapy. Do the various asthma drugs work similarly among all groups? Burchard et al. (2004) found in a study of Mexican and Puerto Rican participants with asthma from San Francisco, New York City, Puerto Rico, and Mexico City that Puerto Ricans had worse lung function and had decreased bronchodilator responsiveness to albuterol compared to Mexicans. The authors speculated that these differences could contribute to the increase in asthma morbidity and mortality reported in Puerto Ricans. Another intriguing piece of evidence is that the treatment responses to various drugs may differ among racial/ethnic groups, comes from a study which looked at T-lymphocyte response to glucocorticoids among whites and blacks with and without asthma. The T-lymphocytes from black asthmatics had significantly lower responsiveness to glucocorticoids as compared to white asthmatics (Federico et al. 2005). In contrast, a study on adults presenting with acute asthma to an emergency room found that albuterol was an equally effective bronchodilator for both blacks and whites. (El-Ekiaby et al. 2006). Two large treatment studies of inner-city children and adolescents reported that excellent control could be achieved in populations by applying guidelines-based asthma therapy with access to medications and reinforcement for adherence (Jones et al. 2007; Szefler et al. 2008).

Genetics

Our understanding of the genetics of asthma has been increasing rapidly. It is worthwhile to examine the genetic differences reported to see if asthma varies genetically among groups. One such target of intense study is the β_2-adrenergic receptor gene. Polymorphisms of this gene are associated with the diagnosis, severity, and response to treatment in non-minority populations (Raby and Weiss 2001). Ethnic variations in this particular gene have been implicated as the underlying cause of the differential bronchodilation that is seen in Puerto Ricans when compared to Mexicans (Choudry et al. 2005b) and to the diagnosis of asthma among Mexican adults (Santillan et al. 2003). Other gene-environment interactions which have been identified in whites are also found in Latinos, such as the interaction of CD14 genotypes and environmental tobacco smoke (Choudhry et al. 2005). Not all implicated asthma genes have been found to be important in minority populations. For example ADAM33, a gene suspected of playing an important role in asthma and airway remodeling, was found not to be associated with asthma in Latinos (Lind et al. 2003). Another approach taken in genetics is to characterize the ancestral background of individuals using ancestry informative markers. Surprisingly, in Mexican Americans, a higher degree of European ancestry was associated with more severe asthma, while in Puerto Ricans no association was found (Salari et al. 2005).

Asthma appears to be governed by many different genes whose expressions are modified by environmental exposure. To date, the various genes implicated in the pathogenesis of asthma do not track well with the various racial and ethnic groups. However, our understanding of the role of genetics is hindered by the lack of reproducibility and contradictory findings of many of the reports.

Asthma Diagnosis

Increased asthma prevalence has long been reported among the various racial/ethnic groups. Prevalence levels can vary greatly among minorities living in a similar environment (Ledogar et al. 2000). Do these differences reflect true differences in disease or simply the differential acquisition of a diagnosis? One approach to this problem is to look at the symptoms of asthma such as wheeze and see how individuals receive the diagnosis of asthma. Akinbami et al. (2005) found evidence that minority children might be over-diagnosed after accounting for wheeze. Differences in active wheeze were found among the various groups, but not to the same extent as the differences in asthma diagnosis. Another study of Philadelphia school children found diagnosed asthma almost twice as high in black children than white children, while the levels of chronic wheeze were equal (Cunningham et al. 1996). When the analyses were restricted to just those reporting chronic wheeze, black children continued to have higher levels of diagnosed asthma. Receiving an asthma diagnosis is related to access to health care. For example, presence of health insurance is associated with increased levels of asthma diagnoses (Freeman et al. 2003). There is no gold standard for the diagnosis of asthma, and in fact one study found that pediatricians often do not know or use national guidelines, and use a variety of clinical factors to make an asthma diagnosis (Werk et al. 2000).

Access to Care

Limited access to quality health care is problematic in poor and minority communities. Many believe that limited access to and use of quality health care contributes, in large part, to the differences in asthma morbidity and mortality among subgroups in the population. The U.S. military offers an opportunity to look at racial and ethnic differences in asthma morbidity and mortality in an environment, where access to care issues are virtually absent or at least well controlled. In the civilian section, blacks have over twice the death rate from asthma than whites. In contrary, the experience in the military finds similar mortality rates in blacks and whites (Ward 1992). Interestingly, when looking at asthma hospitalizations the rate among blacks remained elevated (Gunderson et al. 2005). The lack of difference in mortality may simply reflect the military's not allowing severe asthmatics to enlist or that residual effects of income or education are limited, since the recruits are employed and the income levels of military personnel are not drastically different enough to have effects. The differential in hospitalization may not simply reflect disease differences but behavioral differences in utilization of health care.

Studies have also demonstrated that minority children and children on Medicaid are more likely to use emergency rooms and less likely to use primary care for their ongoing asthma care, even after adjusting for symptom severity, insurance status, and having a usual source of care (Berg et al. 2004; Cohen et al. 2006; Ortega et al. 2001). These findings suggest that medication use patterns and more frequent emergency room use among this population may be related to other factors such as lack of knowledge about the preventative treatment for asthma, potential mistrust of health care providers, and/or medications, perceived convenience and accessibility of services, or specific concerns regarding daily asthma medications.

Is Asthma a Different Disease Among Minorities?

While differences are found in data from pulmonary function tests and certain risk factors such as allergen skin testing, when appropriate treatment is given to inner city asthmatics their disease responds as would be expected in non-minority populations. At this time, there is no clear evidence that asthma is biologically a different disease among the poor and minorities. Thus the differences in prevalence are due in a large part to the differential acquisition of the diagnosis rather than in differences in the disease itself (Gergen 1996). Many of the differences in the morbidity and mortality reflect the inequities within our society, namely less access to quality health care, poor environmental quality and air, and poverty. This conclusion should not dishearten but challenge us with the realization that the differential burden of asthma can be overcome.

Environmental Risk Factors

For the past couple of decades, asthma researchers have tried to understand, which risk factors contribute to higher asthma burden in minorities than whites, in order to develop interventions to reduce the disease and its impact. Epidemiological studies of asthma have largely focused on the role of the environment. Several environmental factors have been implicated in the disease, and they include ozone levels and fine particles, indoor and outdoor allergens (i.e., mold, pet dander, and grass), air contaminants, dust mites, and cockroaches among others (Bakirtas and Turktas 2006; Belanger et al. 2003; Eggleston et al. 1998; Gent et al. 2003; Leaderer et al. 2002).

Studies have also suggested that the environment may explain differences in asthma risk between ethnic and racial minorities and whites (Corburn et al. 2006). A significant proportion of blacks and Latinos, particularly those who live in inner-cities, live in communities that are poor and come from households with low-incomes. Low-income neighborhoods tend to have higher levels of poor indoor and outdoor air quality, and people from such neighborhoods are more likely to be exposed to tobacco smoke (Eggleston et al. 2005; Kattan et al. 2005; Warman et al. 2006) than people from middle or high-income neighborhoods. Housing in low-income neighborhoods are more likely to have poor ventilation and water leaks that foster high concentrations of indoor allergens and infestations of cockroaches, mites and mice (Canino et al. 2006; Rosenstreich et al. 1997).

While many researchers argue that genetic predisposition and the environment play a significant role in the epidemiology of asthma and may contribute to some of the differences in observed risk between minority and non-minority children, other factors deserve attention. In fact, it has been recommended that new community interventions consider additional individual and socio-contextual factors (Canino et al. 2006; Warman et al. 2006). For instance, there has been a growing attention to the roles of psychosocial factors (i.e., stress and violence), mental illness, and physical health co-morbidities in the epidemiology of the disease (Canino et al. 2006; Freeman et al. 2003; Hunninghake et al. 2006; Kwon et al. 2006; Ortega et al. 2004a, 2004b; Wright and Steinbach 2001; Wright et al. 2004).

Psychosocial Factors

Psychosocial factors such as parental stress and community violence have been found to be associated with asthma, in inner-city children. Wright and Steinbach (2001, 2002, 2004) have examined perceived parental stress and violence in inner-city children, and have found modest effects. Clinical studies have demonstrated that parental stress is elevated among youth with asthma and that level of parental stress is related to severity of childhood asthma and use of health services for asthma. It is unclear whether parental stress transmits stress to youth thereby increasing asthma severity, or whether more severe illness in youth leads to increased stress in parents. Wright et al. (2002) have offered the explanation that stress might change parental behaviors such as smoking or breast feeding or may impact child development through pathological processes such as reducing immune response or increasing susceptibility to lower respiratory infection (Wright et al. 2002). Wright (2006) also reviews the literature on community stress such as exposure to crime, violence, poverty, and substandard housing; she posits that violence exposure increases psychological risk which contributes to asthma morbidity.

Other psychosocial factors such as parental worry, which may be related to stress, have been associated with the over use of emergency departments for asthma care and with help seeking for asthma (Carswell et al. 1990; Wakefield et al. 1997), and this is important since minorities, particularly those without insurance or who are under-insured, tend to be high emergency room utilizers. Furthermore, family stress may affect families' knowledge about asthma treatment and perceived severity of the disease (Carswell et al. 1990).

Mental Health and Psychiatric Factors

Consistent with the research on family and community stress and asthma, there have been studies on the associations of psychiatric disorders and asthma and asthma management in minority populations (Ortega et al. 2002b). Parental stress is associated with risk for mental illness and both stress and mental illness are associated with asthma outcomes (Ortega et al. 2002b, 2003, 2004a; Richardson et al. 2006; Wright et al. 2002).

The National Cooperative Inner-City Asthma Study (NCIAS) investigated factors that contribute to asthma morbidity in inner-city children. The study found that children whose caretakers had clinically significant levels of mental health problems were hospitalized for asthma almost twice the rate as children whose caretakers did not have significant mental health problems (Weil et al. 1999). Poor parental mental health is also thought to be associated with less effective parenting styles, inappropriate use of health services, and poor adherence to medications (Bartlett et al. 2004; Weil et al. 1999). Furthermore, Bender et al. (2000) reported that family psychological adaptation is related to parental perception of control of asthma. Less functional families may have difficulty following through with treatment guidelines, which, in turn, may increase children's risk of having severe asthma. For example, Shalowitz et al. (2000) found maternal life stressors and symptoms of depression were associated with high levels of childhood asthma morbidity among children in subspecialty practices.

Asthma is not only associated with mental health problems in parents but also in youth. Associations between parental reports of asthma diagnoses and anxiety and depression were found in island Puerto Rican youth (Ortega et al. 2003). The associations persisted despite adjusting for maternal mental health problems. Island Puerto Rican youth with asthma were 40% more likely to have any psychiatric disorder, 60% more likely to have more than one psychiatric disorder, 40% more likely to have an anxiety disorder, 160% more likely to have an affective disorder, and 210% more likely to have co-morbid anxiety and depression than children without asthma (Ortega et al. 2003). Goodwin et al. (2004, 2005) have also found that asthma is related to depression and anxiety in inner-city community samples, and that psychiatric problems are associated with increased help-seeking for asthma. Most studies have found that asthma is specifically associated with internalizing disorders; this is an important observation, since at least Puerto Ricans have been shown to have higher rates of anxiety and depression than other Latino subgroups (Ortega et al. 2006).

While researchers have observed relationships between asthma and mental health concerns in a variety of settings and populations, little is known about the mechanisms underlying this relationship, even despite recent efforts to explore the prospective relationships between asthma and mental illness (Hasler et al. 2005; Feldman et al. 2006). Several suppositions have been offered. First, psychiatric symptoms (i.e., anxiety attacks) are thought to be part of the development of asthma for some individuals and may lead to exacerbations through hyperventilation (Carr 1998; Carr et al. 1994, 1996). Second, enduring the chronic stress of having asthma may lead to depression (Bender et al. 2000; Mrazek 1997). Third, asthma and mental illness share similar risk factors such as stress (Schmaling et al. 2002; Wright et al. 2002) or genetic predisposition (Slattery et al. 2002; Wamboldt et al. 2002). Fourth, maternal psychopathology may confound the relation between a child's mental health and asthma because parental perception of the child's symptoms may be distorted (Frankel and Wamboldt 1998; Richters 1992; Shalowitz 2001; Wamboldt et al. 1998; Wright et al. 2002). Fifth, some have suggested that confusion over symptoms of anxiety, such as symptoms of panic attacks and separation anxiety, and it could account for elevated rates of co-morbidity between psychiatric disorders and asthma (Davies et al. 2001; Klein 2001; Ortega et al. 2004b). And sixth, studies have found that psychiatric impairment is related to the reduced ability to manage one's (or one's child's) asthma (Bartlett et al. 2004; Bender et al. 2000; Cluley and Cochrane 2001; Weil et al. 1999). Poor asthma management may increase the odds for both morbidity and mortality (Donahue et al. 1997; Suissa et al. 2000). More research is needed to explore directional pathways underlying these associations, and how these relationships may operate in specific ethnic and sub-ethnic groups that may contribute to asthma disparities.

Obesity

Obesity is a nationwide problem, and its increasing prevalence in both adults and children make it a U.S. epidemic (Blanck et al. 2006; Ogden and Tabak 2005). Latinos and blacks are more likely to be obese or overweight than whites (Blanck et al. 2006; Ogden and Tabak 2005). Obesity and overweight are associated with asthma (Gold and Wright 2005). Obesity could impact asthma through a number of different pathways: (1) increasing systemic inflammation through adipose tissue-induced inflammation (Visser et al. 1999) or through a pro-inflammatory diet (i.e., vitamin D intake or high n-6/n-3 polyunsaturated fatty acid ratio) (Mickleborough and Rundell 2005; Troisi et al. 1995); (2) increasing the risk for co-morbid health conditions such as gastro-oesophageal reflux disease (GERD) or sleep-disordered breathing, which are associated with asthma risk (Shore 2006; Gunnbjornsdottir et al. 2004; Sulit et al. 2005); and (3) decreasing lung volume (Shore 2006). The question still remains whether the elevated risk for obesity and poor nutrition among minorities contribute to their asthma risk and helps explaining disparities in asthma.

Culture and Belief Systems

Few studies have examined the association between cultural-related factors and asthma management practices. The impact of culture on asthma morbidity is an area that necessitates further exploration, due to disparate treatment and health outcomes between individuals from racial and ethnic minority and non-Latino white backgrounds. The majority of studies including ethnic minority samples tend to focus on the association of ethnic minority status or racial background and asthma morbidity. Many of these studies conceptualize ethnic or racial background as a "cultural factor," which can be misleading given that these constructs do not represent the specific cultural values or experiences of ethnic minority individuals. In addition, much heterogeneity exists within ethnic groups and subgroups. The interaction between ethnic minority status or racial background and socioeconomic status is often difficult to disentangle, as indicated by findings from research in this area. Some studies have revealed an independent relationship between ethnic minority status and asthma morbidity, even after controlling for socioeconomic status (Lieu et al. 2002). Others indicate that socioeconomic status accounts for a large portion of the disparities in morbidity outcomes between Latino and black individuals and their white counterparts (Miller 2000). One study examined associations among multiple risk factors related to urban poverty and ethnic minority background and asthma morbidity in children, such as acculturative stress and discrimination (Koinis-Mitchell et al. 2007). Results show that multiple risks including those associated with asthma, culture and context account for more morbidity in children than one single risk factor, such as poverty or asthma severity. Since ethnic and racial minority individuals tend to be clustered in urban environments, more work is needed to examine interactions of various experiences related to context and culture that may have a bearing on morbidity for children and adults from specific ethnic groups.

Another line of research including Latino and black children and adults indicates that adherence to controller medication use has been found to be quite low, as studies have reported that, on average, daily controller medications are taken approximately 30% of the time (e.g., Ortega et al. 2002a; Rand et al. 2000; Riekert et al. 2003). Much attention has revolved around identifying the barriers to consistent asthma medication use among this population. Results from some studies widen our understanding of how culture may intersect with medication adherence and two themes appear to emerge. First, beliefs related to the nature of asthma and asthma medications seem to influence medication management practices. Second, studies have found a high use of alternative medications in this population.

An individual's health beliefs should be considered when attempting to understand potential variations in asthma management behaviors among the ethnic minority groups (Flores 2004). Studies that have examined the health beliefs and practices of black and Latino caregivers have shown that the relationships among parents' concerns about their children's medications (e.g., the dangers of dependence or long term effects), the under-use of daily, preventative asthma medications (Butz et al. 2000; Horne and Weinman 1999; Riekert et al. 2003) and lifetime history of asthma hospitalizations (Chen et al. 2003; Conn et al. 2005). These findings are consistent with those of qualitative studies including black adult patients with asthma (George and Apter 2004; George et al. 2003). In this research, the health beliefs and attitudes of adults have been proposed as partial explanations for low adherence to medical therapy and the consequent high burden of morbidity. Health beliefs that influenced adherence included patients' reliance on their assessment of asthma control over that of the health provider and concern about the adverse effects of inhaled corticosteroid therapy. In addition, many participants reported mistrust of the medical establishment. More research is needed to identify specific values and concerns by ethnic group and sub-group that may be associated with non-adherence to prescribed daily medications.

A focus on alternative medication use in ethnic minority populations with asthma has also been highlighted. The question of whether alternative medicines interfere with effective management practices has also been raised. Results indicated a high use of alternative practices (e.g., prayers, rubs and massage) in inner city, black and Latino families with children who have asthma (Braganza et al. 2003). In one study, Dominican families chose remedies derived from folk beliefs about illness and health (Bearison et al. 2002). Results from this study found that Dominican parents frequently use folk remedies instead of their child's prescription medicines (Bearison et al. 2002). Other studies comparing the use of home remedies in Latino ethnic subgroups showed that Puerto Ricans use home remedies less frequently (Ledogar et al. 2000) than other Latino subgroups, while other findings show that Mexican Americans use home remedies frequently but not in place of traditional asthma medications (Wood et al. 1993). Taken together, these results suggest that although some families believe in the biomedical model (e.g., triggers can cause symptoms), they combine this knowledge and practice with locally salient traditional beliefs and practices (e.g., the use of folk remedies). Families' cultural values and beliefs that guide effective treatment behaviors both across and within ethnic groups need to be examined in further depth to inform ethno-medical approaches to asthma care.

Some results have also suggested that aspects of acculturation may be important to consider when identifying potential cultural-related factors, that may contribute to asthma disparities. Language barriers have often been used as an index of acculturation and are associated with lower rates of medication adherence(Apter et al. 1998). In one study, Latino children and adolescents from Spanish-speaking homes had lower rates of peak flow monitoring and poorer asthma knowledge than Latino children and adolescents from English-speaking homes (Chan et al. 2005). The results suggested that language barriers appeared to contribute to poorer asthma management practices and knowledge. Future research should examine other experiences related to acculturation beyond language preference and proficiency that may impact asthma morbidity. It may be that clashes between the value systems of patients and health care providers may have a bearing on management behaviors and subsequently the connection that is developed with providers and the health care center.

Interventions

Logically, narrowly focused interventions focusing on one or two elements of asthma treatment would have less probability of success for families from minority demographic profiles (e.g., versus encouraging consistent medication use, symptom monitoring and trigger control in the context of other stresses families face). For example, a nebulizer-education intervention among children with persistent asthma had no impact on asthma severity or health care use (Butz et al. 2006). Many of the "non-traditional" risk factors do not directly have an impact on the disease but distract the patient and family from paying attention to the disease, such as problems with housing or transportation. Therefore, interventions need to be broad-based. The National Cooperative Inner City Asthma Study (NCICAS) asthma intervention used an asthma counselor (AC) trained in asthma management. The AC usually had a background in social work. The AC worked with the families to better manage their asthma and to deal with other ongoing stresses, which reduced their abilities to focus on their asthma care. This intervention resulted in a reduced number of symptoms, days, and unscheduled health care use, which continued after the intervention ended (Evans et al. 1999). Another successful approach attempted to reduce the allergen burden within inner-city homes. This comprehensive environmental intervention clearly showed that the lower allergen levels were possible in the inner-city and this decrease significantly impacted disease activity (Morgan et al. 2004). These interventions were found to be cost effective (Sullivan et al. 2002; Kattan et al. 2005). An emergency room-based intervention where children and families received a single follow-up clinic visit and self-monitoring, environmental management, and trigger control reduced subsequent unscheduled health care use. (Teach et al. 2006). Interventions can be successful among poor and minority populations. The characteristics of successful interventions are their broad based nature and the involvement of the community.

Resilience in Minority Families: Processes Associated with Optimal Asthma Outcomes

A preponderance of evidence shows how ethnic and racial minority individuals with asthma experience more asthma burden relative to their white counterparts. There is a need for research to identify characteristics of individuals from this demographic profile who are functioning well, despite having asthma and facing other stresses related to the environment and ethnic minority background (Koinis-Mitchell et al. 2004). Many ethnic minority families do cope well in spite of their potential exposure to urban poverty, family stresses, and stresses associated with the complexity of asthma management. However, there is a dearth of research that examines which factors help to guard against adverse asthma outcomes. It should be noted that within the resilience literature, there is an important distinction between simply labeling a process as "protective" and actually demonstrating its moderating effect on an outcome in the face of specific stresses through statistical analyzes. In this regard, the pediatric asthma research has lagged far behind the wider child developmental research, which has employed rigorous methodologies when attempting to identify risk and protective factors associated with resilient developmental outcomes in ethnic and racial minority children (e.g., Koinis-Mitchell et al. 2005; Luthar et al. 2000).

Although this research is sparse, there are some pediatric asthma studies that have focused on identifying protective factors with ethnic minority, inner-city children. The studies have identified characteristics of black and Latino children, their families, and their wider social environment that may buffer their exposure to stresses related to urban living or asthma status, to optimize asthma outcomes (Koinis-Mitchell et al. 2005; Koinis-Mitchell and Murdock 2005; Koinis Mitchell 2004). For example, Koinis-Mitchell et al. (2004) findings showed that higher levels of adaptability (e.g., a more flexible temperament) and perceived control at baseline were related to more optimal asthma management strategies in a sample of urban children one year later, despite the presence of neighborhood disadvantage and asthma symptoms. Ongoing studies by these researchers employ both quantitative and ethnographic approaches to characterize resilient asthma outcomes, and to identify protective family values, beliefs, and practices associated with specific asthma management behaviors in non-Latino black, Dominican, and Puerto Rican families. Other research has shown that aspects of the health care system may be important to consider when attempting to identify potential moderating processes associated with more effective asthma control (Ortega et al. 2002a). It may be that the relationship between the physician and patient is paramount to enhance consistency with asthma-related visits and preventative care. More work demonstrating such protective effects is needed.

An interesting area that also warrants further exploration involves potential protective processes associated with differences in how Latino ethnic subgroups fare in terms of asthma outcomes in the US. Evidence has shown that among Latino ethnic subgroups, Mexican American's have the lowest prevalence of asthma and asthma morbidity in the United States, while Puerto Rican children bear a disproportionate amount of asthma burden (Homa et al. 2000; Lara et al. 2006). Yet, it is unclear what the mechanisms are that account for differences in Latino subgroup outcomes, as they cannot be explained solely by socio-demographic factors. As this review and others (e.g., Canino et al. 2006) indicate, evidence points to a complex interaction between various factors associated with one's genetic makeup, the environment, the health care system, one's psychological functioning and perceptions, and experiences of stress, social experiences (i.e., migration, discrimination, acculturation), and cultural belief systems and practices, that may all contribute to variations in asthma outcomes among Latino ethnic subgroups and blacks.

One recent study examined the relationship between country of birth and acculturation with asthma among a large group of Mexican American youth (using data from the National Health and Nutrition Examination Survey 1999–2002) (Eldeirawi and Persky 2006.). This study found that Mexican American adolescents born in the US and those with high acculturation levels reported significantly higher prevalence rates of asthma and wheezing than their peers with low acculturation levels born in Mexico. Both acculturation and country of birth were linked with the risk of asthma, with acculturation having stronger effects than country of birth. More research is needed to examine how asthma prevalence and morbidity rates among Latino ethnic subgroups may be impacted by migration patterns, acculturation levels, stresses related to acculturation, and the amount of time spent in the US. In addition, moderating processes that may buffer the exposure to stressors related to acculturation and risk for asthma morbidity need to be identified for specific ethnic groups.

Additional work identifying modifiable factors associated with optimal functioning in specific ethnic groups with asthma is needed. Many questions remain unanswered. It is not clear to what extent specific aspects of the health care system, family environment, or community may protect children from different ethnic groups from experiencing asthma morbidity. What is considered a resilient asthma-related outcome for each individual may differ depending upon the level of stresses faced, the duration of the exposure to specific stresses, and the individual's previous level of functioning. In addition, it may be the specific processes such as those associated with the family (e.g., praying, kinship networks) or community (e.g., social support networks, asthma education programs) serve more of a protective function for some families than others, but these processes have not yet been investigated. Future work exploring these questions and identifying the strengths of ethnic minority individuals with asthma would certainly offset the "deficit" emphasis that is commonly illustrated by results from research including this population. Further development of methodologies that capture the cultural uniqueness and hardiness of individuals from specific ethnic groups and subgroups is needed.

Conclusion

Our knowledge and understanding of asthma has increased greatly in the last two decades. This knowledge has changed the way we approach asthma. It was simply believed that asthma affects people due to episodic constrictions of airway smooth muscles. Thus, treatment was focused on episodic use of quick relievers to lessen this constriction. Asthma is now thought to result from a chronic inflammatory process in the lung. Treatments today focus on reducing this inflammation with controller medications such as inhaling steroids. In addition, much work is focused on changing the natural history of asthma by attempting to identify periods during a person's life when addition or removal of certain environmental factors can decrease the risk of developing asthma.

Despite this increase in knowledge, the disparity in asthma morbidity and mortality between whites and minorities remains, and the gap has not significantly decreased in the last decade. To close this continuing disparity among subgroups in the population will require studies specifically addressing these differences, as it appears simply increasing our overall knowledge of asthma will not close these gaps.

Future asthma research, especially in minority populations, must move beyond the traditional biomedical model of agent-disease-host. Research should also explore community, family, individual, psychosocial, and cultural factors and their impact on asthma and asthma management and control. Even if these factors do not change the basic pathophysiology of asthma, if not considered, they do make effective implementation of interventions difficult if not impossible. Identification of risk factors is not enough. Effective, *translatable*, self-sustaining interventions must be developed to change asthma burden in minority populations. Our review points out several interesting areas for further inquiry. More work is needed to determine if asthma is the same disease among ethnic groups in the area of genetics and differential responses to asthma medications. Research and policy on asthma in minority communities needs to focus not only on the reduction of environmental risk factors, but also implement innovative methods and policies to deliver high quality asthma health care, and create a better understanding of cultural values and beliefs around asthma and asthma care among blacks and Latino ethnic subgroups, particularly for Puerto Ricans. And finally, it must never be forgotten that asthma is a disease managed in large part by families at home. Programs must be developed and applied to empower asthmatics and their families to assume a leadership position in the management of the disease.

References

Akinbami LJ, Rhodes JC, Lara M (2005) Racial and ethnic differences in asthma diagnosis among children who wheeze. Pediatrics 115(5):1254–1260

Apter AJ, Reisine ST, Affleck G, Barrows E, ZuWallack RL (1998) Adherence with twice-daily dosing of inhaled steroids. Socioeconomic and health-belief differences. Am J Respir Crit Care Med 157(Pt 1):1810–1817

Arbes SJ, Gergen PJ, Elliott L, Zeldin DC (2005) Prevalences of positive skin test responses to 10 common allergens in the US population: results of the third National Health and

Nutrition Examination Survey. J Allergy Clin Immunol 116(2):377–383

Bakirtas A, Turktas I (2006) Determinants of airway responsiveness to adenosine 5′-monophosphate in school-age children with asthma. Pediatr Pulmonol 41(6):515–521

Bartlett SJ, Krishnan JA, Riekert KA, Butz AM, Malveaux FJ, Rand CS (2004) Maternal depressive symptoms and adherence to therapy in inner-city children with asthma. Pediatrics 113(2):229–237

Bearison DJ, Minian N, Granowetter L (2002) Medical management of asthma and folk medicine in a Hispanic community. J Pediatr Psychol 27(4):385–392

Belanger K, Beckett W, Triche E, Bracken MB, Holford T, Ren P, McSharry JE, Gold DR, Platts-Mills TA, Leaderer BP (2003) Symptoms of wheeze and persistent cough in the first year of life: associations with indoor allergens, air contaminants, and maternal history of asthma. Am J Epidemiol 158(3):195–202

Bender BG, Annett RD, Ikle D, DuHamel TR, Rand C, Strunk RC (2000) Relationship between disease and psychological adaptation in children in the Childhood Asthma Management Program and their Families. CAMP Research Group. Arch Pediatr Adolesc Med 154(7):706–713

Berg J, Wahlgren DR, Hofstetter R, Meltzer SB, Meltzer EO, Matt GE, Martinez-Donate A, Hovell MF (2004) Latino children with asthma: rates and risks for medical care utilization. J Asthma 41(2):147–157

Blanck HM, Dietz WH, Galuska DA, Gillespie C, Hamre R, Kettel Khan L, Serdula MK, Ford ES, Garvin WS, Mokdad AH, Densmore D (2006) State-specific prevalence of obesity among adults – United States, 2005. Morb Mortal Wkly Rep 55(36):985–988

Boudreaux ED, Emond SD, Clark S, Camargo CA Jr (2003a) Race/ethnicity and asthma among children presenting to the emergency department: differences in disease severity and management. Pediatrics 111(5 Pt 1):e615–e621

Boudreaux ED, Emond SD, Clark S, Camargo CA Jr (2003b) Acute asthma among adults presenting to the emergency department: the role of race/ethnicity and socioeconomic status. Chest 124(3):803–812

Braganza S, Ozuah PO, Sharif I (2003) The use of complementary therapies in inner-city asthmatic children. J Asthma 40(7):823–827

Burchard EG, Avila PC, Nazario S, Casal J, Torres A, Rodriguez-Santana JR, Toscano M, Sylvia JS, Alioto M, Salazar M, Gomez I, Fagan JK, Salas J, Lilly C, Matallana H, Ziv E, Castro R, Selman M, Chapela R, Sheppard D, Weiss ST, Ford JG, Boushey HA, Rodriguez-Cintron W, Drazen JM, Silverman EK (2004) Lower bronchodilator responsiveness in Puerto Rican than in Mexican subjects with asthma. Am J Respir Crit Care Med 169(3):386–392

Butz AM, Eggleston P, Huss K, Kolodner K, Rand C (2000) Nebulizer use in inner-city children with asthma: morbidity, medication use, and asthma management practices. Arch Pediatr Adolesc Med 154(10):984–990

Butz AM, Tsoukleris MG, Donithan M, Hsu VD, Zuckerman I, Mudd KE, Thompson RE, Rand C, Bollinger ME (2006) Effectiveness of nebulizer use-targeted asthma education on underserved children with asthma. Arch Pediatr Adolesc Med 160(6):622–628

Canino G, Koines-Mitchell D, Ortega AN, McQuaid EL, Fritz GK, Alegria M (2006) Asthma disparities in the prevalence, morbidity, and treatment of Latino children. Soc Sci Med 63(11):2926–2937

Carr RE (1998) Panic disorder and asthma: causes, effects and research implications. J Psychosom Res 44(1):43–52

Carr RE, Lehrer PM, Hochron SM, Jackson A (1996) Effect of psychological stress on airway impedance in individuals with asthma and panic disorder. J Abnorm Psychol 105(1):137–141

Carr RE, Lehrer PM, Rausch LL, Hochron SM (1994) Anxiety sensitivity and panic attacks in an asthmatic population. Behav Res Ther 32(4):411–418

Carswell F, Heck G, Robinson E, Hallows D, Peters T, Stanton T (1990) Family stress and childhood asthma. Nurs Pract 3(3):10–15

Carter-Pokras OD, Gergen PJ (1993) Reported asthma among Puerto Rican, Mexican-American, and Cuban children. Am J Public Health 83(4):580–582

Chan KS, Keeler E, Schonlau M, Rosen M, Mangione-Smith R (2005) How do ethnicity and primary language spoken at home affect management practices and outcome in children and adolescents with asthma? Arch Pediatr Adolesc Med 159(3):283–289

Chen E, Bloomberg GR, Fisher EGJ, Strunk RC (2003) Predictors of repeat hospitalizations in children with asthma: the role of psychosocial and socioenvironmental factors. Health Psychol 22(1):12–18

Choudhry S, Avila PC, Nazario S, Ung N, Kho J, Rodriguez-Santana JR, Casal J, Tsai HJ, Torres A, Ziv E, Toscano M, Sylvia JS, Alioto M, Salazar M, Gomez I, Fagan JK, Salas J, Lilly C, Matallana H, Castro RA, Selman M, Weiss ST, Ford JG, Drazen JM, Rodriguez-Cintron W, Chapela R, Silverman EK, Burchard EG (2005) CD14 tobacco gene-environment interaction modifies asthma severity and immunoglobulin E levels in Latinos with asthma. Am J Respir Crit Care Med 172(2):173–182

Choudhry S, Ung N, Avila PC et al. (2005) Pharmacogenetic differences in response to atbuterol between Puerto Ricans and Mexicans with asthma. Am J Respir Crit Care Med 171(6):563–570

Cluley S, Cochrane GM (2001) Psychological disorder in asthma is associated with poor control and poor adherence to inhaled steroids. Respir Med 95(1):37–39

Cohen RT, Celedon JC, Hinckson VJ, Ramsey CD, Wakefield DB, Weiss ST, Cloutier MM (2006) Health-care use among Puerto Rican and African-American children with asthma. Chest 130(2):463–471

Conn KM, Halterman JS, Fisher SG, Yoos HL, Chin NP, Szilagyi PG (2005) Parental beliefs about medications and medication adherence among urban children with asthma. Ambul Pediatr 5(5):306–310

Corburn J, Osleeb J, Porter M (2006) Urban asthma and the neighbourhood environment in New York City. Health Place 12(2):167–179

Cunningham J, Dockery DW, Speizer FE (1996) Race, asthma, and persistent wheeze in Philadelphia school children. Am J Public Health 86(10):1406–1409

Davies SJ, Jackson PR, Ramsay LE (2001) Dysfunctional breathing and asthma: panic disorder needs to be considered. Br Med J 323(7313):631

Donahue JG, Weiss ST, Livingston JM, Goetsch MA, Greineder DK, Platt R (1997) Inhaled steroids and the risk of hospitalization for asthma. J Am Med Assoc 277(11):887–891
Eggleston PA, Butz A, Rand C, Curtin-Brosnan J, Kanchanaraksa S, Swartz L, Breysse P, Buckley T, Diette G, Merriman B, Krishnan JA (2005) Home environmental intervention in inner-city asthma: a randomized controlled clinical trial. Ann Allergy Asthma Immunol 95(6):518–524
Eggleston PA, Rosenstreich D, Lynn H, Gergen P, Baker D, Kattan M, Mortimer KM, Mitchell H, Ownby D, Slavin R, Malveaux F (1998) Relationship of indoor allergen exposure to skin test sensitivity in inner-city children with asthma. J Allergy Clin Immunol 102(4 Pt 1):563–570
El-Ekiaby A, Brianas L, Skowronski ME, Coreno AJ, Galan G, Kaeberlein FJ, Seitz RE, Villaba KD, Dickey-White D, McFadden ER Jr (2006) Impact of race on the severity of acute episodes of asthma and adrenergic responsiveness. Am J Respir Crit Care Med 174(5):508–513
Eldeirawi KM, Persky VW (2006) Associations of acculturation and country of birth with asthma and wheezing in Mexican American youths. J Asthma 43(4):279–286
Evans R 3rd, Gergen PJ, Mitchell H, Kattan M, Kerscmar C, Crain E, Anderson J, Eggleston P, Malveaux FJ, Wedner HJ (1999) A randomized clinical trial to reduce asthma morbidity among inner-city children: results of the National Cooperative Inner-City Asthma Study. J Pediatr 135(3):332–338
Federico MJ, Covar RA, Brown EE, Leung DYM, Spahn JD (2005) Racial differences in T-lymphocyte response to glucocorticoids. Chest 127(2):571–578
Feldman JM, Ortega AN, McQuaid EL, Canino G (2006) Comorbidity betweenasthma attacks and internalizing disorders among Puerto Rican children at one-year follow-up. Psychosomatics 47(4):333–339
Flores G (2004) Culture, ethnicity, and linguistic issues in pediatric care: urgent priorities and unanswered questions. Ambul Pediatr 4(4):276–282
Frankel K, Wamboldt MZ (1998) Chronic childhood illness and maternal mental health – why should we care? J Asthma 35(8):621–630
Freeman NC, Schneider D, McGarvey P (2003) The relationship of health insurance to the diagnosis and management of asthma and respiratory problems in children in a predominately Hispanic urban community. Am J Public Health 93:1316–1320
Gent JF, Triche EW, Holford TR, Belanger K, Bracken MB, Beckett WS, Leaderer BP (2003) Association of low-level ozone and fine particles with respiratory symptoms in children with asthma. J Am Med Assoc 290(14):1859–1867
George M, Apter AJ (2004) Gaining insight into patients' beliefs using qualitative research methodologies. Curr Opin Allergy Clin Immunol 4(3):185–189
George M, Freedman TG, Norfleet AL, Feldman HI, Apter AJ (2003) Qualitative research-enhanced understanding of patients' beliefs: results of focus groups with low-income, urban, African American adults with asthma. J Allergy Clin Immunol 111(5):967–973
Gergen P (1996) Social class and asthma – distinguishing between the disease and the diagnosis. Am J Public Health 86(10):1361–1362
Gold DR, Wright R (2005) Population disparities in asthma. Annu Rev Public Health 26:89–113
Goodwin RD, Fergusson DM, Horwood LJ (2004) Asthma and depressive and anxiety disorders among young persons in the community. Psychol Med 34(8):1465–1474
Goodwin RD, Messineo K, Bregante A, Hoven CW, Kairam R (2005) Prevalence of probable mental disorders among pediatric asthma patients in an inner-city clinic. J Asthma 42(8):643–647
Gunderson EKE, Garland CF, Gorham ED (2005) Health surveillance for asthma in the US Navy: experience of 9, 185, 484 person-years. Ann Epidemiol 15(4):310–315
Gunnbjornsdottir MI, Omenaas E, Gislason T, Norman E, Olin AC, Jogi R, Jensen EJ, Lindberg E, Bjornsson E, Franklin K, Janson C, Gulsvik A, Laerum B, Svanes C, Toren K, Tunsater A, Lillienberg L, Gislason D, Blondal T, Bjornsdottir US, Jorundsdottir KB, Talvik R, Forsberg B, Franklin K, Lundback B, Soderberg M, Ledin MC, Boman G, Norback D, Wieslander G, Spetz-Nystrom U, Cashelunge KS, Ryden E (2004) Obesity and nocturnal gastro-oesophageal reflux are related to onset of asthma and respiratory symptoms. Eur Respir J 24(1):116–121
Hankinson JL, Odencrantz JR, Fedan KB (1999) Spirometric reference values from a sample of the general U.S. population. Am J Respir Crit Care Med 159(1):179–187
Hasler G, Gergen PJ, Kleinbaum DG, Ajdacic V, Gamma A, Eich D, Rossler W, Angst J (2005) Asthma and panic in young adults: a 20-year prospective community study. Am J Respir Crit Care Med 171(11):1224–1230
Homa D, Mannino D, Lara M (2000) Asthma mortality in U.S. Hispanics of Mexican, Puerto Rican, and Cuban heritage, 1990–1995. Am J Respir Crit Care Med 161(2 Pt 1):504–509
Horne R, Weinman J (1999) Patients' beliefs about prescribed medicines and their role in adherence to treatment in chronic physical illness. J Psychosom Res 47(6):555–567
Hunninghake GM, Weiss ST, Celedon JC (2006) Asthma in Hispanics. Am J Respir Crit Care Med 173(2):143–163
Jones CA, Clement LT, Morphew T, Kwong KYC, Hanley-Lopez J, Lifson F, Opas L, Guterman JJ (2007) Achieving and maintaining asthma control in an urban pediatric disease management program: the Breathmobile Program. J Allergy Clin Immunol 119(6):1445–1453
Joseph CLM, Ownby DR, Peterson EL, Johnson CC (2000) Racial differences in physiologic parameters related to asthma among middle-class children. Chest 117(5):1336–1344
Kattan M, Stearns SC, Crain EF, Stout JW, Gergen PJ, Evans R 3rd, Visness CM, Gruchalla RS, Morgan WJ, O'Connor GT, Mastin JP, Mitchell HE (2005) Cost-effectiveness of a home-based environmental intervention for inner-city children with asthma. J Allergy Clin Immunol 116(5):1058–1063
Klein DF (2001) Asthma and psychiatric illness. J Am Med Assoc 285(7):881–882
Koinis-Mitchell D, Adams SK, Murdock KK (2005) Associations among risk factors, individual resources, and indices of school-related asthma morbidity in urban, school-aged children: a pilot study. J Sch Health 75(10):375–383
Koinis-Mitchell D, Murdock KK (2005) Identifying risk and resource factors in children with asthma from urban settings: the context-health-development model. J Asthma 42(6): 425–436
Koinis-Mitchell D, Murdock KK, McQuaid EL (2004) Risk and resilience in urban children with asthma. Child Health Care 33:275–298

Koinis-Mitchell D, McQuaid EL, Seifer R, Kopel SJ, Esteban C, Canino G, Garcia-Coll C, Klein R, Fritz GK (2007) Multiple urban and asthma-related risks and their association with asthma morbidity in children. J Pediatr Psychol 32(5): 582–595

Kwon HL, Ortiz B, Swaner R, Shoemaker K, Jean-Louis B, Northridge ME, Vaughan RD, Marx T, Goodman A, Borrell LN, Nicholas SW (2006) Childhood asthma and extreme values of body mass index: the Harlem children's zone asthma initiative. J Urban Health 83(3):421–433

Lara M, Akinbami L, Flores G, Morgenstern H (2006) Heterogeneity of childhood asthma among Hispanic children: Puerto Rican children bear a disproportionate burden. Pediatrics 117(1):43–53

Leaderer BP, Belanger K, Triche E, Holford T, Gold DR, Kim Y, Jankun T, Ren P, McSharry Je JE, Platts-Mills TA, Chapman MD, Bracken MB (2002) Dust mite, cockroach, cat, and dog allergen concentrations in homes of asthmatic children in the northeastern United States: impact of socioeconomic factors and population density. Environ Health Perspect 110(4):419–425

Ledogar R, Penchascadeh A, Iglesias Garden C, Acosta L (2000) Asthma and Latino cultures: different prevalence reported among groups sharing the same environment. Am J Public Health 90(6):929–935

Lester LA, Rick SS, Blumenthal MN, Togias A, Murphy S, Malveaux F, Miller ME, Dunston GM, Solway J, Wolf RL, Samet JM, Marsh DG, Meyers DA, Ober C, Bleecker ER (2001) Ethnic differences in asthma and associated phenotypes: collaborative study on the genetics of asthma. J Allergy Clin Immunol 108(3):357–362

Lieu TA, Lozano P, Finkelstein JA, Chi FW, Jensvold NG, Capra AM, Quesenberry CP, Selby JV, Farber HJ (2002) Racial/ethnic variation in asthma status and management practices among children in managed Medicaid. Pediatrics 109(5):857–865

Lind DL, Choudhry S, Ung N, Ziv E, Avila PC, Salari K, Ha C, Lovins EG, Coyle NE, Nazario S, Casal J, Torres A, Rodriguez-Santana JR, Matallana H, Lilly CM, Salas J, Selman M, Boushey HA, Weiss ST, Chapela R, Ford JG, Rodriguez-Cintron W, Silverman EK, Sheppard D, Kwok PY, Gonzalez Burchard E (2003) ADAM33 is not associated with asthma in Puerto Rican or Mexican populations. Am J Respir Crit Care Med 168(11):1312–1316

Litonjua AA, Celedon JC, Hausmann J, Nikolov M, Sredl D, Ryan L, Platts-Mills TA, Weiss ST, Gold DR (2005) Variation in total and specific IgE: effects of ethnicity and socioeconomic status. J Allergy Clin Immunol 115(4):751–757

Luthar SS, Cicchetti D, Becker B (2000) The construct of resilience: a critical evaluation and guidelines for future work. Child Dev 71(3):543–562

Mannino DM, Homa DM, Akinbami LJ, Moorman JE, Gwynn C, Redd SC (2002) Surveillance for asthma – United States, 1980–1999. Morb Mortal Wkly Rep 51(SS01):1–13

Mannnino DM, Homa DM, Pertowski CA, Ashizawa A, Nixon LL, Johnson CA, Ball LB, Jack E, Kang DS (1998) Surveillance for asthma – United States, 1960–1995. In *CDC Surveillance Summaries,* April 24, 1998. Morb Mortal Wkly Rep 47(No. SS-1):1–27

Mickleborough TD, Rundell KW (2005) Dietary polyunsaturated fatty acids in asthma-and exercise-induced bronchoconstriction. Eur J Clin Nutr 59(12):1335–1346

Miller JE (2000) The effects of race/ethnicity and income on early childhood asthma prevalence and health care use. Am J Public Health 90(3):428–430

Morgan WJ, Crain EF, Gruchalla RS, O'Connor GT, Kattan M, Evans R 3rd, Stout J, Malindzak G, Smartt E, Plaut M, Walter M, Vaughn B, Mitchell H (2004) Results of a home-based environmental intervention among urban children with asthma. N Eng J Med 351(11):1068–1080

Mrazek DA (1997) Psychological aspects in children and adolescents. In: Barnes PJ, Grunstein MM, Leff AR, Woolcock AJ (eds) Asthma. Lippincott-Raven, Philadelphia, pp 2177–2183

Ogden CL, Tabak CJ (2005) Children and teens told by doctors that they were overweight. Morb Mortal Wkly Rep 54(34):848–849

Ortega AN, Belanger KD, Paltiel AD, Horwitz SM, Bracken MB, Leaderer BP (2001) Use of health services by insurance status among children with asthma. Med Care 39(10): 1065–1074

Ortega AN, Calderon JG (2000) Pediatric asthma among minority populations. Curr Opin Pediatr 12(6):579–583

Ortega AN, Feldman JM, Canino G, Steinman K, Alegria M (2006) Co-occurrence of mental and physical illness in US Latinos. Soc Psychiatry Psychiatr Epidemiol 41(12):927–934

Ortega AN, Gergen PJ, Paltiel AD, Bauchner H, Belanger KD, Leaderer BP (2002a) Impact of site care, race, and Hispanic ethnicity on medication use for childhood asthma. Pediatrics 109(1):E1

Ortega AN, Goodwin RD, McQuaid EL, Canino G (2004a) Parental mental health, childhood psychiatric disorders, and asthma attacks in island Puerto Rican youth. Ambul Pediatr 4(4):308–315

Ortega AN, Huertas SE, Canino G, Ramirez R, Rubio-Stipec M (2002b) Childhood asthma, chronic illness, and psychiatric disorders. J Nerv Ment Dis 190(5):275–281

Ortega AN, McQuaid EL, Canino G, Goodwin RD, Fritz GK (2004b) Comorbidity of asthma and anxiety and depression in Puerto Rican children. Psychosomatics 45(2):93–99

Ortega AN, McQuaid EL, Canino G, Ramirez R, Fritz GK, Klein RB (2003) Association of psychiatric disorders and different indicators of asthma in island Puerto Rican children. Soc Psychiatry Psychiatr Epidemiol 38(4):220–226

Perez-Perdomo R, Perez-Cardona C, Disdier-Flores O, Cintron Y (2003) Prevalence and correlates of asthma in the Puerto Rican population: behavioral risk factor surveillance system, 2000. J Asthma 40(5):465–474

Raby BA, Weiss ST (2001) Beta2-adrenergic receptor genetics. Curr Opin Mol Ther 3(6):554–566

Rand CS, Butz AM, Kolodner K, Huss K, Eggleston P, Malveaux F (2000) Emergency department visits by urban African American children with asthma. J Allergy Clin Immunol 105(1 Pt 1):83–90

Rhodes L, Moorman JE, Mannino DM (2003) Self-reported asthma prevalence and control among adults – United States, 2001. Morb Mortal Wkly Rep 52(17):381–384

Richardson LP, Lozano P, Russo J, McCauley E, Bush T, Katon W (2006) Asthma symptom burden: relationship to asthma severity and anxiety and depression symptoms. Pediatrics 118(3):1042–1051

Richters JE (1992) Depressed mothers as informants about their children: a critical review of the evidence of distortion. Psychol Bull 112(3):485–499

Riekert KA, Butz AM, Eggleston PA, Huss K, Winkelstein M, Rand CS (2003) Caregiver-physician medication concordance and undertreatment of asthma among inner-city children. Pediatrics 111(3):e214–e220

Rose D, Mannino DM, Leaderer BP (2006) Asthma prevalence among US adults, 1998–2000: role of Puerto Rican ethnicity and behavioral and geographic factors. Am J Public Health 96(5):880–888

Rosenstreich DL, Eggleston P, Kattan M, Baker D, Slavin RG, Gergen P, Mitchell H, McNiff-Mortimer K, Lynn H, Ownby D, Malveaux F (1997) The role of cockroach allergy and exposure to cockroach allergen in causing morbidity among inner-city children with asthma. N Eng J Med 336(19): 1356–1363

Salari K, Choudhry S, Tang H, Naqvi M, Lind D, Avila PC, Coyle NE, Ung N, Nazario S, Casal J, Torres-Palacios A, Clark S, Phong A, Gomez I, Matallana H, Perez-Stable EJ, Shriver MD, Kwok PY, Sheppard D, Rodriguez-Cintron W, Risch NJ, Burchard EG, Ziv E (2005) Genetic admixture and asthma-related phenotypes in Mexican American and Puerto Rican asthmatics. Genet Epidemiol 29(1):76–86

Santillan AA, Camargo CA Jr, Ramirez-Rivera A, Delgado-Enciso I, Rojas-Martinez A, Cantu-Diaz F, Barrera-Saldana HA (2003) Association between β_2-adrenoceptor polymorphisms and asthma diagnosis among Mexican adults. J Allergy Clin Immunol 112(6):1095–1100

Schmaling KB, McKnight PE, Afari N (2002) A prospective study of the relationship of mood and stress to pulmonary function among patients with asthma. J Asthma 39(6):501–510

Shalowitz MU, Berry CA, Quinn KA, Wolf RL (2001) The relationship of life stressors and maternal depression to pediatric asthma morbidity in a subspecialty practice. Ambul Pediatr 1(4):185–193

Shapiro GG, Stout JW (2002) Childhood asthma in the United States: urban issues. Pediatr Pulmonol 33(1):47–55

Sherman CB, Tollerud DJ, Heffner LJ, Speizer FE, Weiss ST (1993) Airway Responsiveness in young black and white women. Am Rev Respir Dis 148(1):98–102

Shore SA (2006) Obesity and asthma: cause for concern. Curr Opin Pharmacol 6(3):230–236

Slattery MJ, Klein DF, Mannuzza S, Moulton JL 3rd, Pine DS, Klein RG (2002) Relationship between separation anxiety disorder, parental panic disorder, and atopic disorders in children: a controlled high-risk study. J Am Acad Child Adolesc Psychiatry 41(8):947–954

Smith LA, Hatcher-Ross JL, Wertheimer R, Kahn RS (2005) Rethinking race/ethnicity, income, and childhood asthma: racial/ethnic disparities concentrated among the very poor. Public Health Rep 120(2):109–116

Stevenson LA, Gergen PJ, Hoover DR, Rosenstreich D, Mannino DM, Matte TD (2001) Sociodemographic correlates of indoor allergen sensitivity among United States children. J Allergy Clin Immunol 108(5):747–752

Suissa S, Ernst P, Benayoun S, Baltzan M, Cai B (2000) Low-dose inhaled corticosteroids and the prevention of death from asthma. N Eng J Med 343(5):332–336

Sullivan SD, Weiss KB, Lynn H, Mitchell H, Kattan M, Gergen PJ, Evans R (2002) The cost-effectiveness of an inner-city asthma intervention for children. J Allergy Clin Immunol 110(4):576–581

Sulit LG, Storfer-Isser A, Rosen CL, Kirchner HL, Redline S (2005) Associations of obesity, sleep-disordered breathing, and wheezing in children. Am J Respir Crit Care Med 171(6):659–664

Szefler SJ, Mitchell H, Sorkness CA, Gergen PJ, O'Connor GT, Morgan WJ, Kattan M, Pongracic JA, Teach SJ, Bloomberg GR, Eggleston PA, Gruchalla RS, Kercsmar CM, Liu AH, Wildfire JJ, Curry MD, Busse WW (2008) Management of asthma based on exhaled nitric oxid in addition to guideline-based treatment for inner-city adolescents and young adults: a randomized controlled trial. Lancet 372(9643):1065–1072

Teach SJ, Crain EF, Quint DM, Hylan ML, Joseph JG (2006) Improved asthma outcomes in a high-morbidity pediatric population. Arch Pediatr Adolesc Med 160(5):535–541

Troisi RJ, Willett WC, Weiss ST, Trichopoulos D, Rosner B, Speizer FE (1995) A prospective-study of diet and adult-onset asthma. Am J Respir Crit Care Med 151(5):1401–1408

Visser M, Bouter LM, McQuillan GM, Wener MH, Harris TB (1999) Elevated C-reactive protein levels in overweight and obese adults. J Am Med Assoc 282(22):2131–2135

Wakefield M, Staugas R, Ruffin R, Campbell D, Beilby J, McCaul K (1997) Risk factors for repeat attendance at hospital emergency departments among adults and children with asthma. Aust NZ J Med 27(3):277–284

Wamboldt FS, Price MR, Hume LA, Gavin LA, Wamboldt MZ, Klinnert MD (2002) Reliability and validity of a system for coding asthma outcomes from medical records. J Asthma 39(4):29–305

Wamboldt MZ, Fritz G, Mansell A, McQuaid EL, Klein RB (1998) Relationship of asthma severity and psychological problems in children. J Am Acad Child Adolesc Psychiatry 37:943–950

Ward DL (1992) An international comparison of asthma morbidity and mortality in US soldiers 1984 to 1988. Chest 101:613–620

Warman K, Silver EJ, Wood PR (2006) Asthma risk factor assessment: what are the needs of inner-city families? Ann Allergy Asthma Immunol 97(1 Suppl):S11–S15

Weil CM, Wade SL, Bauman LJ, Lynn H, Mitchell H, Lavigne J (1999) The relationship between psychosocial factors andasthma morbidity in inner-city children with asthma. Pediatrics 104(6):1274–1280

Werk LN, Steinbach S, Adams WG, Bauchner H (2000) Beliefs about diagnosing asthma in young children. Pediatrics 105(3 Pt 1):585–590

Wood PR, Hidalgo HA, Prihoda TJ, Kromer ME (1993) Hispanic children with asthma: morbidity. Pediatrics 91(1):62–69

Wright RJ (2006) Health effects of socially toxic neighborhoods: the violence and urban asthma paradigm. Clin Chest Med 27(3):413–421

Wright RJ, Cohen S, Carey V, Weiss ST, Gold DR (2002) Parental stress as a predictor of wheezing in infancy: a prospective birth-cohort study. Am J Respir Crit Care Med 165(3):358–365

Wright RJ, Mitchell H, Visness CM, Cohen S, Stout J, Evans R, Gold DR (2004) Community violence and asthma morbidity: the Inner-City Asthma Study. Am J Public Health 94(4):625–632

Wright RJ, Steinbach SF (2001) Violence: an unrecognizable environmental exposure that may contribute to greater asthma morbidity in high risk inner-city-populations. Environ Health Perspect 109:1085–1089

Chapter 17
Asthma: Interventions in Community Settings

James Krieger and Edith A. Parker

Introduction

Asthma is a complex, heterogeneous condition. Multiple factors contribute to its causation and exacerbation (Eder et al. 2006; Weiss 2002; Martinez 2007; Yeatts et al. 2006). Therefore, prevention and control of asthma requires a multifaceted approach. Interventions that identify people with asthma, assure access to quality medical care, improved self-management, increased social support, reduced exposure to environmental asthma triggers, and address underlying social determinants of health are all necessary. Figure 17.1 depicts a simplified model of how these interventions affect asthma control (Parker et al. 2004; van der Palen et al. 2001; Clark and Valerio 2003; Clark et al. 2001; Wright et al. 2005a; Gold and Wright 2005). Underlying social determinants of health such as discrimination or poverty affect all aspects of asthma control. For example, discrimination may result in sub-optimal medical care or living in substandard housing with high levels of trigger exposure. Transportation policy can affect access to care and exposure to outdoor air pollution.

The model suggests that interventions in community settings are an essential component of a comprehensive approach to asthma control. The goal of this chapter is to review current practice in community-based asthma control and the evidence underlying it. We review the evidence supporting the effectiveness of interventions in homes, social networks, pharmacies, childcare sites, other community settings (e.g., neighborhoods, community organizations, media, asthma camps), and the outdoor environment. We hope that communities will find such a summary useful as they plan and implement asthma interventions.

J. Krieger (✉)
Chronic Disease and Injury Prevention Section,
Public Health - Seattle & King County,
Chinook Building Suite 900, 401 Fifth Ave, 98104,
Seattle, WA, USA
e-mail: james.krieger@kingcounty.gov

Methods

Definition of Community-Based

As noted by Boutilier, community as a setting for interventions can be defined as a venue for health behavior programs (representing the more biomedical and disease prevention orientation), or community can be seen as a locus for organizing efforts to shift broader public and private sector socioeconomic policies and practices (Boutilier et al. 2000). We have included interventions that occur in both contexts. The majority of those included take place in the former context because this is the focus of most current asthma control activity and research. We acknowledge that the larger societal issues affecting asthma, such as housing and air pollution, need more attention.

For the purposes of this chapter, we have defined an intervention strategy as occurring in a community setting if it is implemented outside of a medical setting (with the exception of mobile clinics, which we included because they provide health services in community settings). While school-based interventions met this criterion, Chap. 14 in this volume discusses them in detail and we did not include them. We also did not include worksite interventions (Chap. 18), as they tend to focus on occupational asthma, which is beyond the scope of this chapter.

A. Harver and H. Kotses (eds.), *Asthma, Health and Society: A Public Health Perspective*,
DOI 10.1007/978-0-387-78285-0_17,

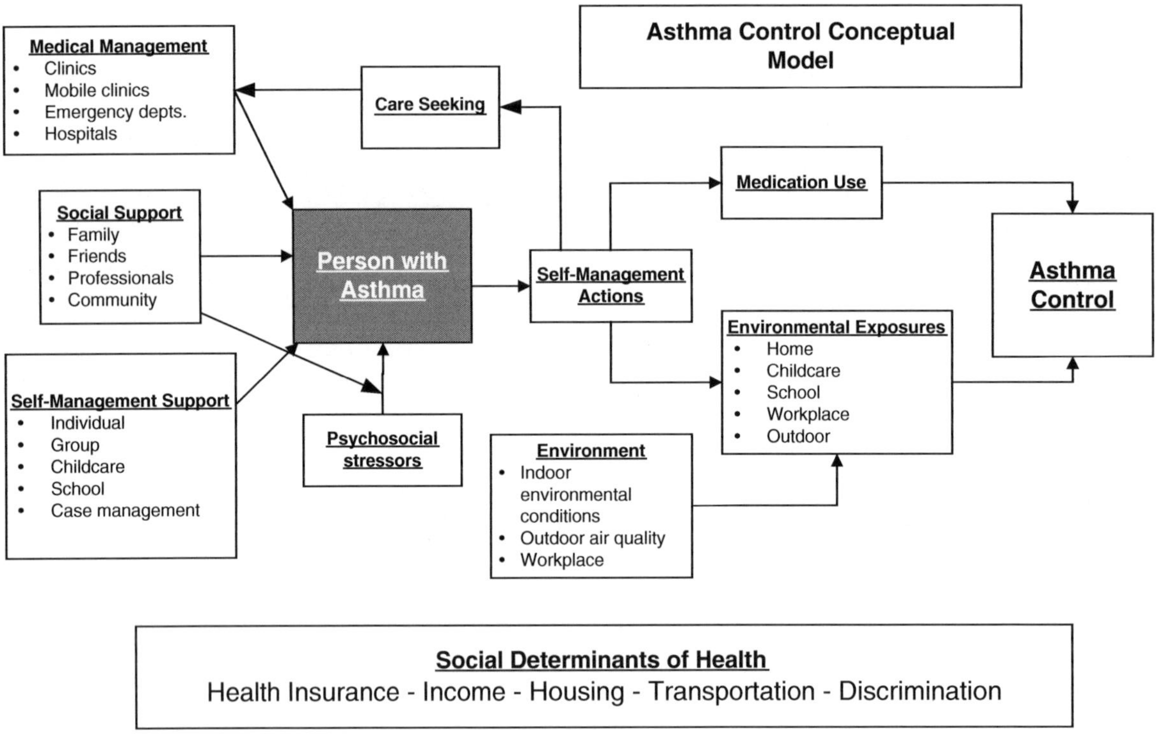

Fig. 17.1 Asthma control conceptual model

Identifying Interventions

We developed a preliminary list of interventions for potential inclusion from our experience in implementing community asthma interventions and by reviewing the action plans of state and local asthma agencies and coalitions (California Strategic Plan for Asthma 2007; Oregon Asthma Leadership 2007; New York State Department of Health 2007; Minnesota Department of Health 2007; New York City Department of Health and Mental Hygiene 2007; Merck Childhood Asthma 2007a; Washington State Department of Health 2005; Boston Urban Asthma 2007; Chicago Asthma 2007; Asthma Coalition of Texas 2007), reading reviews (Thompson et al. 2002; Apter and Szefler 2006; Mathur and Busse 2006) and guidelines (National Asthma Education and Prevention Program 2007a; National Asthma Education and Prevention Program Expert Panel Report 2002; Global Initiative for Asthma 2005; British Thoracic Society and Scottish Intercollegiate Guidelines Network 2007; National Asthma Council of Australia 2007; American Academy of Allergy, Asthma and Immunology 2007), scanning selected websites (Steps to a Healthier US 2007; Centers for Disease Control and Prevention 2007a; National and Lung and Blood Institute 2007; American Academy of Asthma, Allergy and Immunology 2007; California Asthma Public Health 2007; Regional Asthma Management and Prevention 2007; Community Action to Fight Asthma 2007; Allies Against 2007a; New England Regional Asthma 2007; National Conference of State Legislators 2007; Environmental Protection Agency 2007a), and consulting with experts. We used this list to search PubMed for literature published between 1985 and August 2006 using key words for each intervention. We scanned the search results for potentially relevant articles in English, retrieved their abstracts, reviewed them to determine whether they took place in a community setting, obtained the articles and abstracted data into a spreadsheet. We also searched websites with Google™ using the same search terms. Finally, we reviewed the CDC's "Potentially Effective Interventions for Asthma" web page (Centers for Disease Control and Prevention, Environmental Hazards and Health Effects Program 2007).

Criteria for Effectiveness

We used 16 criteria to assess the quality of evidence supporting each intervention, based on the criteria developed by the Consort Group (The Consort 2007), the Cochrane Collaborative (The Cochrane 2007), the United States Preventive Services Task Force (United States Preventive Services Task 2007), and the Community Guide (Centers for Disease Control and Prevention 2007b). Each criterion was given a score of one if adequate and zero if inadequate. The criteria are listed in Table 17.1.

A study was high quality if its score was 11 or higher, low if its score was five or lower, and medium if its score was in between. In reviewing guidelines, we considered a recommendation to be of high quality if it was developed by at least one national panel with recognized expertise using an explicit consensus process with broad stakeholder representation and a well-developed theoretical and evidence base. We included an intervention in this chapter if there was medium-to-high-quality evidence for its effectiveness, based on empirical studies. Lacking such evidence, we also included those recommended by high-quality guidelines. We also included some programs that were neither empirically tested nor recommended by guidelines, but that appeared promising and address areas of asthma control not encompassed by more evidence-based approaches. To be included, a promising program had to focus on a reduction of a trigger known to exacerbate asthma (e.g., indoor smoking bans) and/or use accepted theory or epidemiological evidence as the basis for the intervention.

Table 17.1 Criteria for assessing quality of evidence

Domain	Criteria
Study description	Study population described
	Study site and context described
	Intervention described
Participant selection	Selection universe described
	Clear eligibility criteria
	Selection bias addressed
Randomization	RCT with random number sequence generation
	RCT with concealed allocation
	RCT with blinding of data collection
Sample size	Quantitative justification of sample size and sample size adequate
Measurement	Exposure to intervention measured
	Valid and reliable exposure measurement
	Valid and reliable outcome measurement
Analysis	Appropriate statistical testing
	Appropriate control for differences across groups
Completion rate	At least 80% of participants complete intervention and final data collection

Interventions

Asthma control interventions occur in a variety of community settings. We begin with a discussion of asthma education in homes and neighborhood locations.

Home Visits

Home visitation has become an increasingly popular asthma education strategy in recent years. A growing body of high quality evidence, much published in the last 3 years, suggests that it is a valuable approach. Recruiting people with asthma to traditional asthma education programs (e.g., classes or well-asthma clinic visits) is difficult and many participants drop out. These challenges have led to increasing interest in providing education through home visits. Clients of a home-visit program are more likely to complete participation than those enrolling in classes (Brown et al. 2002).

In-home programs offer some of the same benefits found in traditional individual (as opposed to group) asthma education programs. They provide tailored education and support for improving self-management skills such as using medication and action plans properly, accessing and participating in medical care, communicating with health providers, and becoming more logistically organized for asthma management. They assess family and psychosocial issues, support the client in resolving them, and help them increase mechanisms for coping with stressors (Parker et al. in press). They may also provide resources and referrals for economic and other client needs.

Working in the context of the home provides additional benefits. Home visit programs are better suited to helping participants identify asthma triggers in their homes and take actions to reduce exposures to them, using variations of the "Healthy Homes" approach (Alliance for Healthy Homes 2006; National Center for Healthy Housing 2006; Environmental Protection Agency 2006a). For example, they facilitate client actions to reduce dust mite exposure by lowering humidity through improved ventilation and elimination of moisture intrusion into the home, cleaning bedding and encasing it with allergen-proof covers, and vacuuming and dusting regularly. Some programs arrange for allergy testing to focus exposure reduction activities on allergens to which the client is sensitized. Home visitors build trusting relationships with clients. These relationships enhance the visitor's effectiveness in motivating behavior change. Being in the home allows visitors to reinforce self-management strategies through role modeling (e.g., demonstrating proper cleaning technique or placement of bedding encasements), feedback, and social support. They coordinate care with medical providers by providing them with visit reports that often contain valuable information on asthma status, home conditions or medication adherence only available through direct observation in the home (Group Health Community Foundation Evaluation 2007).

Most home visit programs have served children and their caretakers, while a small number have included all ages or adults only. In general, they have engaged low-income and minority households, often in inner-city settings. The intensity of services in these programs ranges from a single visit to multiple visits over the course of a year. Costs per client range from $200–1,500. Further data regarding cost-effectiveness of home visits in relation to their intensity and also relative to other asthma education approaches are needed. Earlier programs focused on trigger reduction. The emphasis is now moving toward a more holistic approach encompassing all aspects of asthma self-management. Programs have employed several types of home visitors, including community health workers (CHWs), health educators, research assistants, nurses, sanitarians, and even physicians. More evidence comparing the types of home visitors would be welcome.

We believe that CHWs are particularly well suited to serve as home visitors among low-income, ethnically diverse households (Swider 2002a; Butz et al. 1994; Love et al. 1997; Krieger et al. 2002; Friedman et al. 2006; Lewin et al. 2005; Perez et al. 2006). Through sharing community, culture and life experiences with their clients, CHWs effectively establish rapport. They are also less costly than other types of health professionals. CHW programs are becoming widespread. For example, in New York, over 600 CHWs have been trained (Perez et al. 2006), and the Harlem Children's Zone Asthma Initiative is using CHWs to make home visits (Nicholas et al. 2005). Many local health departments and community organizations have developed home visit programs for children with asthma (Hoppin et al. 2006). Protocols for training and program implementation are available (Perez et al. 2006; Public Health – Seattle and King County 2006; http://www.communityhealthworks.org/yeswecan/index.html).

In addition to their home visitation role, CHWs provide additional services, suggesting that may be able to play a broader role in community-based asthma control. In clinics, they offer patient education, cultural mediation, and assistance with appointment scheduling (http://www.communityhealthworks.org/yeswecan/index.html). In the community, they lead asthma classes and support groups, connect people with medical care, and serve as health system navigators. We were unable to find published evaluations of the effectiveness of these types of CHW activities in relation to asthma, although reviews of CHW programs in general suggest they perform these functions effectively (Lewin et al. 2005; Brownstein et al. 2005; Nemcek and Sabatier 2003; Swider 2002b).

Evidence of the effectiveness of in-home interventions among children is supported by several randomized trials of medium to high quality that have demonstrated improved health outcomes, including symptoms, quality of life, and urgent health service utilization (Brown et al. 2002; Krieger et al. 2005; Krieger et al. 2009; Morgan et al. 2004; Dolinar et al. 2000; Eggleston et al. 2005; Bonner et al. 2002; Fisher et al. 2009; Carter et al. 2001). Additional uncontrolled studies have also shown improvements in outcomes (Primomo et al. 2006; Martin et al. 2006; Clougherty et al. 2006; Levy et al. 2006), although the lack of a comparison group weakens these findings. Studies that found limited or no benefit had significant methodological limitations, including high drop-out rates, contamination of control groups, or small sample sizes (Butz et al. 2005; Williams et al. 2006). This evidence has led to recommendations from the Centers for Disease Control and Prevention the Department of Housing and Urban Development (U.S. Department of Housing and Urban Development, Office of Healthy Homes and Lead Hazard Control

2006), the Environmental Protection Agency (Environmental Protection Agency and Air – Indoor Air Quality (IAQ) 2006), and the new National Asthma Education and Prevention Program (National Asthma Education and Prevention Program 2007b) EPR-3 guidelines for implementation of the in-home approach.

Home visitation faces several challenges (Brown et al. 2005). Evidence regarding programs for adults is limited and of low quality; further research is needed (de Blay et al. 2003; Smith et al. 2005; Simpson and Custovic 2005). Recruitment and retention of clients are sometimes issues because not all people with asthma and their families are interested in receiving home visits and those recruited in the programs may grow weary of participation. Development of sustainable funding (e.g., reimbursement by health care payers), even for successful evidence-based home visit programs, remains a challenge. Simplification and standardization of protocols and standard definitions of scope of work and qualifications of home visitors are needed to provide payers with a clearly defined product. A final challenge is the need for better mechanisms to link home visits to other sectors providing asthma management support, such as medical providers and schools.

Group Interventions in the Community Setting

Asthma Classes

An extensive literature of medium to high quality supports the effectiveness of asthma classes for chronic disease management in both acquisition of self-management skills and control of asthma (Powell and Gibson 2002; Gallefoss and Bakke 2000; Cote et al. 2001; Abdulwadud et al. 1997; Lucas et al. 2001; deOliveira et al. 1999; Kotses et al. 1995; Allen et al. 1995). Group interventions can also be used for provision of social support for persons with asthma and/or their caregivers. As most of these studies occurred in clinical settings, the evidence supporting classes is much more robust for clinic-based classes than for community-based ones. In this section, we focus on the latter.

Our literature search for group asthma education interventions (using group asthma interventions OR group asthma education OR asthma support groups as search terms) resulted in few non-clinic based programs. Bryant-Stephens and Li (Bryant-Stephens and Li 2004) conducted a single group pre-post evaluation of a community asthma education program in which peers worked with caregivers of children with asthma in a group setting. They found statistically significant improvements in asthma knowledge, ability to control the child's asthma and asthma-related quality of life. Fisher and colleagues (Fisher et al. 2004) performed a community education study that included group educational programs for parents and children, promotional activities, and individualized support provided by trained neighborhood peer helpers. Findings from this non-randomized, parallel group evaluation found no significant differences in acute care utilization between the intervention and control groups. However, those in the intervention group who had high participation rates in the program showed lower utilization in comparison to both intervention group members with low participation rates and control group members. Thus, evidence for the effectiveness of community-based classes is weak and more research is needed to rigorously compare classes in community vs. clinic settings.

Classes in community settings have some theoretical advantages over those held in medical sites. For example, clinic and hospital-based classes have encountered difficulties in attracting participants through clinician referrals and in retaining participants (Muntner et al. 2001; Yoon et al. 1991; Wood et al. 2006a). To promote participation, community-based organizations and asthma coalitions have been testing community approaches to recruitment such as working with community agencies to recruit their clients, conducting intensive flyering and door-to-door outreach, holding walk-in classes at high-volume community agencies, and case identification at childcare sites and schools. They have used peers as educators to increase retention. Whether these approaches are successful remains to be determined. (Elizabeth Herman, personal communication).

Social Support Groups

Social support can be an enabling factor for people with chronic illnesses and their families as they seek to improve control over the condition (Gallant 2003). For people with asthma, instrumental support may include help with reducing triggers in the home, bringing family members to medical appointments, or helping to increase adherence to prescribed medication. Emotional support may consist of being available to share the stresses and worries of caring for a child with asthma or living with asthma. Interventions designed to enhance social support include peer or community health worker interventions (described previously) and support group interventions.

While some data exist for the effectiveness of support groups for families of children with heterogeneous chronic illnesses, we found very little published evidence on social support interventions specifically for people with asthma. Chernoff et al. (2002) used an experimental design to evaluate a 15-month, community-based, family support intervention designed to reduce risk for poor adjustment and mental health problems in children with one of four chronic illnesses (diabetes, sickle cell anemia, cystic fibrosis, or moderate to severe asthma) and their mothers. The support component of the intervention consisted recruiting and training a group of "experienced" mothers of older children with the same conditions who then worked with mothers of the children in the intervention. The intervention significantly improved the psychosocial adjustment of the participating children.

Asthma clubs may be a promising group intervention strategy for delivery of both education and support for children and their caregivers. A study using a randomized cluster design of schools showed sustained improvements in inhaler technique among club participants (Patterson et al. 2005). A pre-post single group study described increases in knowledge and decreases in emergency department visits as a result of clubs (Alexander et al. 2000).

More research is needed about community-based group interventions that involve community members as peer leaders and instructors, and which foster social support for participants.

Community Pharmacists

Community pharmacists are well positioned to provide asthma self-management support. They can provide asthma education (materials and counseling), peak flow meters and spacers, and asthma action plans. Counseling may occur when customers come to the pharmacy to pick up prescriptions or during specially scheduled visits. They can assess response to medication and side-effects, assess asthma control, and provide customers and their medical providers with feedback.

Numerous investigators have developed and evaluated models of pharmacy-based care for asthma (Bunting and Cranor 2006; Mangiapane et al. 2005; McLean and MacKeigan 2005; Saini et al. 2004; Emmerton et al. 2003; Barbanel et al. 2003; McLean et al. 2003; Weinberger et al. 2002; Stergachis et al. 2002; Cordina et al. 2001; Diamond and Chapman 2001; Schulz et al. 2001; Narhi et al. 2000; Rupp et al. 1997). While sharing a common approach, the models have differed in important details, including the intensity of training of the pharmacists, supervision and quality control of pharmacist activities, level of reimbursement to the pharmacist, duration and intensity of counseling, characteristics of the customers (ages, asthma severity), site of counseling (public vs. private space, on vs. off-site), site of the pharmacy (urban vs. rural, domestic vs. international), extent of disease management data available to the pharmacist, and type of self-monitoring employed (none, diary, peak flow meter).

Given the heterogeneity of programs, differences in communities, and variability in the quality of evaluation methods, it is not surprising that the studies have not reached consistent conclusions. Randomized controlled trials have not found significant benefits. Two in the United States found no impact of pharmacy care on quality of life, peak flow or health services utilization (Weinberger et al. 2002; Stergachis et al. 2002). However, pharmacists in both studies implemented the intervention to a limited extent, perhaps because of the low reimbursement they received for each enrolled customer. Additional implementation barriers included insufficient training, lack of a patient-centered approach, and lack of time and space for counseling. McLean and colleagues conducted a more robust intervention in British Columbia community pharmacies and demonstrated improvements in quality of life, symptoms, and peak flow (McLean et al. 2003). However, evaluation of the program suffered from major flaws, including a high (45%) attrition rate and lack of an intention-to-treat analysis. Another trial in Malta also yielded few, if any benefits (Cordina et al. 2001), while a small pilot study at a single English pharmacy did produce improvement in symptoms (Barbanel et al. 2003).

Studies with weaker evaluation designs have reported more favorable outcomes. Three studies conducted outside of the United States employed a pre-post parallel group design and two showed improved quality of life, but impact on other endpoints was less consistent (Mangiapane et al. 2005; Saini et al. 2004; Schulz et al. 2001).

Two American studies reported benefits in terms of urgent health service utilization, quality of life and symptoms, but employed a single group pre-post evaluation design with its attendant limitations (Bunting and Cranor 2006; Rupp et al. 1997).

Thus the evidence regarding the effectiveness of community pharmacy interventions is inconclusive. Whether a well-implemented, comprehensive program could yield benefits at a reasonable cost remains a question for further research to resolve. Even if effective, this type of intervention may not be feasible. All of these programs encountered substantial obstacles such as difficulty in recruiting and retaining customers and pharmacists, lack of expertise among pharmacists in patient counseling and asthma management, and lack of time and space for pharmacists to provide counseling. McLean has suggested some strategies to overcome these barriers (McLean and MacKeigan 2005).

Mobile Clinic Vans

Many inner-city children with asthma have no regular source of asthma care or receive suboptimal care not meeting current management guidelines (Federico and Liu 2003). Mobile clinics staffed by asthma specialists visit inner city schools to offer evaluation by an asthma specialist including a comprehensive history, physical exam, spirometry, and skin tests; ongoing medical treatment including follow-up visits every 4–8 weeks and (at some sites) medications; family support; education on asthma self-management; assistance in obtaining health insurance; and referral to a primary care medical home and community resources. Each van cares for approximately 1,000 new patients per year. A validated school-based screening process identifies children with poorly controlled asthma for referral to the mobile van. School nurses, safety net clinics, hospitals and emergency departments also refer children. There are mobile clinics in Los Angeles, Orange County, Phoenix, Chicago, and Baltimore (*see* http://www.aafasocal.com/breathmobile.php for links to their websites). Evaluations of these programs have been limited to single group pre-post studies. Results among regular users of the clinic show improved use of controller medications, and decreased symptoms, school absenteeism, and urgent health services utilization (Bollinger et al. 2005; Jones et al. 2000; Liao et al. 2006).

This promising intervention now needs comparison in a randomized trial with a strategy that provides outreach and direct referral to primary care medical homes. Mobile clinics may be most appropriate in communities in which significant numbers of children lack medical homes and rely on episodic urgent care for asthma. Data from several recent studies suggest that in many cities, most children have a medical home (Krieger et al. 2005; Morgan et al. 2004). In such communities, effective mechanisms to link children to primary care through case management and outreach may be effective, less costly, and allow primary care providers to address preventive, anticipatory and other aspects of health care in addition to asthma.

Community-based Asthma Case Detection

An estimated 25–30% of people meeting clinical criteria for asthma are not aware of having the condition (Redline et al. 2004). Many do not recognize a chronic cough or shortness of breath causing them to slow down as potential symptoms of asthma. Community-based case detection may help to identify people with undiagnosed asthma symptoms as well as those with diagnosed but poorly controlled asthma (Lewis et al. 2004; Boss et al. 2003a).

Published case detection efforts have focused on elementary schools (Redline et al. 2004; Jones et al. 2004; Gerald et al. 2004). Detection methods include questionnaires with or without pulmonary function tests. Several investigators have found that questionnaires with three to seven items assessing asthma symptoms have a positive predictive value of 50–70% relative to specialist diagnosis. Sensitivity is approximately 80%. Following up positive questionnaire responses with spirometry increases the positive predictive value to 95%.

What remains to be seen is if case detection results in better health outcomes (Boss et al. 2003b). Yawn and colleagues (Yawn et al. 2003) showed that identification of children with potentially under-treated asthma led to increased physician visits and changes in asthma management, but did not report on health outcomes. Before implementing a case detection program, assuring access to follow-up medical care is necessary. However, it may be difficult to assure such access in some communities (Yawn et al. 2002). In conclusion, school-based case detection may be a reasonable strategy, provided mechanisms (e.g., care coordinators, community health workers, school nurses) are in place to promote follow-up with providers who offer high quality care.

Childcare Sites

Many younger children with asthma spend large portions of their days in childcare settings. Staff often have a limited understanding of asthma management and trigger reduction strategies (Goveia et al. 2005). Most children do not have action plans at their childcare sites. Asthma triggers are common (Fernandez-Caldas et al. 2001; Arbes et al. 2005). Therefore, educating child care providers about creating a safe and supportive environment for their children with asthma is an appealing strategy.

There are many educational resources, asthma management, and environmental assessment tools aimed at childcare providers in print and on-line (Asthma and Allergy Foundation of America and New England 2006; Asthma and Allergy Foundation of America 2006; Connecticut Department of Public Health 2006; Indiana Department of Environmental Management 2006; National Heart and Blood 2006). They cover handling asthma emergencies, using an action plan, understanding asthma medications, and reducing triggers. Local organizations offer asthma management classes and arrange for provision of continuing education credits for participants to facilitate enrollment. California mandated asthma training for childcare providers in 1998 (Emergency Medical Services 2006). Investigators at University of Miami are evaluating on-site training visits with telephone-follow-up by a team of clinicians and educators that promotes implementation of asthma management guidelines (presence of written action plan, tobacco-free environment, and knowledge of medication administration) (Jeffrey Brosco, personal communication). State asthma plans (California Strategic Plan for Asthma 2007) call for developing and implementing model policies and practices for asthma management in childcare facilities.

However, evidence demonstrating the effectiveness of these activities is not available. The benefit of providing asthma education for childcare providers is virtually untested. One group from Australia showed an improvement in knowledge and self-confidence in managing asthma and adoption of self-reported recommended asthma management practices among childcare providers who attended a 2-h workshop (Hazell et al. 2006).

Likewise, the health benefits of improving indoor environmental quality at childcare sites are unknown. Swedish researchers have investigated the low-allergen childcare centers that are present in all municipalities, supported through local government budgets. In a study of single center, extensive renovation, installation of a new ventilation system, replacement of objects likely to serve as allergen reservoirs, and avoidance of contact with pets led to significant decreases in pet allergen exposure (Munir et al. 1996). A recent survey of directors of Swedish "allergen avoidance daycare centers" and "ordinary daycare centers" found fewer reported allergens and irritants (e.g., dampness/mold), fewer dust reservoirs (e.g., curtains, shelves), and higher frequency of allergen reduction activities (e.g., dust control, bedding washing) in the former (Broms et al. 2006). Neither study reported on health outcomes.

Further research is needed to evaluate the effectiveness of asthma education for childcare providers and the value of asthma-friendly childcare facilities.

Asthma Camps

Asthma camps seek to provide children with asthma an opportunity to learn about asthma self-management, increase their self-confidence in engaging in physical activities, meet and learn from other children with asthma, and have fun (Nesvold et al. 2006; Meng 1997; Brazil et al. 1997; Silvers et al. 1992; Lord et al. 2001; Sorrells et al. 1995; Fitzpatrick et al. 1992; Kelly et al. 1998; Punnett and Thurber 1993). There are 121 asthma camps in 43 states in the U.S. (Nesvold et al. 2006). All camps provide self-management education, but differ substantially in terms of age (range 5–18 years), racial/ethnic mix of participants, site of camp (e.g., health club, camp facility), duration of camp (1–7 days), whether campers stay overnight, teaching format and curricula, total hours of self-management instruction (range 0–8+ h), involvement of caretakers, and use of action plans. More than three-quarters are managed by American Lung Association chapters, facilitated by part-time staff and led by volunteer health professionals from multiple disciplines.

Evidence for the effectiveness of camps for reducing asthma morbidity is limited and of low quality. Published evaluations are all single group studies, with the strongest design being a time series study. The study samples are small ($n=34-125$), not able to address Hawthorne and regression to the mean effects, lack robust intervention exposure measures, and often have inadequate statistical methods. Within these significant limitations, the studies have reported decreased urgent health-care utilization (clinic or emergency department or hospital) and decreased school absences. Some reported benefits in secondary outcomes such as decreased anxiety and lower family stress. Others noted improvements in intermediate measures such as correct device use, other self-management behaviors, self-confidence, and asthma knowledge. Surveys of parents and camp directors concluded that the camps are useful for providing intensive asthma education, facilitating peer interaction with resultant improvement in social interaction skills, and increasing the child's independence. More rigorous evaluation is needed before asthma camps can be adopted as an effective strategy.

Indoor Environmental Interventions

Reduction of Individual Asthma Triggers in the Home

While the home visit programs described above emphasize comprehensive interventions that address multiple indoor asthma triggers, there is also a growing body of research that examines the effectiveness of interventions focused on single triggers (Eggleston 2005a). While it is beyond the scope of this chapter to review this literature comprehensively, a few points are worth making. First, it appears focused interventions can successfully reduce exposure to a specific trigger, but that this reduction does not consistently translate into improved asthma control. Second, addressing multiple triggers in the context of a comprehensive home visit program is likely more effective than addressing single exposures (Centers for Disease Control and Prevention 2009; O'Connor 2005; Chapman 2005). Third, behavioral approaches to trigger reduction may be of limited value in the setting of grossly substandard housing conditions.

Dust mites are a common indoor asthma trigger. Numerous interventions to reduce exposure to dust mite allergens have been tested (Sandel et al. 2004a). Although mattress and pillow encasings, washing of bedding, steam cleaning of carpet and upholstered furniture, vacuuming of carpets, and dehumidification can all reduce levels of mite allergen (Vojta et al. 2001; Arlian et al. 2001; Colloff et al. 1995), the clinical benefit of such activities remains controversial. For example, simply placing allergen-impermeable coverings on bedding reduces exposure to mite allergen, but appears not to reduce asthma symptoms (Rijssenbeek-Nouwens et al. 2002; Woodcock et al. 2003). A meta-analysis found no pooled effect of either chemical or physical methods on clinical outcomes (Gotzsche et al. 2004). However, several studies that reduced bedding allergen levels by at least half have shown significant clinical benefits for patients with mite allergy (Halken et al. 2003; Carswell et al. 1996; Ehnert et al. 1992).

Several types of interventions aimed at roaches have produced reductions in dust allergen levels and in roach counts. One model combines professional house cleaning with application of gel bait pesticides (McConnell et al. 2003a; Arbes et al. 2003). A second approach uses peer education to help families reduce roaches' access to food and shelter along with application of boric acid pesticide and bedding covers (McConnell et al. 2005). A third employs professional gel bait application and house cleaning before and after the extermination (Wood et al. 2001). Integrated pest management programs can reduce the number of homes infested with roaches by half (evaluations did not measure dust allergen levels) (Brenner et al. 2003; Wang and Bennett 2006; Miller and Meek 2004). Of interest, application of gel bait pesticide alone may be as effective as more comprehensive interventions (Arbes et al. 2004). Other studies produced less impressive results, perhaps because unlike the more successful programs, they did not emphasize participatory, community-based methods (Gergen et al. 1999). Implementation barriers to be considered include difficulties with recruitment of households, the need to involve multiple household members to sustain a pest-free environment, and severe structural and maintenance problems in older buildings (Kinney et al. 2002). Repeated cleaning up to 6 months after eradication may be necessary to remove residual allergen (Eggleston 2005b).

We had less success in identifying methods that reduce exposure to other common indoor allergens. A single study showed that integrated pest management can reduce levels of mouse allergen in inner city homes, but health outcomes were not assessed

(Phipatanakul et al. 2004). Small patches of mold can be removed by cleansing with detergent, and guidelines are available for removing larger mold-contaminated areas (New York City Department of Health 2000; Storey et al. 2004; Macher 1999), but these approaches have not been rigorously evaluated nor related to health outcomes. Evidence for effective practices to eliminate home environmental tobacco smoke are also lacking, although guidelines recommend smoking outside the home and using a smoking jacket to prevent transport of smoke combustion products into the home (Asthma Initiative of Michigan 2007). Elimination of pet allergens requires removal of the pet from the household, but this is often unacceptable to the patient. Washing the pet, use of air filters and keeping the pet out of the bedroom appear ineffective (Eggleston 2005b).

Addressing Substandard Housing

Living in substandard housing leads to exposure to indoor asthma triggers and higher rates of allergen sensitization, yet educational-only interventions have limited ability to correct the underlying housing conditions that lead to elevated trigger levels (Eggleston 1998a; Wooton and Ashley 2000; Huss et al. 1994a; Christiansen et al. 1996; Willies-Jacobo et al. 1993a; Gelber et al. 1993; Sarpong et al. 1996a; Eggleston 2000a). Remediation of these underlying conditions begins where educational interventions leave off. If leaks and poor ventilation allow excessive moisture or deficits in the building envelope permit entry of pests , interventions focused on behavior change may have limited impact (Krieger and Higgins 2002; Sandel et al. 2004b). Most, but not all, housing intervention studies have found that improving ventilation and reducing humidity with enhanced whole house ventilation can decrease mite levels (Arlian et al. 2001; Somerville et al. 2000; Warner et al. 2000; Harving et al. 1994; Fletcher et al. 1996; Niven et al. 1999). The inconsistency in findings may be due to climate variation across study sites. One study demonstrated clinical improvements (Harving et al. 1994). A recent trial from Cleveland showed that remediation of moisture sources in homes with indoor mold (in conjunction with home-based education and provision of an action plan) led to decreases in mold levels, fewer symptoms and lower emergency department and hospital utilization (Kercsmar et al. 2006). Additional evaluations of structural interventions are needed and at least two are underway (Howden-Chapman et al. 2005; Krieger et al. in press).

Addressing substandard housing requires policy approaches. Advocates in San Diego are urging local government agencies to enforce existing code pertinent to substandard housing conditions (San Diego Regional Asthma 2006). The Boston Urban Asthma Coalition (Boston Urban Asthma 2006) is calling for changes to the Sanitary Code to reflect healthy building and maintenance standards, and submitted changes to the state Building Code (currently under review) that would prevent moisture problems in new construction. It partners with the City of Boston's Inspectional Services Department (ISD) to offer a website for health-care providers and community-based organizations through which they can refer patients with asthma for housing inspections if they suspect substandard housing conditions may be affecting asthma control (City of Boston Inspectional Services Department 2006).

Local asthma coalitions have been collaborating with public housing agencies to assure that residents with asthma live in homes free of triggers. In Seattle, the housing authority, the local health department, community organizations, and housing residents have partnered to develop asthma-friendly housing (Krieger et al. in press; Breathe Easy Homes at High Point 2007) and procedures for transferring residents from units with high levels of asthma triggers. They are exploring additional policies such as expanding smoking restrictions. The Boston coalition convinced local authorities to adopt its healthy home specifications for public housing design, leading to their incorporation into 800 new affordable housing units. Other coalitions have encouraged housing authorities to include asthma triggers and related conditions in property inspections. Many local housing authorities are using integrated pest management approaches. Evidence of the effectiveness of asthma-friendly housing policies and guidelines for best practices is needed.

Completely changing housing and neighborhood conditions may improve asthma outcomes. The Moving to Opportunity project showed that when low-income children with asthma living in public housing in areas with high concentrations of poverty move to higher quality rental housing in more affluent neighborhoods, they have fewer asthma attacks (Katz and Liebman 2001).

At least two additional studies of the impact of moving to healthy housing are in progress (Krieger et al. in press; Wells and Rebecca 2007).

Some communities have addressed private sector housing quality. In Boston, San Diego and elsewhere, advocates provide information to tenants on their rights and assist them in working with landlords to obtain improvements that will reduce trigger levels. Healthy Home checklists and guidelines for residents, buyers, landlords and homebuilders are available (National Center for Healthy Housing 2007). A bill (HR172) in Congress proposes tax credits for homeowners who make improvements leading to better indoor air quality.

Environmental Tobacco Smoke

We discussed exposure to residential indoor asthma triggers above. People with asthma are also exposed to indoor asthma triggers outside their homes. Among triggers in non-residential settings, environmental tobacco smoke is receiving the most attention. Community-level interventions focus on banning smoking from public places, such as restaurants, recreation sites and government buildings. All fifty states and the District of Columbia have smoke-free air provisions restricting smoking in certain places. These restrictions range from simple restrictions (e.g., designated areas in government buildings) to more comprehensive regulations (e.g., prohibiting smoking in all private workplaces, restaurants, and bars) (American Cancer Society 2006a). In addition, several cities in states with limited smoking bans have instituted city or county-wide bans that are more comprehensive in nature and include restaurants, bars, hotel lobbies, and meeting rooms (American Cancer Society 2006b). Smoking bans and restrictions are strongly recommended by the Task Force on Community Preventive Services based on evidence that such measures reduce exposure to tobacco smoke across a wide range of workplace settings and adult populations. These findings hold true whether the measures are applied at different levels of scale or whether they are used alone or as part of a multi-component community or workplace intervention (Task Force on Community Preventive Services 2000). For example, a study on the impact of smoking policy on the respiratory health of food and beverage servers found that the prevalence of irritant and respiratory symptoms among nonsmokers was consistently higher among those who worked in sites in which smoking was permitted (Dimich-Ward et al. 2005). An additional benefit of smoke-free restaurant laws may be their effect on discouraging smoking among adolescents (Siegel et al. 2005). Many communities have formed coalitions to help reduce exposure to environmental tobacco smoke (Cramer et al. 2003).

Outdoor Air Pollution

The link between poor air quality and asthma exacerbations is well-documented, particularly the association between particulate matter (PM) and pulmonary function, but also the associations with ozone and sulfur and nitrogen oxides (McConnell et al. 2003b; Samet et al. 2000). Community and policy interventions to improve air quality have focused on reduction of the pollutant sources (e.g., wood smoke or diesel emissions) or reduction of personal exposure to the pollutant (e.g., avoidance of ozone). There are very few published studies evaluating the asthma-related health effects of such interventions. Thus the following strategies are best viewed as promising approaches.

Wood-Burning Ordinances

A body of scientific literature based on human and animal studies describes an association between wood smoke and pulmonary function (Tesfaigzi et al. 2002; Zelikoff et al. 2002), nasal polyposis (Kim and Hanley 2002), and respiratory symptoms. Particulates (PM) are a major constituent of wood smoke (Mistry et al. 2004). Some studies suggest that in wintertime, as much as 80% of the PM emissions in residential areas are from woodburning devices (Larson et al. 1992; Environmental 2006). Both state and local governments have regulated wood stove use to improve air quality (such as the Colorado Air Quality Control Commission Regulation #4 and municipal ordinances (e.g., Menlo Park, CA)). Wood burning ordinances may prohibit use of uncertified stoves[1] on poor air quality days (with exceptions made for homes in which

[1] Traditional fireplaces or any stove or insert that does not meet the EPA certification of no more than 7.5 grams per hour of particulate emission.

fireplaces are the only source of heat); require installation of EPA-certified wood heaters, fireplaces, natural gas fireplaces, or pellet-fueled wood heaters in new and remodeled construction; or prohibit use of certain fuels, such as garbage and plastics, in a wood-burning appliance (Colorado Department of Public Health and Environment 2006; Bay Area Air Quality Management 2006). We could find no published articles that specifically evaluated the effect of wood-burning regulations on asthma exacerbations.

Anti-Idling Ordinances

To reduce exposure to particulates found in diesel exhaust, many communities and some states have introduced anti-idling regulations that restrict the amount of time a vehicle may stand idle while running its engine. A summary of Anti-Idling Regulations in the United States (Environmental Protection Agency 2006b) notes that 31 states have some type of anti-idling regulation at either the state or the local level. These ordinances regulate heavy diesel vehicles (Arizona), marine terminals or ports (California), and school buses (Connecticut, Minnesota). Idling time-limits range from un-specified periods to 30 min.

Community-wide strategies have encouraged the passage of anti-idling ordinances. They have included letter-writing campaigns and (American Lung Association of Metropolitan Chicago 2006) an anti-idling "day of action." (Community Action to Fight Asthma 2006a) No evidence assessing the effectives of these ordinances and campaigns is available.

Reducing Exposure to High Volume Traffic

High volume traffic located near residential sites may expose people with asthma to significant levels of air pollutants (Gauderman et al. 2007). Communities have taken action to influence policy decisions regarding traffic routing, road siting, locations of intermodal freight and municipal waste truck transfer stations, and placement of bus depots. For example, in New York City in 2000, West Harlem Environmental Action (WEACT) filed a Title VI complaint with the U.S. Department of Transportation against New York's Metropolitan Transportation Authority stating, "the MTA advances a racist, discriminatory policy of disproportionately siting diesel bus depots and diesel bus parking lots in minority neighborhoods in Manhattan" (West Harlem Environmental 2006).

At border crossings in Detroit (Keeler et al. 2002) and Buffalo (Lwebuga-Mukasa et al. 2004) and in the ports of Los Angeles (Hricko 2006), growing international trade has led to an increase in truck, ship, and train traffic with its attendant pollution (Hricko 2006). In Detroit, community groups partnered with the University of Michigan to share results of a local air quality and health effects assessment. They were concerned that proposed transportation-related projects, such as an additional international bridge crossing and an intermodal transfer terminal, would increase particulate exposure in neighborhoods that already exceeded the national standards. The assessment demonstrated negative health effects from exposure to PM for children with asthma (Lewis et al. 2005). They shared summaries of their study with community residents; with local, state and federal elected officials; and with the local advisory boards for the proposed projects (Parker and Salinas 2002). To date, officials have not made a decision about construction of the transfer terminal nor the construction and/or location of an additional bridge.

In southern California, community groups have worked with the Southern California Environmental Health Sciences Center (SCEHSC) to influence transportation-related policies affecting the ports of Los Angeles and Long Beach. SCEHSC researchers have presented data to officials regarding the health effects of air pollution at hearings (Hricko 2004). Community members have discussed their concerns at community forums and meetings with elected officials and port authorities. Community groups, assisted by SCEHSC, have called into question plans to expand intermodal yards (Mongelluzzo 2006).

Other transportation related interventions. The Partnership for a Smog-Free Georgia is the sole commuter behavior intervention that we identified in the peer-reviewed literature. Three large Atlanta-based companies implemented a program to encourage employees to adopt commuter behaviors that would decrease vehicle emissions. Two of the organizations noted a decrease in single-occupancy vehicle commutes and a decrease in the estimated emissions associated commuting. The third organization observed an increase from 20 to 41.5% in the employees who reported participating in the commuting program

(Pierce et al. 2000). However, an editorialist noted concerns about the lack of standard evaluation methods (including lack of comparison groups), the large number of employees who did not participate in alternative commuting activities (50%), and the need to target non-commuting driving behaviors.

Local governments around the country have begun replacing old vehicles with alternative fuel and hybrid (gasoline/electric) vehicles, using lower emission fuels (e.g., ultra-low sulfur diesel), and retrofitting existing diesel vehicles with more effective emission controls in order to lower emissions (Community Action to Fight Asthma 2006b; King County Environmental Purchasing 2007; Creating healthy urban environments for all 2007; News release, Metro Transit earns national Clean Air Excellence Award 2007; News release, Sims: King County will quadruple biodiesel use 2007; City of Seattle 2006).

Poor Air Quality Alert Systems

Many communities use the EPA-sponsored Air Quality Index (AQI) to notify people with asthma when current air quality can adversely affect their health. The AQI is calculated for the five major air pollutants for which there are national air quality standards: ground-level ozone, particulate matter, carbon monoxide, sulfur dioxide, and nitrogen dioxide. The AQI forecasts are often covered by local newspapers, radio and TV stations. Real-time AQI conditions for over 300 cities in the United. States. are available on the website AIRNow (AIRNow 2006). In 2005, the EPA and state and local air quality agencies introduced the EnviroFlash program, which provides the same local air quality information via email or pager notification (AIRNow 2006). Because not all people have the technology to receive such notifications, some state agencies have sought to recruit community service groups and the news media to help spread the word when air quality is poor (DeGuire 2006).

Community Organization

Recent research suggests that neighborhood context (Yen et al. 2006), including attributes such as collective efficacy (Cagney and Browning 2004) and neighborhood violence (Wright et al. 2004), is associated with asthma symptoms and asthma problems. Community organizing has the potential to address these general concerns as well as improve asthma-related issues at the neighborhood level, such as access to health services, housing quality, and outdoor air quality. For example, residents and community-based organizations can unite to promote asthma-friendly policies in schools, indoor public spaces and the outdoor environment. Indeed, community groups using a community organizing approach undertook many of the air pollution interventions mentioned in the section on air quality interventions (Mongelluzzo 2006; Community Action to Fight Asthma 2006c; Brown et al. 2004). Community organizing strategies can also be used to advocate for access to health services (e.g., self-management education, home visits, medications, and medical equipment), to improve access to asthma-friendly housing, and to reduce neighborhood level stressors such as crime.

Lewis and colleagues (Lewis et al. 1996) described a community-organizing intervention to improve the health of Latinos with asthma that employs many of the recognized techniques of community organizing such as network analysis, coalition building, broad-based activities such as recreational and safety activities, and provision of education around asthma. The authors observed a reduction in self-reported asthma health-care utilization among the targeted Latino population, but the analysis did not appear to include a control group. In Detroit, the Community Action Against Asthma project hired community organizers to work with neighborhood residents on reduction of physical and social environmental stressors associated with asthma. Qualitative evaluation results suggested the project increased community awareness and advocacy around environmental health issues and was instrumental in getting proposed public works projects (e.g., transportation related projects) to recognize their impacts on health. However, due to a delay in initial project start-up, the project was unable to link the community organizing activities with ongoing asthma-related health data collection from a "sister" research project and was thus unable to evaluate if the community-organizing intervention resulted in improved asthma-related health (Chung et al. 2006). The project faced the challenge of using a community organizing approach focused on asthma when community members had other priority issues, such as employment or general health care. Another limitation was the short time frame of the study. The trickle-down effect of a community-organizing intervention to reduce neighborhood environmental stressors may take longer to produce changes in asthma outcomes than the 5 years allotted to the study period.

Several ongoing community organizing interventions appear promising but have not yet published results. The Chicago Community Asthma Prevention Project is a partnership of the University of Illinois, the American Lung Association and the Grand Boulevard Federation (a CBO with history of working on economic development and housing issues). The project has trained Federation staff in asthma issues and hired an asthma-focused community organizer and health educators. These staff provide individual services (health education, home visits), offer school and community education, and raise community awareness around issues that affect asthma, such as dust from demolition of buildings and freeway construction. (Personal communication, Victoria Persky, 2006). West Harlem Environmental Action and the Boston Alternatives for Community and Environment use community organizing techniques to increase awareness of environmental health hazards and environmental justice issues around asthma (Brown et al. 2004). The Boston group has accomplished much, including passage of an Environmental Justice policy for the State of Massachusetts; forcing, with its coalition partners, the regional transportation plan to include 100 additional clean fuel buses in its 25-year plan; and persuading the Massachusetts Department of Environmental Protection to install a comprehensive air monitoring station in the Dudley Square area (Alternatives for Community and Environment (ACE) 2007).

In conclusion, there are a few published examples of community organizing interventions and other ongoing projects that show promising results. However, the potential for community organizing in addressing community-level factors that affect asthma remains unexplored and its effectiveness is undocumented.

Community Awareness and Information

Increasing awareness of asthma could yield several benefits. People with undiagnosed asthma might become aware that symptoms they are experiencing could be asthma and seek medical attention. People with asthma and their families could learn of resources to help them better manage asthma. Community members could learn what they can do to support people with asthma. Health providers could be prompted to pay more attention to asthma and deliver effective care. School staff could increase their understanding of how best to support students with asthma. Policy makers could understand the burden of asthma and support asthma control programs and policies. Examples of community awareness and information dissemination efforts abound. We could find no evaluations of their effectiveness in producing these potential benefits. Nonetheless, most guidelines include them.

Awareness Campaigns

Many state asthma plans and community action plans include awareness raising as an objective (California Strategic Plan for Asthma 2007; Oregon Asthma Leadership 2007; Dallas Asthma 2006). Strategies include public relations and marketing campaigns; distribution of culturally appropriate educational materials to health providers, schools and community sites; briefings of public officials; development of websites with asthma resources (including information for people with asthma, best practices for asthma interventions, etc.); placing of information materials in pharmacies, schools, libraries, and other public places; events such as asthma walks (American Lung 2007), cultural events, health fairs, and asthma days (Global Initiative Against 2007; Environmental Protection Agency 2007b); proclamations; resource directories, and even door-to-door outreach (Minnesota Department of Health 2007; New York City Department of Health and Mental Hygiene 2007; Merck Childhood Asthma 2007a; National Asthma Education and Prevention Program 2007a; National Asthma Council of Australia 2007; American Academy of Allergy, Asthma and Immunology 2007; Centers for Disease Control and Prevention 2007a; National and Lung and Blood Institute 2007; American Academy of Asthma, Allergy and Immunology 2007; California Asthma Public Health 2007; Regional Asthma Management and Prevention 2007; Community Action to Fight Asthma 2007; Allies Against 2007a; New England Regional Asthma 2007; Environmental Protection Agency 2007a; Centers for Disease Control and Prevention, Environmental Hazards and Health Effects Program 2007; Public Health – Seattle and King County 2007).

We found only one study that demonstrated positive impacts of an awareness campaign on asthma outcomes. Comino and colleagues (Comino et al. 1997) used four serial cross-sectional population surveys to evaluate the National Asthma Campaign in Australia. The educational campaign used mass media to inform people about new approaches to preventive asthma therapy and why people with symptoms of asthma should talk to their doctors. They described statistically significant increases in awareness of asthma messages in the media, recall of the message, and knowledge about the need to use preventive therapy for asthma.

Asthma Help Lines

A more focused approach seeks to increase awareness of community resources among people with asthma. Asthma coalitions have established "help lines" that provide information, resources, and referrals. For example, eight western counties in New York support a nurse who is a certified asthma educator to staff a toll-free number, link callers to case-management, and offer limited asthma supplies (Western New York Asthma 2007). In Philadelphia, a consortium of health plans, medical providers and the local health department have developed "Link Line." Link Line is a centralized telephone bank staffed by health educators who work with families that include a child with asthma to identify their needs and link them to the city's many asthma programs and services. Link Line staff provide follow-up support and coordination for each family over 4 months to ensure receipt of services (Philadelphia Allies Against 2007). In Seattle, the local asthma coalition took a less intensive approach by establishing toll-free telephone access in three languages to coalition staff who assessed the caller's needs for services and offered relevant referrals. With the caller's permission, staff also contacted service providers, who then followed up with the client. We were unable to find evaluations of any of these types of services.

Coalitions

In the past 25 years, coalitions have gained in popularity as a method for improving community health through improved collaboration among multiple agencies and sectors (Butterfoss et al. 1993; Butterfoss 2007; Zakocs and Edwards 2006; Butterfoss and Kegler 2002). Coalitions focusing on asthma have been part of this trend (Clark et al. 2006; Allies Against 2007b; American College of Chest Physicians 2007). There are currently at least 200 asthma coalitions in the United States (Noreen Clark, personal communication, 2006), increasing from an estimated 44 in 1998 (Schmidt et al. 1999). Review of the roles played by these coalitions in promoting community asthma interventions is beyond the scope of this chapter. In summary, the emerging literature on asthma coalitions and the experience of the authors and others involved in coalition work suggests that coalitions can (Butterfoss and Kegler 2002; Schwartz 2006):

- Bring together agencies and stakeholders who previously had not worked together
- Create a common strategy for improving asthma control in the community
- Generate resources for implementing interventions
- Raise awareness of asthma as an important health issue
- Develop and advocate for policies at the institutional and governmental levels
- Implement focused services and programs
- Promote integration of community asthma activities (*see* below) so that they are consistent, coordinated, and linked

What remains to be seen is if these coalition processes result in improved asthma outcomes at the community level. Evaluations of the outcomes of several coalition efforts are in process (e.g., Allies Against Asthma (Allies Against 2007c), Controlling Asthma in American Cities (Centers for Disease Control and Prevention 2007c), Merck Childhood Asthma Network (Merck Childhood Asthma 2007b), and National Asthma Education and Prevention Program Coaltions (National Asthma Education and Prevention Program 2007c)) but results are not yet available.

Integration of Interventions at the Community Level

We have described many community-based asthma interventions. The effectiveness of these interventions can be enhanced if individual approaches are *integrated*. The Allies Against Asthma coalitions have defined integration as "the alignment of concurrent activities across and within sectors in pursuit of a shared vision and common goals" (Krieger et al. 2006). One aspect of integration focuses on coordination of services to increase accessibility and continuity of care (Agranoff 1991). For example, agencies can link community-based activities such as home visits, self-management education and asthma camps to each other and to clinics through referral and communication mechanisms. They can collaborate on recruiting clients to services. Another dimension of integration relates to advocacy work. Coalitions can connect community and governmental organizations to pursue common policy objectives. Integration of systems, a third aspect of integration, can coordinate agencies to jointly plan and develop community interventions. An article by Krieger, et al. describes integration approaches in more detail (Krieger et al. 2006).

We found few evaluations of the effectiveness of integration efforts. An Australian controlled trial assessed integration of school-based education for parents and children with training of the teachers, community nurses, physicians and pharmacists who cared for these children. Six months after the intervention, bronchial hyper-responsiveness and nocturnal cough decreased and FEV_1 increased relative to baseline and the control group (Toelle et al. 1993).

Community Interventions to Reduce Health Disparities

Community-based interventions provide opportunities to address racial and economic asthma health disparities. Such disparities are well-documented (Gold and Wright 2005; Federico and Liu 2003) and are caused by multiple factors (Grant et al. 1999; Eggleston 1998b; Federico and Liu 2003). For example, living in substandard housing leads to exposure to indoor asthma triggers and higher rates of allergen sensitization (Huss et al. 1994b; Willies-Jacobo et al. 1993b; Sarpong et al. 1996b; Eggleston 2000b). As much as 40% of the excess asthma risk in minority children may be attributable to exposure to residential allergens (Lanphear et al. 2001). People affected by asthma disparities are more likely to live near point sources of pollutants and busy roadways (Mzng et al. 2006; Corburn et al. 2006). Low-income people report high levels of stress, and stress may directly affect airway function (Wright et al. 2005b). Low income people with asthma have difficulties in accessing medical care, medications, and devices.

Many of the interventions we have described and others found in this volume address these and other causes of asthma disparities. Services such as home visits, community health workers, and self-management education and support improve outcomes among low-income and minority people with asthma. Policy initiatives such as improving housing and outdoor environmental quality in minority and low-income neighborhoods tackle some of the underlying determinants of disparities.

Recommendations for Practice

A wide range of interventions is available for use in community settings. Some have convincing evidence of their effectiveness. Others are promising but need further evaluation before widespread adoption. Assessment of the feasibility of disseminating potentially effective interventions is urgently needed. Evidence of effectiveness from a controlled trial does not necessarily guarantee that replication of the intervention in community settings will succeed (Sadof et al. 2006; Wood et al. 2006b; Williams and Redd 2006; Glasgow et al. 2003).

In Table 17.2 we attempt to group the interventions we have discussed according to the quality of the evidence supporting their effectiveness and our assessment of the feasibility of replication in community settings.

Many considerations ultimately affect the interventions a community chooses to implement. Besides effectiveness and feasibility, available funding and other factors affecting the sustainability of the intervention, the prominence of local issues contributing to asthma morbidity, the interests and passions of local advocates and community members for specific approaches, gaps in local programs and policies, and the applicability of the intervention to specific racial and ethnic groups may shape the selection of the interventions. As communities develop community asthma action plans, it is appropriate that each arrive at a blend of interventions suited to local conditions.

Table 17.2 Community interventions, quality of the evidence supporting their effectiveness, and the feasibility of replication in community settings

	Feasibility		
Evidence	Low	Medium	High
High		Group education	Indoor trigger reduction Home visits
Medium	Community pharmacists	Housing quality improvement Mobile clinic	
Low	Housing code revision Community organization Sports Coach training	Support groups Outdoor air quality Community data systems	Camps Awareness Childcare education Case-finding Coalitions

References

Abdulwadud O, Abramson M, Forbes A, James A, Light L, Thien F, Walters EH (1997) Attendance at an asthma educational intervention: Characteristics of participants and non-participants. Respir Med 91:524–529

Agranoff R (1991) Human services integration: Past and present challenges in public administration. Public Adm Rev 51:533–542

AIRNow (2006) Home page. Available at: http://airnow.gov/, Accessed Nov 15, 2006

Alexander J, Divin-Cosgrove C, Faner ML, O'Connell M (2000) Increasing the knowledge base of asthmatics and their families through asthma clubs along the southwest border. J Am Acad Nurse Pract 12:260–266

Allen RM, Jones MP, Oldenburg B (1995) Randomised trial of an asthma self-management programme for adults. Thorax 50:731–738

Alliance for Healthy Homes (2006) Available at http://www.aeclp.org/. Accessed May 9, 2006

Allies Against Asthma (2007a) Available at: http://www.asthma.umich.edu/. Accessed April 9, 2007

Allies Against Asthma (2007b) Available at: http://www.asthma.umich.edu/About_Allies/Program_Summary/prog_sum.html. Accessed Jan 21, 2007

Allies Against Asthama (2007c) Available at: http://www.asthma.umich.edu/About_Allies/Evaluation/findings.html. Accessed Jan 21, 2007

Alternatives for Community and Environment (ACE) (2007) Available at: http://www.ace-ej.org/about#achievements. Accessed March 23, 2007

American Academy of Allergy, Asthma and Immunology (2007) Pediatric asthma: Promoting best practices. Available at: http://www.aaaai.org/members/resources/initiatives/pediatricasthma.stm. Accessed April 9, 2007

American Academy of Asthma, Allergy and Immunology (2007) Available at: http://www.aaaai.org/members/resources/initiatives/pediatricasthma.stm. Accessed April 9, 2007

American Cancer Society (2006a) State legislated action on tobacco issues: Restrictions on smoking in public places. Available at: http://www.cancer.org/docroot/PED/content/PED_10_12_State_Legislated_Actions_on_Tobacco_Issues.asp?sitearea=PED. Accessed Nov 16, 2006

American Cancer Society (2006b) Smoke-free ordinances spreading like wildfire! Available at: http://www.cancer.org/docroot/COM/content/div_TX/COM_4_5x_Smoke-Free_Ordinances_on_a_Roll_in_Texas.asp?sitearea=COM. Accessed Nov 16, 2006

American College of Chest Physicians (2007) A descriptive study of asthma coalitions. Available at: http://www.chestnet.org/patients/guides/asthmaStudy/p01.php. Accessed Jan 21, 2007

American Lung Association (2007) Asthma Walks. Available at: http://www.lungusa.org/site/pp.asp?c=dvLUK9O0E&b=37465. Accessed April 10, 2007

American Lung Association of Metropolitan Chicago (2006) Previous advocacy campaigns from American Lung Association of Metropolitan Chicago. Available at: http://lungaction.org/alaservingillinois/home.html. Accessed Nov 15, 2006

Apter AJ, Szefler SJ (2006) Advances in adult and pediatric asthma. J Allergy Clin Immunol 117:512–518

Arbes SJ Jr, Sever M, Archer J, Long EH, Gore JC, Schal C, Walter M, Nuebler B, Vaughn B, Mitchell H, Liu E, Collette N, Adler P, Sandel M, Zeldin DC (2003) A batement of cockroach allergen in low-income, urban housing: A randomized controlled trial. J Allergy Clin Immunol 112:339–345

Arbes SJ Jr, Sever M, Mehta J, Gore JC, Schal C, Vaughn B, Mitchell H, Zeldin DC (2004) Abatement of cockroach allergens in low-income, urban housing: Month 12 continuation results. J Allergy Clin Immunol 113:109–114

Arbes SJ, Sever M, Mehta J, Collette N, Thomas B, Zeldin DC (2005) Exposure to indoor allergens in day-care facilities: Results from 2 North Carolina counties. J Allergy Clin Immunol 116:133–139

Arlian LG, Neal JS, Morgan MS, Vyszenski-Moher DL, Rapp CM, Alexander AK (2001) Reducing relative humidity is a practical way to control dust mites and their allergens in homes in temperate climates. J Allergy Clin Immunol 107:99–104

Asthma and Allergy Foundation of America (2006) Asthma and allergy essentials for child care providers. Available at: http://

aafa.org/display.cfm?id=4&sub=79&cont=351. Accessed 8/9/06
Asthma and Allergy Foundation of America, New England Chapter (2006) For childcare providers. Available at: http://www.asthmaandallergies.org/Fr_ForChild.html. Accessed Aug 9, 2006
Asthma Coalition of Texas (2007) Texas asthma plan. Available at: http://www.texasasthma.org/pdf/Texas%20Asthma%20Plan%202007%20-%202010.pdf. Accessed April 9, 2007
Asthma Initiative of Michigan (2007) Asthma triggers. Available at: http://www.getasthmahelp.com/asthma_triggers.asp. Accessed April 9, 2007
Barbanel D, Eldridge S, Griffiths C (2003) Can a self-management programme delivered by a community pharmacist improve asthma control? A randomised trial. Thorax 58:851–854
Bay Area Air Quality Management District (2006) Home page. Available at: http://www.baaqmd.gov/. Accessed Nov 22, 2006
Bollinger ME, Foster M, Mebane D, Mudd K et al (2005) Impact of the breathmobile on baltimore city children with asthma (abstract). J Allergy Clin Immunol 115(Suppl 2 Pt 1):S144
Bonner S, Zimmerman BJ, Evans D, Irigoyen M, Resnick D, Mellins RB (2002) An individualized intervention to improve asthma management among urban Latino and African-American families. J Asthma 39:167–179
Boss LP, Wheeler LS, Williams PV, Bartholomew LK, Taggart VS, Redd SC (2003a) Population-based screening or case detection for asthma: Are we ready? J Asthma 40:335–342
Boss LP, Wheeler LS, Williams PV, Bartholomew LK, Taggart VS, Redd SC (2003b) Population-based screening or case detection for asthma: Are we ready? J Asthma 40:335–342
Boston Urban Asthma Coalition (2006) Healthy affordable housing. Available at: http://www.buac.org/healthy_affordable_housing.html. Accessed Oct 12, 2006
Boston Urban Asthma Coalition (2007) Available at: http://www.buac.org/about_us.html. Accessed April 10, 2007
Boutilier M, Cleverly S, Labonte R (2000) Community as a setting for health promotion. In: Poland, Blake D, Green, Lawrence W, Rootman I (eds) Settings for health promotion: Linking theory and practice. Sage, Thousand Oaks, CA pp 250–307
Brazil K, McLean L, Abbey D, Musselman C (1997) The influence of health education on family management of childhood asthma. Patient Educ Couns 30:107–118
Breathe Easy Homes at High Point (2007) Available at: http://www.thehighpoint.com/breatheasy.html. Accessed April 9, 2007
Brenner BL, Markowitz S, Rivera M, Romero H, Weeks M, Sanchez E et al (2003) Integrated pest management in an urban community: A successful partnership for prevention. Environ Health Perspect 111:1649–1653
British Thoracic Society and Scottish Intercollegiate Guidelines Network (2007) British guideline on the management of asthma. Available at: http://www.sign.ac.uk/pdf/sign63.pdf. Accessed April 9, 2007
Broms K, Svardsudd K, Sundelin C, Norback D (2006) A nationwide study of indoor and outdoor environments in allergen avoidance and conventional daycare centers in Sweden. Indoor Air 16:227–235
Brown JV, Demi AS, Wilson SR (2002) Home-based asthma education of young low-income children and their families. J Pediatric Psychol 27:667–688
Brown P, Mayer B, Zavestoski S, Luebke T, Mandelbaum J, McCormick S (2004) Clearing the air and breathing freely: The health politics of air pollution and asthma. Int J Health Serv 34:39–63
Brown JV, Demi AS, Celano MP, Bakeman R, Kobrynski L, Wilson SR (2005) A home visiting asthma education program: Challenges to program implementation. Health Educ Behav 32:42–56
Brownstein JN, Bone LR, Dennison CR, Hill MN, Kim MT, Levine DM (2005) Community health workers as interventionists in the prevention and control of heart disease and stroke. Am J Prev Med 29(Suppl 5, Pt 1):128–133
Bryant-Stephens T, Li Y (2004) Community asthma education program for parents of urban asthmatic children. J Natl Med Assoc 96:954–960
Bunting BA, Cranor CW (2006) The Asheville Project: Long-term clinical, humanistic, and economic outcomes of a community-based medication therapy management program for asthma. J Am Pharm Assoc 46:133–147
Butterfoss FD (2007) Coalitions and Partnerships in Community Health. Jossey-Bass. San Francisco, CA
Butterfoss FD, Kegler MC (2002) Toward a comprehensive understanding of community coalitions: Moving from practice to theory. In: DiClemente RJ, Crosby RA, Kegler MC (eds) Emerging theories in health promotion practice and research. Jossey-Bass, San Franscisco, CA, pp 157–193
Butterfoss FD, Goodman RM, Wandersman A (1993) Community coalitions for prevention and health promotion. Health Educ Res 8:315–330
Butz AM, Malveaux FJ, Eggleston P et al (1994) Use of community health workers with inner-city children who have asthma. Clin Pediat 33:135–141
Butz AM, Syron L, Johnson B, Spaulding J, Walker M, Bollinger ME (2005) Home-based asthma self-management education for inner city children. Public Health Nurs 22:189–199
Cagney KA, Browning CR (2004) Exploring neighborhood-level variation in asthma and other respiratory diseases: The contribution of neighborhood social context. J Gen Intern Med 19:229–236
California Asthma Public Health Initiative (2007) Available at: http://www.betterasthmacare.org/. Accessed April 9, 2007
California Strategic Plan for Asthma (2007) Available at: http://www.dhs.ca.gov/ps/deodc/ehib/asthma/documents/StrategicPlanForAsthma12-01(revised120606).pdf. Accessed April 9, 2007
Carswell F, Birmingham K, Oliver J, Crewes A, Weeks J (1996) The respiratory effects of reduction of mite allergen in the bedrooms of asthmatic children – a double-blind controlled trial. Clin Exp Allergy 26:386–396
Carter MC, Perzanowski MS, Raymond A et al (2001) Home intervention in the treatment of asthma among inner-city children. J Allergy Clin Immunol 108:732–737
Centers for Disease Control and Prevention (2007a) Asthma. Interventions. Available at: http://www.cdc.gov/asthma/interventions.htm. Accessed April 9, 2007
Centers for Disease Control and Prevention (2007b) Guide to community preventive services. Available at: http://www.thecommunityguide.org/. Accessed Jan 4, 2007
Centers for Disease Control and Prevention (2007c) Controlling asthma in American Cities. Available at: http://www.cdc.gov/asthma/aag03.htm#more. Accessed April 10, 2007

Centers for Disease Control and Prevention, Environmental Hazards and Health Effects Program (2007). Potentially effective interventions for asthma. Available at: http://www.cdc.gov/asthma/interventions/default.htm. Jan 4, 2007

Centers for Disease Prevention and Control. The Community Guide. Home-based multi-trigger, multicomponent interventions with an environmental focus. http://www.thecommunityguide.org/asthma/multicomponent.html. Accessed 9/1/09

Chapman MD (2005) Asthma in the third world: Can environmental intervention improve childhood asthma in US inner cities? Ann Allergy Asthma Immunol 95:496–497

Chernoff RG, Ireys HT, DeVet KA, Kim YJ (2002) A randomized, controlled trial of a community-based support program for families of children with chronic illness: Pediatric outcomes. Arch Pediatr Adolesc Med 156:533–539

Chicago Asthma Consortium (2007) Available at: http://www.chicagoasthma.org/site/epage/12590_410.htm. Accessed April 7, 2007

Christiansen SC, Martin SB, Schleicher NC, Koziol JA, Hamilton RG, Zuraw BL (1996) Exposure and sensitization to environmental allergen of predominantly hispanic children with asthma in San Diego's inner city. J Allergy Clin Immunol 98:288–294

Chung L, Parker EA, Israel BA (2006) Paper presented at: The community organizing network for environmental health (CONEH) evaluation

City of Boston Inspectional Services Department (2006) Breathe Easy Program. http://www.cityofboston.gov/isd/housing/bmc/default.asp. Accessed Oct 12, 2006

City of Seattle 2006–2007 action agenda, a global city acting locally (2007) Available at: http://www.seattle.gov/environment/Documents/eaa/2006_Brochure_color.pdf. Accessed Jan 21, 2007

Clark NM, Valerio MA (2003) The role of behavioral theories in educational interventions for pediatric asthma. Pediatr Respir Rev 4:325–333

Clark NM, Gong M, Kaciroti N (2001) A model of self-regulation for control of chronic disease. Health Educ Behav 28:769–782

Clark NM, Doctor LJ, Friedman AR, Lachance LL, Houle CR, Geng X, Grisso JA (2006) Community coalitions to control chronic disease: Allies against asthma as a model and case study. Health Promot Pract 7(Suppl):S14–S22

Clougherty JE, Levy JI, Hynes HP, Spengler JD (2006) A longitudinal analysis of the efficacy of environmental interventions on asthma-related quality of life and symptoms among children in urban public housing. J Asthma 43:335–343

Colloff MJ, Taylor C, Merrett TG (1995) The use of domestic steam cleaning for the control of house dust mites. Clin Exp Allergy 25:1061–1066

Colorado Department of Public Health and Environment (2006) Local residential burning program status. Available at: http://www.cdphe.state.co.us/ap/woodlocal.html. Accessed Nov 22, 2006

Comino EJ, Bauman A, Mitchell CA, Ruffin RE, Antic R, Zimmerman PV, Gutch RC (1997) The Australian national asthma campaign: Effects of public education activities based on mass media. Am J Prev Med 13:251–256

Community Action to Fight Asthma (2006a) Home page. Available at: http://www.CalAsthma.org/. Accessed July 13, 2006

Community Action to Fight Asthma (2006b) Home page. Available at: http://www.CalAsthma.org/. Accessed July 13, 2006

Community Action to Fight Asthma (2006c) Home page. Available at: http://www.CalAsthma.org/. Accessed July 13, 2006

Community Action to Fight Asthma (2007) Available at: http://www.calasthma.org/. Accessed April 9, 2007

Connecticut Department of Public Health (2006) Managing asthma in connecticut child care facilities. Available at: http://www.dph.state.ct.us/BCH/new_asthma/asthma_in_schools.htm. Accessed Aug 6, 2006

Corburn J, Osleeb J, Porter M (2006) Urban asthma and the neighbourhood environment in New York City. Health Place 12:167–179

Cordina M, McElnay JC, Hughes CM (2001) Assessment of a community pharmacy-based program for patients with asthma. Pharmacotherapy 21:1196–1203

Cote J, Bowie DM, Robichaud P, Parent JG, Battisti L, Boulet LP (2001) Evaluation of two different educational interventions for adult patients consulting with an acute asthma exacerbation. Am J Respir Crit Care Med 163:1415–1419

Cramer ME, Mueller KJ, Harrop D (2003) Evaluation informs coalition programming for environmental tobacco smoke reduction. J Community Health Nurse 20:245–258

Creating healthy urban environments for all (2007) Available at http://www.cityofseattle.net/environment/clean_air.htm. Accessed Jan 21, 2007

Dallas Asthma Consortium (2006) Rule of Two Project. Available at: www.dallasasthma.org/index_rule-project.htm. Accessed July 14, 2006

de Blay F, Fourgaut G, Hedelin G, Vervloet D et al (2003) Medical Indoor Environment Counselor (MIEC): Role in compliance with advice on mite allergen avoidance and on mite allergen exposure. Allergy 58:27–33

DeGuire LJ (2006) EnviroFlash: Your environmental news flash – Michigan program. Available at: http://www.deq.state.mi.us/documents/deq-aqd-enviroflash_presentation.pdf. Accessed Nov 15, 2006

deOliveira MA, Feresin SM, Bruno VF, de Bittencourt AR, Fernandes AL (1999) Evaluation of an educational programme for socially deprived asthma patients. Eur Respir J 14:908–914

Diamond SA, Chapman KR (2001) The impact of a nationally coordinated pharmacy-based asthma education intervention. Can Respir J 8:261–265

Dimich-Ward H, Lawson J, Hingston A, Chan-Yeung M (2005) Impact of smoking policy on the respiratory health of food and beverage servers. Scand J Work Environ Health 31:75–81

Dolinar RM, Kumar V, Countu-Wakulcyzk G, Rowe BH (2000) Pilot study of a home-based asthma health education program. Patient Educ Couns 40:93–102

Eder W, Ege MJ, von Mutius E (2006) The asthma epidemic. N Engl J Med 355:2226–2235

Eggleston PA (1998a) Urban children and asthma. Immunol Allergy Clin North Am 18:75–84

Eggleston PA (1998b) Urban children and asthma. Immunol Allergy Clin North Am 18:75–84

Eggleston PA (2000a) Environmental causes of asthma in inner city children. The National Cooperative Inner City Asthma Study. Clin Rev Allergy Immunol 18:311–324

Eggleston PA (2000b) Environmental causes of asthma in inner city children. The national cooperative inner city asthma study. Clin Rev Allergy Immunol 18:311–324

Eggleston PA (2005a) Improving indoor environments: Reducing allergen exposures. J Allergy Clin Immunol 116:122–126
Eggleston PA (2005b) Improving indoor environments: Reducing allergen exposures. J Allergy Clin Immunol 116:122–126
Eggleston PA, Butz A, Rand C, Curtin-Brosnan J, Kanchanaraksa S, Swartz L, Breysse P, Buckley T, Diette G, Merriman B, Krishnan JA (2005) Home environmental intervention in inner-city asthma: A randomized controlled clinical trial. Ann Allergy Asthma Immunol 95:518–524
Ehnert B, Lau-Schadendorf S, Weber A, Buettner P, Schou C, Wahn U (1992) Reducing domestic exposure to dust mite allergen reduces bronchial hyper reactivity in sensitive children with asthma. J Allergy Clin Immunol 90:135–138
Emergency Medical Services Authority (2006) Available at: www.emsa.cahwnet.gov/def_comm/vi_asthma061103.asp. Accessed Aug 9, 2006
Emmerton L, Shaw J, Kheir N (2003) Asthma management by New Zealand pharmacists: A pharmaceutical care demonstration project. J Clin Pharm Ther 28:395–402
Environmental Protection (2006) Agency, T.U.S.E.P. cleaning burning woodstoves and fireplaces. Available at: http://www.epa.gov/airprogm/oar/woodstoves/programs.html. Accessed Feb 23, 2006
Environmental Protection Agency (2007a) Available at: http://www.epa.gov/asthma/programs.html. Accessed April 9, 2007
Environmental Protection Agency (2007b) Asthma awareness month. Available at: http://www.epa.gov/asthma/awm.html. Accessed April 10, 2007
US Environmental Protection Agency (2006a) In-home environmental education. Available at: http://www.epa.gov/asthma/inhome.html. Accessed Aug 22, 2006
US Environmental Protection Agency (2006b) Compilation of state, county, and local anti-idling regulations. Available at: www.epa.gov/smartway. Accessed March 23, 2007
U.S. Environmental Protection Agency, Air – Indoor Air Quality (IAQ) (2006) Available at: http://www.epa.gov/iaq/index.html. Accessed May 9, 2006
Federico MJ, Liu AH (2003) Overcoming childhood asthma disparities of the inner-city poor. Pediatr Clin North Am 50:655–675
Fernandez-Caldas E, Codina R, Ledford DK, Trudeau WL, Lockey RF (2001) House dust mite, cat, and cockroach allergen concentrations in daycare centers in Tampa, Florida. Ann Allergy Asthma Immunol 87:196–200
Fisher EB, Strunk RC, Sussman LK, Sykes RK, Walker MS (2004) Community organization to reduce the need for acute care for asthma among African American children in low-income neighborhoods: The Neighborhood Asthma Coalition. Pediatrics 114:116–123
Fisher EB, Strunk RC, Highstein GR, et al (2009) A randomized controlled evaluation of the effect of community health workers on hospitalization for asthma: the asthma coach. Arch Pediatr Adolesc Med 163(3):225–232
Fitzpatrick SB, Coughlin SS, Chamberlin J (1992) A novel asthma camp intervention for childhood asthma among urban blacks. The pediatric lung committee of the American Lung Association of the District of Columbia (ALADC). Washington, DC. J Natl Med Assoc 84:233–237
Fletcher AM, Pickering CA, Custovic A, Simpson J, Kennaugh J, Woodcock A (1996) Reduction in humidity as a method of controlling mites and mite allergens: The use of mechanical ventilation in British domestic dwellings. Clin Exp Allergy 26:1051–1056
Friedman AR, Butterfoss FD, Krieger JW, Peterson JW, Dwyer M, Wicklund K et al (2006) Allies community health workers: Bridging the gap. Health Promot Pract 7:96S–107S
Gallant MP (2003) The influence of social support on chronic illness self-management: A review and directions for research. Health Educ Behav 30:170–195
Gallefoss F, Bakke PS (2000) Impact of patient education and self-management on morbidity in asthmatics and patients with chronic obstructive pulmonary disease. Respir Med 94:279–287
Gauderman WJ, Vora H, McConnell R, Berhane K, Gilliland F, Thomas D et al (2007) Effect of exposure to traffic on lung development from 10 to 18 years of age: A cohort study. Lancet 369:571–577
Gelber LE, Seltzer LH, Bouzoukis JK, Pollart SM, Chapman MD, Platts-Mills TA (1993) Sensitization and exposure to indoor allergens as risk factors for asthma among patients presenting to hospital. Am Rev Respir Dis 147:573–578
Gerald LB, Grad R, Turner-Henson A, Hains C, Tang S, Feinstein R et al (2004) Validation of a multistage asthma case-detection procedure for elementary school children. Pediatrics 114:459–468
Gergen PJ, Mortimer KM, Eggleston PA, Rosenstreich D, Mitchell H, Ownby D, Kattan M, Baker D, Wright EC, Slavin R, Malveaux F (1999) Results of the National Cooperative Inner-City Asthma Study (NCICAS) environmental intervention to reduce cockroach allergen exposure in inner-city homes. J Allergy Clin Immunol 103(3 Pt 1):501–506
Glasgow RE, Lichtenstein E, Marcus AC (2003) Why don't we see more translation of health promotion research to practice? Rethinking the efficacy-to-effectiveness transition. Am J Public Health 93:1261–1267
Global Initiative Against Asthma (2007) World Asthma Day. Available at: http://www.ginasthma.com/WADIndex.asp. Accessed April 10, 2007
Global Initiative for Asthma (2005) Update: Workshop Report, Global Strategy for Asthma Management and Prevention. Available at: http://www.ginasthma.com/Guidelineitem.asp?l1=2&l2=1&intId=1169. Accessed April 9, 2007
Gold DR, Wright R (2005) Population disparities in asthma. Annu Rev Public Health 26:89–113
Gotzsche PC, Johansen HK, Schmidt LM, Burr ML (2004) House dust mite control measures for asthma. Cochrane Database Syst Rev 4:CD001187
Goveia MG, Shaikh N et al (2005) Asthma-related environmental practices and asthma awareness in California child care centers. Pediatr Asthma Allergy Immunol 18:12–24
Grant EN, Alp H, Weiss KB (1999) The challenge of inner-city asthma. Curr Opin Pulm Med 5:27–34
Group Health Community Foundation Evaluation Team (2007) Evaluation of Seattle/King County Allies Against Asthma. Section 1: Using Community Health Workers to improve asthma knowledge, self-management, home environment and linkages to community resources. Available at: http://www.metrokc.gov/health/asthma/evaluation/section1.pdf. Section 2. Improved Clinic Practices Around Asthma Control http://www.metrokc.gov/health/asthma/evaluation/section4.pdf. Accessed April 8, 2007
Halken S, Host A, Niklassen U, Hansen LG, Nielsen F, Pedersen S, Osterballe O, Veggerby C, Poulsen LK (2003) Effect of mat-

tress and pillow encasings on children with asthma and house dust mite allergy. J Allergy Clin Immunol 111:169–176

Harving H, Korsgaard J, Dahl R (1994) Clinical efficacy of reduction in house-dust mite exposure in specially designed, mechanically ventilated "healthy" homes. Allergy 49:866–870

Hazell J, Henry RL, Francis JL (2006) Improvement in asthma management practices in child care services: An evaluation of a staff education program. Health Promot J Austr 17:21–26

Hoppin P, Jacobs M, Ribble M (2006) Enhancing asthma management using in-home environmental interventions: A review of public health department programs. Asthma Regional Council of New England, Dorchester MA, September 2006. Available at: http://www.asthmaregionalcouncil.org/documents/EnhancingAsthmaManagementUsingIn-HomeEnvironmentalInterventionsHoppin_000.doc. Accessed Oct 12, 2006

Howden-Chapman P, Crane J, Matheson A, Viggers H, Cunningham M, Blakely T et al (2005) Retrofitting houses with insulation to reduce health inequalities: Aims and methods of a clustered, randomized community-based trial. Soc Sci Med 61:2600–2610

Hricko AM (2004) Problems along the new "silk road". Environ Health Perspect 112:A879

Hricko AM (2006) Ships, trucks, and trains: Effects of goods movement on environmental health. Environ Health Perspect 114:204–205

Huss K, Rand CS, Butz AM et al (1994a) Home environmental risk factors in urban minority asthmatic children. Ann Allergy 72:173–177

Huss K, Rand CS, Butz AM et al (1994b) Home environmental risk factors in urban minority asthmatic children. Ann Allergy 72:173–177

Indiana Department of Environmental Management (2006) Protecting Children from Environmental Threats/Self Assessment for Child Care Facilities and 5-Star Environmental Recognition Program. Available at: http://www.in.gov/apps/idem/media/publications/servlet/secondPage?idNumber=735. Accessed Aug 9, 2006

Jones CA, Hanley-Lopez J, Kwong KY, Clement LT et al (2000) Breathmobile program: Two year outcomes. J Allergy Clin Immunol 105(Suppl 1 Pt 2):S103

Jones CA, Morphew T, Clement LT, Kimia T, Dyer M, Li M, Hanley-Lopez J (2004) Breathmobile program. A school-based case identification process for identifying inner city children with asthma: The Breathmobile program. Chest 125:924–934

Katz LF, Liebman JB (2001) Moving to opportunity in Boston: Early years of a randomized mobility experiment. Q J Econ 116:607–654

Keeler GJ, Dvonch T, Yip FY, Parker EA, Israel BA, Marsik FJ et al (2002) Assessment of personal and community-level exposures to particulate matter among children with asthma in Detroit, Michigan, as part of Community Action Against Asthma (CAAA). Environ Health Perspect 110:173–181

Kelly CS, Shield SW, Gowen MA, Jaganjac N, Andersen CL, Strope GL (1998) Outcomes analysis of a summer asthma camp. J Asthma 35(2):165–71. PubMed PMID: 9576142

Kercsmar CM, Dearborn DG, Schluchter M, Xue L et al (2006) Reduction in asthma morbidity in children as a result of a home remediation aimed at moisture sources. Environ Health Perspect 114:1574–1580

Kim J, Hanley JA (2002) The role of woodstoves in the etiology of nasal polyposis. Arch Otolaryngol Head Neck Surg 128:682–686

King County Environmental Purchasing Program (2007) Available at: http://www.metrokc.gov/procure/green/hybrids.htm, Accessed Jan 21, 2007

Kinney PL, Northridge ME, Chew GL, Gronning E, Joseph E, Correa JC, Prakash S, Goldstein I (2002) On the front lines: An environmental asthma intervention in New York City. Am J Public Health 92:24–26

Kotses H, Bernstein IL, Bernstein DI, Reynolds RV, Korbee L, Wigal JK, Ganson E, Stout C, Creer TL (1995) A self-management program for adult asthma. Part I: Development and evaluation. J Allergy Clin Immunol 95:529–540

Krieger J, Higgins DL (2002) Housing and health: Time again for public health action. Am J Public Health 92:758–768

Krieger JK, Takaro TK, Allen C et al (2002) The Seattle-King County Healthy Homes Project: Implementation of a comprehensive approach to improving indoor environmental quality for low-income children with asthma. Environ Health Perspect 110(Suppl 2):311–322

Krieger JW, Takaro TK, Song L, Weaver M (2005) The Seattle-King County Healthy Homes project: A randomized, controlled trial of a community health worker intervention to decrease exposure to indoor asthma triggers. Am J Public Health 95:652–659

Krieger JW, Bourcier E, Lara M, Peterson JW, Rosenthal MP, Taylor-Fishwick JC, Friedman AR, Lachance LL, Doctor LJ (2006) Integrating asthma prevention and control: The roles of the coalition. Health Promot Pract 7(Suppl):S127–S138

Krieger J, Takaro TK, Rabkin J. Breathe easy in Seattle: Addressing asthma disparities through healthier housing. In: Williams RA (ed) Eliminating healthcare disparities in America. Humana Press, Totowa, NJ 313–340

Krieger JW, Takaro T, Song L, Beaudet N, Edwards K (2009) The Seattle-King County Healthy Homes II Project: A Randomized Controlled Trial of Asthma Self-Management Support Comparing Clinic-Based Nurses and In-Home Community Health Workers. Arch of Pediatr Adolesc Med 163:141–149

Lanphear BP, Aligne CA, Auinger P, Weitzman M, Byrd RS (2001) Residential exposures associated with asthma in US children. Pediatrics 107:505–511

Larson TV, Yuen P, Maykut N (1992) Weekly composite sampling of PM2.5 for total mass and trace elements analysis. In: Chow J (ed) Transactions of the air and waste management association specialty conference on PM10 standards and non-traditional particulate source controls, Air & Waste Management Association Pittsburgh, PA, pp 112–130

Levy JI, Brugge D, Peters JL, Clougherty JE, Saddler SS (2006) A community-based participatory research study of multifaceted in-home environmental interventions for pediatric asthmatics in public housing. Soc Sci Med 63:2191–2203

Lewin SA, Dick J, Pond P, Zwarenstein M, Aja G, van Wyk B, Bosch-Capblanch X, Patrick M (2005) Lay health workers in primary and community health care. Cochrane Database Syst Rev 1:CD004015

Lewis MA, Lewis CE, Leake B, Monahan G, Rachelefsky G (1996) Organizing the community to target poor latino children with asthma. J Asthma 33:289–297

Lewis TC, Robins TG, Joseph CL, Parker EA, Israel BA, Rowe Z, Edgren KK, Salinas MA, Martinez ME, Brown RW (2004) Identification of gaps in the diagnosis and treatment of childhood asthma using a community-based participatory research approach. J Urban Health 81:472–488

Lewis TC, Robins TG, Dvonch JT, Keeler GJ, Yip FY, Mentz GB et al (2005) Air pollution associated changes in lung function among asthmatic children in Detroit. Environ Health Perspect 113:1068–1075

Liao O, Morphew T, Amaro S, Galant SP (2006) The breathmobile: A novel comprehensive school-based mobile asthma care clinic for urban underprivileged children. J Sch Health 76:313–319

Lord A, St Leger LH, Ridge DT, Elisha D (2001) The value of asthma camps for young people in Victoria, Australia. Contemp Nurse 11:133–141

Love MB, Gardner K, Legion V (1997) Community health workers: Who they are and what they do. Health Educ Behav 24:510–522

Lucas DO, Zimmer LO, Paul JE, Jones D, Slatko G, Liao W, Lashley J (2001) Two-year results from the asthma self-management program: Long-term impact on health care services, costs, functional status, and productivity. J Asthma 38:321–330

Lwebuga-Mukasa JS, Oyana T, Thenappan A, Ayirookuzhi SJ (2004) Association between traffic volume and health care use for asthma among residents at a U.S.-Canadian border crossing point. J Asthma 41:289–304

Macher J (ed) (1999) Bioaerosols: Assessment and control. American Conference of Governmental Industrial Hygienists, Cinncinati, OH

Mangiapane S, Schulz M, Muhlig S, Ihle P, Schubert I, Waldmann HC (2005) Community pharmacy-based pharmaceutical care for asthma patients. Ann Pharmacother 39:1817–1822

Martin MA, Hernandez O, Naureckas E, Lantos J (2006) Reducing home triggers for asthma: The Latino community health worker approach. J Asthma 43:369–374

Martinez FD (2007) Genes, environments, development and asthma: A reappraisal. Eur Respir J 29:179–184

Mathur SK, Busse WW (2006) Asthma: Diagnosis and management. Med Clin North Am 90:39–60

McConnell R, Jones C, Milam J, Gonzalez P, Berhane K, Clement L et al (2003a) Cockroach counts and house dust allergen concentrations after professional cockroach control and cleaning. Ann Allergy Asthma Immunol 91:546–552

McConnell R, Berhane K, Gilliland F, Molitor J, Thomas D, Lurmann F et al (2003b) Prospective study of air pollution and bronchitic symptoms in children with asthma. Am J Respir Crit Care Med 168:790–797

McConnell R, Milam J, Richardson J, Galvan J, Jones C, Thorne PS, Berhane K (2005) Educational intervention to control cockroach allergen exposure in the homes of hispanic children in Los Angeles: Results of the La Casa study. Clin Exp Allergy 35:426–433

McLean WM, MacKeigan LD (2005) When does pharmaceutical care impact health outcomes? A comparison of community pharmacy-based studies of pharmaceutical care for patients with asthma. Ann Pharmacother 39:625–631

McLean W, Gillis J, Waller R (2003) The BC community pharmacy asthma study: A study of clinical, economic and holistic outcomes influenced by an asthma care protocol provided by specially trained community pharmacists in British Columbia. Can Respir J 10:195–202

Meng A (1997) An asthma day camp. MCN Am J Matern Child Nurse 22:135–141

Merck Childhood Asthma Network (2007a) Program sites. Available at: http://www.mcanonline.org/sites/index.html. Accessed April 9, 2007

Merck Childhood Asthma Network (2007b) Available at: http://www.mcanonline.org/. Access Jan 21, 2007

Miller DM, Meek F (2004) Cost and efficacy comparison of integrated pest management strategies with monthly spray insecticide applications for German cockroach control in public housing. J Econ Entomol 97:559–569

Minnesota Department of Health (2007) Minnesota state asthma plan. Available at: http://www.health.state.mn.us/divs/hpcd/cdee/asthma/StatePlan.html. Accessed April 9, 2007

Mistry R, Wickramasingha N, Ogston S, Singh M, Devasiri V, Mukhopadhya S (2004) Wheeze and urban variation in South Asia. Eur J Pediatr 163:145–147

Mongelluzzo B (2006) Not in my back yard, J Commerce (online). Nov 13, 2006. Accessed 1/21/07

Morgan WJ, Crain EF, Gruchalla RS, O'Connor GT, Kattan M, Evans R III, Stout J, Malindzak G, Smartt E, Plaut M, Walter M, Vaughn B, Mitchell H (2004) Inner-City Asthma Study Group: Results of a home-based environmental intervention among urban children with asthma. N Engl J Med 351:1068–1080

Munir AK, Einarsson R, Dreborg S (1996) Allergen avoidance in a day-care center. Allergy 51:36–41

Muntner P, Sudre P, Uldry C, Rochat T, Courteheuse C, Naef AF, Perneger TV (2001) Predictors of participation and attendance in a new asthma patient self-management education program. Chest 120:778–784

Mzng YY, Rull RP, Wilhelm M, Ritz B et al (2006) Living near heavy traffic increases asthma severity. UCLA Center for Health Policy Research, Los Angeles

Narhi U, Airaksinen M, Tanskanen P, Erlund H (2000) Therapeutic outcomes monitoring by community pharmacists for improving clinical outcomes in asthma. J Clin Pharm Ther 25:177–183

National Asthma Council of Australia (2007) Available at: http://www.nationalasthma.org.au/html/management/home/index.asp. Accessed April 9, 2007

National Asthma Education and Prevention Program (2007a). Expert Panel Report 2: Guidelines for the Diagnosis and Management of Asthma. Available at: http://www.nhlbi.nih.gov/guidelines/asthma/asthgdln.htm. Accessed April 9, 2007

National Asthma Education and Prevention Program (2007b) Available at: http://www.nhlbi.nih.gov/about/naepp/index.htm. Accessed Feb 23, 2007

National Asthma Education and Prevention Program (2007c) Available at: http://hp2010.nhlbihin.net/ast_maps/awardee.html. Accessed Jan 21, 2007

National Asthma Education and Prevention Program Expert Panel Report (2002) Guidelines for the diagnosis and management of asthma update on selected topics-2002. J Allergy Clin Immunol 110:141–219

National Center for Healthy Housing (2006) Available at: http://www.centerforhealthyhousing.org/index.html, Accessed May 9, 2006

National Center for Healthy Housing (2007) Comparing green building guidelines and healthy homes principles: A preliminary investigation. Available at: http://www.centerforhealthyhousing.org/html/green_analysis.htm. Accessed April 9, 2007

National Conference of State Legislators (2007) Asthma-related state legislation and statutes database. Available at: http://www.ncsl.org/programs/environ/envhealth/asthma.cfm. Accessed April 9, 2007

National Heart, Lung, and Blood Institute (2006) How asthma-friendly is your child-care setting? Checklist. Available at: http://www.nhlbi.nih.gov/health/public/lung/asthma/chc_chk.htm. Accessed Aug 22, 2006

National Heart, Lung and Blood Institute (2007) National asthma education and prevention program. Available at: http://hp2010.nhlbihin.net/naepp.htm. Accessed April 9, 2007

Nemcek MA, Sabatier R (2003) State of evaluation: Community health workers. Public Health Nurse 20:260–270

Nesvold JH, Fena PG, Herman J (2006) Consortium On Children's Asthma Camps Board Of Directors. Assessing the value of children's asthma camps. J Asthma 43:273–277

New England Regional Asthma Council (2007) Available at: http://www.asthmaregionalcouncil.org/. Accessed April 9, 2007

New York City Department of Health (2000) Guidelines on assessment and remediation of fungi in indoor environments

New York City Department of Health and Mental Hygiene (2007) Asthma initiative. Available at: http://www.nyc.gov/html/doh/html/asthma/asthma.shtml. Accessed April 9, 2007

New York State Department of Health (2007) Regional Asthma Coalitions in New York State. Available at: http://www.health.state.ny.us/diseases/asthma/coalitions.htm. Accessed April 24, 2007

News release, Metro Transit earns national Clean Air Excellence Award (2007) Available at: http://www.metrokc.gov/exec/news/2006/0405hybrid.aspx. Accessed Jan 21, 2007

News release, Sims: King County will quadruple biodiesel use (2007) Available at: http://www.metrokc.gov/exec/news/2006/0318biodiesel.aspx. Accessed Jan 21, 2007

Nicholas SW, Hutchinson VE, Ortiz B, Klihr-Beall S, et al (2005) Reducing childhood asthma through community-based service delivery. New York, 2001–2004. MMWR 54:11–14

Niven R, Fletcher AM, Pickering AC, Custovic A, Sivour JB, Preece AR, Oldham LA, Francis HC (1999) Attempting to control mite allergens with mechanical ventilation and dehumidification in British houses. J Allergy Clin Immunol 103(Suppl 5 Pt 1):756–762

O'Connor GT (2005) Allergen avoidance in asthma: What do we do now? J Allergy Clin Immunol 116:26–30

Oregon Asthma Leadership Plan (2007) Available at: http://oregon.gov/DHS/ph/asthma/plan/index.shtml. Accessed April 9, 2007

Parker EA, Salinas M (2002) Community-based participatory research interventions for asthma. Paper presented at the American Thoracic Society, Atlanta, GA. May 19, 2002

Parker EP, Baldwin GT, Israel B, Salinas M (2004) Application of health promotion theories and models for environmental health. Health Educ Behav 31:491–509

Parker EA, Lewis TC, Israel BA, Robins TG, Mentz G, Lin X et al (2008) Evaluation of community action against asthma: A community health worker intervention to improve children's asthma-related health by reducing household environmental triggers for asthma. Heal Ed Behav Vol. 35, 3:376–395

Patterson EE, Brennan MP, Linskey KM, Webb DC, Shields MD, Patterson CC (2005) A cluster randomized intervention trial of asthma clubs to improve quality of life in primary school children: The School Care and Asthma Management Project (SCAMP). Arch Dis Child 90:786–791

Perez M, Findley SE, Mejia M, Martinez J (2006) The impact of community health worker training and programs in NYC. J Health Care Poor Underserved 17(Suppl 1):26–43

Philadelphia Allies Against Asthma (2007) LinkLine. Available at: http://www.phillyhealthinfo.org/index.php/general/philadelphia_allies_against_asthma_coalition/. Accessed April 10, 2007

Phipatanakul W, Cronin B, Wood RA, Eggleston PA, Shih MC, Song L, Tachdjian R, Oettgen HC (2004) Effect of environmental intervention on mouse allergen levels in homes of inner-city Boston children with asthma. Ann Allergy Asthma Immunol 92:420–425

Pierce J, Orlando D, Hortman P, Risko T, Powell KE (2000) Corporate action to reduce air pollution – Atlanta, Georgia, 1998–1999. MMWR 4:153–156

Powell H, Gibson PG (2002) Options for self-management education for adults with asthma. Cochrane Database Syst Rev 3:CD004107

Primomo J, Johnston S, DiBiase F, Nodolf J, Noren L (2006) Evaluation of a community-based outreach worker program for children with asthma. Public Health Nurs 23:234–241

Public Health – Seattle & King County (2006) Seattle Healthy Homes Project. Available at: http://www.metrokc.gov/health/asthma/healthyhomes/overview.htm. Accessed Oct 8, 2006

Public Health – Seattle & King County (2007) Asthma. Available at: http://www.metrokc.gov/health/asthma/. Accessed April 10, 2007

Punnett AF, Thurber S (1993) Evaluation of the asthma camp experience for children. J Asthma 30:195–198

Redline S, Gruchalla RS, Wolf RL, Yawn BP, Cartar L, Gan V, Nelson P, Wollan P (2004) Development and validation of school-based asthma and allergy screening questionnaires in a 4-city study. Ann Allergy Asthma Immunol 93:36–48

Regional Asthma Management and Prevention (2007) Available at: http://www.rampasthma.org/. Accessed April 9, 2007

Rijssenbeek-Nouwens LH, Oosting AJ, de Bruin-Weller MS, Bregman I, de Monchy JG, Postma DS (2002) Clinical evaluation of the effect of anti-allergic mattress covers in patients with moderate to severe asthma and house dust mite allergy: A randomized double blind placebo controlled study. Thorax 57:784–790

Rupp MT, McCallian DJ, Sheth KK (1997) Developing and marketing a community pharmacy-based asthma management program. J Am Pharm Assoc NS37:694–699

Sadof MD, Boschert KA, Brandt SJ, Motyl AP (2006) An analysis of predictors of sustainability efforts at the Inner-City Asthma Intervention sites: After the funding is gone. Ann Allergy Asthma Immunol 97(Suppl 1 Pt 1):S31–S35

Saini B, Krass I, Armour C (2004) Development, implementation, and evaluation of a community pharmacy-based asthma care model. Ann Pharmacother 38:1954–1960

Samet JM, Dominici F, Curriero FC, Coursac I, Zeger SL (2000) Fine particulate air pollution and mortality in 20 U.S. cities, 1987–1994. New Engl J Med 343:1742–1749

San Diego Regional Asthma Coalition (2006) Trash, litter, pests, and housing issues. Available at: http://www.calasthma.org/resources/show_resource/312/. Accessed Oct 10, 2006

Sandel M, Phelan K, Wright R, Hynes HP, Lanphear BP (2004a) The effects of housing interventions on child health. Pediatr Ann 33:474–481

Sandel M, Phelan K, Wright R, Hynes HP, Lanphear BP (2004b) The effects of housing interventions on child health. Pediatr Ann 33:474–481

Sarpong SB, Hamilton RG, Eggleston PA, Adkinson NF (1996a) Socioeconomic status and race as risk factors for cockroach allergen exposure and sensitization in children with asthma. J Allergy Clin Immunol 97:1393–1401

Sarpong SB, Hamilton RG, Eggleston PA, Adkinson NF (1996b) Socioeconomic status and race as risk factors for cockroach allergen exposure and sensitization in children with asthma. J Allergy Clin Immunol 97:1393–1401

Schmidt DK, Fulwood R, Lenfant C (1999) The national asthma education and prevention program: Partnering with local asthma coalitions to implement the guidelines. Chest 116(Suppl 4 Pt 1):S235–S236

Schulz M, Verheyen F, Muhlig S, Muller JM, Muhlbauer K, Knop-Schneickert E et al (2001) Pharmaceutical care services for asthma patients: A controlled intervention study. J Clin Pharmacol 41:668–676

Schwartz RH (2006) SOPHE, health promotion practice, and allies against asthma: A special collaboration. Health Promot Pract 7(Suppl):S7

Siegel M, Albers AB, Cheng DM, Biener L, Rigotti NA (2005) Effect of local restaurant smoking regulations on progression to established smoking among youths. Tob Control 14:300–306

Silvers WS, Holbreich M, Go S, Morrison MR, Dennis W, Marostica T, Buckley JM (1992) Champ camp: The Colorado children's asthma camp experience. J Asthma 29:121–135

Simpson A, Custovic A (2005) The role of allergen avoidance in the secondary prevention of atopic disorders. Curr Opin Allergy Clin Immunol 5:223–227

Smith JR, Mildenhall S, Noble MJ, Shepstone L, Koutantji M, Mugford M, Harrison BD (2005) The coping with asthma study: A randomised controlled trial of a home based, nurse led psycho educational intervention for adults at risk of adverse asthma outcomes. Thorax 60:1003–1011

Somerville M, Mackenzie I, Owen P, Miles D (2000) Housing and health: Does installing heating in their homes improve the health of children with asthma? Public Health 114:434–439

Sorrells VD, Chung W, Schlumpberger JM (1995) The impact of a summer asthma camp experience on asthma education and morbidity in children. J Fam Pract 41:465–468

Steps to a Healthier US (2007) Available at: http://www.cdc.gov/steps/steps_communities/index.htm. Accessed April 9, 2007

Stergachis A, Gardner JS, Anderson MT, Sullivan SD (2002) Improving pediatric asthma outcomes in the community setting: Does pharmaceutical care make a difference? J Am Pharm Assoc (Wash) 42:743–752

Storey E, Dangman KH, Schenck P, Yang C et al (2004) Guidance for clinicians on the recognition and management of health effects related to mold exposure and moisture indoors. University of Connecticut Health Center, Center for Environments and Health, Farmington, CT

Swider SM (2002a) Outcome effectiveness of community health workers: An integrative literature review. Public Health Nurs 19:11–20

Swider SM (2002b) Outcome effectiveness of community health workers: An integrative literature review. Public Health Nurs 19:11–20

Task Force on Community Preventive Services (2000) Recommendations regarding interventions to reduce tobacco use and exposure to environmental tobacco smoke. Am J Prev Med 20(Suppl 2):10–15

Tesfaigzi Y, Singh SP, Foster JE, Kubatko J, Barr EB, Fine PM et al (2002) Health effects of subchronic exposure to low levels of wood smoke in rats. Toxicol Sci 65:115–125

The Cochrane Collaboration (2007) Available at: http://www.cochrane.org/index.htm. Accessed Jan 4, 2007

The Consort Group (2007) Available at: http://www.consort-statement.org/, Accessed Jan 4, 2007

Thompson M, Phillips R, Bell J (2002) Fighting childhood asthma: How communities can win. A Policy Link Report. Oakland, CA

Toelle BG, Peat JK, Salmoe CM, Mellis CM et al (1993) Evaluation of a community-based asthma management program in a population sample of school children. Med J Aust 158:742–746

U.S. Department of Housing and Urban Development, Office of Healthy Homes and Lead Hazard Control (2006) Available at: http://www.hud.gov/offices/lead/index.cfm. Accessed May 9, 2006

United States Preventive Services Task Force (2007) Available at: http://www.ahrq.gov/clinic/uspstfix.htm Accessed Jan 4, 2007

van der Palen J, Klein JJ, Zielhuis GA, van Herwaarden CL, Seydel ER (2001) Behavioral effect of self-treatment guidelines in a self-management program for adults with asthma. Patient Educ Couns 43:161–169

Vojta PJ, Randels SP, Stout J, Muilenberg M, Burge HA, Lynn H, Mitchell H, O'Connor GT, Zeldin DC (2001) Effects of physical interventions on house dust mite allergen levels in carpet, bed, and upholstery dust in low-income, urban homes. Environ Health Perspect 109:815–819

Wang C, Bennett GW (2006) Comparative study of integrated pest management and baiting for German cockroach management in public housing. J Econ Entomol 99:879–885

Warner JA, Frederick JM, Bryant TN, Weich C, Raw GJ, Hunter C, Stephen FR, McIntyre DA, Warner JO (2000) Mechanical ventilation and high-efficiency vacuum cleaning: A combined strategy of mite and mite allergen reduction in the control of mite-sensitive asthma. J Allergy Clin Immunol 105(Suppl 1 Pt 1):75–82

Washington State Department of Health (2005) Washington state asthma plan. Available at: http://www.doh.wa.gov/cfh/asthma/state_plan.htm. Accessed April 10, 2007

Weinberger M, Murray MD, Marrero DG, Brewer N, Lykens M, Harris LE et al (2002) Effectiveness of pharmacist care for patients with reactive airways disease: A randomized controlled trial. JAMA 288:1594–1602

Weiss ST (2002) Eat dirt – the hygiene hypothesis and allergic diseases. N Engl J Med 347:930–931

Wells, Rebecca N (2007) Neighborhood design and physical activity: A pre-test/post-test examination. Abstract of work in progress. Available at: http://www.activelivingresearch.org/downloads/wellsabstract.rev.12.05.04.pdf. Accessed April 9, 2007

West Harlem Environmental Action (2006) WEACT history. Available at: http://www.weact.org/history.html, Accessed Nov 3, 2006

Western New York Asthma Coalitions (2007) HelpLine. Available at: http://www.asthmawny.org/helpline.html. Accessed April 10, 2007

Williams SG, Redd SC (2006) From research to reality: From the National Cooperative Inner-City Asthma Study to the inner-city asthma implementation. Ann Allergy Asthma Immunol 97(Suppl 1 Pt 1):S4–S5

Williams SG, Brown CM, Falter KH, Alverson CJ, Gotway-Crawford C, Homa D, Jones DS, Adams EK, Redd SC (2006) Does a multifaceted environmental intervention alter the impact of asthma on inner-city children? J Natl Med Assoc 98:249–260

Willies-Jacobo LJ, Denson-Lino JM, Rosas A, O'Connor RD, Wilson NW (1993a) Socioeconomic status and allergy in children with asthma. J Allergy Clin Immunol 92:630–632

Willies-Jacobo LJ, Denson-Lino JM, Rosas A, O'Connor RD, Wilson NW (1993b) Socioeconomic status and allergy in children with asthma. J Allergy Clin Immunol 92:630–632

Wood RA, Eggleston PA, Rand C, Nixon WJ, Kanchanaraksa S (2001) Cockroach allergen abatement with extermination and sodium hypochlorite cleaning in inner-city homes. Ann Allergy Asthma Immunol 87:60–64

Wood P, Tumiel-Berhalter L, Owen S, Taylor K, Kattan M (2006a) Implementation of an asthma intervention in the inner city. Ann Allergy Asthma Immunol 97(Suppl 1):S20–S24

Wood P, Tumiel-Berhalter L, Owen S, Taylor K, Kattan M (2006b) Implementation of an asthma intervention in the inner city. Ann Allergy Asthma Immunol 97(Suppl 1 Pt 1):S20–S24

Woodcock A, Forster L, Matthews E, Martin J, Letley L, Vickers M, Britton J, Strachan D, Howarth P, Altmann D, Frost C, Custovic A (2003) Medical research council general practice research framework. Control of exposure to mite allergen and allergen-impermeable bed covers for adults with asthma. N Engl J Med 17(349):225–236

Wooton M, Ashley P (2000) Residential hazards: Asthma. Healthy homes initiative background information. US Department of HUD

Wright RJ, Mitchell H, Visness CM, Cohen S, Stout J, Evans R et al (2004) Community violence and asthma morbidity: The Inner-City Asthma Study. Am J Public Health 94:625–632

Wright RJ, Cohen RT, Cohen S (2005a) The impact of stress on the development and expression of atopy. Curr Opin Allergy Clin Immunol 5:23–29

Wright RJ, Cohen RT, Cohen S (2005b) The impact of stress on the development and expression of atopy. Curr Opin Allergy Clin Immunol 5:23–29

Yawn BP, Wollan P, Scanlon P, Kurland M (2002) Are we ready for universal school-based asthma screening?: An outcomes evaluation. Arch Pediatr Adolesc Med 156:1256–1262

Yawn BP, Wollan P, Scanlon PD, Kurland M (2003) Outcome results of a school-based screening program for under treated asthma. Ann Allergy Asthma Immunol 90: 508–515

Yeatts K, Sly P, Shore S, Weiss S, Martinez F, Geller A, Bromberg P, Enright P, Koren H, Weissman D, Selgrade M (2006) A brief targeted review of susceptibility factors, environmental exposures, asthma incidence, and recommendations for future asthma incidence research. Environ Health Perspect 114:634–640

Yen IH, Yelin EH, Katz P, Eisner MD, Blanc PD (2006) Perceived neighborhood problems and quality of life, physical functioning, and depressive symptoms among adults with asthma. Am J Public Health 96:873–879

Yes We Can (2006) Available at: http://www.communityhealthworks.org/yeswecan/index.html. Accessed Oct 8, 2006

Yoon R, McKenzie DK, Miles DA, Bauman A (1991) Characteristics of attenders and non-attenders at an asthma education programme. Thorax 46:886–890

Zakocs RC, Edwards EM (2006) What explains community coalition effectiveness?: A review of the literature. Am J Prev Med 30:351–361

Zelikoff JT, Chen LC, Cohen MD, Schlesinger RB (2002) The toxicology of inhaled woodsmoke. J Toxicol Environ Health B Crit Rev 5:269–282

Kelly CS, Shield SW, Gowen MA, Jaganjac N, Andersen CL, Strope GL (1998) Outcomes analysis of a summer asthma camp. J Asthma 35(2):165–171

Chapter 18
Asthma and the Workplace

Jean-Luc Malo, Catherine Lemière, Denyse Gautrin, Manon Labrecque, and Kim Lavoie

General Considerations

Definitions

The workplace is, apart from smoking, a clearly identified cause for the development of chronic obstructive lung diseases, including asthma (Trupin et al. 2003). Many asthmatic subjects complain that their symptoms are worse at work as related to exposure to their workplace physical and psychological environmental stimuli. Epidemiological studies in the general population show that from 5% to one-third of all asthmatic subjects answer "yes" to the question: "Are your asthmatic symptoms worse at work?" (Blanc and Toren 1999; Johnson et al. 2000). Asthma in the workplace (AWP) encompasses several entities (Fig. 18.1) (Vandenplas and Malo 2003; Bernstein et al. 2006). First, some workplaces can cause asthma, mostly in subjects who, before starting to work, reported no respiratory symptoms. This condition is labelled "occupational asthma" (OA). Two causal mechanisms are implicated. Workers may develop an "allergy" to a product present at work or develop asthmatic symptoms after accidental inhalation of a product generated at abnormally high concentrations. Second, asthmatic subjects may report that their symptoms are aggravated or exacerbated at work although the workplace is not the cause of asthma. Third, several variants of asthma related to the workplace have been described. For instance, some workers in aluminium potrooms develop symptoms that share features of symptoms experienced by asthmatic subjects. Also, a condition that is called occupational eosinophilic bronchitis reproduces the pathologic but not the lung function features of OA.

OA is a type of asthma caused by an agent present in the workplace. It is defined as "a disease characterized by variable airflow limitation and/or airway hyperresponsiveness and/or inflammation due to causes and conditions attributable to a particular occupational environment and not to stimuli encountered outside the workplace" (Bernstein et al. 2006). As regards the allergic type of OA, two categories of causal agents present at work can be identified. Those derived from proteins exert their allergic effect through an IgE-mediated mechanism, a situation similar to the allergic type of common asthma. The other category of agents is chemicals. In this case, the mechanism is rarely IgE-mediated and is still generally unknown. The other type of OA is rarer. It is caused by an irritant accidental exposure at work. This condition is referred to as "irritant-induced asthma" or Reactive Airways Dysfunction Syndrome (RADS) if the accident is unique and not recurrent.

Occupational Asthma

Occupational Asthma with a Latency Period

This condition represents 80–90% of all cases of OA. A worker exposed at work to a potential sensitizer may develop an "allergy" to this product with rhinoconjunctival and respiratory symptoms. The natural history of this condition is illustrated in Fig. 18.2 with a list of factors that may play a role at each step. After acquiring sensitization, some subjects may first develop

J. Malo (✉)
The Axe de recherche en santé respiratoire, Center for Asthma in the Workplace, Hôpital du Sacré-Coeur de Montréal, 5400 West Gouin Blvd, Montreal, QC, Canada, H4J 1C5
e-mail: malojl@meddir.umontreal.ca

A. Harver and H. Kotses (eds.), *Asthma, Health and Society: A Public Health Perspective*,
DOI 10.1007/978-0-387-78285-0_18, © Springer Science+Business Media, LLC 2010

Fig. 18.1 Asthma in the workplace

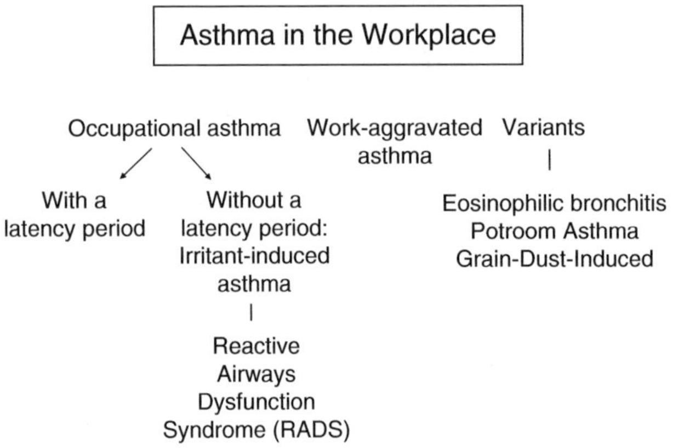

rhinoconjunctival symptoms. We may also hypothesize that some subjects will first develop airway inflammation, followed by airway hyper-responsiveness and changes in airway calibre. Some subjects will develop OA. After removal from exposure, subjects generally improve, but the majority is still left with asthmatic symptoms and abnormalities of airway function and hyper-responsiveness. We know that the shorter the period with symptoms while at work, has been, the more likely subjects are to be cured from asthma, as summarized elsewhere (Becklake et al. 2006). Administration of anti-inflammatory preparations in addition to cessation of exposure may maximize the chance of recovery (Malo et al. 1996).

The list of agents causing OA includes more than 250 high- (proteinaceous) and low- (chemicals) molecular-weight agents. Table 18.1 gives the most frequent causes and occupations. Lists are available on the Web (http://www.asthme.csst.qc.ca and http://www.asmanet.com, both French- and English-language sites). The mechanism of sensitization to high-molecular-weight agents is similar to what is described for ubiquitous allergens, i.e. IgE-mediated (Lemière et al. 2006a). For most low-molecular-weight agents, the mechanism remains unknown.

The diagnosis of OA is based on a decision tree that is shown in Fig. 18.3 (Chan-Yeung and Malo 1995). The clinical history is sensitive but not specific. Symptoms generally considered to be classic, such as improvement of symptoms during weekends and vacations combined with worsening of asthma while at work are not satisfactory predictors of the presence of OA (Vandenplas et al. 2005). For high-molecular-weight agents, nasal and ocular symptoms are most important to document as they often accompany and even precede asthma symptoms and are significant predictors of the presence of OA (Vandenplas et al. 2005). For low-molecular-weight agents, no symptoms have been identified as good predictors of OA. What is important for a physician who sees an asthmatic subject is to always inquire about the subject's type of work and, as importantly, about the nature of products present at work and not only those handled by the patient. Exhaustive lists of agents reported as causing OA have been published on the Web (see http://www.asthme.csst.qc.ca and http://www.asmanet.com, both French-language sites). Safety data sheets (SDS) can help but are not entirely reliable. Many sensitizers present at concentrations lower than 1% are not identified (Bernstein 2002). Every adult-onset asthmatic subject should be questioned about his/her current and past workplaces and, if agents known to cause OA are present, objectively investigated. In OA, the severity of the asthmatic condition is generally worse than for asthma not caused by the workplace (LeMoual et al. 2005). Not only current but also past workplaces should be investigated, as the resulting asthma condition may have been caused by a product to which the worker is no longer exposed. The majority of subjects with OA are indeed left with permanent asthma even after stopping exposure to the agent that caused OA (see below). For high-molecular-weight agents, even if standardized allergens exist, their quality is highly variable. This being said, it would be highly unlikely for a baker with OA not to have positive skin tests to flour or enzymes. The same applies for a laboratory worker exposed to rodents. Therefore, a simple prick test can be used to identify the presence of sensitization, at least for some high-molecular-weight

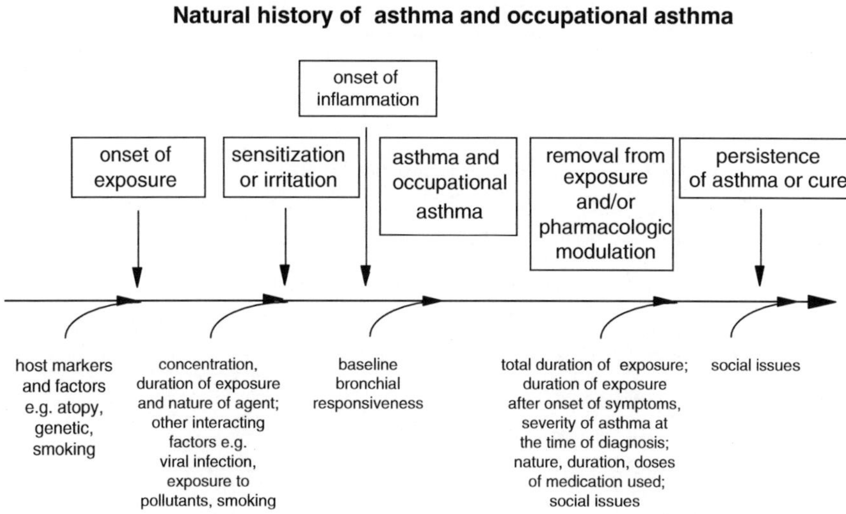

Fig. 18.2 Natural history of asthma and occupational asthma

Table 18.1 Major causes of occupational asthma with a latency period and workers at risk

Agent	Workers at risk
High-molecular-weight agents	
Cereals	Bakers, millers
Animal-derived allergens	Animal handlers
Enzymes	Detergent manufacturers, pharmaceutical workers, bakers
Gums	Carpet makers, pharmaceutical workers
Latex	Health professionals
Seafoods	Seafood processors
Low-molecular-weight agents	
Diisocyanates	Spray painters; insulation installers; manufacturers of plastics, rubbers and foam
Wood dusts	Forest workers, carpenters, cabinetmakers
Anhydrides	Users of plastics, epoxy resins
Amines	Shellac and lacquer handlers, solderers
Fluxes	Electronic workers
Choramine-T	Janitors, cleaners
Dyes	Textile workers
Persulfate	Hairdressers
Formaldehyde, glutaraldehyde	Hospital staff
Acrylate	Adhesive handlers
Drugs	Pharmaceutical workers, health professionals
Metals	Solderers, refiners

allergens. The absence of immunological sensitization in these circumstances makes the diagnosis of OA highly unlikely, unless some other sensitizers are present in the workplace. As shown in Fig. 18.3, the status of immunological sensitization can be assessed for high-molecular-weight agents only.

After examining immunological sensitization, the next step is to verify whether the target organ, in this

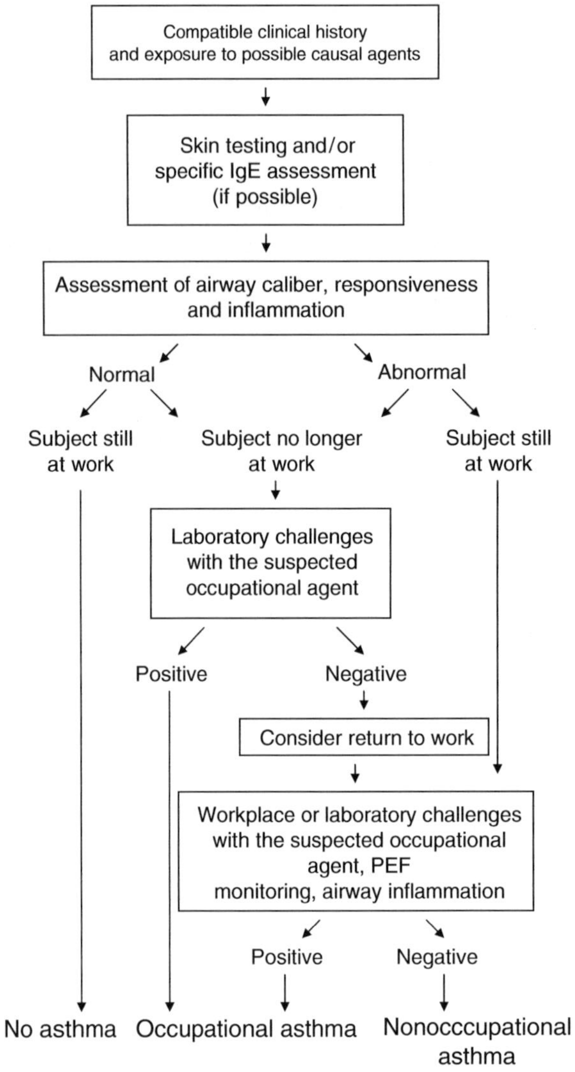

Fig. 18.3 Diagnosis of occupational asthma: Decision tree.

case the bronchi, is involved. This can be done by assessing airway calibre and responsiveness to methacholine, as well by assessing inflammation. This evaluation enables the clinician to find out whether the subject has asthma. Once this is done, the crucial thing to find out is whether asthma is caused by the workplace. This can be done either by exposing the worker in a hospital laboratory to the possible etiological agent by specific inhalation challenges or by returning the worker to his/her workplace and comparing changes in airway function and inflammation for a period at work and off work. For this, serial assessment of peak expiratory flows (PEF) can be used. Also, a technician can go to the workplace and assess airway calibre during a workshift. At the end of the workshift, airway responsiveness and inflammation are reassessed.

As cited by Murphy, "the investigation of allergic problems requires the inquisitiveness of a Sherlock Holmes, the genius of Thomas Edison, the patience of Diogenes and the optimism of an idiot" (Murphy 1976).

Occupational Asthma Without a Latency Period: Irritant-Induced Asthma and Reactive Airways Dysfunction Syndrome

The consequences of accidental inhalation injuries were recognized in the early twentieth century, during World War I. Exposures to war gases such as mustargen caused acute lung injury and edema, which were more frequent causes of death than bronchial damage. However, not until mid-century was bronchial damage documented, especially in civil populations living close to railways who were accidentally exposed to spills producing irritant vapours such as chlorine (Das and Blanc 1993) and ammonia. Assessment of bronchial responsiveness to pharmacological agents was more routinely carried out in the investigation of cases. The Bhopal accident, which exposed the civilian population to monoisocyantes (Nemery 1996), and, more recently, the World Trade Center disaster (Scanlon 2002), during which firefighters inhaled a vast amount of a mixture of dry particles, aerosols and vapours, represented major occurrences of the so-called Reactive Airways Dysfunction Syndrome (acronym = RADS), a label proposed by Brooks and colleagues (Brooks et al. 1985) in 1985.

The more general term of irritant-induced asthma, which was more recently proposed for this syndrome, may encompass not only RADS, which is related to a single accident, but also instances of recurrent episodes, sometimes in workers exposed to lower but still irritant concentrations of a gas, vapour or dust (Gautrin et al. 2006a).

The diagnosis is based on the clinical history of a subject free of respiratory diseases who is acutely exposed to an agent (most often a vapour) generated at high concentrations and who presents an intense nasal burn (Meggs 1994) with important coughing and, less consistently or at a later stage, shortness of breath and wheezing. Reversible airway obstruction or hyperresponsiveness is documented in the hours or days following the accident. Examination of bronchial biopsies obtained from sufferers and animals close to the inhalational accident shows important desquamation of the epithelium followed by more important thickening of the submucosal space than what is found in asthma and in OA with a latency period (Gautrin et al. 1994; Demnati et al. 1998a; Martin et al. 2003), which explains lesser reversibility of airway obstruction to an inhaled bronchodilator. As for OA with a latency period, this syndrome leaves permanent asthmatic sequelae (Malo et al. 1994). Approximately one-quarter of affected subjects are cured around 2 years after the inhalational accidents (Malo et al. 1994), a proportion similar to that found in OA with a latency period. In an animal model, early administration of steroids soon after the inhalational accident has been shown to be beneficial (Demnati et al. 1998b). Administration of parenteral and inhaled steroids is also recommended in humans (Lemière et al. 1997).

Work-Aggravated Asthma

Work-aggravated asthma (WAA) is defined as pre-existing or concurrent asthma that is exacerbated by workplace exposure (Wagner and Wegman 1998; Vandenplas and Malo 2003; Bernstein et al. 2006), implying that the workplace triggers but does not induce asthma.

According to epidemiologic studies that used various definitions of WAA based on self-reports, 18–34% of the respondents reported worsening of asthma in association with work (Saarinen et al. 2003; Axon et al. 1995; Tarlo 2000; Blanc and Toren 1999; Goe et al. 2004; Johnson et al. 2000). Henneberger not only defined WAA based on a self-reported symptom-work association, but also required that the participant was likely to be exposed to agents liable to cause asthma at work, as determined by researchers who reviewed self-reported details about the participant's job (Henneberger et al. 2006). In this study, 24% of the employed adults with asthma met the symptom and exposure criteria for WAA.

Differentiating OA from WAA is often difficult in clinical practice. Workers with WAA tend to show functional characteristics similar to those shown by subjects with OA (Girard et al. 2004). However, subjects with OA show eosinophilic airway inflammation when exposed to a specific agent at their workplace, whereas subjects with WAA show neutrophilic airway inflammation (Girard et al. 2004). Although subjects with OA tend to improve after removal from exposure, subjects with WAA do not show significant improvement in their respiratory function (Lemière et al. 2006b).

Few data are available regarding the socio-economic consequences of WAA. However, WAA seems to be associated with substantial socio-economic consequences.

Labarnois et al. evaluated the socio-economic outcome of subjects experiencing work- related asthma symptoms (Larbanois et al. 2002). Although the rate of job change or work loss was seen to be higher in OA subjects, they found that the rates of work disruption and income loss were similar among both OA and WAA subjects, indicating that WAA and OA may have a similar socio-economic impact.

Variants

Eosinophilic Bronchitis

Eosinophilic bronchitis is a condition identified in 1989 in subjects complaining of chronic cough (Gibson et al. 1989). Eosinophilic bronchitis has been shown to be the cause of 12% of cases of chronic cough (Brightling et al. 1999). This condition was also reported in the occupational setting in a subject who developed respiratory symptoms on exposure to cyanoacrylates (Lemière and Hargreave 1999). This condition has been reported with several other occupational agents. Diagnostic criteria have been proposed (Quirce 2004): isolated chronic cough (lasting more than 3 weeks) that worsens at work, sputum eosinophilia greater than 2.5% in either spontaneous or induced sputum, increases in sputum eosinophilia related to exposure to the offending agent (either at work or after a specific inhalation challenge in the laboratory), spirometry parameters within normal limits and not significantly affected by exposure to the offending agent, absence of airway hyper-responsiveness to methacholine both at work and away from work, and other causes of chronic cough ruled out. This condition is likely to be underestimated since induced sputum is not routinely performed in many centers. Although it is not known whether subjects with occupational eosinophilic bronchitis will develop OA if they stay exposed to the offending agent, it would seem medically prudent to remove symptomatic subjects from the workplace.

Aluminium Potroom Asthma

Workers in aluminium potrooms often suffer from respiratory symptoms with some wheezing. Although reversible airway obstruction and hyper-responsiveness can be demonstrated in these symptomatic workers, changes in airway calibre during a workshift do not generally, except in rare cases (Desjardins et al. 1994), reach levels that are considered significant to diagnose OA, which is a 20% fall in FEV1 (Bernstein and Merget 2006).

Grain-Dust Induced Asthma

Exposure to grain dust can cause a variety of respiratory symptoms, including OA as such and asthma-like syndromes and non-allergen-induced airflow obstruction (Chan-Yeung et al. 2006). In addition, exposure to grain dust is often accompanied by the development of fixed chronic airway obstruction.

As a Burden to Health

Medico-Legal Considerations

OA is an accepted medico-legal condition in most countries (Dewitte et al. 1994; Bersntein et al. 2006). Workers can therefore apply to their respective national agencies for compensation, provided that they have access to such insurance. Many workers fail to apply because the social and financial benefits they may derive are minimal, as in the U.K. or France. Application may even make the situation worse since workers may suffer employment prejudice. Too often, the diagnosis is not based on objective evidence (Moscato et al. 2002; Ameille et al. 2003; Nicholson et al. 2005). A compatible history is considered sufficient in most instances, which should not be the case since clinical history is sensitive but not specific (see above). Making a wrong diagnosis has major social and financial consequences for workers, employers and medico-legal agencies. On the one hand, advising a worker (in most instances, these are young workers) to leave his/her job often results in retraining and unemployment. On the other hand, telling a worker not to leave his/her job if he/she suffers from OA will result in more severe asthma (deaths have been reported in subjects who remain at their workplace (Ortega et al. 2002)) and less likelihood of being free of asthmatic sequelae, since the longer the symptoms last, the more likely asthma will persist (Becklake et al. 2006).

Ideally, workers should not remain exposed to the agent that caused OA. The main focus should be placed on rehabilitation programs with financial compensation and not on financial compensation alone, because affected workers are generally young and can be retrained in a new job. If this is not achievable, at least reducing exposure should be the aim. Although long-term assessment of workers who are less exposed has not been carried out, there are documented short-term advantages (Slovak et al. 1985; Vandenplas et al. 1995). Workers should be encouraged to take inhaled anti-inflammatory preparations to hasten improvement (Malo et al. 1996). The cost of medications used to control asthma should be covered by the medico-legal agencies.

Medico-legal considerations should also include the possibility of allocating impairment/disability since permanent sequelae are the rule more often than not. Studies of the natural history of OA show that the rate of improvement is greater in the two first years or so after leaving work with some improvement thereafter, though at a slower rate (Malo and Ghezzo 2004). For practical reasons, it has been suggested that workers be re-assessed for permanent impairment/disability approximately 2 years after stopping exposure.

Impairment represents a loss in function, whereas disability is the impact of this loss on the worker's life (Bersntein et al. 2006). To assess the former, a scaling system has been advocated (American Medical 2001) based on recommendations made by the American Thoracic Society (American Thoracic Society 1993) that include key elements, i.e. airway calibre and hyper-responsiveness, as well as the need for medication to control asthma as proposed in Quebec in 1984 (Dewitte et al. 1994). One of several tools used to assess disability is to evaluate answers to a disease-specific questionnaire on quality of life with asthma (Juniper et al. 1999). This questionnaire was administered to nearly 100 workers who were accepted by the Quebec medico-legal agency and seen 2 years after cessation of exposure. Most were employed. Quality of life was minimally affected (Malo et al. 1993). The same conclusion was reached more recently in a small group of workers from Ontario, Canada, with OA due to latex, who found alternative jobs (Al-Otaibi et al. 2005).

Prevention Issues

Since reducing or even eliminating possible harmful exposures is a key issue in the prevention of OA, all prevention programs should first be focused on industrial hygiene measures. It has been demonstrated in many epidemiological studies that exposure is the single most important determinant of OA (Becklake et al. 2006). There is general agreement that atopic workers (i.e. those with documented allergies to general ubiquitous inhaled allergens such as house dust, mites, pollens, pets, and moulds) should not be excluded from at-risk workforces. Although they are at greater risk of developing sensitization to high-molecular-weight agents, the risk is not high enough (ORs in the order of 2–4 depending on the study) to justify such interventions. Moreover, since 50% of young individuals are atopic (Gautrin et al. 1997), it would be impractical to exclude 50% of possible workers from specific workplaces.

We do not know for sure whether medical primary (before symptoms start) or secondary (pre-clinical status, in this instance once sensitization has occurred) prevention programs in high-risk workplaces are efficient and cost-effective (Tarlo and Liss 2005). How useful is performance in allergy skin tests to flour and enzymes in bakers and to rodent proteins in workers exposed to laboratory animals? How useful is the assessment of bronchial responsiveness and repeating this test serially? What is sure is that once the disease is present (tertiary prevention), early removal from exposure is crucial as discussed above.

Epidemiology

General Considerations

Epidemiology is a discipline that studies the distribution and determinants of health-related states and disease in populations (Last 1995). The determinants include environmental and personal host factors. In the context of an occupational disease, environmental factors are those encountered in the workplace and include exposure to various types of contaminants, physical stress and factors related to workplace organization (Becklake et al. 2006). A determinant has been defined as "any physical, biological, social, cultural or behavioural factor that can influence the study outcome" (e.g. work-related asthma) (Last 1995).

Occupational exposures to airborne particulates, gases and vapours are measured to assess exposure–response relationships. Such relationships are useful to (1) determine a link of causality between suspected exposure and the disease, in this context, work-related asthma, and (2) provide objective evidence to control exposure levels in the workplace.

Epidemiological studies of OA may be conducted with different objectives in mind, using different designs and in different populations, and the definition of OA may differ accordingly (Becklake et al. 2006). Because the definition does not conform to the clinical definition, terms such as "asthma-like" and "probable OA" have been used (Manfreda et al. 1993; Gautrin et al. 2001a).

Study approaches and design in the context of investigations of OA have been described and discussed in terms of strengths and weaknesses by Becklake et al. (2006). These designs include randomized control trials, longitudinal (cohort) studies, case-control (case-referent) studies, cross-sectional (prevalence) studies and clinical case reports. The selection of the most appropriate design should be based on the purpose of answering a study question as discussed by McDonald (1995). Other considerations in choosing a study design include more practical issues, such as the availability of a suitable population, appropriate instruments to measure the study outcome and exposure, and resources. Randomized clinical trials are usually not feasible in the context of the study of OA, except when the effect of a treatment on recovery from OA is examined (Malo et al. 1996). Cross-sectional studies have been widely used to determine the prevalence of OA (Gautrin et al. 2003; Mapp et al. 2005). This type of design is likely to provide underestimates of the rates of the disease due to survivor bias (caused by attrition from the workforce for health reasons) (Newman-Taylor and Venables 1984; Becklake et al. 2006). Prospective cohort studies are used to estimate the incidence and determinants of work-related asthma; this approach has been used, for example, in cohorts of apprentices entering a program in which they are exposed to known sensitizers (De Zotti and Bovenzi 2000; Gautrin et al. 2000, 2001a; Archambault et al. 2001; Rodier et al. 2003; El-Zein et al. 2003; Walusiak et al. 2004), in specific workforces (Brisman et al. 2004) and among members of a health maintenance organization (Vollmer et al. 2005). Case-control (retrospective) studies are designed to examine the role of environmental (exposure) and host risk factors; nested case-control analysis within a cohort offers the advantage that cases can be compared with controls with similar exposure when host determinants, including genetic polymorphisms, are studied, or alternatively with controls with similar socio-cultural, economic and education backgrounds to study the effect of occupational exposure (Cullinan et al. 2001; Brisman et al. 2003).

Methodological issues of importance in epidemiological studies include measurement of outcomes and risk factors. As pointed out by Becklake et al. (2006), the tools used to measure health outcomes are similar to those used in the clinical setting; in a chapter of Asthma in the Workplace, the authors discuss the importance of using a standardized approach with all measuring instruments, including those used to assess symptoms, immunological status, lung function and bronchial responsiveness to "minimize differential across comparison groups" (Becklake et al. 2006). Similar precautions need to be taken for measurements of exposure.

Depending on the objective of the epidemiological study, the size of the study population and the resources available, the methods used for case identification may be more or less exhaustive. Questionnaires have been used as the only method of assessment for a number of workforce-based or community-based studies to assess the prevalence of work-related asthma; however, questionnaires are very sensitive and poorly specific. For example, in a workforce-based study of workers exposed to guar gum in the carpet industry, 23/162 had symptoms suggestive of OA, but only two had a confirmed diagnosis of OA using specific challenge tests (Malo et al. 1990), considered the gold standard for the diagnosis of OA (Vandenplas et al. 2006). An algorithm has been proposed for the investigation of OA in epidemiological studies including the following measures (1) questionnaire, (2) skin prick tests and/or immunological testing with the suspected specific etiologic agent, when feasible, (3) assessment of non-specific bronchial responsiveness, (4) serial peak flow monitoring and/or specific inhalation tests (Chan-Yeung and Malo 1995). When participants in an epidemiological study take part in an investigation beyond a questionnaire, one or more of the above mentioned measures are added. Toelle et al. suggested that in epidemiological studies, ascertainment of asthma and of OA should be based on a questionnaire and confirmed bronchial hyper-responsiveness using challenge tests to non-specific pharmacological agents (Toelle et al. 1992) that have been used safely for field studies (Troyanov et al. 2000). In prospective studies conducted in apprentices exposed to high-molecular-weight allergens, the diagnosis of "probable OA" was based on immunological evidence and objective testing for bronchial responsiveness (Gautrin et al. 2001a; Archambault et al. 2001) on the assumption that 80% of subjects with skin reactivity to a specific allergen and confirmed bronchial hyper-responsiveness would react to a specific challenge test with the appropriate inhalant (Cockcroft et al. 1987).

Frequency and Determinants

The frequency of asthma in the workplace can be assessed by several means. Surveys in the general population propose figures that are higher (5% up to one-third of all asthmatic subjects) than those obtained from sentinel projects where potential cases are reported by physicians and medicolegal statistics, especially for countries that accept cases based on diagnostic confirmation through objective evidence (10–15 cases/million workers in Quebec).

Prevalence

The prevalence of work-related respiratory symptoms suggestive of OA and of OA has been investigated in several different workplace surveys and among workers in the same occupational groups, e.g. laboratory-animal facilities, large bakeries, snow-crab and other seafood processing plants, food processing plants, farms, silk works, latex-glove manufacturing plants, carpet manufacturing plants, the pharmaceutical industry, plastic and varnish production plants and/or utilization, spray-painting, hairdressing, production of resins, sawmill, welding, textile (dyes), hospitals, greenhouses, etc. (Becklake et al. 2006). These results are helpful in providing information about the scope of the problem in high-risk workplaces, although they are potentially prone to survivor bias. The well-known survivor effect (selection "out") is probably the most important bias affecting prevalence estimates from cross-sectional surveys in individual workplaces. Observed differences in the prevalence of OA due to the same agent may be accounted for, at least in part, by particular conditions at a given site, such as exposure to other asthmagenic agents or respiratory irritants. Large discrepancies in the prevalence of work-related symptoms and OA between workforces exposed to different agents of low molecular weight (e.g. isocyanates) or high molecular weight (e.g. flour, laboratory animals) have been reported. One might question whether these are entirely attributable to the agents themselves or to other circumstances, for instance, ascertainment of cases of OA, country, differential effect of other factors such as work practice, and potential identified/non-identified biases. An additional source of controversy in the ascertainment of OA is that it can be defined as either new-onset asthma or WAA (Toren et al. 2000).

Prevalence studies in workforce-based studies remain useful for the evaluation of interventions to control exposure to a specific contaminant, as was the case for enzyme detergents. Prevalence rates of respiratory symptoms and skin reactivity have successively decreased from 50% in the 1960s (Mitchell and Gandevia 1971) but rose again in the late 1990s (Cullinan et al. 2000; Vanhanen et al. 2000); these variations have led researchers to identify various causes that were followed by changes in formulation processes.

Incidence

A few prospective cohort studies have been designed in selected high-risk professions to assess the incidence and determinants of probable OA among apprentices newly exposed to high-molecular-weight agents (De Zotti and Bovenzi 2000; Gautrin et al. 2001a, b, 2002; Archambault et al. 2001; Brisman et al. 2003; Walusiak et al. 2004), and low-molecular-weight sensitizers (El-Zein et al. 2003; 2005). A summary of key features of the prospective studies carried out in apprentices by Gautrin and coworkers is presented in Table 18.2. The cumulative incidence of probable OA (work-related new chest symptoms and increase in bronchial hyper-responsiveness) over an average period of 15 months of intermittent exposure to welding fumes while training to become a welder was 13.8% (32/232) (El-Zein et al. 2003). In comparison, the incidence of the outcome (new work-related chest symptoms) in

Table 18.2 Features of prospective studies carried out in apprentices by Gautrin and coworkers

A. High-molecular-weight agents

Assessment of 769 apprentices starting training in Animal Health, Pastry-making and Dental Hygiene:

1. On entry into the apprenticeship, a significant proportion (up to 7.4%) of apprentices show signs of immunological sensitization to a work-related allergen (Gautrin et al. 1997)
2. The risk of sensitization during the training program was higher for apprentices exposed to animal-derived allergens than for those exposed to flour and latex. There was no excess of sensitization to flour in bakers, compared to that in the other groups not exposed to this allergen at work (Gautrin et al. 2000)

Incidence of program-related sensitization (Gautrin et al. 2000)

	Animal health	Pastry-making	Dental hygiene
	(n=395)	(n=186)	(n=109)
No. of incident cases	85	8	7
Proportion by number at risk	21.5%	4.3%	6.4%
Rate by person-years	7.9%	4.2%	2.5%

3. In apprentice animal technicians exposed to laboratory animals:
   - Atopy (Rate Ratio (RR)=2.20, 95%CI: 1.4–3.91), respiratory symptoms in the pollen season (RR=5.19, 95% CI: 1.68–16.05) and spending more than 52 h exposed to rodents (RR=2.51, 95% CI: 1.32–4.76) were significantly associated with incident specific sensitization to a laboratory animal-derived allergen adjusting for possible confounders (Gautrin et al. 2000)
   - The rate of sensitization was higher in the first 2 years (of a total of 4 years) of training (10.3% and 10.7% for years 1 and 2, respectively); work-related rhinoconjonctivitis was more frequent in the first 2 years of training (12.5% and 13.9%), whereas respiratory symptoms took longer to appear (maximum incidence of 3.2% and 2.5% in years 2 and 3, respectively, of the program) (Gautrin et al. 2001b)
   - The incidence of probable OA was 2.7% (28/1043 person-years). Baseline immediate skin reactivity to pets (RR=4.1, 95% CI: 1.6–10.8), and bronchial responsiveness (RR=2.5, 95% CI: 1.0–5.8) were risk factors for probable OA; a higher FEV1 was mildly associated with an increased risk of probable OA (RR=1.74, 95% CI: 1.29–2.34) (Gautrin et al. 2001a)
4. In apprentices exposed to latex, the cumulative incidences of skin sensitization, probable occupational rhinoconjunctivitis and OA to latex were 6.4%, 1.8% and 4.5%, respectively. Sensitized subjects were more likely to be atopic and to have a previous history of asthma and respiratory symptoms on exercise than were nonsensitized subjects (Archambault et al. 2001)
5. In apprentice-pastry-makers, work-related rhinoconjonctivitis was common (16.1% of subjects; 13.1/100 person-years) but rarely associated with skin sensitization to flour (3/186=1.6%) (Gautrin et al. 2002).

B. Low-molecular weight agents

1. Welding fumes

Cohort of 286 apprentice welders:

- 13.8% developed at least one welding-related respiratory symptom suggestive of work-related asthma, 11.8% at least one immediate skin reaction to a metallic salt solution, and 11.9% a significant increase in bronchial responsiveness (El-Zein et al. 2003)
- 3.1% developed probable OA(at least one welding-related respiratory symptom and a significant change in bronchial responsiveness) (El-Zein et al. 2005).

2. Hexamethylene diisocyanates

Cohort of342 apprentice car-painters:

- 13 (4.8%) subjects developed at least one work-related respiratory symptom, 15 (5.6%) showed an increase in bronchial responsiveness and 8 (3%) apprentices presented immunological sensitization (IgE- and/or IgG-dependent) to HDI (Dragos M et al., submitted)

bakers' studies varied between 12% (Brisman et al. 2004) and 4.2% (Cullinan et al. 2001), which appeared to be somewhat lower.

Estimates of the incidence of OA have mainly been made using National and Regional Disease Registers, Surveillance Systems and medico-legal statistics, although these systems were not primarily intended for that purpose. The Sentinel Event Notification System for Occupational Risk (SENSOR) was introduced in several states in the United States in the 1980s, based on mandatory or voluntary reporting of work-related diseases (Matte et al. 1990). This system was mainly developed to identify and investigate workplaces at risk and implement interventions. In the United Kingdom, two voluntary reporting schemes have been set up since 1989. The Surveillance of Work-related and Occupational Respiratory Diseases (SWORD) is based on voluntary reporting from selected specialists in occupational or respiratory medicine in the country (McDonald et al. 2005). The other system, a Surveillance Scheme of OA in the West Midlands Region, was designed to study the incidence of OA in this specific area (Gannon and Burge 1993). Recent figures from SWORD show stabilization and even a reduction in the number of new cases of OA (McDonald et al. 2005). Similar surveillance systems have been initiated in the Canadian provinces of Quebec (Provencher et al. 1997) and British Columbia (Contreras et al. 1994), in France (Ameille et al. 2003) and in South Africa (Hnizdo et al. 2001). Other sources used to derive estimates of the incidence of OA include Medico-legal Statistics in the province of Quebec (Lagier et al. 1990) and in Finland (FROD) (Reijula et al. 1996), as well as self-reporting systems as in Sweden (Toren 1996). There are large differences between countries in the estimates of incidence of OA derived from these sources, ranging from 20 per million per year in the United Kingdom to 187 per million per year in Finland, as illustrated and discussed by Becklake et al. (Becklake et al. 2006). These differences may be attributed to methodological differences (in case ascertainment and classification of job), the type of industries, as well as differences in reporting. Within a country, differences in time are useful to indicate trends in incidence rates overall and for specific causal agents (such as isocyanates or latex). Despite some weaknesses of these schemes for obtaining valid estimates of the incidence of OA, they have been successfully used to derive information on the distribution of the disease by occupational categories and the frequency of afflicted workers by agent.

Adult-Onset Asthma Attributable to Work Exposures: Population Attributable Risk (PAR%)

Since the 1990s, there has been increased interest in the proportion of adult-onset asthma that could be attributable to work exposure. Blanc and Toren (1999), in a review of studies that used different epidemiological designs, arrived at a median estimate of 9% of attributable risk of asthma to work exposure, and 15% when only high-quality studies were considered. Estimates of PAR% have been derived from community-based surveys and population-based incidence studies. In community-based studies in large populations (more than 1,000 and up to several thousand) of male and female adults in countries around the world (Europe, Canada, the United States, New Zealand and Singapore), consistent associations were found between wheezing complaints or asthma diagnosed by a physician, and those being exposed at work to non-specific agents or to dust alone or to dust with fumes and/or gases (irritants). Becklake et al. (2006) reviewed selected studies in which the PAR% ranged from 3% in studies from Spain (Kogevinas et al. 1996) and New Zealand (Fishwick et al. 1997), to 23% in Canada (Becklake et al. 1996) and 33% in Singapore (Ng et al. 1994). Becklake et al. (2006) also discussed the strength of these studies, which involve not only the population of workers currently exposed, but also all those who have ever been exposed in workplaces at risk, thus reducing survivor effects.

A population-based incidence study included the entire employed Finnish population. The cohort was followed for 10 years, using two registers, one of clinically established persistent asthma, the other of census data (for information on employment) (Karjalainen et al. 2001). A total of 49,575 incident cases of asthma were recorded, and the fraction attributable to work was 29% for males and 17% for females. The proportion attributable to work according to the Finnish Register of Occupational Diseases was ~5% (Reijula et al. 1996). As discussed earlier (Gautrin et al. 2003), this discrepancy in the PAR% figures between the two sources of data may be due to failure to recognize association with work exposure, or physicians' failure to submit workers for evaluation. The Finnish study also found excess risk of asthma in workplaces associated with exposure to irritants such as dust, welding and soldering fumes, disinfectants, traffic, exhaust combustion and cold air (Karjalainen et al. 2002). Other community-based studies have found increased risks of asthma in jobs associated with irritant exposures but not habitually with OA, for example among construction and textile workers (Ng et al. 1994), cleaners (Kogevinas et al. 1999; Karjalainen et al. 2000), shoemakers, metal-plating workers and electrical machinery workers (Arif et al. 2002).

Exposure–Response Relationships

In cohort studies investigating the incidence and determinants of OA, time spent in contact with the responsible agent has been used as a surrogate of exposure when objective measurements were not available. In a cohort of apprentices exposed to laboratory animals, a dose–response relationship was shown between the number of hours of contact with rodents in the laboratory and the incidence of specific skin reactivity to rodent urinary proteins independently of host factors (atopy, pre-exposure respiratory symptoms during the pollen season); the risk was 2.5 times greater in subjects exposed to the longest compared to the shortest of three duration categories (Gautrin et al. 2000). Prospective studies of laboratory-animal workers (Cullinan et al. 1999), flour mill and bakery workers (Cullinan et al. 2001) and acid anhydride workers (Barker et al. 1998) performed in the United Kingdom were reviewed by Newman-Taylor (Newman Taylor 2002). They all showed evidence of exposure–response relationships between direct measures of exposure and the risk of developing work-related chest symptoms. Another study using a case-control design found an exposure–response relationship between measurements of isocyanate and OA (McDonald et al. 2000). As noted earlier, such studies provide strong evidence for developing preventive strategies (Gautrin et al. 2003) for agents that are responsible for a substantial number of cases of OA.

Sociopsychological Impacts

Not only is OA a multifactorial lung disease that is associated with significant health impacts, but it also has important personal, financial and sociopsychological impacts.

Quality of Life Impacts

Once a diagnosis of OA has been confirmed and patients' are removed from the workplace, this does not guarantee a swift recovery. In fact, respiratory symptoms may persist for years, even following cessation of exposure (Becklake et al. 2006). It has been estimated that as many as 70% of patients experience persistent symptoms and nonspecific airway hyper-responsiveness, and the majority of patients who develop OA with or without a latency period do not recover. It is therefore not surprising that patients with OA may suffer a significantly reduced quality of life following diagnosis. A study by Malo and coworkers found that patients with OA with a latency period report having significantly reduced quality of life in at least four life domains (activity limitations, asthma symptoms, management of environmental triggers, and emotional distress) 2 years after cessation of exposure (Malo et al. 1993). The impact was, however, mild, and this can be explained by the fact that only 8% of them were still unemployed at the time of the study. Moreover, this study found that patients with OA suffered from worse asthma-related quality of life than non-OA patients matched for disease severity. This suggests that the quality of life impacts of OA may exceed those of 'traditional' asthma, and highlights the magnitude of this diagnosis' impact on functional status (Al-Otaibi et al. 2005).

Psychological Impacts

The idea that asthma may be related to psychological factors is not new. Negative emotions have long been considered important asthma triggers, with references to asthma as being "passion-induced" and related to mood dating back as far as 200 BC (Gregerson 2003). By the late nineteenth and early twentieth centuries, Sir William Osler viewed asthma as a "neurotic affection" in which imbalances of the nervous system and emotional factors played a fundamental role (Osler 1892). Since then, a growing number of studies have provided evidence of a link between various psychosocial factors and asthma (Gregerson 2003). Data from both clinical and community settings suggest that psychiatric disorders, and mood and anxiety disorders in particular, are disproportionately more prevalent among asthmatics relative to the general population. Point prevalence rates of anxiety disorders (e.g., panic disorder, generalized anxiety disorder, and social phobia) and mood disorders (e.g., major and minor depressive disorder) are especially high among asthmatics, ranging from 16–52% for anxiety disorders(Goodwin et al. 2003; Naciemento et al. 2002; Perna et al. 1997) and 14–41%

for mood disorders (Goodwin et al. 2003; Naciemento et al. 2002; Perna et al. 1997; Goldney et al. 2003; Netjeck et al. 2001). A recent study by Lavoie and coworkers including over 500 asthma outpatients indicated that 31% of asthmatics meet criteria for one or more *current* mood (20%) or anxiety (23%) disorders (Lavoie et al. 2006). Rates of certain disorders (i.e., panic disorder and major depressive disorder) are as much as *six times* more prevalent among asthmatics relative to the general population. However, the extent to which patients with OA suffer as much (if not more) psychiatric comorbidity at the time they are still exposed at work and are affected with asthmatic symptoms is not yet known, and future studies are needed to assess this.

Not only is psychological stress common in asthmatic subjects, but there is a vast literature linking symptoms of psychological stress to increased asthma morbidity. For example, symptoms of anxiety and depression have been associated with increased asthma severity, increased use of emergency services, increased symptom reporting, poorer pulmonary function, lengthier hospital stays, and increased use of reliever medication (Rimington et al. 2001; Janson et al. 1994; Kaptein 1982; Kolbe et al. 1996).To date, relatively few studies have evaluated associations between actual psychiatric disorders (which imply experiencing psychological stress at a level that is clinically significant and impairs daily functioning) and asthma morbidity. However, the few studies conducted have yielded similar results. For example, one study found associations between major depressive disorder (assessed using the Primary Care Evaluation for Mental Disorders, PRIME-MD) and worse nocturnal asthma symptoms, worse waking asthma symptoms, and worse asthma-related quality of life (Goldney et al. 2003). A related study found that asthmatics identified as having a psychiatric disorder (according to the Structured Clinical Interview for DSM-III-R) were more likely to have poorly controlled asthma, demonstrate worse medication adherence, and have greater drop-out rates from asthma management programs relative to patients without a psychiatric disorder (Kolbe et al. 1996). A study by Lavoie and coworkers also found evidence of an association between psychiatric disorders and greater asthma morbidity (Lavoie et al. 2005). Collectively, these studies indicate a strong association between both psychological stress and psychiatric disorders and increased asthma morbidity.

Despite strong associations between psychiatric disorders, high levels of psychological stress, and asthma morbidity, these associations remain unexplored in patients with OA. When one also considers the scope of the burden associated with non-OA and applies those potential impacts to patients who were for years disease-free, an additional psychological burden associated with OA that surpasses that of non-OA can be hypothesized. High job-specific stress is common and associated with worse health outcomes in patients with several chronic illnesses (e.g., hypertension and cardiovascular disease). For example, perceived job stress (defined as severity and frequency of stressful job tasks), job strain (defined as high job demands and low decision latitude), job insecurity, and threat of unemployment have been associated with increased risk of cardiovascular disease (Kang et al. 2005), incident hypertension (Markovitz et al. 2004; Levenstein et al. 2001), and non-fatal myocardial infarction (Lee et al. 2004).

We are aware of only one study to date to specifically assess levels of psychological stress in patients with OA after removal from exposure (Yacoub et al. submitted). In this study, psychological distress levels were assessed using two self-report instruments: the Psychiatric Symptom Index (PSI) (Illfeld 1976) and Millon Clinical Multiaxial Inventory (MCMI) (Millon 1994) in 40 workers with OA 2 years after cessation of exposure. This study found that levels of anxiety, depression, and cognitive dysfunction were all in the clinical range according to the PSI, suggesting that not only are the psychological consequences of OA significant but they may affect a range of psychological factors. It is noteworthy that psychological distress levels were measured at least 2 years after workers received their diagnosis and after they had been removed from the workplace, suggesting that psychological distress in these patients may persist beyond receiving the diagnosis and beyond withdrawal from the workplace. Certain psychiatric disorders were also found to be common in this sample, with anxiety disorders and dysthymia (a chronic form of depression) affecting approximately 35% and 22.5% of patients, respectively. Though preliminary and in need of replication, these results suggest that patients with OA are anxious and many are chronically depressed, a finding that is consistent with previous studies in subjects with non-OA (Goodwin et al. 2003; Lavoie et al. 2005). However, it is noteworthy that rates of anxiety disorders and dysthymia in Yacoub et al.'s study were much higher than those observed in previous studies with non-occupational asthmatics (e.g., 35% vs. 23%) (Yacoub et al. submitted), which suggests that the psychological consequences (like quality of life impacts) of OA, may exceed those of non-OA.

Social and Financial Costs

General Considerations

Asthma is a common medical condition and a frequent cause of work disability. Unlike many chronic medical conditions that primarily affect older persons, asthma disproportionately affects those of working age. Because it is prevalent during ages of peak participation in the workforce and because its impact can be severe, asthma is one of the leading medical conditions associated with work limitations and work loss. A study done between 1983 and 1985 showed that 326,000 adults in the United States between the ages of 18 and 44 were limited in their ability to work by asthma (Laplante 1988). This represents approximately 10% of all persons with asthma in this age group (Ries 1986). Indeed, 21% of asthmatic subjects complain of worsening of their asthma when they are at work (Saarinen et al. 2003). The estimated asthma-related cost of lost work days for persons 18 years and older in the workforce is $284.7 million per annum alone (Weiss et al. 1992). Costs can be estimated using PAR estimates (Leigh et al. 2002). Leigh et al. used a PAR of 15% for both asthma and COPD to calculate costs, with the human capital method that breaks down costs into direct categories, such as medical expenses, as well as indirect categories, such as lost earnings and lost home production. The 15% PARs result in costs of $1.6 billion for asthma, 74% direct and 26% indirect. These estimates are conservative, since costs associated with pain and suffering as well as the value of care rendered by family members were not included.

Concerning risk factors for work disability among adults with asthma, in a cross-sectional survey of 698 registered patients of pulmonary and allergy internal medicine subspecialists, Blanc et al. (1996) showed that the severity of asthma score predicted both complete disability (odds ratio –OR-, 7.9; 95% CI, 4.2–15 per 10-point increment) and partial disability (OR 2.6; 95% CI, 1.6–4.2), and taking illness severity into account, job conditions, occupation, and work exertion carried a combined disability OR of 3.9 (95% CI, 1.7–8.6). Blanc et al. (1996) concluded that work disability is common among adults with asthma receiving specialist care. Severity of disease is a powerful predictor, but not the sole predictor of disability in this group. Working conditions, including job-related exposures, are associated with added disability risk even after taking illness severity into account.

Social Impact

Occupational Asthma with a Latency Period

From an international perspective, although OA is a condition that is under the jurisdiction of medico-legal authorities, in most countries, examination of cases is often unsatisfactory and takes time. The protection offered to workers is generally inadequate. Affected workers frequently continue to be exposed or encounter serious socio-economic losses (Gannon et al. 1993; Ameille and Descatha 2005; Larbanois et al. 2002). Although a study published on the outcome of workers who stayed at the same job with pharmacologic treatment after a diagnosis of OA found no significant differences in any of the morbidity outcomes (FEV1, PD20, PEF variability, use of rescue salbutamol, respiratory symptom score) as compared to baseline or run-in values after 3 years of follow up in 20 workers (Marabini et al. 2003), this study has many limitations: small number of subjects and lack of power of the analysis, uncontrolled study, and selection of workers who had mild-to-moderate and not moderate to severe persistent asthma. Although none of the subjects deteriorated, none recovered from asthma even if they wore respiratory protection at work. Therefore, there is a consensus that workers with OA should not remain in the same job after diagnosis.

OA with a latency period generally affects young workers. This is different from standard pneumoconiosis such as silicosis and asbestosis, in which a very long latency period is generally the rule and compensation agencies deal with older workers. For OA, workers generally get sensitized in the first few years after starting exposure, even more generally so in the case of high-molecular-weight proteinaceous agents (Malo et al. 1992). It is therefore mandatory to offer rehabilitation programs adapted to these young workers. Rather than offering a lump sum, emphasis should be put on retraining these workers in a new job in which they will no longer be exposed to the agent causing OA. Although most workers with OA will still have asthma even after stopping exposure, asthma is generally mild and most workers are able to carry on almost any type of work. If the emphasis is put on adequate 1–2-year rehabilitation programs (this is generally long enough to retrain young workers into a new job) with financial compensation, very few workers are unable to find another job. In a study of 134 workers carried out in Quebec 2 years after cessation of exposure, only 8% were still unemployed (Dewitte et al. 1994). Moreover, workers generally report a satisfactory quality of life (see above).

Irritant-Induced Asthma

There is little published information about the socio-economic consequences of RADS, time lost from work, and the outcome. Some authors have reported a worse prognosis in workers exposed to spills without prior history of disease (Gautrin et al. 2006b). It is also relevant to distinguish work-exacerbated asthma (with a history of previous asthma) from irritant-induced asthma. Workers with the latter condition have more prolonged symptoms after exposure and seem less likely to have returned to the same work environment in comparison with workers with work-exacerbated asthma (Chatkin et al. 1999; Tarlo et al. 1995). In a descriptive epidemiological study of work-related cases of RADS, Henneberger et al. found more information on the outcome of these workers (Henneberger et al. 1993). In that study, cases of work-related asthma were identified in four states in the United States during 1993–1995 as part of the Sentinel Event Notification Systems for Occupational Risks (SENSOR) program. Information gathered by follow-back interview was used to describe 123 work-related RADS cases and compare them to 301 other work-related asthma cases in which the onset of disease was associated with a known asthma inducer. RADS represented 14% of all new-onset work-related cases identified by the state SENSOR surveillance systems. RADS cases had significant adverse medical and occupational outcomes identified by follow-back interview. In particular, 89% still had breathing problems, 78% had sought emergency care and 39% had been hospitalized for work-related breathing problems; 54% had applied for worker compensation benefits; and 41% had left the company where they experienced onset of asthma. These values were equal to or higher than the comparable figures for those work-related OA cases in which onset was attributed to a known inducer. The authors concluded that RADS cases represent a minority of all work-related asthma cases, but the adverse health impact of this condition appears to equal that of cases of OA with a latency period, a conclusion also reached in a study carried out by Malo and coworkers (Malo et al. 1994).

Work-Aggravated Asthma

Despite its immense medical and societal importance, very little is known about the importance of asthma-related work disability and the prognosis of these workers compared to workers with true OA. Two recent studies explored this topic. Larbanois et al. investigated the socio-economic outcomes of subjects who experienced WAA symptoms in the absence of demonstrable OA and compared these outcomes with those of subjects with documented OA (Larbanois et al. 2002). Subjects ($n = 157$) who were being investigated for work-related asthma were surveyed. Of these, 86 had OA, ascertained by a positive specific inhalation challenge (SIC), and 71 had a negative SIC response. After a median interval of 43 months (range 12–85 months), the subjects were interviewed to collect information on employment status, income changes, and asthma-related work disability. Rates of work disruption and income loss at follow-up were similar in subjects with negative SIC (46% and 59% respectively) and in those with OA (38% and 62%). The median loss as a percentage of initial income was 23% in subjects with negative SIC and 22% in subjects with OA. Asthma-related work disability, defined as any job change or work loss due to asthma, was slightly more common in subjects with OA (72%) than in those with negative SIC (54%). More recently, Lemière et al. (2006b) conducted a cross-sectional study in subjects previously investigated for work-related asthma within 1–4 years of their original diagnosis of OA or WAA. Subjects were considered to have OA if they showed a positive specific inhalation challenge to an occupational agent, whereas subjects were considered as having WAA if they reported a worsening of their asthma symptoms when at work but showed a negative specific inhalation challenge to occupational agents. Clinical, functional, inflammatory and occupational characteristics were reassessed in both classes of subjects. Eighteen subjects with OA and 10 with WAA were assessed. All subjects with OA had to change their work environment, except one worker who had developed OA due to exposure to an occupational sensitizer used by a colleague working next to him. No subjects with WAA remained in the same workplace post-diagnosis. These two studies therefore show that, even in the absence of demonstrable OA, work-related asthma symptoms are associated with considerable socio-economic consequences.

Costs

Compensation

In the context of OA, provisions for temporary and permanent disability should be applied (see above) (Bersntein et al. 2006). These result in significant costs. Once the diagnosis is confirmed, the subject should be considered 100% impaired on a permanent basis in terms of the job that caused the illness, as well as other jobs entailing exposure to the same causative agent. It is important for subjects with OA with a latency period to no longer be exposed to the causal agent, as further exposure will increase the risk of deterioration of asthma (Côté et al. 1990; Moscato et al. 1999). In subjects with OA with a latency period, the threshold level of exposure for developing symptoms, airway obstruction and/or hyper-responsiveness is very much lower than that required for "sensitization." Subjects may react to a minute amount of the causative agent, which precludes any further exposure to the product. Financial compensation should be offered in every instance where there is a loss of earning power. Workers should be re-assessed 2 years after leaving exposure for permanent disability/impairment (see above). Compensation is not the same in all countries; most compensation systems are administered by national agencies (Dewitte et al. 1994; Bersntein et al. 2006). However, in the United States, disputes are usually settled through litigation in an adversarial setting. Evidence from witnesses is presented. Once a claim is accepted, complete medical care is provided and medical expenses are paid either by the privately insured employer or by the state compensation fund for workers who qualify under various programs (Bersntein et al. 2006). In most U.S. states, workers' compensation wage replacement equals two-thirds of workers' pre-disability wages, up to a maximum determined from the statewide average weekly wage for the duration of disability.

In Quebec, it has been estimated that a case of OA with a latency period accepted by the provincial medico-legal agency costs an average of $50,000 CAN in the late 1980s (Dewitte et al. 1994). There was an increase to $75,000 CAN since, with a plateau thereafter (Table 18.3). Approximately 80% of that sum is allocated as temporary indemnities insuring a full salary for the period of 1–2 years required for finding a new job with or without retraining. The rest is allocated for permanent disability indemnities.

Surveillance Program in High-Risk Workplaces

A consensus statement in 1995 suggested that "routine surveillance be performed in all workers with exposure to agents known to cause asthma and especially if cases of work-related asthma have occurred at a particular worksite" (Chan-Yeung 1995). Surveillance decisions in occupational settings must often be made without evidence of relative benefits and costs. A surveillance program with workers exposed to diisocyanates in Ontario coupled an industrial hygiene approach, by which levels of exposure were reduced, and a medical surveillance. Although this has resulted in a reduction of cases after a few years, it is not known if these gains were principally due to the industrial hygiene program or the medical surveillance, or both (Tarlo et al. 1997a), (b) in a period during which cases of OA due to diisocyanates diminished worldwide, even in countries where no surveillance programs were applied.

Using the example of diisocyanate-induced OA, the most common type of OA with a latency period, Wild et al. recently published a model-based approach to evaluate the costs and benefits of surveillance from the perspectives of both employers and society (Wild et al. 2005). The authors used a mathematical simulation model of diisocyanate-induced OA to compare annual surveillance to passive case finding. Outcome measures included symptom-free days, quality adjusted life years (QALY), direct costs, productivity losses, and incremental

Table 18.3 Summary of cost for occupational asthma in Québec, 1989–1999

Year	Temporary indemnities	Permanent disability indemnities	Total[a]
1988	31,400 (390–36,600)	8,900 (2,000–13,200)	41,000 (420–49,500)
1989	41,100 (500–45,700)	14,800 (2,000–13,700)	61,000 (700–63,000)
1990	50,900 (270–60,200)	13,400 (2,300–17,400)	63,700 (400–80,800)
1991	61,900 (4,200–101,700)	9,100 (2,100–14,000)	71,300 (3,800–125,000)
1992	54,700 (5,000–74,300)	13,600 (4,700–18,500)	70,400 (15,300–92,000)
1993	52,900 (3,600–80,800)	14,800 (4,300–20,400)	70,900 (11,600–111,600)
1994	49,900 (2,200–66,000)	14,300 (6,50–20,600)	62,100 (2,700–79,400)
1995	47,600 (21,200–54,400)	11,800 (2,100–18,700)	72,100 (33,000–84,500)
1996	54,800 (3,500–82,600)	11,400 (2,300–16,500)	75,600 (21,600–122,200)
1997	53,600 (15,400–79,800)	13,700 (2,400–20,100)	77,600 (31,200–104,400)
1998	51,100 (11,600–73,200)	13,100 (3,700–20,800)	77,200 (22,200–132,300)
1999	49,600 (1,100–62,700)	11,800 (2,400–18,000)	71,800 (35,600–90,100)

[a]The total also includes medical fees and drug reimbursement

cost effectiveness ratio (CER), measured from both perspectives. For 100,000 exposed workers, surveillance resulted in 683 fewer cases of disability over 10 years. Surveillance conferred benefits at an incremental cost of $24,000/QALY (employer perspective; $13.33/SFD) and was a cost saving from the societal perspective. Baseline results placed the CER for surveillance for diisocyanate-induced OA within the acceptable range. Costs from the societal and employer perspectives differed substantially, with a more attractive CER from the societal perspective, suggesting opportunities for employer/societal cost-sharing.

Conclusion

Asthma in the workplace can have important health and socio-economic consequences (Vandenplas et al. 2003). As regards health issues, workers should be investigated by objective means, not by questionnaires alone. If the workplace is shown to be the cause of the asthma (referred to as "occupational asthma with a latency period," see above), workers should ideally be removed from exposure, as this always has a beneficial effect, including complete cure from asthma, whereas continuing exposure leads to worsened asthma. As regards socio-economic impact, workers with asthma caused by the workplace should be offered satisfactory rehabilitation programs so as to minimize impairment/disability. If there is no cure for the asthma as a result of cessation of exposure, compensation should be offered.

References

Al-Otaibi S, Tarlo SM, House R (2005) Quality of life in patients with latex allergy. Occup Med 55:88–92
Ameille J, Descatha A (2005) Outcome of occupational asthma. Curr Opin Allergy Clin Immunol 5:125–128
Ameille J, Pauli G, Calastreng-Crinquand A, Vervloët D, Iwatsubo Y, Popin E, Bayeux-Dunglas MC, Kofperschmitt-Kubler MC (2003) ONAP and the corresponding members of the. Reported incidence of occupational asthma in France, 1996–99. Occup Environ Med 60:136–142
American Medical Association (2001) In: Cocchiarella L, Andersson GBJ (eds) Guides to the evaluation of permanent impairment, 5th edn. American Medical Association, Chicago, IL
American Thoracic Society (1993) Guidelines for the evaluation of impairment/disability in patients with asthma. Am Rev Respir Dis 147:1056–1061
Archambault S, Malo JL, Infante-Rivard C, Ghezzo H, Gautrin D (2001) Incidence of sensitization, symptoms and probable occupational rhinoconjunctivitis and asthma in apprentices starting exposure to latex. J Allergy Clin Immunol 107:921–923
Arif AA, Whitehead LW, Delclos GL, Tortolero SR, Lee ES (2002) Prevalence and risk factors of work related asthma by industry among United States workers: data from the third national health and nutrition examination survey (1988–94). Occup Environ Med 59:505–11
Axon EJ, Beach JR, Burge PS (1995) A comparison of some of the characteristics of patients with occupational and non-occupational asthma. Occup Med 45:109–111
Barker RD, van Tongeren MJ, Harris JM, Gardiner K, Venables KM, Newman Taylor AJ (1998) Risk factors for sensitisation and respiratory symptoms among workers exposed to acid anhydrides: a cohort study. Occup Environ Med 55:684–691
Becklake M, Ernst P, Chan-Yeung M, Manfreda J, Dimich-Ward H, Sears M, Siersted H (1996) The burden of asthma attributable to work exposures in Canada. Am J Respir Crit Care Med 153:A433
Becklake MR, Chan-Yeung M, Malo JL (2006) Epidemiological approaches in occupational asthma. In: Bernstein IL, Chan-Yeung M, Malo JL, Bernstein DI (eds) Asthma in the workplace, 3rd edn. Taylor & Francis, New York, 37–85
Bernstein JA (2002) Material safety data sheets: are they reliable in identifying human hazards? J Allergy Clin Immunol 110:35–8

Bernstein IL, Chan-Yeuno M, Malo JL, Merget R, Bernstein OI eds (2006) Metals. In: Asthma in the workplace, 3rd edn. Taylor & Francis, New York, pp 525–554

Bernstein IL, Chan-Yeung M, Malo JL, Berstein DI (2006) Asthma in the workplace, 3rd edn. Taylor & Francis, New York

Bersntein IL, Keskinen H, Blanc PD, Chan-Yeung M, Malo JL (2006) Medicolegal aspects, compensation aspects, and evaluation of impairment/disability. In: Bernstein IL, Chan-Yeung M, Malo JL, Bernstein DI (eds) Asthma in the Workplace, 3rd edn. Taylor & Francis, New York, pp 319–351

Blanc PD, Toren K (1999) How much asthma can be attributed to occupational factors? Am J Med 107:580–587

Blanc PD, Cisternas M, Smith S, Yelin EH (1996) Asthma, employment status, and disability among adults treated by pulmonary and allergy specialists. Chest 109:688–696

Brightling CE, Ward R, Goh KL, Wardlaw AJ, Pavord ID (1999) Eosinophilic bronchitis is an important cause of chronic cough. Am J Respir Crit Care Med 160:406–410

Brisman J, Lillienberg L, Belin L, Ahman M, Jarvholm B (2003) Sensitization to occupational allergens in bakers' asthma and rhinitis: a case-referent study. Int Arch Occup Environ Health 76:167–170

Brisman J, Nieuwenhuijsen MJ, Venables KM (2004) Exposure–response relations for work related respiratory symptoms and sensitisation in a cohort exposed to alpha-amylase. Occup Environ Med 61:551–553

Brooks SM, Weiss MA, Bernstein IL (1985) Reactive airways dysfunction syndrome (RADS); persistent asthma syndrome after high level irritant exposures. Chest 88:376–84

Chan-Yeung M (1995) Assessment of asthma in the workplace. Chest 108:1084–1117

Chan-Yeung M, Malo JL (1995) Occupational asthma. N Engl J Med 333:107–112

Chan-Yeung M, Bernstein IL, Essen Von S, Singh J, Schwartz DA (2006) Acute airway diseases due to organic dust exposure. In: Bernstein IL, Chan-Yeung M, Malo JL, Bernstein DI (eds) Asthma in the workplace, 3rd edn. Taylor & Francis, New York, pp 641–682

Chatkin CJM, Tarlo SM, Liss G, Banks D, Broder I (1999) The outcome of asthma related to workplace exposures. Chest 116:1780–1785

Cockcroft DW, Murdock KY, Kirby J, Hargreave F (1987) Prediction of airway responsiveness to allergen from skin sensitivity to allergen and airway responsiveness to histamine. Am Rev Respir Dis 135:264–7

Contreras GR, Rousseau R, Chan-Yeung M (1994) Occupational respiratory diseases in British Columbia, Canada in 1991. Occup Env Med 51:710–712

Côté J, Kennedy S, Chan-Yeung M (1990) Outcome of patients with cedar asthma with continuous exposure. Am Rev Respir Dis 141:373–6

Cullinan P, Cook A, Gordon S, Nieuwenhuijsen MJ, Tee RD, Venables KM, McDonald JC, Newman Taylor AJ (1999) Allergen exposure, atopy and smoking as determinants of allergy to rats in a cohort of laboratory employees. Eur Respir J 13:1139–1143

Cullinan P, Taylor AJ, Taylor Newman AJ, Hole AM, Jones M, Barnes F, Jolliffe G (2000) An outbreak of asthma in a modern detergent factory. Lancet 356:1899–1900

Cullinan P, Cook A, Nieuwenhuijsen MJ, Sandiford C, Tee RD, Venables KM, McDonald JC, Taylor Newman AJ (2001) Allergen and dust exposure as determinants of work-related symptoms and sensitization in a cohort of flour-exposed workers; a case-control analysis. Ann occup hyg 45:97–103

Das R, Blanc PD (1993) Chlorine gas exposure and the lung: a review. Toxicol Ind Health 9:439–455

De Zotti R, Bovenzi M (2000) Prospective study of work related respiratory symptoms in trainee bakers. Occup Environ Med 57:58–61

Demnati R, Fraser R, Ghezzo H, Martin JG, Plaa G, Malo JL (1998a) Time-course of functional and pathological changes after a single high acute inhalation of chlorine in rats. Eur Respir J 11:922–928

Demnati R, Fraser R, Martin JG, Plaa G, Malo JL (1998b) Effects of dexamethasone on functional and pathological changes in rat bronchi caused by high acute exposure to chlorine. Toxicol Sci 45:242–246

Desjardins A, Bergeron JP, Ghezzo H, Cartier A, Malo JL (1994) Aluminium potroom asthma confirmed by monitoring of forced expiratory volume in one second. Am J Respir Crit Care Med 150:1714–1717

Dewitte JD, Chan-Yeung M, Malo JL (1994) Medicolegal and compensation aspects of occupational asthma. Eur Respir J 7:969–980

El-Zein M, Malo JL, Infante-Rivard C, Gautrin D (2003) Incidence of probable occupational asthma and of changes in airway calibre and responsiveness in apprentice welders. Eur Respir J 22:513–518

El-Zein M, Infante-Rivard C, Malo JL, Gautrin D (2005) Is metal fume fever a determinant of welding related respiratory symptoms and/or increased bronchial responsiveness? A longitudinal study. Occup Environ Med 62:688–694

Fishwick D, Pearce N, D'Souza W, Lewis S, Town I, Armstrong R, Kogevinas M, Crane J (1997) Occupational asthma in New Zealanders: a population based study. Occup Environ Med 54:301–306

Gannon PF, Burge PS (1993) The SHIELD scheme in the West Midlands Region, United Kingdom. Midland Thoracic Society Research Group. Br J Ind Med 50(9):791–796

Gannon PFG, Weir DC, Robertson AS, Burge PS (1993) Health, employment, and financial outcomes in workers with occupational asthma. Br J Ind Med 50:491–496

Gautrin D, Boulet LP, Boutet M, Dugas M, Bhérer L, L'Archevêque J, Laviolette M, Côté J, Malo JL (1994) Is reactive airways dysfunction syndrome a variant of occupational asthma? J Allergy Clin Immunol 93:12–22

Gautrin D, Infante-Rivard C, Dao TV, Magnan-Larose M, Desjardins D, Malo JL (1997) Specific IgE-dependent sensitization, atopy and bronchial hyperresponsiveness in apprentices starting exposure to protein-derived agents. Am J Respir Crit Care Med 155:1841–1847

Gautrin D, Ghezzo H, Infante-Rivard C, Malo J-L (2000) Incidence and determinants of IgE-mediated sensitization in apprentices: a prospective study. Am J Respir Crit Care Med 162:1222–1228

Gautrin D, Infante-Rivard C, Ghezzo H, Malo JL (2001a) Incidence and host determinants of probable occupational asthma in apprentices exposed to laboratory animals. Am J Respir Crit Care Med 163:899–904

Gautrin D, Ghezzo H, Infante-Rivard C, Malo JL (2001b) Natural history of sensitization, symptoms and diseases in apprentices exposed to laboratory animals. Eur Respir J 17:904–908

Gautrin D, Ghezzo H, Infante-Rivard C, Malo JL (2002) Incidence and host determinants of work-related rhinoconjunctivitis in apprentice pastry-makers. Allergy 57:913–918

Gautrin D, Newman-Taylor AJ, Nordman H, Malo JL (2003) Controversies in epidemiology of occupational asthma. Eur Respir J 22:551–559

Gautrin D, Bernstein IL, Brooks SM, Henneberger PK (2006) Reactive airways dysfunction syndrome and irritant-induced asthma. In: Bernstein IL, Chan-Yeung M, Malo JL, Bernstein DI (eds) Asthma in the Workplace, Taylor & Francis, New York, 581–629

Gautrin D, Bernstein IL, Brooks SM, Henneberger PK (2006) Reactive airways dysfunction syndrome and irritant-induced asthma. In: Bernstein IL, Chan-Yeung M, Malo JL, Bernstein DI (eds) Asthma in the workplace, 3rd edn. Taylor & Francis, New York, pp 579–627

Gibson PG, Dolovich J, Denburg J, Ramsdale EH (1989) Chronic cough: Eosinophilic bronchitis without asthma. Lancet 1:1346–1348

Girard F, Chaboillez S, Cartier A, Côté J, Hargreave FE, Labrecque M, Malo JL, Tarlo S, Lemière C (2004) An effective strategy for diagnosing occupational asthma. Induced sputum. Am J Respir Crit Care Med 170:845–850

Goe SK, Henneberger PK, Reilly MJ, Rosenman KD, Schill DP, Valiante D, Flattery J, Harrison R, Reinisch F, Tompowsky C, Filios MS (2004) A descriptive study of work aggravated asthma. Occup Environ Med 61:512–517

Goldney RD, Ruffin R, Fisher LJ, Wilson DH (2003) Asthma symptoms associated with depression and lower quality of life: a population survey. Med J Aust 178:437–441

Goodwin RD, Jacobi F, Thefeld W (2003) Mental disorders and asthma in the community. Arch Gen Psychiatry 60:1125–1130

Gregerson MB (2003) The historical catalyst to cure asthma. In: Brown ES (ed) Asthma: social and psychological factors and psychosomatic syndromes. Basel, Karger, pp 16–41

Henneberger PK, Ferris Jr, BG, Sheehe PR (1993) Accidental gassing incidents and the pulmonary function of pulp mill workers. Am Rev Respir Dis 148:63–67

Henneberger PK, Derk SJ, Sama SR, Boylstein RJ, Hoffman CD, Preusse PA, Rosiello RA, Milton DK (2006) The frequency of workplace exacerbation among health maintenance organisation members with asthma. Occup Environ Med 63:551–557

Hnizdo E, Esterhuizen TM, Rees D, Lalloo UG (2001) Occupational asthma as identified by the Surveillance of Work-related and Occupational Respiratory Diseases programme in South Africa. Clin Exp Allergy 31:32–39

Illfeld FW (1976) Further validation of a psychiatric symptom index in a normal population. Psychol Rep 39:1215–1228

Janson C, Bjornsson E, Hetta J, Boman G (1994) Anxiety and depression in relation to respiratory symptoms and asthma. Am J Respir Crit Care Med 149:930–934

Johnson AR, Dimich-Ward HD, Manfreda J, Becklake MR, Ernst P, Sears MR, Bowie DM, Sweet L, Chan-Yeung M (2000) Occupational asthma in adults in six Canadian communities. Am J Respir Crit Care Med 162:2058–2062

Juniper EF, Buist AS, Cox FM, Ferrie PJ, King DR (1999) Validation of a standardized version of the asthma quality of life questionnaire. Chest 115:1265–1270

Kang MG, Koh SB, Cha BS, Park JK, Baik SK, Chang SJ (2005) Job stress and cardiovascular risk factors in male workers. Prev Med 40:583–588

Kaptein AA (1982) Psychological correlates of length of hospitalization and rehospitalization in patients with acute, severe asthma. Soc Sci Med 16:725–729

Karjalainen A, Kurppa K, Virtanen S, Keskinen H, Nordman H (2000) Incidence of occupational asthma by occupation and industry in Finland. Am J Ind Med 37:451–458

Karjalainen A, Kurppa K, Martikainen R, Klaukka T, Karjalainen J (2001) Work is related to a substantial portion of adult-onset asthma incidence in the Finnish population. Am J Resp Crit Care Med 164:565–568

Karjalainen A, Kurppa K, Martikainen R, Karjalainen J, Klaukka T (2002) Exploration of asthma risk by occupation-extended analysis of an incidence study of the Finnish population. Scand J Work Environ Health 28:49–57

Kogevinas M, Anto JM, Soriano JB, Tobias A, Burney P (1996) The risk of asthma attibutable to occupational exposures: A population-based study in Spain. Spanish Group of the European Asthma Study. Am J Respir Crit Care Med 154:137–143

Kogevinas M, Anto JM, Sunyer J, Tobias A, Kromhout H, Burney P (1999) Group and the European Community Respiratory Health Survey Study. Occupational asthma in Europe and other industrialised areas: a population-based study. Lancet 353:1750–1754

Kolbe J, Vamos M, Fergusson W, Elkind G, Garrette J (1996) Differential influences on asthma self-management knowledge and self-management behavior in acute severe asthma. Chest 110:1463–1468

Lagier F, Cartier A, Malo JL (1990) Statistiques médico-légales sur l'asthme professionnel au Québec de 1986 à 1988. Medico-legal statistics on occupational asthma in Quebec between 1986 and 1988. Rev Mal Respir 7:337–341

Laplante M (1988) Data on disability from the National Health Interview Survey 1883–1985. InfoUsed Report. US National Institute on Disability and Rehabilitation Research, Washington, DC

Larbanois A, Jamart J, Delwiche JP, Vandenplas O (2002) Socioeconomic outcome of subjects experiencing asthma symptoms at work. Eur Respir J 19:1107–1113

Last JM (1995) A dictionary of epidemiology, 3rd edn. Oxford University Press, Oxford, pp 1–180

Lavoie KL, Cartier A, Labrecque M, Bacon SL, Lemière C, Malo JL, Lacoste G, Barone S, Verrier P, Ditto B (2005) Are psychiatric disorders associated with worse asthma control and quality of life in asthma patients? Respir Med 99:1249–1257

Lavoie KL, Bacon SL, Cartier A, Barone S, Ditto B, Labrecque M (2006) What's worse for asthma control and quality of life: depressive disorders, anxiety disorders, or both? Chest 130:1039–1047

Lee S, Colditz GA, Berkman LF, Kawashi I (2004) Prospective study of job insecurity and coronary heart disease in US women. Ann Epidemiol 14:24–30

Leigh JP, Romano PS, Schenker MB, Kreiss K (2002) Costs of occupational COPD and asthma. Chest 121:264–72

Lemière C, Hargreave FE (1999) Occupational eosinophilic bronchitis without asthma. Can J Allergy Clin Immunol 4:332–335

Lemière C, Malo JL, Boutet M (1997) Reactive airways dysfunction syndrome due to chlorine: sequential bronchial biopsies and functional assessment. Eur Respir J 10:241–244

Lemière C, Biagini RE, Zeiss CR (2006) Immunological and inflammatory assessments. In: Bernstein IL, Chan-Yeung M, Malo JL, Bernstein DI (eds) Asthma in the workplace, 3rd edn. Taylor & Francis, New York, 179–197

Lemière C, Pelissier S, Chaboillez S, Teolis L (2006b) Outcome of subjects diagnosed with occupational asthma and work-aggravated asthma after removal from exposure. J Occup Environ Med 48:656–659

LeMoual N, Siroux V, Pin I, Kauffmann F, Kennedy SM (2005) (EGEA) on behalf of the epidemiological study on the genetics and environment of asthma. Asthma severity and exposure to occupational asthmogens. Am J Respir Crit Care Med 172:440–445

Levenstein S, Smith MW, Kaplan GA (2001) Psychosocial predictors of hypetension in men and women. Arch Inter Med 161:1341–1346

Malo JL, Ghezzo H (2004) Recovery of methacholine responsiveness after end of exposure in occupational asthma. Am J Respir Crit Care Med 169:1304–1307

Malo JL, Cartier A, L'Archevêque J, Ghezzo H, Soucy F, Somers J, Dolovich J (1990) Prevalence of occupational asthma and immunological sensitization to guar gum among employees at a carpet-manufacturing plant. J Allergy Clin Immunol 86:562–9

Malo JL, Ghezzo H, D'Aquino C, L'Archevêque J, Cartier A, Chan-Yeung M (1992) Natural history of occupational asthma: relevance of type of agent and other factors in the rate of development of symptoms in affected subjects. J Allergy Clin Immunol 90:937–944

Malo JL, Dewitte JD, Cartier A, Ghezzo H, L'Archevêque J, Boulet LP, Côté J, Bédard G, Boucher S, Champagne F, Tessier G, Contandriopoulos AP (1993) Quality of life of subjects with occupational asthma. J Allergy Clin Immunol 91:1121–1127

Malo JL, Cartier A, Boulet LP, L'Archevêque J, Saint-Denis F, Bhérer L, Courteau JP (1994) Bronchial hyperresponsiveness can improve while spirometry plateaus two to three years after repeated exposure to chlorine causing respiratory symptoms. Am J Respir Crit Care Med 150:1142–1145

Malo JL, Cartier A, Côté J, Milot J, Leblanc C, Paquette L, Ghezzo H, Boulet LP (1996) Influence of inhaled steroids on the recovery of occupational asthma after cessation of exposure: an 18-month double-blind cross-over study. Am J Crit Care Respir Med 153:953–960

Manfreda J, Becker AB, Wang PZ, Roos LL, Anthonisen NR (1993) Trends in physician-diagnosed asthma prevalence in Manitoba between 1980 and 1990. Chest 103:151–157

Mapp CE, Boschetto P, Maestrelli P, Fabbri LM (2005) Occupational asthma. Am J Respir Crit Care Med 172:280–305

Marabini A, Siracusa A, Stopponi R, Tacconi C, Abbritti G (2003) Outcome of occupational asthma in patients with continuous exposure: a 3-year longitudinal study during pharmacologic treatment. Chest 124:2372–6

Markovitz JH, Matthews KA, Whooley M, Lewis CE, Greenlund KJ (2004) Increases in job strain are associated with incident hypertension in the CARDIA study. Ann Behav Med 28:4–9

Martin JG, Campbell HR, Iijima H, Gautrin D, Malo JL, Eidelman DH, Hamid Q, Maghni K (2003) Chlorine-induced injury to the airways in the mouse. Am J Respir Crit Care Med 168:568–574

Matte TD, Hoffman RE, Rosenman KD, Stanbury M (1990) Surveillance of occupational asthma under the SENSOR model. Chest 98:173S–178S

McDonald JC (1995) Methodology. Study design. In: McDonald JC (ed) Epidemiology of work related diseases. BMJ:325–351

McDonald JC, Keynes HL, Meredith SK (2000) Reported incidence of occupational asthma in the United Kingdom, 1989–97. Occup Environ Med 57:823–829

McDonald JC, Chen Y, Zekveld C, Cherry NM (2005) Incidence by occupation and industry of acute work related respiratory diseases in the UK, 1992–2001. Occup Environ Med 62:836–842

Meggs WJ (1994) RADS and RUDS-The toxic induction of asthma and rhinitis. J Toxicol Clin Toxicol 32:487–501

Millon T (1994) Millon multiaxial inventory, 3rd edn. National Computer Systems, Minneapolis, MN

Mitchell CA, Gandevia B (1971) Respiratory symptoms and skin reactivity in workers exposed to proteolytic enzymes in the detergent industry. Am Rev Respir Dis 104:1–12

Moscato G, Dellabianca A, Perfetti L, Brame B, Galdi E, Niniano R, Paggiaro P (1999) Occupational asthma. A longitudinal study on the clinical and socioeconomic outcome after diagnosis. Chest 115:249–256

Moscato G, Dellabianca A, Maestrelli P, Paggiaro P, Romano C, de Zotti R, Marabini A, Voltolini S, Crippa M, Previdi M, Bramé B, Benzon R, Siracusa A (2002) Features and severity of occupational asthma upon diagnosis: an Italian multicentric case review. Allergy 57:236–242

Murphy RLH (1976) Industrial diseases with asthma. In: Weiss EB, Segal MS (eds) Bronchial asthma, Little, Brown and Cie, Boston, pp 517–536

Naciemento I, Nardi AE, Valenca AM, Lopes FL, Mezzasalma MA, Nascentes R, Zin WA (2002) Psychiatric disorders in asthmatic outpatients. Psychiatry Res 110:73–80

Nemery B (1996) Late consequences of accidental exposure to inhaled irritants: RADS and the Bhopal disaster. Eur Respir J 9:1973–1976

Netjeck V, Brown E, Khan D, Moore J, Wagner J, Perantie D (2001) Prevalence of mood disorders and relationship to asthma severity in patients at an inner-city asthma clinic. Ann Allergy Asthma Immunol 87:129–133

Newman Taylor A (2002) Asthma and work. Ann Occup Hyg 46:563–574

Newman-Taylor AJ, Venables KM (1984) Clinical and epidemiological methods in investigating occupational asthma. Clin Immunol Allergy 4:3–17

Ng TP, Hong CY, Goh LG, Wong ML, Koh KTC, Ling SL (1994) Risks of asthma associated with occupations in a community-based case-control study. Am J Ind Med 25:709–718

Nicholson PJ, Cullinan P, Newman TAJ, Burge PS, Boyle C (2005) Evidence based guidelines for the prevention, identification, and management of occupational asthma. Occup Environ Med 62:290–299

Ortega HG, Kreiss K, Schill DP, Weissman DN (2002) Fatal asthma from powdering shark cartilage and review of fatal occupational asthma literature. Am J Ind Med 42:50–54

Osler W (1892) The principles and practice of medicine. D. Appleton & Cie, New York, Special Edition Copyright 1978, The Classics of Medicine Library, Birmingham, AL

Perna G, Bertani A, Politi E, Colombo G, Bellodi L (1997) Asthma and panic attacks. Biol Psychiatry 42:625–630

Provencher S, Labrèche FP, De GL (1997) Physician based surveillance system for occupational respiratory diseases: the experience of PROPULSE, Québec, Canada. Occup Env Med 54:272–276

Quirce S (2004) Eosinophilic bronchitis in the workplace. Curr Opin Allergy Clin Immunol 4:87–91

Reijula K, Haahtela T, Klaukka T, Rantanen J (1996) Incidence of occupational asthma and persistent asthma in young adults has increased in Finland. Chest 110:58–61

Ries P (1986) Current estimates from the National health Interview Survey: United States, 1984. National Health Survey, Series 10, no 156. DHHS Publication (PHS), Washington, DC

Rimington LD, Davies DH, Lowe D, Pearson MG (2001) Relationship between anxiety, depression, and morbidity in adult asthma patients. Thorax 56:266–271

Rodier F, Gautrin D, Ghezzo H, Malo JL (2003) Incidence of occupational rhinoconjunctivitis and risk factors in animal-health apprentices. J Allergy Clin Immunol 112:1105–1111

Saarinen K, Karjalainen A, Martikainen R, Uitti J, Tammilehto L, Klaukka T, Kuppa K (2003) Prevalence of work-aggravated symptoms in clinically established asthma. Eur Respir J 22:305–309

Scanlon PD (2002) World Trade Center cough – A lingering legacy and a cautionary tale. N Engl J Med 347:840–842

Slovak AJM, Orr RG, Teasdale EL (1985) Efficacy of the helmet respirator in occupational asthma due to laboratory animal allergy (LAA). Am Ind Hyg Assoc J 46:411–5

Tarlo SM (2000) Workplace respiratory irritants and asthma. Occup Med: State Art Rev 15:471–483

Tarlo SM, Liss GM (2005) Prevention of occupational asthma–practical implications for occupational physicians. Occup Med (Lond) 55:588–594

Tarlo SM, Liss G, Corey P, Broder I (1995) A workers' compensation claim population for occupational asthma. Chest 107:634–641

Tarlo SM, Liss GM, Banks DE (1997a) Assessment of the relationship between isocyanate exposure levels and occupational asthma. Am J Ind Med 32:517–521

Tarlo SM, Banks D, Liss G, Broder I (1997b) Outcome determinants for isocyanate induced occupational asthma among compensation claimants. Occup Environ Med 54:756–761

Toelle BG, Peat JK, Salome CM, Mellis CM, Woolcock AJ (1992) Toward a definition of asthma for epidemiology. Am rev Respir Dis 146:633–637

Toren L (1996) Self reported rate of occupational asthma in Sweden 1990–2. Occup Environ Med 53:757–761

Toren K, Brisman J, Olin AC, Blanc PD (2000) Asthma on the job: work-related factors in new-onset asthma and in exacerbations of pre-existing asthma. Respir Med 94:529–535

Troyanov S, Malo JL, Cartier A, Gautrin D (2000) Frequency and determinants of exaggerated bronchoconstriction during shortened methacholine challenge tests in epidemiological and clinical set-ups. Eur Respir J 16:9–14

Trupin L, Earnest G, SanPedro M, Balmes JR, Eisner MD, Yelin E, Katz PP, Blanc PD (2003) The occupational burden of chronic obstructive pulmonary disease. Eur Respir J 22: 462–469

Vandenplas O, Malo JL (2003) Definitions and types of work-related asthma: a nosological approach. Eur Respir J 21:706–712

Vandenplas O, Delwiche JP, Depelchin S, Sibille Y, Vande Weyer R, Delaunois L (1995) Latex gloves with a lower protein content reduce bronchial reactions in subjects with occupational asthma caused by latex. Am J Respir Crit Care Med 151:887–891

Vandenplas O, Toren K, Blanc P (2003) Health and socioeconomic impact of work-related asthma. Eur Respir J 22:689–697

Vandenplas O, Ghezzo H, Munoz X, Moscato G, Perfetti L, Lemière C, Labrecque M, L'Archevêque J, Malo JL (2005) What are the questionnaire items most useful in identifying subjects with occupational asthma? Eur Respir J 26:1056–1063

Vandenplas O, Cartier A, Malo JL (2006) Occupational challenge tests. In: Bernstein IL, Chan-Yeung M, Malo JL, Bernstein DI (eds) Asthma in the workplace, 3rd edn. Taylor & Francis, New York, 227–252

Vanhanen M, Tuomi T, Tiikkainen U, Tupasela O, Voutilainen R, Nordman H (2000) Risk of enzyme allergy in the detergent industry. Occup Environ Med 57:121–125

Vollmer WM, Heumann MA, Breen VR, Henneberger PK, O'connor EA, Villnave JM, Frazier EA, Buist AS (2005) Incidence of work-related asthma in members of a health maintenance organization. J Occup Environ Med 47: 1292–1297

Wagner GR, Wegman DH (1998) Occupational asthma: Prevention by definition. Am J Ind Med 33:427–429

Walusiak J, Hanke W, Gorski P, Palczynski C (2004) Respiratory allergy in apprentice bakers: do occupational allergies follow the allergic march? Allergy 59:442–450

Weiss KB, Gergen PJ, Hodgson TA (1992) An economic evaluation of asthma in the United States. N Engl J Med 327:571–572

Wild DM, Redlich CA, Paltiel AD (2005) Surveillance for isocyanate asthma: a model based cost effectiveness analysis. Occup Environ Med 62:743–749

Chapter 19
The Cost of Asthma

Adam Atherly

Introduction

Asthma is one of the most costly chronic illnesses in both the developed and developing world. Asthma is a significant factor in the use of health care services, particularly emergency departments and prescription medications. In the United States, asthma is the 13th most costly medical condition and the 7th leading cause of work-loss days (Druss et al. 2002). The cost for patients with asthma in Western countries ranges from $300 to $1,300 per capita per year (Braman 2006). In the future, costs are expected to substantially increase.

The purpose of this chapter is to discuss the cost of asthma to society and to evaluate the role of cost in individual access to care. The impact of cost on societies differs from that on individuals. For societies, the economic burden of an illness can help to prioritize the use of economic resources. Understanding which illnesses, from a societal perspective, use the most resources can suggest illnesses where treatments can be potentially cost saving.

Higher costs can represent a barrier to care. For individuals, the cost of care at the point of service is the important element – and the total cost is unimportant if another payer finances the residual cost. The danger with chronic illnesses such as asthma is that higher cost sharing – which typically leads to reduced use of services – may actually result in greater overall expenditures. For example, individuals may forgo relatively inexpensive services such as medications and preventive care but later require expensive services, such as hospital or emergency department services. Higher cost sharing may also lead to reduced health outcomes if costs serve as a barrier to access to care.

The Cost of Asthma to Societies

Cost of illness studies are frequently published in the academic literature, as are critiques of these studies that question their value. Cost of illness studies are criticized on a number of grounds (Koopmanschap 1998; Shiell et al. 1987). First, cost of illness studies provide no guidance on the effectiveness of healthcare spending. Cost of illness studies provide the gains that would be associated with the elimination of the illness – a goal that is usually unattainable. This is in contrast to cost effectiveness studies, which quantify the gains associated with a particular intervention. Because cost of illness studies are not associated with interventions, they cannot establish value (Drummond 1992). That an illness is costly does not necessarily imply that there are effective interventions available that could reduce spending. Shiell et al. argue that the use of cost of illness studies is to prioritize illnesses where spending is already potentially inefficient – the less effective the spending, the more costly the illness, the greater justification for more spending if spending is prioritized according to cost of illness studies.

The value of cost of illness studies lies in their ability to prioritize diseases for future economic evaluation (Koopmanschap 1998; Hodgson 1994). Although costly diseases are not necessarily amenable to treatment, it is reasonable to examine the most costly illnesses for potential cost savings. Much as the famous bank robber

A. Atherly (✉)
Department of Health Systems, Management, & Policy, Colorado School of Public, 13001 E. 17th Place, B119, Bldg. 500, Room E3315, Aurora, CO, 80045, USA
e-mail: adam.atherly@ucdenver.edu

A. Harver and H. Kotses (eds.), *Asthma, Health and Society: A Public Health Perspective*,
DOI 10.1007/978-0-387-78285-0_19, © Springer Science+Business Media, LLC 2010

Willie Sutton, when asked why he robbed banks, replied "Because that's where the money is," trying to control spending by focusing on the most costly illnesses is inherently reasonable. Cost of illness studies can show which of the cost components are most important for particular illnesses. Also, by projecting disease costs into the future based on demographics or epidemiological trends, illnesses that will be priorities in the future can be prospectively identified. Bloom et al. (2001) suggest that the three primary purposes of cost of illness studies are to estimate current costs, measure changes over time and generate new research hypotheses.

Methodological Issues

Differences in estimates of the cost of a particular illness, such as asthma, can be caused by differences in perspective, in focus, in time or in methodology. For methodological differences, there are a series of key methodological choices that lead to different estimates. First, there is the decision of what costs to include. Cost of illness studies typically include direct medical care costs, such as hospital care, medications, physician services and other costs directly related to the provision of care. But studies are less consistent in their treatment of indirect costs. Indirect costs are costs associated with the illness that are not directly borne by the health care system. Examples include costs associated with work loss, reduced productivity, and time costs due to missed school and disease mortality. Previous studies have found that estimates of indirect costs for particular illnesses can vary by a factor of seven (Bloom et al. 2001).

The perspective of the study is also important. The standard is to adopt the societal perspective (Gold et al. 1996). The societal perspective is the broadest possible perspective, and it considers all costs and benefits, regardless of source. The reason for this preference is that other perspectives may be misleading. For example, an intervention that refused to pay for asthma medications could be cost reducing for an insurance company or government payer while imposing substantial costs on individuals in the form of higher prices for prescription drugs and on employers in the form of increased worker absenteeism.

The Cost of Asthma

There have been many studies estimating the cost of asthma. However, these studies have varied widely in their estimates of the cost of asthma, even within particular countries. The variability is caused by differences in methodology, data sources (commercial vs. government), timeframe (as costs increase, new medications are developed and the incidence rate changes), sample (elderly vs. working adults vs. children vs. a representative sample) and the costs included (direct, indirect, medications, emergency room visits). Comparing different estimates of the cost of asthma requires consideration of all these factors. Overall, on average, asthma accounts for 1–2% of total health care costs in developed countries (Sennhauser et al. 2005). The key numbers most studies of the cost of asthma try to quantify are the amount and components of direct costs and the amount and components of indirect costs.

Three relatively recent studies have estimated the cost of illness in the United States. Colice et al. (2006) found that employers in the United States spend, on average, $1,680 more per year for individuals with asthma on asthma specific care (Table 19.1) (Colice et al. 2006). The total increased spending for all medical care was found to be $3,567, with the primary cost being prescription drugs ($1,656) and outpatient care ($1,015). Indirect costs were $924 per person, with the bulk of the costs being associated with absenteeism ($779).

In a similar population, Birnbaum et al. (2002) found that asthmatic patients have approximately three times higher medical claims than the average beneficiary in an employer population, and total average annual per capita employer expenditures (including indirect costs) were approximately 2.5 times higher ($5,385 vs. $2,121). The bulk of the costs were associated with medical care (59%), followed by prescription drugs (25%) and work loss (16%). Notably, the direct cost of asthma care was $1,119, with the remainder of the increased expenditures for asthma being associated with the treatment of non-asthma diagnoses. However, the overall cost of asthma per capita ($3,264) was not dissimilar to that reported by Colice et al. (2006).

A slightly different estimate was calculated by Cisternas et al. (2003) in a cross-sectional survey data from a community-based panel from northern

Table 19.1 The cost of asthma

Excess cost per capita	Sample	Location	Year(s) of data	Author(s)
$4,214	Employer, including retirees and dependents	USA	2002–2003	Colice et al. (2006)
$497 (direct costs only)	Children in a managed care organization	USA	1992	Lozano et al. (1999)
$3,265	Employer claims	USA	1998	Birnbaum et al. (2002)
$4,912	Physicians claims for pulmonologists, allergist-immunologists, and family practitioners	USA	1998–1999	Cisternas et al. (2003)
$756	Nationally survey	USA	1994	Weiss et al. (1992, 2000)
$791	Children	USA	1996	Wang et al. (2005)
CHF 2,797	Physician practices	Switzerland	1996–1997	Szucs et al. (1999)
741€	Young adults in seven centers	Italy	2000	Accordini et al. (2006)
1,260€	Multicenter study in hospital-based asthma clinics	Italy	1999	Antonicelli et al. (2004)
$2,879	Asthma patients who sought care	Spain	1994–1995	Serra-Batlles et al. (1998)
$1,465	Physician sample	Turkey	2002	Celik et al. (2004)
$238	National survey	Singapore	1992–1993	Chew et al. (1999)

California pulmonologists, allergist-immunologists and family practitioners. Total per-person annual costs of asthma were estimated at $4,912. The majority of costs were direct costs ($3,180 or 65% of the total) with indirect costs equal to $1,732 (35%). Half of the direct costs were attributable to prescription drugs ($1,605) followed by hospital admissions ($463) and non-emergency department ambulatory visits ($342). For indirect costs, the majority of the costs were associated with total cessation of work ($1,062 or 61%), followed by work loss for those who remained employed ($486 or 28%). Costs were dramatically higher for those with severe asthma ($12,813) compared to those with moderate ($4,530) or mild ($2,646) asthma.

Older estimates of the cost of illness related to asthma in the United States include a 1990 estimate of $6.2 billion (Weiss et al. 1992). This study found that 43% of the economic impact was associated with emergency room use, hospitalization and death, with the cost of inpatient hospital services estimated to be $1.6 billion; thirty eight percent of total costs were indirect, led by reduced productivity due to loss of school days with a cost of nearly $1 billion in 1990. Similarly, the total cost of asthma in 1987 (in 1994 dollars) was estimated to be $5.8 billion, with direct costs representing 88% of the total (Smith et al. 1997). Hospitalizations accounted for more than half of all expenditures. Finally, Weiss et al. (2000) estimated that the total cost of asthma in 1994 was $10.7 billion (Table 19.1). Of these, direct medical expenditures accounted for 57% of total costs ($6.1 billion), with prescription drugs accounting for the largest direct medical expenditure ($2.5 billion). For indirect costs, 45% of the $4.6 billion expenditure ($2.07 billion) was attributable to loss of work productivity through disability.

Comparable data are available for other countries. For example, total annual costs associated with asthma in Switzerland were estimated at approximately CHF 1,200 million per year (Szucs et al. 1999). Of these, 61% (CHF 762 million) were for direct medical expenditures and the remainder for indirect costs. The bulk of the indirect costs (75%) was associated with home care for asthmatic patients.

In Italy, the mean annual cost per patient was 741€ (Accordini et al. 2006), with 43% of the total cost associated with direct costs and 57% with indirect costs. Medication costs represented 47% of direct medical expenditures and were followed in importance by hospitalizations (23%). But the mean annual cost per patient ranged from only 379€ for well-controlled asthmatics to 1,341€ for poorly controlled cases. The poorly controlled cases accounted for 46% of the total costs.

More recently, among adult patients in Italy, the total cost of asthma was estimated to be 1,260€ (Antonicelli et al. 2004). Total costs were distributed as follows: drug costs (16%), physician costs (12%), emergency service and hospitalization costs (20%) and indirect costs (52%).

Annual costs varied by disease severity: 720€ for intermittent asthma, 1,046€ for mild persistent asthma, 1,535€ for moderate persistent asthma and 3,328€ for patients with severe persistent asthma.

The per capita annual total cost of asthma in Spain was estimated at $2,879 (Serra-Batlles et al. 1998). The proportion of total costs included $885(31%) for direct costs including prescription medications (45%; $400) and hospitalizations (33%; $289). Indirect costs ($1,993) were led by costs associated with work loss. But the cost varied by disease severity; for patients with mild asthma, the total average annual cost was $1,336. For those with moderate asthma, it rose to $2,407, and it rose further to $6,393 for those with severe asthma. In the Netherlands, the top expenditure for asthma is prescription medications (Rutten van-Molken and Feenstra 2001). Annual per capita direct medical care expenditures in 1993 were estimated to be $499 (Rutten-van Molken et al. 1999).

The ratio of direct to indirect costs varies widely internationally (Fig. 19.1). The variability likely reflects both the difficulty in estimating indirect costs and real differences in indirect costs. Direct medical expenditures can typically be estimated using payment or claims data. In contrast, indirect costs involve factors such as work loss or school days missed, which are often not available on standardized data sources. But there is little controversy that asthma imposes substantial costs on workers and on their employers. More than 20% of persons with asthma reported one or more complete or partial work days lost per month (Blanc et al. 2001). In a careful assessment of productivity loss in Canada, workers with asthma lost an average of 12 days of work per year due to asthma (Ungar and Coyte 2000). Most productivity loss is due to restricted days rather than absence, on days when the worker is present but productive at a much lower rate ("presenteeism"). However, a study conducted in the United Kingdom found that the cost of presenteeism ($658 annually) is roughly equivalent to that of absenteeism ($597 annually) (Joshi et al. 2006).

The ratio of direct-to-indirect costs ranges from a high of 87% of total costs being associated with direct costs (in a U.S. worker population) to a low of 25% (in Germany) (Stock et al. 2005). The size of the German estimate may be a function of the pension system in Germany. Of the estimated indirect costs, 58% were associated with payment of sick benefits through sickness funds. The highly formalized German system is in contrast to the less formalized U.S. system, which not only complicates data collection but also likely changes the extent of sick leave taken. Indeed, the top three estimates of the proportion of total costs associated with direct costs are all from the United States (with direct costs constituting 87%, 85% and 65% of total costs, respectively). In Canada 61% of the total cost of asthma was associated with direct medical costs (Krahn et al. 1996). However, many of the estimates are near 50%, including those from Italy, Singapore and another United States estimate focusing on children.

The Cost of Asthma in Children

Children have been a particular area of emphasis for cost of illness studies. Typically, children are healthy and relatively low cost. However, caring for children with asthma can be costly. The United Kingdome spends 0.15% of their total health care budget treating children of age 1–5 with "wheezing disorders" (Stevens et al. 2003). Children with asthma use 88% more health care services, including 2.8 times more prescription drugs, 65% more outpatient visits and 2 times more inpatient days than children without asthma (Lozano et al. 1997). Another estimate suggests that children with asthma in the United States use 2.8 times more medical care than children without asthma, including 3.1 times more prescriptions, 1.9 times more ambulatory provider visits, 2.2 times more emergency department visits and 3.5 times more hospitalizations (Lozano et al. 1999).

In the United States, children with asthma used $615 more services per year than children without asthma, including both asthma and non-asthma health care. Yet, failure to diagnose asthma may be even more costly. Stempel et al. (2006) found that children without an asthma diagnosis, but with a prescription for asthma controller or reliever medication, have considerably higher costs than those with both an asthma diagnosis and a prescription for asthma controller or reliever medication. Children with asthma were three times more likely to have co-morbidity than children without asthma (Grupp-Phelan et al. 2001). Children with asthma had a 47% probability of being in the highest total cost quintile, compared to 29% once adjusted for comorbidities.

Among children, the total per capita economic impact of asthma in school-age children was estimated

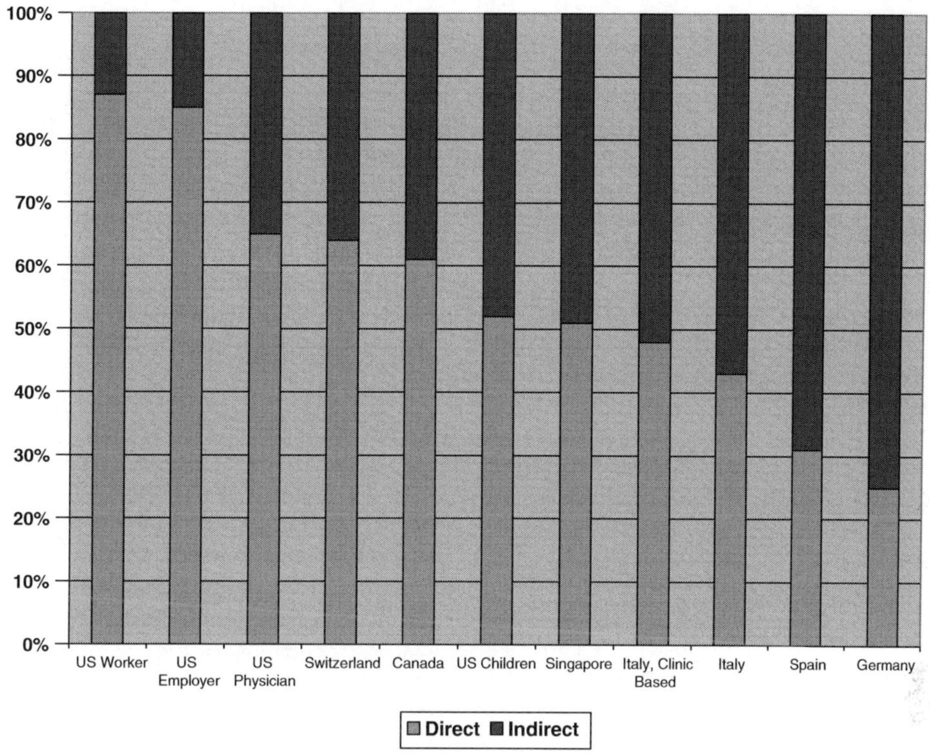

Fig. 19.1 Ratio of direct to indirect costs internationally

to be $791 per child with asthma (Wang et al. 2005). This includes $401 per child in direct medical expenditures (prescribed medicine, hospital inpatient stay, hospital outpatient care, emergency room visits, office-based visits). Children miss, on average, 2.5 days of school per year, and parents' loss of productivity from asthma-related school absence days was valued at $285 per child. Additionally, early death from asthma imposed a societal burden of $105 per child with asthma. However, the long term impact may not be that dire. A recent review of the literature revealed that although asthma limits children's daily activities and adversely affects social activities, there is little evidence of major, adverse long-term social and economic impacts of children's asthma (Milton et al. 2004).

Asthma Severity

One area of recent interest is the impact of asthma severity on cost (Table 19.2). Several studies have examined this question in different countries and found similar results. A recent study in France found that costs were substantially higher for patients with poor asthma control (Van Ganse et al. 2002). Direct medical costs for asthma were found to be 1,451€ for poorly controlled patients, but 746€ for moderately controlled patients and only 550€ for well-controlled patients (a ratio of 1.4 and 2.6, respectively). In Hungary, the cost of care, relative to good asthma control, was 1.4 times higher for adults with moderate control and 2.4 times higher for adults with poor control (Herjavecz et al. 2003). In Switzerland, direct asthma costs were 2.5 times higher in the highest severity groups, compared to the lowest severity group, if no asthma exacerbations were present (Schwenkglenks et al. 2003). In the USA, the costs associated with severe asthma were 1.3 times the cost of a patient with moderate asthma and 1.7 times the cost of a patient with mild asthma (Colice et al. 2006) Indeed, more than 80% of resources were used by the most expensive 20% of the patients (Smith et al. 1997) But this may be because high cost asthmatics are more likely to be in fair or poor health (Malone et al. 2000).

Asthma is a problem not just in the developed world, but also in poorer countries. In Turkey, mean

Table 19.2 Ratio of costs among asthmatics with moderate and poor control versus good control

Country	Moderate control	Poor control
France	1.4	2.6
Hungary	1.4	2.4
Switzerland		2.5
United States	1.3	1.7

annual direct medical costs of asthma were $1,465, with prescription medications comprising 81% of total direct costs (Celik et al. 2004). Similarly, in Estonia, 53% of asthma treatment costs were associated with prescription medications (Kiivet et al. 2001). In Singapore, hospitalizations were the leading source of direct costs, while indirect costs were largely attributable to productivity losses (Chew et al. 1999). Finally, in India, median spending on asthma medications for children with mild or moderate persistent asthma was equivalent to one-third of average monthly per capita income, highlighting the profound difficulties faced by poorer countries (Lodha et al. 2003).

The Cost of Asthma to Individuals

The impact of financing mechanisms on cost, access and quality of care has been a topic of considerable interest. Increased cost sharing has the effect of potentially reducing costs for payers (either health insurers or governments) by shifting the responsibility for paying for care to the individual. However, if the individual then forsakes prescription drugs or preventive care, this not only has a potentially deleterious effect on the individual's health, but may also lead to increased spending by the payer in the form of emergency department visits or hospitalizations. Alternatively, by rewarding high quality care with higher payments, payers can potentially improve the quality of care provided.

The annual cost to the healthcare system of nonadherence to prescribed medications (including asthma) has been estimated at $300 billion (Bender and Rand 2004). Since 1991, the National Institutes of Health has recommended that children with even moderate asthma may benefit from daily treatment with anti-inflammatory drugs. In the Florida Medicaid program, the proportion of children receiving at least one prescription for a preventive drug rose from 27% of children in 1990–1992 to 53% in 1997–1998, an approximate doubling in the proportion who received a prescription for a daily anti-inflammatory drug; but low adherence rates were evident even among those with the severest asthma (David 2004).

Asthmatics who visit the emergency department are likely to be adults with daily or weekly asthma symptoms who are in fair or poor health status, and who delay care for asthma because of cost or insurance issues (Meng et al. 2006). Similarly, children without health insurance are not less likely to be diagnosed with asthma, but are less likely to be prescribed asthma medications (Freeman et al. 2003). This suggests that the key to reducing the use of emergency departments is to control asthma symptoms and to reduce delays in receiving asthma care. Data from the nationally representative Behavioral Risk Factor Surveillance System (BRFSS) showed that individuals with asthma having interruptions in health insurance coverage were at greater risk of using urgent or emergency care (Markovitz and Andresen 2006). However, the association disappeared when controlling for race/ethnicity, employment status, gender, age and other independent variables, suggesting that there may be other factors that explain both lack of insurance and increased risk of using urgent or emergency care.

This increased risk of high utilization of emergency departments is also true among Medicaid children with asthma despite the absence of cost sharing. Children on Medicaid use the emergency department more than privately insured children, even after controlling for asthma-related primary care visits, use of asthma specialists, age, gender, use of medication and symptomatology (Ortega et al. 2001). Individuals with Medicaid insurance are also more likely to use the emergency department as their usual source of care for problems with asthma (Ferris et al. 2002).

If the differences are not due to structural, enabling or need factors, then why do Medicaid children use more high cost services? One study found that the high usage of these services was concentrated among a small percentage of provider practices and patients (Fredrickson et al. 2004). The parents of these children expressed a preference for primary care treatment, but had trouble contacting their primary care physicians and obtaining urgent appointments and believed their physicians preferred that they use emergency services in place of primary care. Although the children had multiple risk factors, the parents had no memory of their health care provider explaining asthma risk factors during primary care visits. The parents also reported a lack of continuity of care and difficulties in obtaining medications. This suggests that the children were receiving sub par asthma care, despite the removal of financial barriers. A similar result was found among a Medicaid population in Kentucky with asthma: nonadherence to expert asthma guidelines was common; less than 10% of patients who received rescue medications used inhaled steroids regularly (Piecoro et al. 2001). However, one study found that higher hospitalization rates among inner-city children in Rochester, New York were due to higher incidence of severe acute asthma exacerbations (McConnochie et al. 1999).

In Canada, where universal health insurance is provided without cost sharing, there is mixed evidence regarding the impact of income on asthma medication adherence (Blais et al. 2006). Although low and high income adolescents (ages 13–17) had similar rates of medication adherence, low income children (ages 5–12) had lower rates of medication adherence when a stricter definition of adherence was used and had similar rates of adherence when an alternative definition with lower thresholds was used. Along the same lines, very poor, poor and nonpoor groups had similar number of office visits for asthma, but very poor children were more likely to use emergency services (Sin et al. 2003).

Together, these observations suggest that although insurance may play a role in determining how asthmatics use health care, there are other factors at work that are at least as important as the financing mechanism. For example, in Spain, patients with asthma were more likely to use the emergency department than those in France or Italy (Van Ganse et al. 2006). This result was found despite few differences between the individuals with asthma in the three countries in terms of either asthma burden or use of prescription medications. The rate of asthma hospitalizations was also similar across the three countries, but the cost of emergency care in all asthma severity categories was up to ten times higher in Spain than in France or Italy. The authors conclude that the results are likely driven by unseen attributes of the Spanish health care system.

Access to insurance matters; in the USA, quality of care is lower for the uninsured. Among patients in emergency departments for acute asthma, uninsured patients received poorer quality of care on seven (out of seven) quality measures than insured patients (Ferris et al. 2002). In a multivariate analysis, uninsured patients had lower quality of care on five of seven measures and had lower initial peak expiratory flow. Despite differences in indicators of quality of care between types of insurance, short term patient outcomes were similar across all insurance types.

Generally, private insurance plans cover recommended asthma services. An analysis of 98 health plans from every state and the District of Columbia found that most plans provided coverage for all recommended health services for asthma, although the coverage tended to be better in managed care products versus preferred provider organizations (Fox et al. 2003). Despite this, there are large, systematic differences between health plans in terms of the rate of compliance of plan members with asthma to recommended guidelines for asthma care (Eisenberg 2004). In the previously mentioned analysis of patients in the emergency departments for acute asthma, managed care patients were more likely to have used inhaled steroids in the month prior to arrival in the emergency department than indemnity-insured patients, and they received the best overall care (Ferris et al. 2002). However, patients hospitalized for asthma from managed care plans had both shorter average length of stays and higher readmission rates (Ather et al. 2004).

In the United States, employer claims files show that the controller-to-reliever ratio rose steadily over from 1995 to 2000, suggesting that the quality of care was improving (Crown et al. 2004). On the other hand, out-of-pocket payments for asthma medications also increased, with larger increases for controllers than relievers. After controlling for other independent variables, the authors found that mean plan-level out-of-pocket copayments did not have a statistically significant effect on patient-level asthma treatment patterns. However, the prescribing patterns of physicians and physician practices strongly influenced treatment patterns. Similarly, in Sweden, large variations in costs across different primary health clinics were found even after controlling for asthma severity (Arnlind et al. 2006). And in Switzerland, costs were higher for patients treated by nonspecialists, for those without supplementary insurance, and for those treated in rural areas and in French-speaking cantons (Szucs et al. 2000).

Can insurance or payment mechanisms be used to either improve the quality of care or reduce the cost of care? One challenge is that these may be contradictory goals; increased compliance leads to fewer asthma attacks and better asthma control, but is likely to increase primary-care costs (Dasgupta and Guest 2003). However, in some high cost populations, inhaled corticosteroids are cost effective and lead not only to significant clinical improvement but also to savings in both direct and indirect costs (Navarro and Parasuraman 2005). These populations are the focus of disease management programs.

There are a number of suggestive studies of disease management that show the promise of reducing the cost of care while simultaneously improving quality. For example, a small randomized trial of young women hospitalized with an asthma exacerbation found that intervention by asthma nurse specialist decreased hospitalizations by 60% and readmissions for asthma by 54%, and led to reductions in health care costs (direct and indirect) of $6,462 per patient (Castro et al. 2003). Similarly, in a Medicaid based disease management program, the intervention group exhibited 18% lower costs as compared to a matched control group (Tinkelman and Wilson 2004). Another program in a Medicaid managed care plan improved quality of life and reduced utilization (Jowers et al. 2000). Case management has also been found to have a positive impact on a number of case studies (Anonymous 2002). Finally, an asthma disease management program that helped physicians manage asthma in a fee-for-service primary care case management program reduced the rate of emergency visit claims by 23% and increased the rate of prescribing reliever drugs by 25% (Rossiter et al. 2000). The project suggested a return-on-investment of $3–$4 for every incremental dollar spent. But these studies are fraught with difficulties in replication and specificity of the particular population studied. Methodologically, controlling for issues such as regression to the mean is challenging. However, it seems likely that such programs can be effective for certain high cost populations.

Conclusion

Asthma is a costly illness, regardless of country, payment system, population characteristics or timeframe. Asthma is expensive for children, the elderly and working age populations. Asthma imposes high costs for the healthcare system, in the form of direct medical costs, and on employers and asthmatics in the form of work loss, days with reduced health and school days lost.

The causes of direct medical care expenditures for asthma are variable. Traditionally, hospital costs have been the most expensive element of care. This observation provided inspiration for policy makers to improve care because asthma hospitalizations are viewed as potentially avoidable, and in many of the studies reviewed, hospitalizations were the most expensive element of care. However, in several studies prescription drugs were found to be more expensive than hospital care. This is partially due to sample selection issues; in populations with less severe asthma, prescription drug expenditures will likely outweigh hospital expenditures. However, reduced hospital expenditures may reflect improving care and a concomitant reduction in hospitalizations due to asthma.

From the individual standpoint, it is clear that payment rules matter. Asthmatics without health insurance experience barriers accessing care, tend to delay seeking services, are less likely to use asthma medications and are more likely to end up in costly settings such as emergency departments. However, there is also tremendous variability in the quality of care provided within more uniform national health care systems, such as France, Sweden, Canada and Switzerland, and within the relatively uniform Medicaid system. Creating more even financial access to care may mitigate differences in access, but significant differences will remain. Even when use of primary care services is uniform across different income groups, adherence to prescribed medications and use of emergency and urgent care services is not. Further research into understanding critical socio-demographic and cultural differences in care seeking behavior among asthmatics is warranted.

It appears that there is some potential in using payment systems to provide improved care. For example, managed care plans are able to demonstrate differences in quality of care, and efforts to reward better care may yield intended results. Related evidence indicates that disease management programs may be able to improve outcomes and reduce costs in certain high cost populations.

Standard asthma care is well covered by most insurance plans, in the United States, Canada and Europe. However, there are many potentially valuable additional services that could be covered by health insurance such as home environmental modification. For insurers, a concern emerges that paying for services that are beneficial for those with severe symptoms may lead to substantial costs if the services are utilized more generally.

Chernew et al. (2007) proposes to replace the standard insurance design with a "Value Based Insurance Design" whereby cost-sharing and benefit design is driven not just by costs, but also by evidence of clinical benefits. This can be done most easily by targeting particular clinical services that are "high value," such as controller medications. Under this scheme, exceptions to the standard benefit package would be made for these high value services to encourage their use. The drawback to this approach is that it may lead to increases in use by both those for whom there is high clinical value and by some for whom there is less value.

A more challenging alternative is to alter the design of the insurance based on diagnosis. For example, if a person were diagnosed with severe asthma, a set of additional benefits would become available. This could include not just medications, but also such benefits as home environmental modification. Such an approach has already been successfully piloted at the University of Michigan for diabetics (Chernew et al. 2007), suggesting that a similar approach for asthma may be possible.

References

Accordini S, Bugiani M, Arossa W, Gerzeli S, Marinoni A, Olivieri M, Pirina P, Carrozzi L, Dallari R, De Togni A, de Marco R (2006) Poor control increases the economic cost of asthma. A multicentre population-based study. Int Arch Allergy Immunol 141(2):189–198

Anonymous (2002) Diverse approaches to asthma DM succeed in Medicaid populations. Dis Manag Advis 8(5):71–77

Antonicelli L, Bucca C, Neri M, De Benedetto F, Sabbatani P, Bonifazi F, Eichler HG, Zhang Q, Yin DD (2004) Asthma severity and medical resource utilisation. Eur Respir J 23(5):723–729

Arnlind MH, Nokela M, Rehnberg C, Jonsson EW (2006) The relationship between pharmaceutical costs, disease severity, and health-related quality of life in asthmatics in Swedish primary care. J Asthma 43(8):585–591

Ather S, Chung KD, Gregory P, Demissie K (2004) The association between hospital readmission and insurance provider among adults with asthma. J Asthma 41(7):709–713

Bender BG, Rand C (2004) Medication non-adherence and asthma treatment cost. Curr Opin Allergy Clin Immunol 4(3):191–195

Birnbaum H, Berger W, Greenberg P, Holland M, Auerbach R, Atkins K, Wanke L (2002) Direct and indirect costs of asthma to an employer. J Allergy Clin Immunol 109(2):264–270

Blais L, Beauchesne MF, Levesque S (2006) Socioeconomic status and medication prescription patterns in pediatric asthma in Canada. J Adolesc Health 38(5):607.e9–607.e16

Blanc PD, Trupin L, Eisner M, Earnest G, Katz PP, Israel L, Yelin EH (2001) The work impact of asthma and rhinitis: findings from a population-based survey. J Clin Epidemiol 54(6):610–618

Bloom B, Bruno D, Maman D, Jayadevappa R (2001) Usefulness of US cost-of-illness studies in healthcare decision making. Pharmacoeconomics 19(2):207–213

Braman SS (2006) The global burden of asthma. Chest 130(1):4S–12S

Castro M, Zimmermann NA, Crocker S, Bradley J, Leven C, Schechtman KB (2003) Asthma intervention program prevents readmissions in high healthcare users. Am J Respir Crit Care Med 168(9):1095–1099

Celik GE, Bavbek S, Paaolu G, Mungan D, Abadolu O, Harmanci E, Misirligil Z (2004) Direct medical cost of asthma in Ankara, Turkey. Respiration 71(6):587–593

Chernew M, Rosen A, Fendrick AM (2007) Value-based insurance design. Health Aff 26(2):w195–w203

Chew FT, Goh DY, Lee BW (1999) The economic cost of asthma in Singapore. Aust N Z J Med 29(2):228–233

Cisternas MG, Blanc PD, Yen IH, Katz PP, Earnest G, Eisner MD, Shiboski S, Yelin EH (2003) A comprehensive study of the direct and indirect costs of adult asthma. J Allergy Clin Immunol 111(6):1212–1218

Colice G, Wu E, Birnbaum H, Daher M, Marynchenko M, Varghese S (2006) Healthcare and workloss costs associated with patients with persistent asthma in a privately insured population. J Occup Environ Med 48(8):794–802

Crown WH, Berndt ER, Baser O, Finkelstein SN, Witt WP, Maguire J, Haver KE (2004) Benefit plan design and prescription drug utilization among asthmatics: do patient copayments matter? Front Health Policy Res 7:95–127

Dasgupta R, Guest JF (2003) Factors affecting UK primary-care costs of managing patients with asthma over 5 years. Pharmacoeconomics 21(5):357–369

David C (2004) Preventive therapy for asthmatic children under Florida Medicaid: changes during the 1990s. J Asthma 41(6):655–661

Drummond M (1992) Cost of illness studies: a major headache? Pharmacoeconomics 2(1):1–4

Druss B, Marcus SC, Olfson M, Pincus A (2002) The most expensive medical conditions in America. Health Aff 21(4):105–111

Eisenberg SS (2004) Building the case for asthma as a disease management program. Dis Manag 7(3):202–215

Ferris TG, Blumenthal D, Woodruff PG, Clark S, Camargo CA, MARC Investigators (2002) Insurance and quality of care for adults with acute asthma. J Gen Intern Med 17(12):905–913

Fox HB, McManus MA, Reichman MB (2003) Private health insurance for adolescents: is it adequate? J Adolesc Health 32(6 Suppl):12–24

Fredrickson DD, Molgaard CA, Dismuke SE, Schukman JS, Walling A (2004) Understanding frequent emergency room use by Medicaid-insured children with asthma: a combined quantitative and qualitative study. J Am Board Fam Pract 17(2):96–100

Freeman NC, Schneider D, McGarvey P (2003) The relationship of health insurance to the diagnosis and management of asthma and respiratory problems in children in a predominantly Hispanic urban community. Am J Public Health 93(8):1316–1320

Gold M, Siegel J, Russell L, Weinstein M (1996) Cost-effectiveness in health and medicine. Oxford University Press, Oxford

Grupp-Phelan J, Lozano P, Fishman P (2001) Health care utilization and cost in children with asthma and selected comorbidities. J Asthma 38(4):363–373

Herjavecz I, Nagy GB, Gyurkovits K, Magyar P, Dobos K, Nagy L, Alemao E, Ben-Joseph R (2003) Cost, morbidity, and control of asthma in Hungary: The Hunair Study. J Asthma 40(6):673–681

Hodgson T (1994) Cost of illness in cost-effectiveness analysis: a review of the methodology. Pharmacoeconomics 6(6):536–552

Joshi AV, Madhavan SS, Ambegaonkar A, Smith M, Scott VG, Dedhia H (2006) Association of medication adherence with workplace productivity and health-related quality of life in patients with asthma. J Asthma 43(7):521–526
Jowers JR, Schwartz AL, Tinkelman DG, Reed KE, Corsello PR, Mazzei AA, Bender DR, Lochhead RA (2000) Disease management program improves asthma outcomes. Am J Manag Care 6(5):585–592
Kiivet RA, Kaur I, Lang A, Aaviksoo A, Nirk L (2001) Costs of asthma treatment in Estonia. Eur J Public Health 11(1):89–92
Koopmanschap M (1998) Cost of illness studies. Useful for health policy? Pharmacoeconomics 14(2):143–148
Krahn MD, Berka C, Langlois P, Detsky AS (1996) Direct and indirect costs of asthma in Canada, 1990. CMAJ 154(6):821–831
Lodha R, Puranik M, Kattal N, Kabra SK (2003) Social and economic impact of childhood asthma. Indian Pediatr 40(9):874–879
Lozano P, Fishman P, VonKorff M, Ad Hecht J (1997) Health care utilization and cost among children with asthma who were enrolled in a health maintenance organization. Pediatrics 99(6):757–764
Lozano P, Sullivan SD, Smith DH, Weiss KB (1999) The economic burden of asthma in US children: estimates from the National Medical Expenditure Survey. J Allergy Clin Immunol 104(5):957–963
Malone DC, Lawson KA, Smith DH (2000) Asthma: an analysis of high-cost patients. Pharm Pract Manag Q 20(1):12–20
Markovitz BP, Andresen EM (2006) Lack of insurance coverage and urgent care use for asthma: a retrospective cohort study. BMC Public Health 6:14
McConnochie KM, Russo MJ, McBride JT, Szilagyi PG, Brooks AM, Roghmann KJ (1999) Socioeconomic variation in asthma hospitalization: excess utilization or greater need? Pediatrics 103(6):e75
Meng YY, Babey SH, Brown ER, Malcolm E, Chawla N, Lim YW (2006) Emergency department visits for asthma: the role of frequent symptoms and delay in care. Ann Allergy Asthma Immunol 96(2):291–297
Milton B, Whitehead M, Holland P, Hamilton V (2004) The social and economic consequences of childhood asthma across the lifecourse: a systematic review. Child Care Health Dev 30(6):711–728
Navarro RP, Parasuraman B (2005) Cost effectiveness of asthma controller therapies: influence of disease severity and other variables. Manag Care Interface 18(6):31–40
Ortega AN, Belanger KD, Paltiel AD, Horwitz SM, Bracken MB, Leaderer BP (2001) Use of health services by insurance status among children with asthma. Med Care 39(10):1065–1074
Piecoro LT, Potoski M, Talbert JC, Doherty DE (2001) Asthma prevalence, cost, and adherence with expert guidelines on the utilization of health care services and costs in a state Medicaid population. Health Serv Res 36(2):357–371
Rossiter LF, Whitehurst-Cook MY, Small RE, Shasky C, Bovbjerg VE, Penberthy L, Okasha A, Green J, Ibrahim IA, Yang S, Lee K (2000) The impact of disease management on outcomes and cost of care: a study of low-income asthma patients. Inquiry 37(2):188–202
Rutten van-Molken MP, Feenstra TL (2001) The burden of asthma and chronic obstructive pulmonary disease: data from The Netherlands. Pharmacoeconomics 19(Suppl 2):1–6
Rutten-van Molken MP, Postma MJ, Joore MA, Van Genugten ML, Leidl R, Jager JC (1999) Current and future medical costs of asthma and chronic obstructive pulmonary disease in The Netherlands. Respir Med 93(11):779–787
Schwenkglenks M, Lowy A, Anderhub H, Szucs TD (2003) Costs of asthma in a cohort of Swiss adults: associations with exacerbation status and severity. Value Health 6(1):75–83
Sennhauser FH, Braun-Fahrlander C, Wildhaber JH (2005) The burden of asthma in children: a European perspective. Paediatr Respir Rev 6(1):2–7
Serra-Batlles J, Plaza V, Morejon E, Comella A, Brugues J (1998) Costs of asthma according to the degree of severity. Eur Respir J 12(6):1322–1326
Shiell A, Gerard K, Donaldson C (1987) Cost of illness studies: an aid to decision-making? Health Policy 8:317–323
Sin DD, Svenson LW, Cowie RL, Man SF (2003) Can universal access to health care eliminate health inequities between children of poor and nonpoor families?: a case study of childhood asthma in Alberta. Chest 124(1):51–56
Smith DH, Malone DC, Lawson KA, Okamoto LJ, Battista C, Saunders WB (1997) A national estimate of the economic costs of asthma. Am J Respir Crit Care Med 156(3):787–793
Stempel DA, Spahn JD, Stanford RH, Rosenzweig JR, McLaughlin TP (2006) The economic impact of children dispensed asthma medications without an asthma diagnosis. J Pediatr 148(6):819–823
Stevens CA, Turner D, Kuehni CE, Couriel JM, Silverman M (2003) The economic impact of preschool asthma and wheeze. Eur Respir J 21(6):1000–1006
Stock S, Redaelli M, Luengen M, Wendland G, Civello D, Lauterbach KW (2005) Asthma: prevalence and cost of illness. Eur Respir J 25(1):47–53
Szucs T, Anderhub H, Rutishauser M (1999) The economic burden of asthma: direct and indirect costs in Switzerland. Eur Respir J 13:281–286
Szucs TD, Anderhub HP, Rutishauser M (2000) Determinants of health care costs and patterns of care of asthmatic patients in Switzerland. Schweiz Med Wochenschr 130(9):305–313
Tinkelman D, Wilson S (2004) Asthma disease management: regression to the mean or better? Am J Manag Care 10(12): 948–954
Ungar WJ, Coyte PC (2000) Measuring productivity loss days in asthma patients. The Pharmacy Medication Monitoring Program and Advisory Board. Health Econ 9(1):37–46
Van Ganse E, Laforest L, Pietri G, Boissel JP, Gormand F, Ben-Joseph R, Ernst P (2002) Persistent asthma: disease control, resource utilisation and direct costs. Eur Respir J 20(2): 260–267
Van Ganse E, Antonicelli L, Zhang Q, Laforest L, Yin DD, Nocea G, Sazonov Kocevar V (2006) Asthma-related resource use and cost by GINA classification of severity in three European countries. Respir Med 100(1):140–147
Wang LY, Zhong Y, Wheeler L (2005) Direct and indirect costs of asthma in school-age children. Prev Chronic Dis 2(1):A11
Weiss KB, Gergen PJ, Hodgson TA (1992) An economic-evaluation of asthma in the United-States. N Engl J Med 326(13):862–866
Weiss KB, Sullivan SD, Lyttle CS (2000) Trends in the cost of illness for asthma in the United States, 1985–1994. J Allergy Clin Immunol 106(3):493–499

Chapter 20
Asthma, Public Health, and Policy

Noreen M. Clark

Introduction

Asthma is one of America's most perplexing public health problems. It is a ubiquitous and costly disease of society, as well as individuals. This chapter examines asthma in the larger context of public health by discussing different but related aspects of disease management and control. We will consider the way the characteristics of the society affect the extent and severity of the disease, and how asthma affects important public health indicators of well-being. We will review examples of interventions, some that have focused on clinical settings and some that have ventured into the community to relieve the burden of asthma more broadly. We will suggest how these efforts can be directed to generate a wider change. We will discuss ways to modify the impact of the condition through policy. Finally, we will consider the problems in our current approaches to asthma control and suggest alternative directions.

The Public Health Burden of Asthma

Asthma exacts a toll not only for the person with the disease, but those closest to him or her. In addition, extant evidence suggests that the public health impact of asthma is substantial and that characteristics of the society themselves conspire to create a disease that is more prevalent and more serious than an alternative set of conditions .

N.M. Clark (✉)
Center for Managing Chronic Disease, University of Michigan, School of Public Health, 109 Observatory Street, Ann Arbor, MI, 48109-2029, USA
e-mail: nmclark@umich.edu

Asthma costs the society greatly. Over 15 million people suffer from asthma, and it affects children and adolescents more than any other illness (Sondik 2008). Each year in the U.S., there are 5,000 deaths, 500,000 hospitalizations, and 2 million ED visits for asthma. In 1998, health care costs were approximately $12.7 billion. Just over 58% of asthma-related health care costs were direct medical care costs of which 45% comprised hospitalizations, outpatient hospital visits, and ED visits. Over 40% were the costs indirectly associated with the illness (Sondik 2008). Adults with asthma have more days of poor health, as well as more days with limited activity than adults who do not have asthma. Adults who have children with asthma accrue more work absence days and restricted days than parents of children where asthma is not present (Goldfarb et al. 2004). Asthma annually accounts for 14 million school absence days and 14.5 million work absence days.

Societal Influences on Asthma

Perhaps, the most well-documented society-wide features associated with more severe asthma are the economic, social, and demographic factors reflected in a community and seen specifically in income, education, age, race/ethnicity, sex, physical environment, stress, and obesity.

Income

Income disparities among populations have long been shown to produce a negative picture of health status in public health data in general (Kaplan et al. 1996) and

A. Harver and H. Kotses (eds.), *Asthma, Health and Society: A Public Health Perspective*,
DOI 10.1007/978-0-387-78285-0_20, © Springer Science+Business Media, LLC 2010

in asthma specifically (Weiss et al. 1992). The extent to which income is a proxy for other related characteristics of a population such as education and race/ethnicity has been discussed. One or two studies have indicated that the contribution of race, specifically the African American, to asthma prevalence, morbidity and mortality is independent of income (Grant et al. 2000). Others contend that the two are so interrelated as to confound efforts to consider them separately (Weiss et al. 1992). Regardless, being poor is hazardous to one's health and results in severity and premature mortality for people with asthma which is more than twice as common than in those of higher income (Volmer 2001).

The way in which low income leads to more burdensome asthma frequently has been discussed. Access to a requisite level of quality of clinical care has been identified (National Asthma Education and Prevention Program, 2007). For example, children in a community where the average family income is less than $20,000 per annum have been shown to be on clinical regimens for asthma that fall far below the National Asthma Education and Prevention Program (NAEPP) standard of care (Cabana et al. 2004; Clark et al. 2002). Emergency department data (Radeos et al. 2001) illustrate that income is closely associated with the lack of follow-up care subsequent to an urgent asthma ED visit.

Interestingly, studies have suggested that the majority of poor asthma patients, especially children, have some form of insurance coverage that would give them access to a health care provider (Clark et al. 2004). However, two glaring problems greatly reduce one's optimism about this apparent fact. First is the previously mentioned questionable quality of care that may be provided. Second is the well-documented fact that 20 million Americans (conservatively speaking, 10% of whom have a respiratory condition) have no health insurance and, frequently, avoid seeking health care even in urgent situations (Ayanian et al. 2000; Becker 2001; Sudano and Baker 2003). African American and Latino/Hispanic people are more likely not to have health insurance [American Diabetes Association (ADA) 2008]. Effective clinical care is the frontline of defense for managing asthma. The presence of large numbers of citizens who have no care or receive inadequate care guarantees the failure of public health disease control efforts.

The cost of asthma drugs is another route for producing ill effects for the poor. For example, Ungar et al. (2005) showed that at a cost of $300–$3,000 a year, paying for asthma medicine reduces the ability of families to pay for other essentials, e.g. food and housing, as well as "nonessentials" such as recreation. These costs were also shown to detract from vital long-term family investments; for example, the child's future education, home mortgages, etc. Stealing from the future helps perpetuate poverty and ill health for asthma sufferers.

Race/Ethnicity

Despite the discussion of race/ethnicity as a confounder with income, one's racial and ethnic identification has frequently been associated with asthma (Gupta et al. 2006) and the asthma disparities observed between minority and nonminority groups. For example, mortality data indicate that young, African American men are particularly susceptible to death from asthma (McFadden and Warren 1997; Weitzman et al. 1998). Krishnan et al. (2006) subsequent to a study of patients hospitalized for asthma concluded that the overall higher risk of death from asthma in black patients compared with white patients is not explained by race differences in hospital deaths and is attributable to factors preceding hospitalization. Research has also found that young children of African American and Latino/Hispanic families admitted to the hospital for asthma were less likely to have received optimum preventive therapy and experienced lower quality discharge planning compared to white patients (Finkelstein et al. 1995). Epidemiologic data suggest that asthma prevalence in predominantly Latino/Hispanic areas such as Puerto Rico are far above national averages (Lara et al. 2006; Sondik 2008). Data also indicate that asthma in pregnancy worsens most significantly for African American women (Carroll et al. 2005).

An interesting study by Cunningham et al (1996) suggests another way that race may play out in asthma. They found that minority patients were more likely than others to receive a diagnosis of asthma. On the other hand, race did not influence the higher presence of asthma symptoms. No definitive explanation is available for this contradiction, although one speculation is that clinicians may be responding to the epidemiological data suggesting that minorities are more susceptible to the disease.

The glaring reality in such studies is that whether there is some unexplained causative factor in race/ethnicity or whether these variables actually represent lower income in the populations studied, minority people with asthma have been shown to be more vulnerable as far as prevalence, incidence, and burden of the diseaseare concerned.

Education, Age, and Sex

Education too has predicted asthma outcomes. Educational background has been shown to enable (when at a higher level) or detract (when lower) from an asthma patient's ability to access specialized asthma care (Finnvold 2006). Education, defined as a low level of health literacy, has been shown to predict poor longitudinal asthma outcomes (Mancuso and Rincon 2006). It has also been shown to be independent of income in predicting negative consequences of asthma for African Americans (Grant et al. 2000).

Age and sex are influential in asthma. Most Americans are aware that the general population is aging. By 2030, it is estimated that about 20% of the U.S. population will be 65 years of age or older (Centers for Disease Control 2003). Currently, older individuals comprise 10% of the population of asthma sufferers, and this growing population of individuals over time is likely to require more hospitalizations and longer stays for asthma (Cortes et al. 2004). As noted earlier, adolescent age puts some individuals with asthma at greater mortality risk. Further, young children have consistently accounted for the highest number of emergency department visits for asthma in the U.S. (Centers for Disease Control 2002).

Sex, too, plays a role. Asthma clearly predominates in boys in childhood and in women in adulthood (Mannino et al. 2002; Schatz et al. 2006). Somewhere around puberty, asthma makes the epidemiological transition from favoring males to favoring females. Quite likely, hormonal factors play an important role in this shift, but the particular mechanisms are not well understood. Nonetheless, in childhood, more boys than girls have a diagnosis and symptoms and are taken for health care services although the proportionate differences are not always great (Schatz et al. 2006). In adulthood, however, significantly more women are burdened with asthma. They have 30% higher prevalence, 50% higher outpatient care use, a 35% higher hospitalization rate, a 6% higher ED use rate, and a 40% higher death rate than men (Sondik 2008)

Stress, Depression, and Violence

There are a range of other complex societal features that have been explored as influences on the prevalence of asthma and public health efforts to control the disease. These include the levels of stress, depression, and violence in a community.

Some of the most interesting works regarding these aspects of asthma have been done by Wright and colleagues. For example, their group has provided persuasive evidence that psychological stress is associated with atopy in predisposed children (Wright et al. 2005; Wright et al. 2004a) and that higher parental levels of stress predict wheezing in infants (Wright et al. 2002). As one might expect, stress has been identified at particularly high levels in low income communities (Ampon et al. 2005). Depression (some say the major chronic condition of the 21st century) has been shown to be associated with lower levels of asthma-related quality of life (Kullowatz et al. 2006), and one study has indicated that its effects may be additive in producing an adverse quality of life (Opolski and Wilson 2005). Likely of little surprise to any reader are the data that illustrate low income mothers of children with asthma report more symptoms of depression and the presence of more life stressors than those of higher income (Shalowitz et al. 2006) and that mental health is a significant factor in predicting asthma morbidity (Weil et al. 1999).

Wright et al. (2004b) and Wright and Steinbach (2001) have also shown the complex picture that exposure to violence draws for children with asthma. Their study illustrated that the higher the level of exposure to violence, the greater the number of days with asthma symptom for the child and the more nights the child's caretaker lost sleep. When stress levels were controlled in the analyses, the gradient of increase in the outcomes was somewhat attenuated. In short, however, one can say that neither stress nor exposure to violence is good for any child, and this fact is especially clear for a child with asthma.

On the other hand, those with circumstance, reason, or predisposition to be optimistic appear to have a different disease trajectory. Kubzansky et al. (2002) in a longitudinal study of older men with asthma illustrated that their level of optimism about their life and health was significantly associated with better FEV_1 (forced expiratory volume) and forced vital capacity.

Obesity and Asthma

As public health data and public attention have increasingly concerned the rising levels of obesity and overweight in the U.S., their associations with asthma have been discussed (Chinn et al. 2006; Flaherman and Rutherford 2006; Hendler et al. 2006). Cogent arguments for the role of leptin in obesity and asthma have been made (Mancuso et al. 2004; Shore et al. 2005). One review (Ford 2005) suggested that in adults obesity was higher in those with asthma. Among children and adolescents, study results were less consistent. Prospective studies have found a link between higher BMI (body mass index) at baseline and an increased risk for asthma in adults; however, again, data were inconclusive regarding children. Reports show particularly high levels of overweight and obesity among female patients with asthma (Clark et al. 2003) and illustrate increased symptoms in these women compared to those of normal weight (Clark et al. 2003). Two or three studies suggest that weight loss reduces asthma symptoms (see in: (Ford 2005)). However, the chicken or egg question about asthma and overweight has not been answered. Are overweight people more susceptible to asthma or does being overweight exacerbate a problem that was already there? Regardless of the answer, it would appear that being overweight or obese gives rise to problems with managing asthma. These problems are on the rise, and, in part, are viewed as a social-cultural phenomenon. Our current understanding of day to day management of asthma does not stretch to the special problems of the overweight.

Physical Environment

Yet another set of public health concerns is the physical environment of a community. At least two aspects of the environment, indoor and outdoor conditions, have been discussed as essential to asthma control. Further, the interaction of the physical and social environments as a predictor of more asthma symptoms has been considered (Levy et al. 2006). In two reports, the Institute of Medicine (IOM) (Institute of Medicine 2000, 2004) has described factors in the indoor physical environment associated with asthma. In "Clearing the Air," the IOM provides evidence to support the presence of cat dander, cockroach antigen, house dust mites, and environmental tobacco smoke (ETS) as causally related to the development of asthma. In "Damp Indoor Spaces," dampness, usually a function of inadequate building construction, is viewed as precipitating respiratory symptoms in sensitized persons and people with asthma. All these factors (except ETS) have been associated with low income.

A number of studies have connected air pollution, i.e. particulate matter in the air, to asthma symptoms. For example, levels of air pollutants above the National Ambient Air Quality standards have been shown to adversely affect lung function of susceptible children with asthma (Lewis et al. 2005). However, the data are not definitive regarding the aspects of air of matter that are most troublesome in asthma, nor the underlying mechanisms that produce ill effects. As a result, policy action is made more difficult. Further, the standards that may apply to adults may be different for children, and the policy actions to control pediatric asthma deserve more concerted attention (Goldman et al. 2004).

In summary, asthma is a significant public health problem. In reciprocal fashion, the nature of the society regarding its economic, social, and psychosocial features exerts influence on asthma prevalence and burden, and asthma detracts significantly from the public's health. One can argue that to realize a dramatic downturn in negative asthma outcomes, for example, reduction in asthma disparities evident across populations in the U.S., fundamental economic changes are needed to eliminate the pockets of poverty associated with these disparities. This position has been well formed by a number of observers (Kaplan et al. 1996). Another part of the problem may be the ways in which we conceive of helping those with asthma control the effects of the disease. Control, that is, full functioning with no (or rare) symptoms, is the benchmark of success as long as we are unable to cure or prevent asthma.

Interventions for Asthma Control

Public health efforts to achieve control over asthma have tended to be directed toward therapies (see, for example, (Paltiel et al. 2001)) and more effective organization and delivery of health services (Weiss et al. 1992). There is little doubt in the mind of an informed observer that these are needed fixes. However, in our vision of intervention, we have usually ignored or avoided a locus of power for real change in asthma outcomes: effective management by the person himself or herself who has the disease. Further, we have failed to recognize that the major task of everyone else in the circles of influence of such an individual is assisting the person to manage optimally. Excellent therapies are a needed element of control. Members of the health system must be the guides and advisors of patients and families. But, the power is in the hands of the individual and the resources available to that person, as well as the efforts of those surrounding him or her, who enable or deter effective management.

Figure 20.1 presents the concentric circles of influence in asthma control. It shows that at the center of all efforts is the patient whose capacity for day to day management must be at an optimum level to enable full functioning and quality of life. Families must positively support the one managing the disease. The responsible clinician must guide and recommend appropriate actions for the person and family, and do so within a health system that is effectively and efficiently organized to enable the clinician to help the patient. The neighborhood or community must be aware of the problem and nurture and sustain the person and family in their efforts. The physical environment must be one that fosters health. Policies must be conducive to effective asthma management and control.

If our collective efforts focus on this vision of capacity, they are likely to be more successful in reaching the goals of fewer symptoms, more appropriate health care use, full functioning of patients, and families that reach their optimum level of asthma-related quality of life.

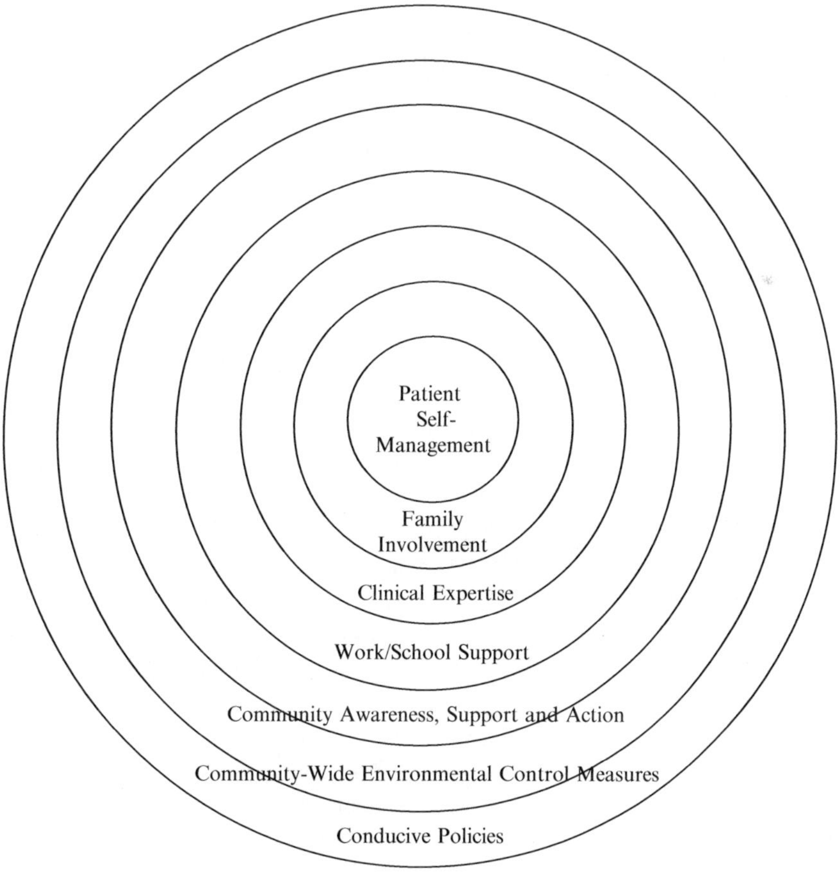

Fig. 20.1 Concentric circles of influence in asthma control

Management by People with Asthma and their Families

Indeed, we have examples of a number of types of interventions that appear to have built capacity for effective asthma management. A fair number of clinical trials have been directed at the center of the circles of influence: management by individual patients. Many have shown positive results. For example, Gibson et al. (2000) in a systematic Cochrane review showed that self-management interventions for adult patients resulted in changes in symptoms, health care use, and quality of life. Wolf and colleagues in another Cochrane review (Wolf et al. 2003) showed similar results for interventions directed at children with asthma. This form of capacity building is widely accepted as important (National Asthma Education and Prevention Program, 2007) to asthma control. Yet, the quality and quantity of programs that are actually available and accessible for individual patients have been called into question. Proven models have not been replicated, modes of wide spread distribution have not been found, and financial support for interventions to enhance patient self-management is not widely available.

There are far fewer studies that show us how to build capacity in the other circles of influence, that is, beyond the individual's management abilities. Some, however, hold promise, for example, capacity building programs for families (Hindi-Alexander and Cropp 1984; Melnyk et al. 2004; Wilson et al. 1996). Family involvement is crucial when the patient is a child, and these caretakers have been the target of effective interventions to enhance their capacity to support and, as needed, undertake management on behalf of the child (Wilson et al. 1996). For example, studies illustrate that parents can be directly helped through an educational intervention to manage a child's asthma better (Clark et al. 2004) and a program for children that indirectly involves parents also can enhance their management (Evans et al. 1987).

Management by Clinicians and the Health System

A small but important body of work has concerned the capacity of clinicians and of the health care system to organize and deliver effective support to the person managing asthma. For example, brief interventions to build the capacity of physicians to provide guideline-recommended therapies, communicate with, and educate their patients have been shown to significantly improve physician performance, patients' health care use, and family ratings of the care they received (Cabana et al. 2006; Clark et al. 1998, 2000). Nurses deployed to provide follow-up care to asthma patients have been shown to be effective and comprise the equivalent of physician follow up care (Nathan et al. 2006). Community health workers have been successfully utilized to extend asthma clinical care to high risk individuals (Perez et al. 2006). Emphasizing, as part of emergency department services, the need for continuity of asthma care has been shown to increase subsequent visits by patients to a primary care physician (Sockrider et al. 2006; Zorc et al. 2003), and ED information systems have been used to track action plan use and use of controller medicine (Boychuck et al. 2006). System-wide interventions to improve disease management for asthma within a facility have been shown to increase physician adherence to asthma guidelines for diagnosis and treatment and to reduce health care use (Cloutier et al. 2005). Physician information systems, case management, and quality improvement activities have been associated with positive outcomes (Sullivan et al. 2005). Nonetheless, these interventions have rarely been replicated, tested for generalizability, or disseminated beyond the initial research site.

Communities and Coalitions

The same might be said for community-based efforts: reaching those with asthma through schools, work sites, and in other community settings. However, a number of excellent prototypes do exist (Clark et al. in press). For example, a number of investigators have examined models for school-based programs to build the capacity of children, their parents, and those in the school system to manage asthma. These efforts have been undertaken in elementary schools (Clark et al. 2004; Levy et al. 2006; Splett et al. 2006) and in high schools (Shah et al. 2001) with positive results related to the child's asthma symptoms, activity levels, and academic performance. At least one study has shown that hospitals are willing and effective partners in school based programs (Byrne et al. 2006) and that school-based programs can be disseminated to additional school sites (Johnstone et al. 2006).

Community coalitions for asthma control (there are more than 200 asthma coalitions in the U.S. alone) have proven effective in mobilizing important organizations and constituencies to work collaboratively. The means by which they organize and carry out their work has been closely examined (Clark et al. 2006). The contribution of asthma coalitions to community organization, development of leadership, and creation of new collaborations has been documented (Butterfoss et al. 2006; Clark et al. 2006; Krieger et al. 2006; Nicholas et al. 2006; Wandersman 2003; Wandersman et al. 1996). The promise of the community coalitions is great, currently there is limited information about their ultimate impact on the health status of individual asthma patients or benefits for their families. Although the available data are promising suggesting that both policy change and improved asthma status for children can result from the work of coalitions (Clark et al. 2009). Work sites, churches, recreational facilities, and other community venues have not been examined regarding their effectiveness and efficacy for supporting management by asthma patients, but they may well hold potential.

Interventions designed to enable people with asthma to control indoor environments have been shown to reduce the presence of dust mites, dander, and cockroach antigen; however, subsequent changes in asthma symptoms or exacerbations have not been well documented (Institute of Medicine 2000), and/or studies have not separated environmental changes from other social and behavioral efforts (Kercsmar et al. 2006). Careful examination of changes in health associated with remediation of building dampness has not been undertaken, although there is consensus that constructing buildings to resist dampness should be the standard of practice (Institute of Medicine 2004).

Changing standards for clean air (U.S. Clean Air Act Amendments 1990) have been examined for their impact on the health of children. Prospective analyses suggest that the benefits of such change would greatly outweigh the costs (Wong et al. 2004), although data regarding specific asthma outcomes are scarce.

The utility and impact of interventions across the circles of influence on asthma management, such as the ones described here, ultimately depend on the extent to which they (and other successful innovations for asthma control) become regular practice as usual in families, health systems, and communities in the country. No doubt, sustaining and disseminating effective asthma programs and services are do-able; however, this result is likely possible only with organizational, institutional, community, and public policies that specifically support capacity building and effective practice.

National Public Health Effort

The control of asthma requires a national response, and the efforts of a number of agencies have been important to local through nation-wide public health. The Centers for Disease Control and Prevention (CDC) has instituted surveillance in most US states and maintains a database of prevalence and incidence statistics and associated demographic factors. The Behavioral Risk Factors Survey of the CDC includes a number of asthma-related items, and data are compiled periodically to describe behaviors associated with prevention and management of the disease.

Most state health authorities have risen to the asthma challenge. Many have initiated surveillance in addition to those they conduct in concert with the CDC. Further, many state health departments have engaged in efforts to coordinate and assist asthma awareness and intervention programs, as well as to enhance service delivery. In many states, these efforts have been carried out in collaboration with asthma coalitions.

The National Heart, Lung and Blood Institute has been at the forefront for national asthma control activities. It not only sponsors research into respiratory disease, but is responsible for the National Asthma Education and Prevention Program (NAEPP). NAEPP comprises all the major national organizations with interest in asthma (see Table 20.1 for a list). These organizations through the NAEPP undertake information and education activities targeted at people with asthma and their families, as well as clinicians and other health care providers. The Science Base Committee of NAEPP has generated the National Guidelines for Diagnosis and Treatment of Asthma (NAEPP 2007), the gold standard for clinical care. The NAEPP has also promulgated a Guidelines Implementation Plan (NAEPP 2008) describing strategies to ensure adherence to NAEPP clinical recommendations.

Table 20.1 Elements of the blueprint for policy action (Lara et al. 2002)

1. Develop and implement primary care performance measures for childhood asthma care
2. Teach all children with persistent asthma and their families a specific set of self-management skills
3. Provide care management to high risk children
4. Extend continuous health insurance coverage to all uninsured children
5. Develop model-benefit packages for essential childhood asthma services
6. Educate health care purchasers about asthma benefits
7. Establish public health grants to foster asthma friendly communities and home environments
8. Promote asthma friendly schools and school-based asthma programs
9. Launch a national asthma public education campaign
10. Develop a national asthma surveillance system
11. Develop and implement national agenda for asthma prevention research

The NAEPP has also issued other important guidelines: for example, concerning asthma in pregnancy (NAEPP 2004) and, in concert with the American Academy of Pediatrics, asthma in childhood (NAEPP 2007).

National voluntary organizations also work toward asthma control through providing information, education, and supporting research. The American Lung Association is perhaps the most well known and works through approximately 50 local and state affiliates and chapters. The Asthma and Allergy Foundation is another major provider of asthma information and services.

The Role of Policy in Asthma Control

A number of conferences, workshops, and studies have delved into the question of needed public health-related policies. One fairly comprehensive report is an investigation using a nominal group process involving asthma experts conducted by the Rand corporation (Lara et al. 2002) and resulting in a policy action blueprint. This report posited that national public health efforts are essential to turning around the discouraging data regarding asthma morbidity, mortality, and disparities across population groups. The study advisors conceived of "Asthma Friendly Communities" where proven services and programs were evident and available for all those needing assistance. A number of blueprint recommendations attempted to get at the underlying causes of negative asthma outcomes for the poor or otherwise disadvantaged. Advisors called for financing for universally available primary care, self management education and case management in childhood asthma. They believed expanded coverage and improved benefits were vital to reach and help the underserved. They posited that a strengthened public health infrastructure is necessary to achieve asthma friendly communities, that is, a system that provides resources for schools, public education campaigns, and a fully national surveillance system. They included a call for a national agenda for asthma prevention research.

The specific elements of the Blueprint for Policy Action paper are presented in Table 20.1. Although these recommendations focus on pediatric asthma, the proposals are generalizable to asthma in all age groups. That being said, other areas, e.g. policy related to environmental conditions, work settings, research regarding asthma's interaction with obesity, sex and gender role, race and ethnicity, and the implications for management deserve policy attention.

These important observations notwithstanding, a number of problems and issues precede the formulation of sound asthma-related local, state, and national public health policy. One is the lack of standardization of approaches to asthma therapy and service delivery obvious across the country, as well as a lack of conclusive evidence about the effectiveness of many of the clinical approaches utilized (Buxton et al. 2004; Paltiel et al. 2001; Silber et al. 2003). One of the most influential efforts to address this problem is the Guidelines for the Diagnosis and Treatment of Asthma of the National Asthma Education and Prevention Programs of the National Heart, Lung, and Blood Institute. These guidelines draw on the best evidence and collective judgment in the asthma field. The newest guidelines [2007] incorporate evidence and expert opinion to recommend clinical practice to enhance disease control. Nonetheless, studies have shown that in general and specifically in asthma, use of guidelines is not as robust as we might wish. Particularly in low-income communities, care has been shown to fall below NAEPP standards (Clark et al. 2002; Halm et al. 2005) In considering the problem of use of guidelines for respiratory disease, a distinguished group of experts called for exploration of more effective ways to communicate key asthma information both to clinicians and patients and promote appropriate management of the disease (Boulet et al. 2006).

Another challenge for policy making is the ongoing debate about the role of nonclinical factors in asthma exacerbations e.g. social factors, income (Brown et al. 2004; Kramer et al. 2006; Rogge and Combs-Orme 2003), the rights of asthma sufferers etc. (Jones and Wheeler 2004; Joseph et al. 2006).

Further, there are looming questions regarding conventional wisdom in asthma, that is, assumptions that guide policy and practice that have not been proven. For example, as noted previously, a number of environmental studies show it is possible to reduce environmental triggers to asthma in the home (Martin et al. 2006), however, rarely have changes in health status been clearly documented from such modifications (Kattan et al. 1997; Kercsmar et al. 2006). Although a number of interventions have attempted to ensure that high risk children see a primary care physician after an asthma emergency, subsequent change in the child's health status has not been examined and at least one study says that such follow-up does not change outcomes for patients (likely because the PCP continues to do the same thing that did not work in the first place) (Cabana et al. 2003). A number of studies have shown that community health workers can be trained and deployed to extend clinical care to the disadvantaged asthma patients, but changes in health status for individuals reached by these workers have not been extensively documented (Krieger et al. 2006). As discussed earlier, we do not know if more severe asthma is a result of obesity and requires special therapies, although we do know that overweight individuals have more asthma-related management problems than those of normal weight (Clark et al. 2003). Further, we are still in the dark regarding the onset of asthma and, therefore, its prevention or cure. For example, Marks et al. (2006) tried allergen avoidance and diet modification in newborns over five years to see if these interventions eliminated or reduced the effects of asthma, wheeze, eczema, or atopy. No differences were observed. The gaps in our conventional wisdom about asthma are many and wide. Some actually may be deterring control and are not wise choices at all. Some may be worthy of continuing. Only data can tell.

Conclusion

Reflecting on the example problems and solutions described in this chapter leads one to a few conclusions. If we are serious about controlling asthma as a public health problem, the effects of asthma on the society and the effects of the society on asthma, we need to think differently about our fundamental approach. Several things come to mind: (1) One is to recognize that in asthma there are interactions among environmental, social, behavioral, neural, endocrine, and immune processes that produce disease and affect interventions (Wright et al. 2004a). This suggests that new models for research are needed that can describe and explicate these interactions. (2) Another is to advocate for intervention research that illuminates how to build capacity across the circles of influence of the individual managing the condition. We need to keep that person in the center of our efforts and emphasize that he or she is the primary manager (not act as if clinicians or health faculties are). We must see health professionals and health systems as crucial advisors and facilitators who direct all their actions to one end: enabling effective management efforts of the patient. Similarly, families, communities, and policy makers – all must be recognized as enablers of good management and encouraged to do their part. (3) We need to explore conventional wisdom in asthma to discover if our assumptions about how to control it are sound ones. In short, we need to explore not only what we do not know but also what we think we know but have not examined closely. (4) The means to widely apply what we do know about asthma control and effective interventions must be found. In other words, replication of promising models and dissemination research are requisite for positive change. (5) The societal attention span (reflected in media, policy, practice) is short and many health problems vie for the spotlight. Although currently we know more about treating asthma than we have ever known, we are not seeing dramatic downward changes in data that indicate the high level of burden of the disease. A concerted voice and continuous effort are needed to remind patients, the clinical community, politicians, and policymakers how serious and costly asthma is and what they can do to help.

References

American Diabetes Association (2008) Economic costs of diabetes in the U.S. in 2007. Diabetes Care 31:1–20

Ampon RD, Williamson M, Correll PK, Marks GB (2005) Impact of asthma on self-reported health status and quality of life: a population based study of Australians aged 18–64. Thorax 60:735–739

Ayanian JZ, Weissman JS, Schneider EC, Ginsburg JA, Zaslavsky AM (2000) Unmet health needs of uninsured

adults in the United States. J Am Med Assoc 284(16): 2061–2069
Becker G (2001) Effects of being uninsured on ethnic minorities' management of illness. West J Med 175(1):19–23
Boulet L, Becker A, Bowie D, McIvor A, Hernandez P, Rouleau M et al (2006) Implementing practice guidelines: a workshop on guidelines dissemination and implementation with a focus on asthma and COPD. Can Respir J 13(Suppl A):5–47
Boychuck RB, DeMesa CJ, Kiyabu KM, Yamamoto F, Yamamoto LG, Sanderson R et al (2006) Change in approach and delivery of medical care in children with asthma: results from a multicenter emergency department educational asthma management program. Pediatrics 117(4):S145–S151
Brown P, Mayer M, Zavestoski S, Luebke T, Mandelbaum J, McCormick S (2004) Clearing the air and breathing freely: the health politics of air pollution and asthma. Int J Health Serv 34(1):39–63
Butterfoss FD, Gilmore LA, Krieger JW, Lachance LL, Lara M, Meurer JR et al (2006) From formation to action: how allies against asthma coalitions are getting the job done. Health Promot Pract 7(2 Suppl):34s–43s
Buxton MJ, Sullivan SD, Andersson LF, Lamm CJ, Liljas B, Busse WW et al (2004) Country-specific cost-effectiveness of early intervention with budesonide in mild asthma. Eur Respir J 24(4):568–574
Byrne J, Schreiber ME, Nguyen TQ (2006) Community hospital-school partnership to treat asthma episodes at school and improve management. J Sch Health 76(6):336–339
Cabana MD, Bruckman D, Bratton SL, Kemper AR, Clark NM (2003) Association between outpatient follow-up and pediatric emergency department asthma visits. J Asthma 40(7): 741–749
Cabana MD, Slish KK, Evans D, Mellins RB, Brown R, Lin X et al (2006) Impact of physician asthma care education on patient outcomes. Pediatrics 117(6):2149–2157
Cabana MD, Slish KK, Lewis TC, Brown R, Nan B, Lin X et al (2004) Parental management of asthma triggers within a child's environment. J Allergy Clin Immunol 114:352–357
Carroll KN, Griffin MR, Gebretsadik T, Shintani A, Mitchel E, Hatert TV (2005) Racial differences in asthma morbidity during pregnancy. Obstet Gynecol 106:66–72
Centers for Disease Control (2002) Surveillance for asthma – United States, 1980–1999. MMWR Surveill Summ 51:1–13
Centers for Disease Control (2003) Public Health and Aging: Trends in Aging -- United States and Worldwide. In: MMWR (ed) *MMWR Weekly* (February 14, 2003 edn, Vol. 52). CDC, Atlanta, pp 101–106
Chinn S, Downs SH, Anto JM, Gerbase MW, Leynaert B, deMarco R et al (2006) Incidence of asthma and net change in symptoms in relation to changes in obesity. Eur Respir J 28:763–771
Clark NM, Brown R, Joseph CL, Anderson EW, Liu M, Valerio M (2004) Effects of a comprehensive school-based asthma program on symptoms, parent management, grades, and absenteeism. Chest 125(5):1674–1679
Clark NM, Brown R, Joseph CL, Anderson EW, Liu M, Valerio M et al (2002) Issues in identifying asthma and estimating prevalence in an urban school population. J Clin Epidemiol 55(9):870–881
Clark NM, Doctor LJ, Friedman AR, Lachance LL, Houle CR, Geng X et al (2006) Community Coalitions to Control Chronic Disease: Allies Against Asthma as a Model and Case Study. Health Promot Pract 7(Suppl):44s–55s
Clark NM, Doctor LJ, Gilmore L, Kelly C, Krieger J et al (2009) Policy and system change and community coalitions outcomes from allies against asthma. Manuscript submitted for publication
Clark NM, Gong M, Schork MA, Evans D, Roloff D, Hurwitz M et al (1998) Impact of education for physicians on patient outcomes. Pediatrics 101(5):831–836
Clark NM, Gong M, Schork MA, Kaciroti N, Evans D, Roloff D et al (2000) Long-term effects of asthma education for physicians on patient satisfaction and use of health services. Eur Respir J 16:15–21
Clark NM, Gong M, Yu J, Lin X, Valerio M, Bria W et al (2003) Impact of overweight in women with asthma. European Respiratory Society Annual Congress, Vienna
Clark NM, Lachance LL, Friedman, AR, Stoll SC, Awad DA (in press) Characteristics of successful asthma programs. Public Health Rep
Cloutier MM, Hall CB, Wakefield DB, Bailit H (2005) Use of asthma guidelines by primary care providers to reduce hospitalizations and emergency department visits in poor, minority, urban children. J Pediatr 146(5):591–597
Cortes T, Lee A, Boal J, Mion L, Butler A (2004) Using focus groups to identify asthma care and education issues for elderly urban-dwelling minority individuals. Appl Nurs Res 17(3):207–212
Cunningham J, Dockery DW, Speizer FE (1996) Race, asthma, and persistent wheeze in Philadelphia schoolchildren. Am J Public Health 86(10):1406–1409
Evans D, Clark NM, Feldman CH, Rips J, Kaplan D, Levison MJ et al (1987) A school health education program for children with asthma aged 8–11 years. Health Educ Q 14(3):267–279
Finkelstein JA, Brown RW, Schneider LC, Weiss ST, Quintana JM, Goldmann DA et al (1995) Quality of care for preschool children with asthma: the role of social factors and practice setting. Pediatrics 95(3):389–394
Finnvold JE (2006) Access to specialized health care for asthmatic children in Norway: the significance of parents' educational background and social network. Soc Sci Med 63(5):1316–1327
Flaherman V, Rutherford GW (2006) A meta-analysis of the effect of high weight on asthma. Arch Dis Child 91:334–339
Ford E (2005) The epidemiology of obesity and asthma. J Allergy Clin Immunol 115(5):897–909
Gibson P, Coughlan J, Wilson A, Abramson M, Bauman A, Hensley M et al (2000) Self-management education and regular practitioner review for adults with asthma . Cochrane Database Syst Rev. 2000;(2):CD001117
Goldfarb N, Weston C, Hartmann C, Sikirica M, Crawford A, He H et al (2004) Impact of appropriate pharmaceutical therapy for chronic conditions on direct medical costs and workplace productivity: a review of the literature. Dis Manag 7(1):61–75
Goldman L, Falk H, Landrigan PJ, Balk SJ, Reigart JR, Etzel RA (2004) Environmental pediatrics and its impact on government health policy. Pediatrics 113(4):1146–1157
Grant EN, Lyttle CS, Weiss KB (2000) The relation of socioeconomic factors and racial/ethnic differences in US asthma mortality. Am J Public Health 90(12):1923–1925

Gupta RS, Carriòn-Carire V, Weisse KB (2006) The widening black/white gap in asthma hospitalizations and mortality. J Allergy Clin Immunol 117(2):351–358

Halm EA, Wisnivesky JP, Leventhal H (2005) Quality and access to care among a cohort of inner city adults with asthma. Chest 128:1943–1950

Hendler I, Schatz M, Momirova V, Wise R, Landon M, Mabie W et al (2006) Association of obesity with pulmonary and nonpulmonary complications of pregancy in asthmatic women. Obstet Gynecol 108(1):77–82

Hindi-Alexander MC, Cropp GJ (1984) Evaluation of a family asthma program. J Allergy Clin Immunol 74(4 pt 1):505–510

Institute of Medicine (2000) Clearing the air: asthma and indoor air exposures. Institute of Medicine, Washington, DC

Institute of Medicine (2004) Damp indoor spaces and health. Washington, DC, National Academies Press

Johnstone E, Knight J, Gilham K, Campbell E, Nicholas C, Wiggers J (2006) System-wide adoption of health promotion practices by schools: evaluation of a telephone and mail-based dissemination strategy in Australia. Health Promot Int 21(3):209–218

Jones SE, Wheeler L (2004) Asthma inhalers in schools: rights of students with asthma to a free appropriate education. Am J Public Health 94(7):1102–1108

Joseph CL, Williams LK, Ownby DR, Saltzgaber J, Johnson CC (2006) Applying epidemiological concepts of primary, secondary, and tertiary prevention to the elimination of racial disparities in asthma. J Allergy Clin Immunol 117(2): 233–240

Kaplan G, Pamuk ER, Lynch JW, Cohen RD, Balfour JL (1996) Inequality in income and mortality in the United States: analysis of mortality and potential pathways. Br Med J 312:999–1003

Kattan M, Mitchell H, Eggleston P, Gergen PJ, Crain E, Redline S et al (1997) Characteristics of inner-city children with asthma: the National Cooperative Inner-City Asthma Study. Pediatr Pulmonol 24(4):253–262

Kercsmar CM, Dearborn DG, Schluchter M, Xue L, Kirchner HL, Sobolewski J et al (2006) Reduction in asthma morbidity in children as a result of home remediation aimed at moisture sources. Environ Health Perspect 114(8):1564–1580

Kramer CB, Cullen AC, Faustman EM (2006) Policy implications of genetic information on regulation under the Clean Air Act: the case of particulate matter and asthmatics. Environ Health Perspect 114(3):313–319

Krieger JW, Bourcie E, Lara M, Peterson JW, Ronsenthal MP, Taylor-Fishwick JC et al (2006) Integrating asthma prevention and control: the roles of the coalition. Health Promot Pract 7(2 Suppl):127S–138S

Krishnan V, Diette GB, Rand CS, Bilderback AL, Merriman B, Hansel NN et al (2006) Mortality in patients hospitalized for asthma exacerbations in the United States. Am J Respir Crit Care Med 174:633–638

Kubzansky LD, Wright RJ, Cohen S, Weiss ST, Rosner B, Sparrow D (2002) Breathing easy: a prospective study of optimism and pulmonary function in the normative aging study. Ann Behav Med 24(4):345–353

Kullowatz A, Kanniess F, Dahme B, Magnussen H, Ritz T (2006) Association of depression and anxiety with health care use and quality of life in asthma patients. Respir Med 2007 Mar:101(3):638–44. Epub 2006 Aug 7.

Lara M, Akinbami L, Flores G, Morgenstern H (2006) Heterogeneity of childhood asthma among Hispanic children: Puerto Rican children bear a disproportionate burden. Pediatrics 117(1):43–53

Lara M, Rosenbaum S, Rachelefsky G, Nicholas W, Morton SC, Emont S et al (2002) Improving childhood asthma outcomes in the United States: a blueprint for policy action. Pediatrics 109(5):919–930

Levy JI, Brugge D, Peters JL, Clougherty JE, Saddler SS (2006) A community-based participatory research study of multifaceted in-home environmental interventions for pediatric asthmatics in public housing. Soc Sci Med 63:2191–2203

Lewis T, Robins TG, Dvonch JT, Keeler GJ, Yip FY, Mentz GB et al (2005) Air pollution-associated changes in lung function among asthmatic children in Detroit. Environ Health Perspect 113(8):1068–1075

Mancuso CA, Rincon M (2006) Impact of health literacy on longitudinal asthma outcomes. J Gen Intern Med 21(8):813

Mancuso P, Canetti CA, Gottschalk A, Tithof PK, Peters-Golden M (2004) Leptin enhances macrophage leukotriene synthesis by augmenting arachidonic acid release and $cPLA^2v$ protein expression. Am J Physiol Lung Cell Mol Physiol 287: L497–L502

Mannino DM, Homa DM, Akinbami L, Moorman JE, Gwynn C, Redd SC (2002) Surveillance for asthma – United States, 1980–1999. MMWR 51:1–13

Marks GB, Mihrshahi S, Kemp AS, Tovey ER, Webb K, Almqvist C et al (2006) Prevention of asthma during the first 5 years of life: a randomized controlled trial. J Allergy Clin Immunol 118(1):53–60

Martin MA, Hernandez O, Naureckas E, Lantos J (2006) Reducing home triggers for asthma: the Latino community health worker approach. J Asthma 43(5):369–374

McFadden ER, Warren EL (1997) Observations on asthma mortality. Ann Intern Med 127(2):142–147

Melnyk BM, Alpert-Gillis L, Feinstein NF, Crean HF, Johnson J, Fairbanks E et al (2004) Creating opportunities for parent empowerment: program effects on the mental health/coping outcomes of critically ill young children and their mothers. Pediatrics 113(6):e597–607

Nathan JA, Pearce L, Field C, Dotesio-Eyres N, Sharples LD, Cafferty F et al (2006) A randomized controlled trial of follow-up of patients discharged from the hospital following acute asthma. Chest 130:51–57

National Asthma Education and Prevention Program (2004) Managing asthma during pregnancy: recommendations for pharmacologic treatment. Retrieved October, 2006, from www.nhlbi.nih.gov/health/prof/lung/asthma/astpreg/astpreg_full.pdf

National Asthma Education and Prevention Program (2007) Guidelines for the diagnosis and management of asthma (No. 07-4051). National Heart, Lung and Blood Institute, Bethesda, Maryland

National Asthma Education and Prevention Program (2008) Expert panel report 3 – guidelines for the diagnosis and management of asthma: partners putting guidelines into action (No. 09-6147). National Heart, Lung and Blood Institute

Nicholas EA, Dwyer M, Murphy A, Taylor-Fishwick JC, Cohn JH, Kelly CS et al (2006) Coalition-based approaches for addressing environmental issues in childhood asthma. Health Promot Pract 7(2 Suppl):108S–116S

Opolski M, Wilson I (2005) Asthma and depression: a pragmatic review of the literature and recommendations for future research. Clin Pract Epidemol Ment Health 1:18

Paltiel AD, Fuhlbrigge AL, Kitch BT, Liljas B, Weiss ST, Neumann PJ et al (2001) Cost-effectiveness of inhaled corticosteroids in adults with mild-to-moderate asthma; results from the asthma policy model. J Allergy Clin Immunol 108(1):39–46

Perez M, Findley SE, Mejia M, Martinez J (2006) The impact of community health worker training and programs in New York City. J Health Care Poor Underserved 17(1 Suppl):26–43

Radeos MS, Leak LV, Lugo BP, Hanrahan JP, Clark S, Camargo CA (2001) Risk factors for lack of asthma self management knowledge among ED patients not on inhaled steroids. Am J Emerg Med 19(4):253–259

Rogge ME, Combs-Orme T (2003) Protecting children from chemical exposure: social work and US social welfare policy. Soc Work 48(4):439–450

Schatz M, Clark S, Camargo CA (2006) Sex differences in the presentation and course of asthma hospitalizations. Chest 129(1):50–55

Shah S, Peat JK, Mazurski EJ, Wang H, Sindhusake D, Bruce C et al (2001) Effect of peer led programme for asthma education in adolescents: cluster randomised controlled trial. Br Med J 322:583–585

Shalowitz MU, Mijanovich T, Berry CA, Cark-Kauffman E, Quinn KA, Perez EL (2006) Context matters: a community-based study of maternal mental health, life stressors, social support, and children's asthma. Pediatrics 117(5): e940–e948

Shore SA, Schwartzman IN, Mellema MS, Flynt L, Imrich A, Johnston RA (2005) Effect of leptin on allergic airway responses in mice. J Allergy Clin Immunol 115(1):103–109

Silber JH, Rosenbaum PR, Even-Shoshan O, Shabbout M, Zhang X, Bradlow ET et al (2003) Length of stay, conditional length of stay, and prolonged stay in pediatric asthma. Health Serv Res 38(3):867–886

Sockrider MM, Abramson S, Brooks E, Caviness AC, Pilney S, Koerner C et al (2006) Delivering tailored asthma family education in a pediatric emergency department setting: a pilot study. Pediatrics 117(4):S135–S144

Sondik EJ (2008, May) Focus area 24 respiratory diseases progress review. Presented at the National Center for Health Statistics, Hyattsville, MD

Splett PL, Erickson CD, Belseth SB, Jensen C (2006) Evaluation and sustainability of the healthy learners asthma initiative. J Sch Health 76(6):276–282

Sudano JJ, Baker DW (2003) Intermittent lack of health insurance coverage and use of preventive services. Am J Public Health 93(1):130–137

Sullivan SD, Lee TA, Blough DK, Finkelstein JA, Lozano P, Inui TS et al (2005) A multisite randomized trial of the effects of physician education and organizational change in chronic asthma care: cost-effectiveness analysis of the Pediatric Asthma Care Patient Outcomes Research Team II (PAC-PORT II). Arch Pediatr Adolesc Med 159(5):428–434

Ungar WJ, Macdonald T, Cousins M (2005) Better breathing or better living? A qualitative analysis of the impact of asthma medication acquisition on standard of living in low-income families of children with asthma. J Pediatr Health Care 19(6):354–362

Volmer T (2001) The socio-economics of asthma. Pulm Pharmacol Ther 14(1):55–60

Wandersman A (2003) Community science: bridging the gap between science and practice with community-centered models. Am J Community Psychol 31(3–4):227–242

Wandersman A, Valois R, Ochs L, Cruz DSdl, Adkins E, Goodman RM (1996) Toward a social ecology of community coalitions. Am J Health Promot 10(4):299–307

Weil CM, Wade SL, Bauman LJ, Lynn H, Mitchell H, Lavigne J (1999) The relationship between pyschosocial factors and asthma morbidity in inner-city children with asthma. Pediatrics 104(6):1274–1280

Weiss KB, Gergen PJ, Hodgson TA (1992) An economic evaluation of asthma in the United States. N Eng J Med 326(13):862–866

Weitzman JB, Kanarek NF, Smialek JE (1998) Medical examiner asthma death autopsies: a distinct subgroup of asthma deaths with implications for public health preventive strategies. Arch Pathol Lab Med 122(8):691–699

Wilson SR, Latini D, Starr NJ, Fish L, Loes LM, Page A et al (1996) Education of parents of infants and very young children with asthma: a developmental evaluation of the Wee Wheezers Program. J Asthma 33(4):239–254

Wolf FM, Guevara JP, Grum CM, Clark NM (2003) Educational interventions for asthma in children. Cochrane Database Syst Rev 2003;(1): CD000326.

Wong EY, Gohlke J, Griffith WC, Farrow S, Faustman EM (2004) Assessing the health benefits of air pollution reduction for children. Environ Health Perspect 112(2):226–232

Wright RJ, Cohen RT, Cohen S (2005) The impact of stress on the development and expression of atopy. Curr Opin Allergy Clin Immunol 2005 Feb; 5(1):23–29

Wright RJ, Cohen S, Carey V, Weiss ST, Gold DR (2002) Parental stress as a predictor of wheezing in infancy: a prospective birth-cohort study. Am J Respir Crit Care Med 165(3):358–365

Wright RJ, Finn P, Contreras JP, Cohen S, Wright RO, Staudenmayer J et al (2004a) Chronic caregiver stress and IgE expression, allergen induced proliferation, and cytokine profiles in a birth cohort predisposed to atopy. J Allergy Clin Immunol 113(6):1051–1057

Wright RJ, Mitchell H, Visness CM, Cohen S, Stout J, Evans R et al (2004b) Community violence and asthma morbidity: the inner-city asthma study. Am J Public Health 94(4):625–632

Wright RJ, Steinbach SF (2001) Violence: an unrecognized environmental exposure that may contribute to greater asthma morbidity in high risk inner city populations. Environ Health Perspect 109(10):1085–1089

Zorc JJ, Scarfone RJ, Li Y, Hong T, Harmelin M, Grunstein L et al (2003) Scheduled follow-up after a pediatric emergency department visit for asthma: a randomized trial. Pediatrics 111(3):495–502

Index

H

I

L

M

N

O

P